FORDNEY'S
MEDICAL
INSURANCE
AND BILLING

FORDNEY'S MEDICAL INSURANCE AND BILLING

16TH EDITION

LINDA M. SMITH
CPC, CPC-I, CEMC, CMBS

Training and Consulting
MedOffice Resources
Greene, New York

ELSEVIER

Elsevier
3251 Riverport Lane
St. Louis, Missouri 63043

FORDNEY'S MEDICAL INSURANCE AND BILLING,   ISBN: 978-0-323-79535-7
SIXTEENTH EDITION

Notices

Practitioners and researchers must always rely on their own experience and knowledge in evaluating and using any information, methods, compounds or experiments described herein. Because of rapid advances in the medical sciences, in particular, independent verification of diagnoses and drug dosages should be made. To the fullest extent of the law, no responsibility is assumed by Elsevier, authors, editors or contributors for any injury and/or damage to persons or property as a matter of products liability, negligence or otherwise, or from any use or operation of any methods, products, instructions, or ideas contained in the material herein.

Library of Congress Control Number: 2021946514

Senior Content Strategist: Linda Woodard
Content Development Specialist: Brooke Kannady
Director, Content Development: Laurie Gower
Publishing Services Manager: Shereen Jameel
Senior Project Manager: Umarani Natarajan
Design Direction: Amy L. Buxton

Printed in India

Last digit is the print number: 9 8 7 6 5 4 3 2 1

Working together
to grow libraries in
developing countries

www.elsevier.com • www.bookaid.org

Linda M. Smith has worked in the health care industry for more than 40 years. She started her career as a medical assistant and journeyed through the health care industry, spending time in various positions. Throughout that time, the health care industry went through dramatic changes. Health care providers experienced a multitude of billing and reimbursement changes, while also facing the challenges of an ever-increasing focus on regulatory guidelines and compliance. Simultaneously, the need for trained staff and resources to assist with billing, reimbursement, and compliance issues increased, which led her to found her own company, MedOffice Resources, in 2000. MedOffice Resources provides training to health care organizations and to various business and technical schools. She and her associates provide training in the areas of medical ethics, medical terminology, anatomy and physiology, medical coding and billing, and value-based incentive programs. Billing, coding, and auditing services are also offered to health care organizations. Health care facilities, practices, providers, and their office staff have been using the services of MedOffice Resources for the past 20 years to strengthen their staff's skills and strengthen their organizations.

Ms. Smith is a certified professional coder (CPC). She has also earned the credentials E/M coding specialist (CEMC) and is an approved professional medical coding curriculum instructor (CPC-I) through the American Academy of Professional Coders (AAPC). Additionally, Ms. Smith holds the credential of certified medical billing specialist (CMBS) through the Medical Association of Billers.

Ms. Smith was given the opportunity to work with Marilyn Fordney, the original author of the *Insurance Handbook for the Medical Office*. She worked with Fordney as a contributor to the textbook. After Ms. Fordney's retirement, Smith took on the editor position for the 15th and 16th editions.

ACKNOWLEDGMENTS

I would like to acknowledge and dedicate this 16th edition of the *Insurance Handbook* to Marilyn Fordney, the original author of this textbook. Marilyn published the first edition of the *Insurance Handbook* in 1977 and has followed it through the many changes in our health care industry. It has served as the training tool and building block for so many of us in the field. The publication's longevity speaks for itself.

It was a privilege to have been asked to be a contributor in the 13th and 14th editions of the *Handbook*, but an even greater honor to be asked to follow in Marilyn's footsteps as the primary editor of the 15th and 16th editions. Marilyn is a remarkable woman with a beautiful heart. Thank you, Marilyn, for all you have contributed to our field.

I would also like to give special thanks to Cheryl Fassett, who has been an outstanding partner in this project and a contributor in eight chapters of this 16th edition. Cheryl's expertise in our field, coupled with her outstanding talent and love for writing, has made this experience even more enjoyable. Cheryl's work is both remarkable and exemplary. I can't think of anyone else I would rather take this ride with.

And to the former owner of Practicare Medical Management, Hal Harkavy, a sincere thank you for asking me to join you in your journey into the world of outsourced medical billing so many years ago. There is so much that you taught me for which I will always be thankful.

Thank you to the many students who have given me the opportunity to share my knowledge of the medical billing and coding field. I can only hope that you will find the passion for it that will provide you with all the opportunities I have had the pleasure of. You have been my motivation and my reward.

I am indebted to many individuals on the staff at Elsevier for encouragement and guidance. Thank you to all the experts in the field who served as reviewers of the 15th edition and guided us with their recommendations. I express special appreciation to Linda Woodard, senior content strategist, and Brooke Kannady, content development specialist at Elsevier.

And lastly, thank you to my husband, John Wells, and my family who always support and encourage me. You are my reason for everything.

Linda M. Smith, CPC, CPC-I, CEMC, CMBS

CONTRIBUTOR

Cheryl Fassett, CPC, CPMA, CRC, CDEO, CPB, CPPM, CPC-I
Practice Manager
Riverside Associates in Anesthesia, PC
Binghamton, New York

REVIEWERS

Christine L. Berard, CPT
Coordinator/Instructor
Medical Billing & Coding, 911Programs
Warwick, Rhode Island

Rita Courier, MA, CCA
Account Representative/Billing & Coding Instructor
Hospital Community College
Munson Healthcare Otsego Memorial Hospital
North Central Michigan Community College
Gaylord, Michigan, Petoskey, Michigan

Nadinia Davis, MBA, RHIA, CHDA, FAHIMA
Adjunct Instructor
Delaware Technical Community College
Wilmington, Delaware

Melissa De Leon, NRCCS, NRCAHA
Medical Coding and Billing Program Director
Medical Office Specialist Program Director
The College of Health Care Professions
McAllen, Texas

Nancy J. Gammons, MS, CCS-P, CHSP, CHLP
AHIMA-approved ICD-10-CM/PCS Trainer
Certified Coding Specialist—Physician Based
Certified HIPAA Security Professional
Certified Health IT Leadership Proficiency
Professor HIT Programs
Allied Health Department
Shawnee Community College
Ullin, Illinois

Sandra J. Hertkorn, UC Davis Coder Academy
Director of Operations
Administration
All Inclusive Medical Services
Adult Ambulatory Clinic
Carmichael, California

Jennifer K. Jones, CPC, CPC-I, OHCC, CCS, CPMA
Columbia, Alabama

This textbook was first published by Marilyn Fordney as the *Insurance Handbook* in 1977. At that time, few people were aware of how important the subject of health insurance would become. I am confident that Marilyn Fordney had no idea that her textbook would become the basis of knowledge for so many of us in the field. Marilyn Fordney is a dedicated professional and a forward thinker whose work provided a strong foundation to many of us entering the field.

Forty-four years after that first publication, the textbook is celebrating its 16th edition. The longevity of this publication speaks for itself, and through the years, Fordney's textbook has been the leader in its field. The textbook is widely accepted across the nation among educators and those working in the health care industry.

Originally, the *Insurance Handbook* was designed primarily for students who planned to seek employment in the outpatient setting (such as a physician's office or clinic). The name of the publication was changed to *Fordney's Medical Insurance and Billing* at the 15th edition of the textbook and changes were made to expand the textbook beyond the world of professional billing and into facility billing. With this expansion, the textbook now provides a strong foundation to students who may also seek employment in a hospital, nursing home, or other type of health care facility.

To remain at the forefront of the industry and because of the ever-changing nature of health care, *Fordney's Medical Insurance and Billing* is revised every 2 years to keep the information current. Reviewing and revising the 16th edition has been as challenging and exciting as all of the publications before it.

PURPOSE

The goals of this textbook are to prepare students to excel as insurance billing specialists and to increase efficiency and streamline administrative procedures for one of the most complex tasks of the health care industry: insurance coding and billing.

Why Is This Book Important to the Profession?

In the past several decades, health care professionals and the community have witnessed the emergence of an administrative medical specialty known variously as insurance billing specialist, medical biller, or reimbursement specialist. Thus *Fordney's Medical Insurance and Billing* has been written to address the specialty of medical billing as another branch of the administrative medical assistant profession.

As the complexity of the health care field increased, the need for both basic and advanced training has become essential. There are national organizations offering certification in the field, which has quickly become the method of attaining higher recognition for advanced skill levels. *Fordney's Medical Insur-*

ance and Billing will serve as a training tool to establish a strong foundation of knowledge and will help bridge the learning process into the more advanced levels of expertise.

Insurance claims are being submitted for patients on the recommendation of management consultants to control cash flow, obtain correct reimbursement amounts, honor insurance contracts, compete with other health care organizations, and maintain a good relationship with patients. Even health care organizations that do not routinely complete insurance claims for patients make exceptions for elderly patients or patients with mental incompetence, illiteracy, diminished eyesight, or a poor command of the English language. When the amount of the bill is hundreds or thousands of dollars or when a surgical report is required, the health care organization should submit the bill to obtain maximum reimbursement. Individuals who administer the federal government's Medicare program increasingly promote electronic transmission of insurance claims for medium-sized and large medical practices. Because of these factors, as well as federal mandates to document care electronically, the amount of knowledge and skills that one must have has substantially increased. This textbook addresses all clerical functions of the insurance billing specialist, and illustrations throughout the text feature generic forms created to help simplify billing procedures.

Who Will Benefit From This Book?

Many colleges are now offering associate degree programs in medical billing and coding. At the same time, schools and colleges also offer 1-year certificate programs for those interested in a career as an insurance billing specialist. The student may find programs that offer medical insurance as a full-semester, 18-week course on campus or as a hybrid course (mix of online and face-to-face classroom instruction). Some schools include medical billing and coding as part of a medical assisting program's curriculum, so the individual has knowledge in all administrative functions of a health care organization. *Fordney's Medical Insurance and Billing* may be used as a learning tool and resource guide in all of those programs as well as in vocational or commercial training institutes. *Fordney's Medical Insurance and Billing* is recommended for use as a text for in-service training in health care organizations or it can be used for independent home study if no formal classes are available in the community. The layperson who is not pursuing a career in the medical field will find the textbook useful when working with a claims assistance professional or for billing his or her insurance plans. Insurance companies and their agents have found *Fordney's Medical Insurance and Billing* to be a valuable reference tool when answering clients' questions. Finally, the textbook may be used as a stand-alone reference source or as an educational tool to increase the knowledge of someone currently working as an insurance billing specialist in any health care setting.

CONTENT

General Features

Each chapter has been updated to reflect current policies and procedures.

- All chapters have been completely restructured for better organization and flow of content, with legal information included where applicable to insurance billing and coding. The information presented is not a substitute for legal advice, and the health care organization and their insurance billing specialists should always seek legal counsel about specific questions of law as they relate to their organization.

The unique color-coded icons have been visually updated and are featured throughout the textbook to denote and clarify information specific to each type of payer. This system makes the learning process more effective by helping students to identify each insurance payer with a specific color and graphic. These icons follow:

! COMPLIANCE ALERT

- Compliance Alerts are interspersed throughout all chapters for emphasis.
- Objectives are provided at the beginning of each chapter, sequenced to match the technical content, and help to guide instructors in preparing lecture material and inform readers about what material is presented.
- By reviewing the key terms that introduce each chapter, students are alerted to important words for the topic. Key abbreviations follow the key terms; spell-outs of the abbreviations are provided in a section that follows the Glossary near the back of the textbook.
- Boxed examples are provided throughout each chapter.
- Key points are presented at the end of each chapter, summarizing and emphasizing the most important technical information in the chapter.
  Many experts in the field reviewed the chapters in previous editions so that improvements in content, clarity of topics, and deletions could be considered.

 ## INSIGHTS FROM THE FIELD

- Each chapter includes "Insights From the Field," which is a short interview with an insurance billing specialist with experience in the field, who provides a snapshot of their career path and advice to the new student.

 ## QUICK REVIEW QUESTIONS

- Quick review questions have been added within each chapter to facilitate learning of key points.

DISCUSSION POINTS

- Discussion points at the end of each chapter will provide the opportunity for students and instructors to participate in interesting and open dialogue related to information provided.

 ## PRIVATE INSURANCE

The Blue plans and private insurance.

 ## ♥ MANAGED CARE

All managed care organizations.

 ## ◎ MEDICARE

Federal Medicare programs, Medicare/Medicaid, Medicare/Medigap, and Medicare Secondary Payer (MSP).

 ## ◎ MEDICAID

State Medicaid programs.

 ## ▶ MILITARY PLANS

TRICARE plans and the Civilian Health and Medical Program of the Department of Veterans Affairs.

⚡ WORKERS' COMPENSATION

State workers' compensation programs.

ORGANIZATION

Unit 1: Career Role and Responsibilities

- Chapters 1 through 3 are included under Unit 1, Career Role and Responsibilities, which explains the role of the insurance billing specialist and provides the student with a thorough understanding of the associated responsibilities. Because of the strong base of knowledge that the insurance billing specialist will need to understand the federal and state guidelines associated with the industry, Chapters 2 and 3 have in-depth information surrounding privacy, security, and health care fraud and abuse legislation. This is coupled with a strong emphasis on the compliance process and the insurance billing specialist's obligation to comply in all situations.

Unit 2: Introduction to Health Insurance

- Chapters 4 through 10 make up Unit 2, Introduction to Health Insurance. This unit will provide the student with an introduction into health insurance. The chapters in this unit are intended to build the learners' foundation of the basics of health care and introduce them to the various types of insurance carriers they will most likely encounter. Thorough, up-to-date information is presented for Medicare, Medicaid, TRICARE, private plans, workers' compensation, managed care plans, disability income insurance, and disability benefit programs.

Unit 3: Documentation and Coding for Professional Services

- Chapters 11 to 13 are included under Unit 3, Documentation and Coding for Professional Services. Medical documentation and the electronic health record have become essential components of the medical billing process. The insurance billing specialist must be knowledgeable of federal and industry-wide documentation requirements to assist providers and to ensure compliance in billing. Furthermore, the student will learn and develop diagnostic coding and procedural coding skills.

Unit 4: Claims Submission in the Medical Office

- Chapters 14 and 15 make up Unit 4 and will teach students the claims submission process. The textbook offers a unique block-by-block approach for completion of a paper insurance claim form in Chapter 14. In Chapter 15, the student will learn the electronic claims process and the advantages of electronic claim submission. They will learn federal legislation that governs the electronic claims process and the standard requirements for electronic claims submission.

Unit 5: Revenue Cycle Management

- Unit 5 is titled Revenue Cycle Management and includes Chapters 16 and 17. These chapters focus on the skills necessary to receive and process payments for health care services. Chapter 16 provides problem-solving techniques to use when dealing with insurance carriers. Chapter 17 provides the student with office and insurance collection strategies.

Unit 6: Health Care Facility Billing

- Chapter 18, Introduction to Health Facilities and Ambulatory Surgery Centers, was renamed in the 16th edition and expanded to introduce the student to many types of health care facilities they may be associated with throughout their career. The chapter describes the different types of health care facilities, rules, and guidelines specific to facility billing and the many types of reimbursement systems that health care facilities work with. Chapter 19, Billing for Health Care Facilities, was also renamed in the 16th edition. This chapter now outlines the billing process used by health care facilities and claim form completion. Furthermore, the chapter presents coding guidelines specific to facility billing and information about the *International Classification of Disease, Tenth Revision, Procedure Classification System (ICD-10-PCS)*. Step-by-step procedures are stated for processing a new patient for admission and to verify insurance benefits. Both Chapters 18 and 19 have been updated to provide the most current issues impacting insurance billing specialists in the facility setting.

Unit 7: Employment

- Chapter 20, Seeking a Job and Attaining Professional Advancement, provides insight into the insurance billing career field and lists employment opportunities for those seeking a position after their training. The chapter covers the job search, application, and interview processes. Information regarding advanced job opportunities, certification and the importance of professional organizations, networking, and mentoring are offered.

ANCILLARIES

Workbook

For students, the *Workbook* that accompanies the textbook is a practical approach to learning insurance billing. It progresses from easy to more complex issues within each chapter and advances as new skills are learned and integrated.

The *Workbook* that accompanies this edition of the textbook contains the following features:

- Each chapter has performance objectives for assignments that indicate to students what will be accomplished.
- Key terms are repeated for quick reference when studying.
- Key abbreviations followed by blank lines are listed alphabetically so that students can assemble their own reference list for each chapter, thus reinforcing the abbreviations' spell-outs.
- Assignments which include fill-in-the-blank, multiple-choice, mix-and-match, and true/false review questions.
- Some assignments give students hands-on experience in completing insurance claims on the CMS-1500 and UB-04 claim forms using standardized guidelines.
- Patients' medical records, financial accounting statements, and encounter forms are presented as they might appear in the health care organization's files so that students may learn how to abstract information to complete claim forms properly and accurately.
- Patient records and ledgers have been completely updated for technical clinical content and reworded to correspond with the 2021 CPT procedural and ICD-10-CM diagnostic code books.
- Easily removable forms and other sample documents are included in the *Workbook* for completion and to enhance keying skills.
- A final test section at the end of the *Workbook* to provide a complete, competency-based educational program.
- Answers to *Workbook* assignments have been put into the Instructor Resources that are available on the companion Evolve website.

Special appendixes are included at the end of the *Workbook*. These include a simulated practice, the College Clinic, with a group of physicians who employ the student. The appendix may be used as reference tools to complete workbook problems. These appendixes include the following:

- Appendix A details information for a simulated practice called *College Clinic*. Information is provided about the group of physicians and a mock fee schedule is included with codes and fees (including Medicare).

Evolve Companion Website (for Instructors)

Evolve is an interactive learning environment that works in coordination with the textbook. It provides internet-based course management tools that instructors can use to reinforce and expand on the concepts delivered in class. It can be used for the following:

- To publish the class syllabus, outline, and lecture notes
- To set up "virtual office hours" and e-mail communication

- To share important dates and information through the on-line class calendar
- To encourage student participation through chat rooms and discussion boards

The *TEACH Instructor's Resource Manual* is also available on the Evolve site. This resource allows instructors the flexibility to quickly adapt the textbook for their individual classroom needs and to gauge students' understanding. The *TEACH Instructor's Resource Manual* features the following:

- Announcements and content updates that become available.
- Lesson plans for each chapter.
- Power point slides and handouts for each chapter.
- Answer keys to the *Workbook* and Student Software Challenge assignments and tests with rationales, optional codes, and further explanations for most of the code problems
- Test banks for each chapter.

Evolve Companion Website (for Students)

Evolve also provides online access to free Learning Resources designed specifically to give students the information they need to quickly and successfully learn the topics covered in this textbook. These Learning Resources include the following:

- Announcements and content updates that become available.
- Blank CMS-1500 claim forms with the instructions for completion by the National Uniform Claims Committee (NUCC).
- Blank UB-04 claim forms with guidance for completion of both paper and electronic claims.
- Student 1500 Software Challenge simulates realistic experience by having students gather necessary documents and extract specific information to complete the CMS-1500 insurance claim form.
- Performance Evaluation Checklists for each chapter.
- Self-assessment quizzes and final exam to evaluate students' mastery through multiple-choice, true/false, fill-in-the-blank, and matching questions. Instant scoring and feedback are available at the click of a button.

Medical Insurance Online for Fordney's Medical Insurance and Billing

Medical Insurance Online for Fordney's Medical Insurance and Billing provides supplementary content and engaging activities to help students master the information presented in *Fordney's Medical Insurance and Billing, 16e*. Gradable case studies and assessments measure student progress and comprehension of the essential and challenging concepts that health insurance professionals face in the industry today. This course meets 508 and WCAG 2.0 accessibility criteria.

SUMMARY

Fordney's Medical Insurance and Billing and its ancillaries provide a complete competency-based educational program. The textbook and workbook learning and performance objectives, assignments, tests, Student Software Challenge, and incorporation of lesson plans and suggested classroom activities from the *TEACH Instructor's Resource Manual* ensure that students know everything they need to succeed in the workforce. Escalating costs of medical care, the effect of technology, and the multitude of insurance types have affected insurance billing procedures and claims processing and have necessitated new legislation for government and state programs. Therefore, it is essential that all medical personnel who handle claims continually update their knowledge. This may be accomplished by reading bulletins from state agencies and regional insurance carriers, speaking with insurance representatives, or attending insurance workshops offered at local colleges or local chapters of professional associations, such as those mentioned in Chapters 1 and 20. It is hoped that this textbook will resolve any unclear issues pertaining to current methods and become the framework on which the insurance billing specialist builds new knowledge as understanding and appreciation of the profession are attained.

Linda M. Smith, CPC, CPC-I, CEMC, CMBS
Greene, New York

CONTENTS

Career Role and Responsibilities

1

Role of an Insurance Billing Specialist

Linda M. Smith

OBJECTIVES

After reading this chapter, you should be able to:

1. Identify the background and importance of accurate insurance claims submission, coding, and billing.
2. Assess the various roles and responsibilities assigned to insurance billing specialists.
3. Name and discuss the office procedures performed in a health care organization during a workday that may affect billing.
4. Specify the educational requirements for a job as an insurance billing specialist and a coder.
5. Describe the variety of career advantages open to those trained as insurance billing specialists.
6. List qualifications, attributes, and skills necessary to be an insurance billing specialist.
7. Determine an appropriate dress code that would provide an image of confidence and professionalism.
8. Describe professional behavior when working as an insurance billing specialist.
9. Differentiate between professional ethics and medical etiquette.
10. Specify instances when an employer, an employee, or an independent contractor can be liable when billing for medical services.
11. Identify common practices and limitations of a claims assistance professional's scope of practice to his or her clients.
12. Explain how insurance knowledge and medical knowledge can be kept current.

KEY TERMS

accounts receivable
American Medical Association
cash flow
claims assistance professional
claims examiners
cycle
dress code
electronic mail
emoticons
encounter
errors and omissions insurance

ethics
etiquette
facility billing
health record
independent contractor
insurance billing specialist
management service organizations
medical billing representative
medical record
non-physician practitioner
personal health record

physician extender
professional billing
professional liability insurance
reimbursement specialist
respondeat superior
revenue
self-pay patient
senior billing representative
text speak

KEY ABBREVIATIONS

AMA	CAP	MSO	NPP
ASHD	e-mail		

Melissa A.: Certified Professional Coder (CPC) and Billing/Coding Consultant

I started into health care 36 years ago, as a transport specialist. From there I worked as a phlebotomist, operating room scheduling secretary, and medical office assistant where I learned medical billing and became very proficient at it. I went on to get my coding certification and all of this led me to where I am today. Currently, I am employed by a large health care organization where I perform coding for their skilled nursing facility. I also provide consulting services to medical practices. In my opinion, the most valuable skills an individual can have in this field are perseverance and determination. It's my job to bring the money in. I have always taken my role very personally whether I was working for a private practice or a large organization. If I am not successful in my role, the health care organization may not survive.

BACKGROUND OF INSURANCE CLAIMS, CODING, AND BILLING

Welcome to the world of medical billing, an exciting, ever-changing, and fast-growing career field. To help focus on important terms and definitions, the key words in this and subsequent chapters appear in **bold** or *italic* type.

Insurance billing specialists are nonclinical medical staff who work in all types of health care organizations. Their primary goals are to help patients obtain maximum insurance plan benefits for the services they received while ensuring the cash flow of their organization through revenue cycle management. Revenue is the total income produced by a medical practice or health care organization, and the cycle is the regularly repeating set of events for producing it.

Over the years, medical billing has become extraordinarily complex. The charge for a baby being born in the late 1960s could have been as little as $250. This was a flat fee that covered a 3-day hospital stay and a doctor's fee. The receipt for the birth typically looked like a receipt from a hardware store and contained the name of the patient, the total cost of care, and three options for payment (cash, check, or money order). Today, the average cost for giving birth is estimated to be between $5000 and $11,000 for an uncomplicated vaginal delivery. The estimated average cost for a cesarean birth can range from $7500 to $14,500 while complications during birth may further increase the charge. These prices include the total duration of care, the obstetrician's fee, the anesthesiologist's fee, and the hospital care fee. And as the charge for services has increased, so has the complexity of billing for them. There are numerous payers that the billing specialist must be familiar with, each with their own guidelines. In addition, health care organizations use electronic medical records, electronic health records, and personal health records which the insurance billing specialist must be familiar with and learn to use.

- Medical records refer to patient charts which includes notes and information collected by and for the clinicians in that specific health care provider's office or organization.
- Health records refer to information collected from *all* of the clinicians involved in a patient's care. Clinicians can be authorized to access the patient's health record to assist them in providing care to that patient. Health records could include such things as laboratory and radiology reports or consultations with other providers.
- Personal health records are designed to be set up, accessed, and managed by the patient. The records typically contain information such as diagnoses, medications, immunizations, family medical histories, and provider contact information.

The insurance billing specialist must also have strong computer skills and learn to use the various software programs used for medical billing. Patient conditions and services must be coded which is a skill that individuals must excel in. Additionally, there are various methods of reimbursement for the services that the insurance billing specialist must be familiar with. It is often difficult for health care organizations to obtain maximum payment for services. The health care industry is one of the most heavily regulated industries in the United States. There are laws that must be followed and many billing and coding guidelines. Physicians and health care organizations rely on professional insurance billing specialists to handle this complex part of their business. An insurance billing specialist must be knowledgeable of the health care system and all of the components, interrelationships, and interdependencies, such as hospitals, outpatient laboratories, insurance companies, federal government, patients, patient families, other health care professionals, and co-workers.

In medical billing, there are two different types of billing: facility billing and professional billing. Facility billing is charging for services done in hospitals, acute care hospitals, skilled nursing or long-term care facilities, rehabilitation centers, or ambulatory surgical centers. Professional billing is charging for services performed by physicians or non-physician practitioners (NPPs). An NPP is a provider of health care services, such as a physician assistant, nurse practitioner, advanced registered nurse practitioner, certified nurse anesthetist, physical therapist, speech therapist, licensed clinical social worker, or certified registered nurse practitioner, who has not obtained a medical degree but is allowed to see patients and prescribe medications. These professionals are sometimes referred to as physician extenders. Professional billing is also relevant to other ancillary providers such as ambulance services, radiology and laboratory services, and physical therapists. This textbook will address both facility billing and professional billing. Although there are significant differences in the processing of claims between facility and professional billing, the basic setup of a business office encompasses the following units or combined departments:

- reception of the patient,
- rendering of medical services,
- documentation of the services, and
- financial accounting.

The insurance billing specialist must understand the function of each department in relation to the business office and the health care organization as a whole and how they affect the revenue cycle. The flow of information between departments is one of the most vital components of an organization.

In the health care organization, office procedures performed throughout a workday include the following:

- *Scheduling appointments* involves assigning time slots for patient encounters. An encounter is defined as an interaction between a patient and a health care provider for the purpose of providing health care services or assessing the patient's health

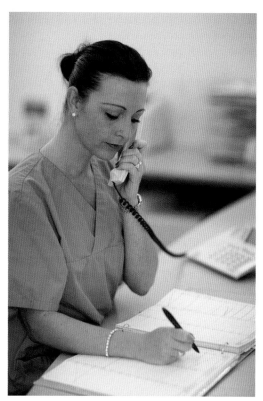

Fig. 1.1 Health care staff scheduling an appointment. (Copyright © iStock.com/fotografixx.)

status. Canceling and rescheduling may also be involved. If the time is not properly assigned, there may be an influx or low volume of patients at a given time. Paperwork required for the encounter must also be produced. It is important to record why the patient requires health care services. See Fig. 1.1.

- *Registering patients* may involve preregistration for visits by using a questionnaire referred to as a *patient registration form*. Financial and personal data are collected and accurately recorded (input) in a timely manner. Incorrect information affects the submission and payment of claims.
- *Documenting* pertinent clinical notes for assignment of a diagnosis and service code to the patient's encounter is done by the provider of service. The notes in the patient's medical record include the reason for the encounter, history, physical examination, diagnostic tests, results, diagnosis, and plan of treatment. The insurance billing specialist may be required to contact the insurance company to obtain authorization for treatment by secondary providers. He or she must also ensure that forms are properly completed, and data are input into the system. Both proper documentation and assignment of the correct code for service affect the revenue cycle.
- Posting (inputting) a *charge entry* for patient care service rendered into the billing system by the charge entry staff member. The insurance biller must make certain that the insurance is correct in the system and must ensure that the diagnosis coincides with the service rendered. For example, an obstetrics/gynecology encounter should not have a diagnosis related to ophthalmology. Many times, individuals have the same names, so billing service dates and the name of the patient seen must be accurate. The charge entry staff member must ensure that the correct charge is assigned to the correct

patient. Proper charge entry ensures timely billing and reimbursement.
- *Bookkeeping and accounting* is the posting of payments received (cash, checks, electronic funds transfer, or debit and credit cards) to patients' financial accounts. The bookkeeper or accountant must pay special attention to adjustments, denials, and write-offs. These entries may require investigation for validation. He or she may also receive insurance payer remittance advices and may be assigned to follow up on denials.

> ### 1.1 QUICK REVIEW
> Question: What is the difference between facility billing and professional billing?

ROLE OF THE INSURANCE BILLING SPECIALIST

Several job titles are associated with medical billing personnel. The professional title used may depend on the region within the United States. Some of the most popular titles include insurance billing specialist, electronic claims processor, medical biller, reimbursement specialist, medical billing representative, and senior billing representative. In large health care organizations it is common to find a billing department made up of many people; within the department, each position is specialized, such as Medicare billing specialist, Medicaid billing specialist, coding specialist, insurance counselor, collection manager, and revenue cycle manager. In this handbook the title *insurance billing specialist* will be used throughout to represent this broad spectrum of titles.

Insurance carriers also employ insurance billing specialists who may serve as claims examiners. Claims examiners are also referred to as claims adjustors or claims representatives. Their role is to analyze and process incoming claims, checking them for validity and determining if the services were reasonable and necessary.

Some health care organizations contract with management services organizations (MSOs), which perform a variety of business functions, such as accounting, billing, coding, clinical documentation improvement, collections, computer support, compliance oversight, legal advice, marketing, payroll, and management expertise. An insurance billing specialist may find a job working for an MSO as a part of this team.

Individuals called claims assistance professionals (CAPs) work for the consumer. They help patients organize, file, and negotiate health insurance claims of all types; assist the consumer in obtaining maximum benefits for the health care services they received; and tell the patient how much to pay the health care organization to make sure there is no overpayment. It is possible for someone who has taken a course on insurance billing to function in this role.

Job Responsibilities

Whether employed by a medical practice, a hospital, or other health care organization as an insurance billing specialist, the individual should be able to perform any and all duties related to the business office. All health care staff, regardless as to whether they work in scheduling, registration, charge posting, or accounting, must work together to ensure a strong revenue cycle and appropriate reimbursement. Health care organizations have job descriptions to outline the job duties, skills, and requirements for insurance billing specialists and other related job titles. See Figs. 1.2 and 1.3.

GENERIC JOB DESCRIPTION FOR ENTRY LEVEL INSURANCE BILLING SPECIALIST

Knowledge, skills, and abilities:
1. Minimum education level consists of certificate from 1-year insurance billing course, associate degree, or equivalent in work experience and continuing education.
2. Knowledge of basic medical terminology, anatomy and physiology, diseases, surgeries, medical specialties, and insurance terminology.
3. Ability to operate computer, printer, photocopy, and calculator equipment.
4. Written and oral communication skills including grammar, punctuation, and style.
5. Ability and knowledge to use procedure code books.
6. Ability and knowledge to use diagnostic code books.
7. Knowledge and skill of data entry.
8. Ability to work independently.
9. Certification in billing and/or coding is preferred.

Salary:
Employer would list range of remuneration for the position.

Job responsibilities:	Performance standards:
1. Abstracts health information from patient records.	1.1 Uses knowledge of medical terminology, anatomy, diseases, surgeries, and medical specialties. 1.2 Consults reference materials as needed. 1.3 Meets accuracy and production requirements. 1.4 Verifies with physician any vague information for accuracy.
2. Exhibits an understanding of ethical and medicolegal responsibilities related to insurance billing programs.	2.1 Observes policies and procedures related to federal privacy regulations, health records, release of information, retention of records, and statute of limitations for claim submission. 2.2 Meets standards of professional etiquette and ethical conduct. 2.3 Recognizes and reports problems involving fraud, abuse, embezzlement, and forgery to appropriate individuals.
3. Follows employer's policies and procedures.	3.1 Punctual work attendance and is dependable. 3.2 Answers routine inquiries related to account balances and insurance forms submitted.
4. Transmits insurance claims accurately.	4.1 Updates insurance registration and account information. 4.2 Processes payments and posts to accounts accurately. 4.3 Handles correspondence related to insurance claims. 4.4 Reviews encounter forms for accuracy before submission to data entry. 4.5 Inserts data for generating insurance claims accurately. 4.6 Codes procedures and diagnoses accurately. 4.7 Telephones third-party payers with regard to delinquent claims. 4.8 Traces insurance claims. 4.9 Files appeals for denied claims.
5. Enhances knowledge and skills to keep up to date.	5.1 Attends continuing education activities. 5.2 Keeps abreast and maintains files of current changes in coding requirements from Medicare, Medicaid, and other third-party payers. 5.3 Assists with updating fee schedules and encounter forms with current codes. 5.4 Assists in the research of proper coding techniques.
6. Employs interpersonal expertise to provide good working relationships with patients, employer, employees, and third-party payers.	6.1 Works with employer and employees cooperatively as a team. 6.2 Communicates effectively with patients and third-party payers. 6.3 Executes job assignments with diligence and skill. 6.4 Assists staff with coding and reimbursement problems. 6.5 Assists other employees when needed.

Fig. 1.2 Generic job description for an insurance billing specialist.

GENERIC JOB DESCRIPTION FOR
AN ELECTRONIC CLAIMS PROCESSOR

Knowledge, skills, and abilities:
1. Minimum education level consists of certificate from 1-year insurance billing course, associate degree, or equivalent in work experience and continuing education.
2. Knowledge of basic medical terminology, anatomy and physiology, diseases, surgeries, medical specialties, and insurance terminology.
3. Ability to operate computer and printer, as well as photocopy and calculator equipment.
4. Written and oral communication skills including grammar, punctuation, and style.
5. Ability and knowledge to use procedure code books.
6. Ability and knowledge to use diagnostic code books.
7. Knowledge and skill of data entry.
8. Ability to work independently.
9. Certification in electronic claims processing is preferred.

Salary:
Employer would list range of remuneration for the position.

Job responsibilities:	Performance standards:
1. Acts as a link between the medical provider or facility and third-party payers.	1.1 Uses knowledge of medical terminology, anatomy, diseases, surgeries, and medical specialties. 1.2 Understands computer applications and equipment required to convert and transmit patient billing data electronically. 1.3 Consults reference materials as needed. 1.4 Meets accuracy and production requirements.
2. Converts patient billing data into electronically readable formats.	2.1 Inputs data and transmits insurance claims accurately, either directly or through a clearinghouse. 2.2 Answers routine inquiries related to insurance data transmitted to third-party payers. 2.3 Updates and maintains software applications as needed.
3. Uses software that eliminates common claim filing errors, provides clean claims to third-party payers expedites payments, and follows, up on delinquent or denied claims.	3.1 Codes procedures and diagnoses accurately. 3.2 Telephones third-party payers about delinquent claims. 3.3 Traces insurance claims. 3.4 Files appeals for denied claims.
4. Exhibits an understanding of ethical and medicolegal responsibilities related to insurance billing programs and plans.	4.1 Observes policies and procedures related to federal privacy regulations, health records, release of information, retention of records, and statute of limitations for claim submission. 4.2 Meets standards of professional etiquette and ethical conduct. 4.3 Recognizes and reports problems involving fraud, abuse, embezzlement, and forgery to appropriate individuals.
5. Follows employer's policies and procedures.	5.1 Must have punctual work attendance and be dependable.
6. Enhances knowledge and skills to keep up to date.	6.1 Attends continuing education skills activities. 6.2 Obtains current knowledge applicable to transmission of insurance claims. 6.3 Keeps abreast and maintains files of current changes in coding requirements from Medicare, Medicaid, and other third-party payers. Assists in the research of proper coding techniques to maximum reimbursement.
7. Employs interpersonal expertise to provide good working relationships with patients, employer, employees, and third-party payers.	7.1 Works with employer and employees cooperatively as a team. 7.2 Communicates effectively with patients and third-party payers. 7.3 Executes job assignments with diligence and skill. 7.4 Assists staff with coding and reimbursement problems. 7.5 Assists other employees when needed.

Fig. 1.3 Generic job description for an electronic claims processor.

Administrative office duties have gained in importance in the medical billing process. In some health care organizations, an insurance billing specialist may act as an insurance counselor, taking the patient to a private area of the office before being seen by the provider. The insurance counselor will discuss the health care organization's financial policies and review the patient's insurance coverage. The counselor confirms with the insurance company any fees the patient is responsible for and verifies whether any preauthorization, precertification, or second-opinion requirements exist. Insurance counselors help to obtain payment in full when expensive procedures are necessary. Insurance counselors ensure that the health care organization will be paid for services rendered and to develop good communication lines.

Front desk staff are responsible for collecting payment from self-pay patients. Self-pay patients are those who do not have any medical insurance and are liable for the entire bill. Front desk staff are also responsible for collecting any copayments or deductible amounts from the patient at each encounter before the patient is treated.

After the patient has been treated, the insurance billing specialist should confirm that documentation of services has been completed by the health care provider. Documentation of services is vital to good patient care and must be done comprehensively and timely for proper reimbursement. A coding specialist may review or assign diagnostic and procedural coding which must be supported in the documentation.

Federal and state insurance programs require the provider of services to submit claims for the patient. Other insurance payers may see claim submission as the patient's obligation, although most health care organizations submit all claims for patients as a courtesy. The insurance billing specialist must submit insurance claims promptly, ideally within 1 to 5 business days, to ensure continuous cash flow. Cash flow is the amount of actual money generated and available for use by the health care organization within a given period. Without money coming in, overhead expenses such as salaries, rent, supplies, and insurance cannot be met and an organization will face financial difficulties.

In some organizations the insurance biller may act as a collection manager, who answers routine inquiries related to account balances and insurance submission dates; assists patients in setting up a payment schedule that is within their budget; follows up on delinquent accounts; and traces denied, "adjusted," or unpaid claims (Fig. 1.4).

The accounts receivables for a health care organization is the total amount of money owed to them for health care services rendered to patients. Having a large accounts receivables is often a direct result of failure to verify insurance plan benefits, obtain authorization or precertification, or collect fees from patients or inadequate claims filing. The rush to get a claim "out the door" cannot be justified when an organization has thousands or millions of dollars in unpaid or denied claims. Accounts receivables will be low and revenue high if the organization takes the extra time to ensure that the claim is 100% accurate, complete, and verified.

Educational and Training Requirements

A high school diploma or equivalent and previous experience in a health care setting may not always be enough for positions as an insurance billing specialist. Typically a postsecondary

Fig. 1.4 Insurance biller talking to a patient on the telephone about copayment required for an office encounter under the patient's insurance plan.

certificate or an associate's degree is required to enter the field. Postsecondary certificates and associate's degree programs usually include courses in medical terminology, anatomy and physiology, insurance claims completion, procedural and diagnostic coding, health care reimbursement methods, ethics and medicolegal knowledge, computer skills, and general office skills. Completion of an accredited program for coding certification or an accredited health information technology program is necessary for a job as a coder.

The curriculum that might be offered in an online certificate program for a medical insurance specialist is shown in Fig. 1.5. A 2-year educational course can result in obtaining an associate's degree. Many accredited programs include an externship, which is a training program with private businesses that gives students brief practical experience in their field of study. It is usually short term but allows the student to gain firsthand insight into the field.

Experience and a moderate to high degree of knowledge of the health insurance business are necessary if the individual's goal is to become a self-employed insurance billing specialist or CAP. In addition to insurance terminology, claims procedures, and coding, a CAP must know commercial insurance payers' requirements as well as Medicare and state Medicaid policies and regulations. Proficiency in running a business, including marketing and sales expertise is also essential.

To reach a professional level of billing or coding expertise, certification is available from many national associations, depending on the type of certification desired. Refer to Chapter 20 for more information on this topic.

Career Advantages

According to the US Bureau of Labor Statistics,[1] employment in the field is expected to grow faster than jobs in other occupations. The demand for health services and related jobs is expected to increase over the next 10 years as the population ages. Jobs are available in every state, ranging from entry level to management positions. Insurance billing specialists can receive a salary of $8000 part-time to $50,000 full-time or more per year, depending on knowledge, experience, duties, responsibilities, locale, and size of the employing institution. Jobs are available with insurance and managed care companies, medical clearinghouses, ambulatory

Medical Billing and Coding Program Curriculum

Curriculum Description:
Students learn the fundamentals of medical billing and coding and are prepared to take the Certified Billing and Coding Specialist (CBCS) exam from the National Healthcareer Association, the Certified Professional Coder (CPC exam) from the American Academy of Professional Coders (AAPC) and the Certified Coding Associate (CCA) exam from the American Health Information Management Association (AHIMA). Program topics include medical terminology, insurance plans, medical ethics, HIPAA, diagnostic and procedural coding, coding compliance and auditing, physician and hospital billing, Medicare, Medicaid and TRICARE. Students receive training on ICD-10-CM/PCS, CPT and HCPCS code assignment.

LESSON GROUPS

Group 1: Introduction to Allied Health • Allied Health Careers	Group 2: Law, Ethics, and Confidentiality in Allied Health • Law in Allied Health • Ethics in Allied Health • Confidentiality in Allied Health
Group 3: Medical Billing and Health Insurance • Reimbursement Methodologies • Comprehensive Health Insurances	Group 4: Medical Office Procedures • Basic Math for Allied Health • Basic Grammar for Allied Health • Professional Communications • Basic Microsoft® Word and Excel
Group 5: Body Systems and Terminology • Introduction to Medical Terminology • Cardiovascular and Hematologic Systems • Respiratory and Endocrine Systems • GI, Urinary, and Reproductive Systems	Group 6: Body Systems and Terminology • Integumentary and Musculoskeletal Systems • Sensory Organs and Nervous System Immune System, HIV, and Cancer
Group 7: Pathology and Pharmacology • Introduction to Pharmacology • Pharmacology • Introduction to Pathology • Pathology	Group 8: Electronic Medical Records • Electronic Health Records and Security • Administrative and Clinical Use of the EHR • Reimbursement and Personal Health Records • Electronic Medical Records Final Exam • Electronic Medical Records Graded Project
Group 9: Basic Medical Coding • Introduction to Coding • Diagnosis Coding with ICD-10-CM • Guidelines for Using ICD-10-CM • Procedure Coding with ICD-10-PCS • Basic Medical Coding Graded Project	Group 10: Intermediate Medical Coding • Introduction to CPT • Evaluation and Management and Anesthesia Coding • Surgical CPT Coding, Part 1 • Surgical CPT Coding, Part 2 • Surgical CPT Coding, Part 3 • Intermediate Medical Coding Graded Project
Group 11: Billing and Coding Professional Certification Exam Review • Anatomy, Terminology and Pathophysiology • CPT Coding • HCPCS Coding and Reimbursement • ICD-10-CM Coding • Post-Exam	

Fig. 1.5 Example of an online medical billing certificate course curriculum. (Reprinted with permission from Ashworth College.)

surgical centers, clinics, hospitals, multispecialty medical groups, and private physicians' practices. Many insurance billing specialists will have the good fortune to advance their careers and move into higher paying positions that come with additional learning, certifications, and experience. These positions may be with consulting firms, instructors at educational facilities, lecturers, or consumer advocates. Other branches of the advanced career field include specialty coding, auditing, compliance, and documentation improvement specialists. These advancement opportunities and certifications will be discussed further in Chapter 20.

Self-Employment or Independent Contracting

After gaining experience, many people establish independently owned and self-operated businesses within their communities as medical insurance billing specialists, coders, claim assistance professionals, collectors, or consultants. However, the responsibilities are greater in this area because such work demands a full-time commitment, a lot of hard work, long hours to obtain clients, and the need to advertise and market the business. The self-employed insurance billing specialist is responsible for everything: advertising, billing, bookkeeping, and other general business tasks.

Flexibility

The nature of medical billing lends itself to flexible hours and flexible job options. The medical insurance billing specialist may want to come in early to transmit electronic claims during off-peak hours or stay late to make collection calls. Many times, medical billing positions have various combinations of work flexibility such as telecommuting, part-time, contract, and work-at-home opportunities. There is an increase in the number of employers who will provide a work-at-home option to highly competent billers and coders who have proven their technical skills and work ethic. In most cases where working from home is allowed, it will be on a hybrid basis, which allows the employees to complete part of their work from home but be required to spend time in the office as well. The availability of work-from-home jobs varies on a case-by-case basis and depends on the employer's policy. Many employers see this type of arrangement as a way to save time, money, and overhead costs while building productivity and increasing job satisfaction.

Disabled Workers

A career as an insurance billing specialist or a collector of delinquent accounts can be rewarding for persons with disabilities. The revenue cycle management responsibilities and other jobs involving telephone communications are an opportunity for someone who is visually impaired because he or she is usually a good listener when properly and specifically trained. Special equipment, such as a Braille keyboard, magnified computer screen, audible scanner, or digital audio recorder, may be necessary to enhance job performance.

Working independently from a home office may appeal to a physically disabled person when there is no need to commute to the health care organization on a daily basis. Accessing information remotely via the computer is a manageable method for success. However, it is important first to gain experience before trying to establish a work-at-home situation.

Qualifications and Attributes

An individual must have a variety of characteristics or qualities to function well as an insurance billing specialist. Strong critical thinking and reading skills with good comprehension are a must. Being a logical and practical thinker, as well as a creative problem solver, is important. Being meticulous and neat makes it easier to get the job done at the workstation. A person with good organizational skills who is conscientious and loyal is always an asset to the employer. Because a large amount of specific data must be obtained, this work requires an individual who is detail oriented. A person with a curious nature will dig deeper into an issue and not be satisfied with an answer unless the "whys" and "whats" are defined. This also helps one to grow while on the job and not become stagnant. Equally important are time management and social skills.

Skills

A person who completes insurance claims must have many skills. One needs the following skills to be proficient Table 1.1:

TABLE 1.1	Skills Application
Skill	**Application**
Solid foundation and working knowledge of medical terminology, including anatomy, physiology, disease, and treatment terms, as well as the meanings of abbreviations.	Interpretation of patient's chart notes and code manuals. For example, the diagnosis which is documented is ASHD. **ASHD** must be translated to arteriosclerotic hear disease.
Expert use of procedural and diagnostic code books and other related resources.	Code manuals, official coding guidelines, and other reference books are used to assign accurate codes for each case billed.
Precise reading skills.	Differentiate between the technical descriptions of two different but similar procedures. Example: Procedural (CPT) code 43352 Esophagostomy (fistulization of esophagus, external; cervical approach) and Procedural (CPT) code 43020 Esophagotomy (cervical approach, with removal of foreign body). Note that the addition of the letter s to the surgical procedure in the first part of the example changes the entire procedure.
Basic mathematics.	Calculate fees and adjustments on the insurance claim forms and enter them into the patient accounts. It is essential that the figures be accurate
Knowledge of medicolegal rules and regulations of various insurance programs.	Avoid filing of claims considered fraudulent or abusive because of code selection and program policies.
Knowledge of compliance issues.	Federal privacy, security, and transaction rules in addition to fraud, waste, and abuse.

Continued

TABLE 1.1	Skills Application—cont'd
Skill	**Application**
Basic keyboarding and computer skills.	Good keyboarding and data entry skills and knowledge of computer programs are essential in an industry which utilizes various software programs for management of electronic medical records, management of the revenue cycle, and electronic claims submission
Proficiency in accessing information through the internet.	Obtain federal, state, and commercial insurance regulations and current information as needed through the internet. Sign on as a member of an electronic mailing list where questions may be posted. Find one composed of working coders to obtain answers on how to code complex care, or difficult medical cases.
Knowledge of billing and collection techniques.	Use latest billing and collection ideas to keep cash flow constant and avoid delinquent accounts.
Expertise in the legalities of collection on accounts.	Avoid lawsuits by knowing state and federal collection laws as they apply to medical collection of accounts receivable.
Ability to generate insurance claims with speed and accuracy.	Independent medical claims and billing specialists are often paid according to the amount of paid claims the health care practice is reimbursed. Because they rely on volume for income, the more expeditious they become, the more money they earn. Therefore accuracy in selecting the correct codes and data entry and motivation in completing claims also become marketable skills.
Excellent communication skills	Insurance billing specialists communicate with health car eproviders and other professionals to collect accurate information for billing purposes. The communicate with patients and insurance carriers to collect fees and resolve pending and denied claims. Many specialists also communicate with health care administrative professionals as part of revenue cycle management. Having a pleasant tone and friendly attitude are important skills for an effective communicator. Insurance billing specialists must have empathy when communicating with patients and confidence when working with health care professionals and insurance carriers. In all cases, communications should be clear and concise.

Fig. 1.6 Male and female medical personnel who project a clean, fresh, and professional image.

Personal Image

To project a professional image, the insurance billing specialist must be attentive to apparel and grooming (Fig. 1.6). Health care professionals are expected to present themselves in an appropriate and professional manner that portrays an image of confidence and security to the patient. Appearance and perception play a key role in patient service.

When hired, it is important to request the organization's dress-code policy. A **dress code** is a set of guidelines identifying what is appropriate for the employee to wear to work. The insurance billing specialist might be expected to wear scrubs or business attire that is conservative and frequently referred to as *business casual*. Distracting items in appearance or dress, low-cut clothing, exposed midriff, T-shirts, or sheer clothing are typically considered unacceptable. It is absolutely necessary for health care professionals to present neat and clean in the professional setting. Fingernails should be carefully manicured and appropriate to the dress code. Employers may also have guidelines regarding body piercings and tattoos. Keep in mind that fragrances can be offensive or cause allergies to some co-workers and patients; therefore, use good judgment. An example of a dress code policy is shown in (Fig. 1.7).

Behavior

Many aspects make an individual a true professional: getting along with people rates high on the list, as does maintaining confidentiality of patients' health information. An insurance billing specialist depends on many co-workers for information needed to bill claims; therefore it is necessary to be a team player and treat patients and co-workers with courtesy and respect. Consider all co-workers' duties as important because they are part of the team, working together to reach the goal of processing the billing and obtaining maximum reimbursement for the patient and the health care organization. Communicate effectively. Be honest, dependable, and on time. Never take part in office gossip or politics.

 1.2   **QUICK REVIEW**
Question: What is cash flow and why is it important?

XYZ Medical Practice

Dress Code Policy
Insurance Billing Specialist

Introduction:
Appearance and perception play a key role in patient services. Dress, grooming and personal cleanliness standards contribute to the morale of all employees and affect the professional image we present to patients and visitors.

The XYZ Medical Practice's dress code policy is designed to provide our staff with consistent and appropriate guidance as we strive to maintain a professional appearance at all times. The goal is to provide an image of confidence and security to our patients.

Designated Staff: Insurance Billing Specialist

Policy:
- Employees are expected to dress in scrubs or business casual attire. Business casual includes: dress pants, Docker-type pants, khakis, slacks, casual skirts or dresses of appropriate length, shirts with collars, blazers, sports coats, sweaters, golf shirts/polo shirts and blouses.
- Blue jeans are not permitted with the exception of "jean day" to raise money for charity.
- Inappropriate attire includes (but is not limited to): shorts, sweatpants, spandex leggings, wind suits, miniskirts and spaghetti strap tops and sundresses.
- Clothing with offensive or inappropriate designs or stamps are not allowed.
- Clothing should not be too revealing
- Employees must always present a clean and professional appearance. Staff should be well-groomed and wear clean clothing.
- Hair should be clean, combed and neatly trimmed. This includes sideburns, mustaches and beards.
- Due to possible allergies of co-workers and patients, it is requested that staff do not wear fragrances.
- ID badges should be worn in a visible place above the waist at all times.

Dress Code Violations:
The guidelines established in this policy cannot be all-inclusive. Therefore, management will make the final decision as to the appropriateness of work attire as needed.

Office managers are responsible for ensuring appearance is appropriate and are expected to inform staff when they are violating the dress code. Staff in violation are expected to immediately correct the issue. This may include having to leave work to change clothes. Repeated violations or violations that have major repercussions may result in disciplinary action being taken up to and including termination.

Fig. 1.7 Example of a dress code policy for an insurance billing specialist.

MEDICAL ETIQUETTE

Before beginning work as an insurance billing specialist, it is wise to have a basic knowledge of medical etiquette as it pertains to the medical profession, the insurance industry, and the medical coder. Medical etiquette has to do with how medical professionals conduct themselves, their behavior. Customs, courtesy, and manners of the medical profession can be expressed in three simple words: *consideration for others.*

In every business that interacts with customers or clients, the focus begins with good customer service. Co-workers and patients should always be acknowledged with a smile, a nod, or a greeting. Patients may arrive for their appointments ill or injured and suffering from a lot of negativity. If a mistake is made, there is power in an apology given at the first sign of trouble. Attentiveness and a helpful, friendly atmosphere can smooth out the kinks and wrinkles of stressful and negative situations. All people have the need to feel special and they gravitate toward individuals who make them feel that way. All of these personal skills mean good customer service and satisfaction and can lead to professional success for the insurance billing specialist and the health care organization.

Several points about medical etiquette bear mentioning, as follows:

1. Always connect another health care provider who is calling on the telephone to the provider immediately, asking as few questions as possible.
2. Follow the basic rules of etiquette with co-workers while working in the office, such as acknowledging people entering the work area and by saying, "I'll be with you in a moment."
3. Clearly identify yourself when placing or receiving calls.
4. Do not use first names unless permission to do so has been given.
5. Maintain a professional demeanor and a certain amount of formality when interacting with others. Remember to be courteous and always project a professional image.
6. Observe rules of etiquette when sending e-mail messages and placing or receiving cellphone calls.
7. Practice cultural awareness by understanding and respecting the differences of others. Be sensitive to differences in attitudes, values, and perceptions.

Proper etiquette may make the difference between a highly satisfied patient and a disgruntled patient. Proper etiquette lets the patient know that you value them and that your organization is happy to help them.

EXAMPLE 1.1   Electronic Mail Address

Electronic mail (e-mail) address mason@gmail.com means:
Mason individual user (Mason)

@	at
gmail	site (an online service provider)
com	type of site (commercial business)

Electronic Mail Etiquette

Electronic mail (e-mail) is the transmitting, receiving, storing, and forwarding of text, voice messages, attachments, or images by computer from one person to another. Every computer user subscribing to an online service may establish an e-mail address (Example 1.1).

Because this is a more cost-effective and efficient method of sending a message to someone and obtaining a quicker response, insurance billing specialists frequently compose, forward, and respond via e-mail with staff in other locations, with patients, and with insurance billers (Fig. 1.8). It is important to set some standards to follow when communicating via e-mail. The messages sent are a reflection of an individual's professional image.

1. Compose the message in a clear and concise manner using good grammar and proper spelling. Make sure it cannot be misconstrued.
2. Clearly identify the reason for the message in the subject line. If a reply changes the topic, then change the subject line.
3. Do not put confidential information in an e-mail message (e.g., patient-identifiable information).
4. Encrypt (code) all files about patients and e-mail attachments and limit the size of attachments.

Address → To: apcconsulting@gmail.com
Subject Line → Subj: **anesthesia modifiers**
Date → Date: Friday, April 17, 2020
Sender Address → From: brownm@xyz.org
Salutation → Dear Madam or Sir:
Left → Question: Is conscious sedation considered anesthesia in
Justified   relationship to modifier -73 and -74? A speaker at a recent
Brief Message   conference said "yes" but another said it had not yet been
With Proper   clarified by CMS. Our fiscal intermediary manual has an
Grammar   example that said modifier -52 would be used in conjunction
   with a colonoscopy with conscious sedation. What is correct?

Complimentary
Closing → Sincerely,
Signature Line → Mary Brown
Title → Insurance Billing Specialist
Location → XYZ Ambulatory Surgery Center
E-mail address → brownm@xyz.org

Confidentiality
Statement → IMPORTANT WARNING: This e-mail (and any attachments) is only intended for the use of the person or entity to which it is addressed, and may contain information that is privileged and confidential. You, the recipient, are obligated to maintain it in a safe, secure and confidential manner. Unauthorized re-disclosure or failure to maintain confidentiality may subject you to federal and state penalties. If you are not the intended recipient, please immediately notify us by return e-mail, and delete this message from your computer.

Fig. 1.8 Electronic mail message sent to an ambulatory surgical center consultant asking a question about the use of modifiers.

5. Recognize that all e-mail is discoverable in legal proceedings, so be careful with content and choice of words.
6. Do not use all capital letters for more than one word.
7. Insert a blank line between paragraphs.
8. Surround URLs (long web addresses) with angle brackets [] to avoid problems occurring at the end of a line because of the word wrap feature.
9. Do not use variable text styles (bold or italic) or text colors.
10. Quote sparingly when automatically quoting the original message in replies. Quotation marks should be inserted to differentiate original and new text.
11. Avoid sending or forwarding junk messages (e.g., welcome messages, congratulation messages, jokes, chain messages).
12. Avoid "**emoticons**," a short sequence of keyboard letters and symbols used to convey emotion, gestures, or expressions (e.g., "smiley" [(;:–)]).
13. Avoid "**text speak**," which is the process of shortening words and using abbreviations that do not follow standard grammar, spelling, and punctuation. (e.g. "TY" for "thank you" or "IMO" for "in my opinion".
14. Do not respond immediately to e-mails that result in negative emotions or anger. Put the message aside until the next day and then answer it diplomatically.
15. Do not write anything that is racially or sexually offensive.
16. A short signature at the end of the message should be inserted that includes the sender's name, affiliation, and e-mail and/or URL address.
17. When replying to emails with multiple addresses, make sure to respond only to the desired individual.

1.3 QUICK REVIEW

Question: What are three simple words that can be used to express customs, courtesy, and manners of any medical professional?

PROFESSIONAL ETHICS

Ethics are not laws but standards of conduct generally accepted as moral guides for behavior. Ethics should be relied upon as the insurance billing specialist relates with patients, health care providers, co-workers, the government, and insurance companies. Insurance billing specialists are entrusted with holding patients' medical information in confidence, collecting money for their health care organization, and being a reliable resource for co-workers. To act with ethical behavior means carrying out responsibilities with integrity, decency, honesty, competence, consideration, respect, fairness, trust, and courage.

The earliest written code of ethical principles and conduct for the medical profession originated in Babylonia about 2500 BC and is called the *Code of Hammurabi*. Then, about the fifth century BC, Hippocrates, a Greek physician who is known as the "Father of Medicine," conceived the Oath of Hippocrates.

In 1980 the **American Medical Association (AMA)** adopted a modern code of ethics, called the *Principles of Medical Ethics*, for the benefit of the health professional and to meet the needs of changing times. The Principles of Medical Ethics of the AMA (Box 1.1) guide physicians' standards of conduct for honorable behavior in the practice of medicine.

BOX 1.1 Principles of Medical Ethics of the American Medical Association

Preamble

The medical profession has long subscribed to a body of ethical statements developed primarily for the benefit of the patient.

As a member of the profession, a physician must recognize responsibility to patients first and foremost, as well as to society, to other health professionals, and to self. The following principles adopted by the AMA are not laws, but standards of conduct that define the essentials of honorable behavior for the physician.

I. A physician shall be dedicated to providing competent medical service with compassion and respect for human dignity and rights.
II. A physician shall uphold the standards of professionalism, be honest in all professional interactions, and strive to report physicians deficient in character or competence, or engaging in fraud or deception to appropriate entities.
III. A physician shall respect the law and also recognize a responsibility to seek changes in those requirements which are contrary to the best interests of the patient.
IV. A physician shall respect the rights of patients, of colleagues, and of other health professionals, and shall safeguard patient confidences and privacy within the constraints of the law.
V. A physician shall continue to study, apply, and advance scientific knowledge, maintain a commitment to medical education, make relevant information available to patients, colleagues, and the public; obtain consultation; and use the talents of other health professionals when indicated.
VI. A physician shall, in the provision of appropriate patient care, except in emergencies, be free to choose whom to serve, with whom to associate, and the environment in which to provide medical care.
VII. A physician shall recognize a responsibility to participate in activities contributing to the improvement of the community and the betterment of public health.
VIII. A physician shall, while caring for a patient, regard responsibility to the patient as paramount.
IX. A physician shall support access to medical care for all people.

Revised June 2001. Permission granted to reproduce by the American Medical Association.

It is the insurance billing specialist's responsibility to inform administration or their immediate supervisor if unethical or possibly illegal billing or coding practices are taking place. Illegal activities are subject to penalties, fines, and/or imprisonment and can result in loss of morale, reputation, and the goodwill of the community.

The following are principles of ethics for the insurance billing specialist:
- Never make critical remarks about a health care organization or provider to a patient or anyone else. Maintain dignity; never belittle patients.
- Notify a supervisor if it is discovered that a patient may have questionable issues of care, conduct, or treatment with the health care organization or another provider.

Maintain a dignified, courteous relationship with all persons in the office—patients, staff, and health care providers—as well as with insurance adjusters, pharmaceutical representatives, and others who come into or telephone the office (Fig. 1.9).

It is *illegal* to report incorrect information to government-funded programs, such as Medicare, Medicaid, and TRICARE.

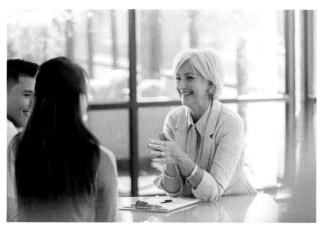

Fig. 1.9 A mental health professional working in a dignified manner with patients. (Copyright © iStock/SDI Productions.)

Federal legislation has been passed on fraud and abuse issues that relate to federal health care programs. However, private insurance payers operate under different laws and it is *unethical but may not be illegal, depending on state laws,* to report incorrect information to private insurance payers. Incorrect information may damage the individual and the integrity of the database, allow reimbursement for services that should be paid by the patient, or deny payment that should be made by the insurance company.

Most professional organizations for insurance billing specialists or coders have established a code of ethics for their members to follow. A sample code of ethics is shown in Fig. 1.10.

In the final analysis, most ethical issues can be reduced to right and wrong with the focus being the moral dictum to do no harm.

American Health Information Management Association

STANDARDS OF ETHICAL CODING

Coding professionals should:

1. Apply accurate, complete and consistent coding practices that yield quality data.

2. Gather and report all data required for internal and external reporting, in accordance with applicable requirements and data set definitions.

3. Assign and report, in any format, only the codes and data that are clearly and consistently supported by health record documentation in accordance with applicable code set and abstraction conventions, and requirements.

4. Query and/or consult as needed with the provider for clarification and additional documentation prior to final code assignment in accordance with acceptable healthcare industry practices.

5. Refuse to participate in, support, or change reported data and/or narrative titles, billing data, clinical documentation practices, or any coding related activities intended to skew or misrepresent data and their meaning that do not comply with requirements.

6. Facilitate, advocate, and collaborate with healthcare professionals in the pursuit of accurate, complete and reliable coded data and in situations that support ethical coding practices.

7. Advance coding knowledge and practice through continuing education, including but not limited to meeting continuing education requirements.

8. Maintain the confidentiality of protected health information in accordance with the Code of Ethics.

9. Refuse to participate in the development of coding and coding related technology that is not designed in accordance with requirements.

10. Demonstrate behavior that reflects integrity, shows a commitment to ethical and legal coding practices, and fosters trust in professional activities.

11. Refuse to participate in and/or conceal unethical coding, data abstraction, query practices, or any inappropriate activities related to coding and address any perceived unethical coding related practices.

Revised and approved by AHIMA's House of Delegates December 12, 2016

Fig. 1.10 American Health Information Management Association (AHIMA) Standards of Ethical Coding, revised and adopted by AHIMA House of Delegates, 2016. (Copyright © 2018 American Health Information Management Association. All rights reserved. Permission granted to reproduce.)

1.4 QUICK REVIEW

Question: What moral dictum can an insurance billing specialist rely upon when faced with an ethical issue?

SCOPE OF PRACTICE AND LIABILITY

Most health care professions have a well-defined scope of practice that easily draws a boundary on things that professionals can do and things they are not supposed to do. The field of medical billing and coding does not have such a well-defined scope of practice. Instead, professionals in this field are guided by job descriptions, codes of ethics, coding policies, internal compliance policies, insurance carrier policies, and health care regulations. Regardless of whether they are involved in facility or professional billing, they must be aware of their own liability.

Employer Liability

As mentioned, insurance billing specialists can be either self-employed or employed by physicians, clinics, hospitals, or ancillary service providers. The health care organization that employs the insurance billing specialist is legally responsible for its own conduct and any actions of its employees performed within the context of their employment. This is referred to as *vicarious liability*, also known as respondeat superior, which literally means "let the master answer." However, this does not mean that an employee cannot be sued or brought to trial. Actions of the insurance biller may have a definite legal ramification on the employer, depending on the situation. For example, if an employee knowingly submits a fraudulent Medicare or Medicaid claim at the direction of the employer and subsequently the business is audited, both the employer and employee can be brought into litigation by the state or federal government. An insurance biller always should check with their employer to determine whether they are included in the medical professional liability insurance policy, otherwise known as malpractice insurance. If not included, he or she could be sued as an individual. It is the health care organization's responsibility to make certain all staff members are protected.

Employee Liability

Billers and coders can be held personally responsible under the law for billing errors and have been listed as defendants in billing-fraud lawsuits. An insurance billing specialist who knowingly submits a false claim or allows such a claim to be submitted can be liable for a civil violation. If they conceal information or fail to disclose it to obtain payment, they can be held liable. Even if they did not prepare the false claim, the individual who mails or electronically files the claim may also be implicated in mail or wire fraud. Fraud will be covered in greater detail in Chapter 3.

If any staff member within a health care organization, or any provider of services, asks the insurance biller to do something that is the least bit questionable, such as writing off patient balances for certain patients automatically, it is recommended that the biller contact their supervisor and make sure they have a legal document or signed waiver of liability relieving them of the responsibility for such actions. When such problems are noted, it is the insurance billing specialist's responsibility to correct it and to document their actions in writing.

Independent Contractor Liability

Independent contractors are those who may have decided to establish their own self-operated business as a medical insurance billing specialist, coder, or consultant. These individuals perform services for health care organizations under contract and are not covered under the organization's professional liability insurance.

Independent contractors should purchase errors and omissions insurance, which provides protection against loss of money caused by failure through error or unintentional omission on the part of the individual or service involved in any aspect of preparation or submission of an insurance claim. Independent contractors can often purchase errors and omission insurance though professional organizations they may belong to.

Claims Assistant Professional Liability

An individual who works as a CAP acts as an informal representative of patients, helping them to obtain insurance reimbursement. A CAP reviews and analyzes existing or potential policies, renders advice, and offers counseling, recommendations, and information. A CAP may not interpret insurance policies or act as an attorney. The legal ability of a CAP to represent a policyholder is limited. When a claim cannot be resolved after a denied claim has been appealed to the insurance company, the CAP must be careful in rendering an opinion or advising clients that they have a right to pursue legal action. State regulations should always be checked to see whether there is a scope of practice. In some states, a CAP could be acting outside the scope of the law by giving advice to clients on legal issues, even if licensed as an attorney but not practicing law full time. If the client wishes to take legal action, it is their responsibility to find a competent attorney specializing in contract law and insurance. In some states, giving an insured client advice on purchase or discontinuance of insurance policies is construed as being an insurance agent.

A number of states require CAPs to be licensed, depending on the services rendered to clients. CAPs who perform only the clerical function of filing health insurance claims do not have to be licensed. Check with the state's department of insurance and insurance commissioner to determine whether licensing is required.

1.5 QUICK REVIEW

Question: Can billers and coders be held personally responsible under the law for billing errors?

FUTURE CHALLENGES

An insurance billing specialist must remember that they are expected to manage a health care organization's financial affairs accurately; otherwise, they will not be considered qualified for this position. Subsequent chapters contain valuable information to help develop the knowledge and skills necessary to help achieve this goal. Insurance billing specialists will be expected to do the following:

- Know billing regulations for each insurance program in which the health care organization is a participant.
- Know the aspects of compliance rules and regulations.
- State various insurance rules about treatment and referral of patients.
- Become proficient in computer skills and use of various medical software packages.
- Learn electronic billing software and the variances of each payer.
- Develop diagnostic and procedural coding expertise.
- Know how to interpret insurance carrier's remittance advice summary reports, explanation of benefit documents, or both.
- Attain bookkeeping skills necessary to post, interpret, and manage patient accounts.
- Keep current and stay up to date by reading the latest health care industry association publications, participating in e-mail listserv discussions, joining a professional organization for networking, and attending seminars on billing and coding.
- Insurance billing specialists should train to also become familiar with other aspects of the health care organization.
- Discover opportunities for career advancement.

- Strive toward becoming certified as an insurance billing specialist and/or coder and, once certified, seek continuing education credits to become recertified.

Becoming an insurance billing specialist is the first step into an exciting career that has endless opportunities. Chapter 20 will provide information into some of the more advanced roles that the billing specialist can work toward and the professional organizations that offer certification.

DISCUSSION POINT

Describe why you are training to become an insurance billing specialist?

PROCEDURE 1.1 Analyze Professional Ethics and Medical Etiquette

Objectives: To analyze how professional ethics and medical etiquette are essential qualities for insurance billing specialists
Directions:
1. Review and identify the difference between professional ethics and medical etiquette.
2. With a classmate, make a list of ways the insurance billing specialist could observe rules of medical etiquette when discussing claims with patients.
3. With a classmate, make a list of ways the insurance billing specialist could practice professional ethics when discussing claims with patients.
4. With a classmate, role-play a situation in which the insurance billing specialist is being challenged by a frustrated and angry patient who has an outstanding bill with the health care organization.

KEY POINTS

This is a brief chapter review, or summary, of the key issues presented.

1. The medical insurance billing specialist's primary goal is to help patients obtain maximum insurance plan benefits for the services they received while ensuring the cash flow of their organization through revenue cycle management.
2. The health care industry is one of the most heavily regulated industries in the U.S. which contributes to the complexities of medical billing.
3. The person who does facility or professional billing has become a proficient specialist known by a number of job titles, such as insurance billing specialist or reimbursement specialist.
4. Insurance claims must be promptly submitted to ensure continuous cash flow for a health care organization. If not, overhead expenses cannot be met and the organization will face financial difficulties.
5. Because of the increased technical knowledge that a biller must have, education and training must be more comprehensive and skills must be developed in coding and claims completion. When proficiency is reached, a person can work for a health care organization or may possibly set up their own billing service. In this career, jobs can be rewarding for persons with disabilities.
6. Individuals who do billing and complete insurance claims must have many skills, such as knowledge of medical ter-

minology and abbreviations, expert use of procedural and diagnostic code books, precise reading skills, ability to perform basic mathematic calculations, knowledge of medicolegal rules and regulations of various insurance programs, ability to understand and apply compliance issues, basic computer skills (keyboarding and software applications), proficiency in accessing information via the internet, ability to carry out billing and collection techniques, expertise in the legalities of collection on accounts, and ability to generate insurance claims expediently and accurately.
7. Becoming a professional is a gradual process and one must project an appropriate image and develop themselves as a courteous and respectful team player.
8. Etiquette in a medical setting must be adhered to routinely. The insurance billing specialist must display customs, courteousness, and manners that always show consideration of others.
9. A health care organization that employs an insurance billing specialist is legally responsible for any actions its employees perform within the context of their employment. This is referred to as vicarious liability, also known as *respondeat superior.*
10. Remember, ignorance of the law is not a protection for anyone working in a health care organization, so one must stay up to date and well informed on state and federal statutes.

STUDENT ASSIGNMENT

Read the Introduction in the *Workbook,* which explains how you will be working as an insurance billing specialist during this course.

- Study Chapter 1.
- Complete all exercises in the *Workbook* to reinforce the theory learned in this chapter.

- Turn to the Glossary at the end of this book for a further understanding of the key terms and key abbreviations used in this chapter.

Privacy, Security, and HIPAA

Cheryl Fassett

OBJECTIVES

After reading this chapter, you should be able to:

1. Name the two provisions of the Health Insurance Portability and Accountability Act (HIPAA) that relate most to health care.
2. Explain the difference between *Title I: Health Insurance Reform* and *Title II: Administrative Simplification*.
3. Define and discuss HIPAA roles, relationships, and key terms, including HIPAA in the practice setting.
4. Describe the Privacy Rule under HIPAA.
5. Define and discuss protected health information (PHI).
6. Illustrate the difference between privileged and nonprivileged information.
7. Identify the difference between disclosure and use of PHI and discuss exceptions to HIPAA.
8. State the guidelines for HIPAA privacy compliance.
9. Explain patient rights under HIPAA.
10. Explain responsibilities of the health care organization to protect patient rights under HIPAA.
11. Define the provisions of the Health Information Technology for Economic and Clinical Health Act (HITECH Act).
12. Discuss the Security Rule and how it relates to coding and billing.
13. List the three major categories of security safeguards under HIPAA.
14. Explain the purpose of the HIPAA Omnibus Rule.
15. List consequences of noncompliance with HIPAA and the HITECH Act.
16. Discuss how HIPAA affects all areas of the health care office, including the organization and staff responsibilities in protecting patient rights.

KEY TERMS

administrative safeguards
American Recovery and
    Reinvestment Act
authorization
authorization form
breach
business associate
clearinghouse
confidential communication
confidentiality
consent
covered entity
designated record sets
disclosure
electronic protected health
    information
employer identification number

health care organization
health care provider
The Health Information Technology
    for Economic and Clinical Health
    Act
Health Insurance Portability and
    Accountability Act
HIPAA Omnibus Rule
incidental use and disclosure
individually identifiable health
    information
Minimum Necessary Rule
mitigation
National Provider Identifier
nonprivileged information
Notice of Privacy Practices
Office of Inspector General

Patient Protection and Affordable
    Care Act of 2010
physical safeguards
portability
preexisting condition
privacy
privacy officer, privacy official
privacy rule
privileged information
protected health information
psychotherapy notes
security officer
Security Rule
state preemption
technical safeguards
transaction
use

KEY ABBREVIATIONS

ARRA	FBI	IIHI	PHI
CMS	FTP	NPI	PO
DHHS	HHS	NPP	P&P
EIN	HIPAA	OCR	PPACA
ePHI	HITECH	OIG	TPO

INSIGHTS FROM THE FIELD

Cindy B.: Certified Professional Coder (CPC), Certified Professional Medical Auditor (CPMA)

I started as an Emergency Department Services coder in 2006 and am a Clinical Coding Supervisor. I oversee medical coding for various services provided by the hospital and nursing facilities. I also manage physician educators who balance reimbursement and compliance.

I think being inquisitive is the most valuable skill. Never be afraid to question anything! The hardest part of joining this field is accepting that many of the concepts are not just black and white. Having a solid understanding of the basics and the foundation of coding allows each of us to justify our coding decisions, and defend ourselves in audits. I try to stress this to any of my newer coders; they will continue to build their skills, but there is no shortcut to learning the basics.

HEALTH INSURANCE PORTABILITY AND ACCOUNTABILITY

One of the most important pieces of legislation to have an impact on health care organizations, health care workers, and patients is the Health Insurance Portability and Accountability Act (HIPAA) of 1996. The Act is made up of five titles. Among these five titles, there are two provisions that relate most to health care: *Title I: Health Insurance Reform* and *Title II: Administrative Simplification*. The goals of HIPAA were as follows:
- Assure health insurance portability
- Enforce standards for health information
- Reduce health care fraud and abuse
- Guarantee security and privacy of an individual's health information

The Department of Health and Human Services (DHHS or HHS) is the US government's principal agency for protecting the health of all Americans and providing essential human services. HIPAA legislation required the DHHS to establish national standards and identifiers for electronic transactions as well as to implement privacy and security standards.

The Office of E-Health Standards and Services, a division of the Centers for Medicare and Medicaid Services (CMS), enforces the insurance portability and transaction and code set requirements for Medicare and Medicaid programs.

The Office for Civil Rights (OCR) enforces privacy and security rules. It is a part of DHHS. The OCR protects our rights under nondiscrimination laws and HIPAA privacy laws. It investigates violations of these rights as well as patient safety issues.

The projected long-term benefits of HIPAA legislation include the following:
- Lowered administrative costs
- Increased accuracy of data
- Increased patient and customer satisfaction
- Reduced revenue cycle time, and
- Improved revenue cycle management

Title I: Health Insurance Reform

The primary purpose of HIPAA *Title I: Health Insurance Reform* is to provide insurance portability, or continuous insurance coverage for workers and their dependents when they change or lose jobs. Under this provision, an employee has the right to maintain health care benefits under a group health plan when leaving a job. The former employee has the option to continue their group health plan benefits; however, he or she is responsible for the *total* cost of the benefit.

Previously, when an employee left or lost a job and changed insurance coverage, coverage was limited for preexisting conditions. A preexisting condition is an illness or injury that began prior to when the insurance went into effect. HIPAA now limits the use of preexisting condition exclusions. It also prohibits discrimination for past or present medical conditions, and guarantees certain individuals the right to purchase new health insurance coverage after losing a job. HIPAA also allows renewal of health insurance coverage regardless of an individual's health condition.

It is also important to understand what HIPAA *Title I* does *not* do. HIPAA does not force employers to offer health insurance. It also does not regulate how much insurance companies can charge for premiums.

Title II: Administrative Simplification

HIPAA *Title II: Administrative Simplification* focuses on reducing administrative costs and burdens for health care organizations. Standardizing electronic transmissions of billing and payment information reduces the number of forms and methods used in processing claims. This reduces the effort needed to process paper or nonstandard electronic claims.

Additional provisions are meant to ensure the privacy and security of an individual's health data. *Title II* also focuses on reducing fraud, waste, and abuse in health care by increasing both the funding to combat fraud and abuse and the penalties associated with fraudulent activities.

There are four main parts of HIPAA *Title II* that directly pertain to health care organizations:
- Standard Transactions and Code Sets
- Unique Identifiers
- Privacy and Confidentiality
- Security of Health Transactions

2.1 QUICK REVIEW
Question: What were the four main goals of HIPAA legislation?

TRANSACTION AND CODE SETS

HIPAA requires the use of standard code sets to represent health care concepts and procedures. This reduces the number of forms and standardizes the method used to process claims. It allows providers, facilities, and other health care organizations to code and submit claims in the exact same format for every payer, thereby reducing cost and effort. This was not the case before HIPAA when every health plan could require a different format and additional nonstandard information. It made the billing process time consuming and difficult.

The standard code sets required in HIPAA include the following:

- International Classification of Disease, Tenth Revision, Clinical Modification (ICD-10-CM, Volumes I and II) for diagnosis coding
- International Classification of Disease, Tenth Revision, Procedure Coding System (ICD-10-PCS) for hospital and facility procedure coding
- Current Procedural Terminology (CPT) for professional health care procedure coding
- Healthcare Common Procedure Coding System (HCPCS) for nonphysician services and supply coding
- Current Dental Terminology (CDT) for dental procedure coding

CMS refers to a *transaction* as the electronic exchange of information between two parties to carry out financial or administrative activities related to health care. These data exchanges include information that completes the insurance claim process and are discussed later in the text. These transactions are typically done in an electronic format, though paper claims processing is still an option.

HIPAA electronic transaction standards require all covered entities to use the same format. All payers are then required to communicate payment, denial, and pended claims in the same format as well. These transaction and code set standards create a common language among health care providers and payers, thereby increasing the efficiency of the claims process. Types of transactions that transmit sensitive data are as follows:

- Claims and encounter information
- Payment and remittance advice
- Claims status
- Eligibility
- Enrollment and disenrollment
- Referrals and authorizations
- Coordination of benefits, and
- Premium payments

 2.2   QUICK REVIEW
Question: What are the standard code sets required by HIPAA?

NATIONAL IDENTIFIERS

HIPAA *Title II* also mandates the creation of a National Identifier system. This assigns unique identifiers to every health care organization, employer, health plan, and patient. The purpose of the identifiers is to further standardize electronic transmissions of claim data.

While the first two types of identifiers were implemented after HIPAA became law, the health plan identifiers were not officially mandated until the Patient Protection and Affordable Care Act of 2010 (PPACA). Patient identifiers are still in the discussion phase. Proponents claim the use of unique patient identifiers will increase patient safety and help with the digitizing of health care data. Those who are against it raise concerns over privacy.

The Internal Revenue Service assigns employer identifier numbers (EINs) to employers. Also known as tax identification numbers (TINs), they identify an employer in all electronic transactions from payroll to health plan enrollment.

National Provider Identifiers (NPIs) are unique identifiers assigned to every health care organization, employer, health plan, and patient. These are used to submit and process health care claims. If a billing specialist submits a claim for a provider in a health care organization, both the provider's NPI and the health care organization's NPI must appear on the claim.

 2.3   QUICK REVIEW
Question: What is an NPI?

THE PRIVACY RULE: CONFIDENTIALITY AND PROTECTED HEALTH INFORMATION

Federal and state regulations, professional standards, and ethics all address patient privacy. In the past, health care organizations simply locked health records in file cabinets and often refused to share patient health information. Now, under HIPAA, patients have specific rights regarding how their health information is used and disclosed. Knowledge of and attention to the rights of patients are important to being compliant in a health care organization.

Health care staff are entrusted with private information that can identify a person such as name, date of birth, and social security number. They also have access to private health information and are expected to recognize when certain health information can be used or disclosed. Health care organizations and their employees can be held accountable for using or disclosing patient health information inappropriately. Following privacy and security procedures prevents the misuse of health information.

Computers are essential to health care organizations. Confidential health data is now sent across networks and e-mailed over the internet. Sometimes few safeguards are taken to protect data and prevent information from being lost or intercepted by hackers. With the implementation of standardized electronic transactions of health care information, the use of technology poses new risks for privacy and security. HIPAA addresses these concerns.

Regulations now closely govern how the industry handles its electronic activities. The HIPAA Privacy Rule establishes national standards to protect individuals' health records and other personal health information. It applies to all covered entities that conduct health care transactions electronically.

The HIPAA Privacy Rule has three main objectives:

1. to protect patient information from being used and disclosed inappropriately
2. to give patients greater control over sharing of information, and
3. to increase patient access to information.

Privacy, Confidentiality, Use, and Disclosure

Privacy is the condition of being secluded from the presence or view of others. Confidentiality is using discretion in keeping information secret. An employee must have strong moral principles and integrity and must be committed to protecting the privacy and rights of the health care organization's patients.

Health care organizations and their staff use and disclose health information on a regular basis. Use means the sharing, application, utilization, examination, or analysis of health information within the organization. For example, when a patient's billing record is accessed to review the claim submission history, the individual's health information is in use. Records are also shared between providers in the course of patient care; information is released to health plans to process claims.

Disclosure means the release, transfer, provision of access to, or divulging information to people or entities outside the health care organization. An example of a disclosure is a scheduler giving information about a patient when setting them up for a procedure to the health care facility's outpatient surgery center. See Table 2.1 for examples of uses and disclosures of PHI.

TABLE 2.1 Title II: Administrative Simplification: Uses and Disclosures of Protected Health Information

Permitted Disclosures (No Authorization Required)	What It Means for a Health Care Organization
Disclose PHI to patient	A health care provider may discuss the patient's own medical condition with him or her. **Doing so does not require signed authorization from the patient.**
Disclose PHI for treatment	Treatment includes speaking with the patient, ordering tests, writing prescriptions, coordinating their care, and consulting with another health care provider about the patient. **"Treatment" does not require signed authorization from the patient.**
Disclose PHI for payment	Payment includes obtaining the patient's eligibility or benefits coverage information from the insurance payer, obtaining preapproval for treatment, and billing and managing the claims process. **"Payment" does not require signed authorization from the patient.**
Disclose PHI for health care operations	Do not confuse this with performing surgery. The term *health care operations* refers to the business activities in which the organization participates. Examples include case management, certification, accreditation, medical reviews, and audits to detect fraud and abuse. **"Operations" do not require signed authorization from the patient.**
Disclose PHI for public purposes	PHI may be disclosed for public health purposes, such as reporting a communicable disease, injury, child abuse, domestic violence, judicial and administrative proceedings, law enforcement, coroner or medical examiner, or research purposes, if PHI is "de-identified." This is not an all-inclusive list, but **these examples do not require signed authorization from the patient.**
Disclose PHI for workers' compensation	A billing specialist may disclose PHI as authorized by the laws relating to workers' compensation. Such disclosures to programs that provide benefits for work-related injuries or illness **do not require signed authorization from the patient.**
Disclosures That Require Patient's Opportunity to Agree or Object Disclose PHI to persons involved with the patient	**What It Means for a Health Care Organization** An organization must provide patients with an opportunity to object to sharing PHI with family, friends, or others involved with their care. The health care provider can use professional judgment when disclosing PHI to a person involved with the patient's care when the patient is not present. **This requires the patient to have the opportunity to agree or object.**
Disclosures (Authorization Required) Disclose psychotherapy notes	**What It Means for a Health Care Organization** Psychotherapy notes may not be disclosed without authorization except for use by the notes' originator (therapist) for treatment. **Signed authorization *is* required.**
Disclose PHI to a child's school for permission to participate in sports	A health care organization may not disclose a child's PHI to a school to permit the student's participation in a sports activity. **Signed authorization *is* required.**
Disclose PHI to employer	A health care organization may not disclose PHI to a patient's employer unless the information is necessary to comply with OSHA, MSHA, or other state laws. **With certain exceptions, signed authorization *is* required.**
Disclose PHI to insurer	A health care organization may not disclose PHI to an insurer for underwriting or eligibility without authorization from the patient (for example, if the patient is trying to obtain a life insurance policy). **Signed authorization *is* required.**
Disclose PHI for fundraising or marketing	If the health care organization does fundraising or marketing activities, it may not disclose PHI without prior authorization from the patient. **Signed authorization *is* required.**

MSHA, Mine Safety and Health Administration; *OSHA,* Occupational Safety and Health Administration; *PHI,* protected health information.

Covered Entities

Under HIPAA, a covered entity is any health care provider, health care organization, health plan, or clearinghouse that transmits health information in electronic form for any number of transactions. The covered entity may be (1) a health plan carrier, such as Medicare or Blue Cross/Blue Shield; (2) a health care clearinghouse through which claims are submitted; or (3) a health care provider, such as a primary care physician, hospital, or laboratory.

A health care provider is a person trained and licensed to provide care to a patient or a place that is licensed to give health care. A provider may work in a hospital, skilled nursing facility, inpatient/outpatient rehabilitation facility, home health agency, hospice program, physician, diagnostic department, outpatient physical or occupational therapy department, or rural clinic or with a home dialysis supplier. A provider may be a physician, physician's assistant, nurse practitioner, social worker, chiropractor, dentist, and so on.

HIPAA's definition of a health care organization extends to entities that provide health care services to a patient. In addition to provider groups, this includes hospitals, ambulance service providers, clinics, nursing homes, pharmacies, and others.

A health care clearinghouse is an organization that acts as a go-between for a health care organization and the entity to which health care information is transmitted. It is an independent organization that receives insurance claims from the health care organization, performs software edits, and reformats data as needed into proper format. It then sends the claims electronically to various third-party payers.

HIPAA requires the designation of a privacy officer or privacy official (PO). A PO is an individual who is tasked with helping the health care organization remain in compliance by setting policies and procedures (P&P) and by training and managing the staff regarding HIPAA and patient rights. The PO is usually the contact person for questions and complaints. This advisory role in larger organizations may be filled by an attorney or other professional with extensive compliance experience. In smaller health care organizations such as individual or small groups of health care providers, the PO may be an employee who consults with an attorney as needed.

A security officer protects the computer and networking systems within the health care organization and implements protocols such as password assignment, backup procedures, firewalls, virus protection, and contingency planning for emergencies. Larger organizations such as hospital systems may have an entire information technology (IT) department working in coordination with the security officer. A smaller organization may assign the role of security officer to the practice manager who may be supported by an outside IT consultant.

Business Associates

A business associate is a person or entity that performs certain functions or activities using health care information on behalf of a covered entity. It is considered an extension of the health care organization and is held to the same standards under HIPAA. A business associate performs or assists in the performance of a function or activity involving the use or disclosure of health information. These functions include claims processing or administration, data analysis, processing or administration, utilization review, quality assurance, billing, benefit management, practice management, and repricing. For example, if a health care provider contracts with an outside billing company to manage its claims and accounts receivable, the billing company would be a business associate of the provider (the covered entity).

Covered entities should have a business associate agreement in place with all entities that work with them. The agreement needs to specifically outline how the business associate complies with HIPAA legislation. If a health care provider either transmits directly or uses a business associate, such as a billing company or clearinghouse, to send information electronically for any of the transactions listed, all parties are a covered entity and must comply with HIPAA.

Protected Health Information

Protected health information (PHI) is any information that identifies an individual and describes their health status, age, sex, ethnicity, or other demographic characteristics, whether that information is stored or transmitted electronically. It refers to any part of the patient's health information that is transmitted by electronic media, maintained or stored in electronic form, or in any other form or medium. See Example 2.1 for examples of PHI. Traditionally, privacy focused on protecting paper health records that held patient's health information, such as laboratory results and radiology reports. HIPAA Privacy Rule expands these protections to apply to PHI. The individual's health information is protected regardless of the type of medium in which it is maintained. This includes paper, the organization's computerized medical billing system, spoken words, and x-ray films.

EXAMPLE 2.1   Examples of Protected Health Information

- Name
- Address
- Telephone Number
- Social Security Number
- Health Record Number
- Driver's License Number
- Account Number
- Health Plan ID Number
- Date of Birth
- Dates of admission/discharge
- Date of Death
- Email Address
- Biometric Identifiers (i.e. fingerprint)
- Photographic Images

Individually Identifiable Health Information

Individually identifiable health information (IIHI) is any part of an individual's health information, including demographic information, collected from the individual by a covered entity. This information relates to the individual's past, present, or future physical or mental health or condition; the provision of health care to the individual; or the past, present, or future payment for the provision of health care. IIHI data identify the individual or establish a reasonable basis to believe that the information can be used to identify the individual. For example, if a health care provider is talking to an insurance representative, they will likely give information such as the patient's date of birth and last name. These pieces of information would make it reasonably easy to identify the patient. Conversely, if a staff member in a health care organization is talking to a pharmaceutical representative about a drug assistance program that covers a new pill for heartburn and says that the organization has a patient living in a particular town who is indigent and has stomach problems, the staff member is not divulging information that would identify the patient.

Other requirements relating to uses and disclosures of PHI focus on information that does not identify an individual or leaves no reasonable basis to believe that the information can be used to identify an individual. This de-identified information is no longer considered to be individually identifiable health information (IIHI). The regulations give specific directions on how to ensure that all pieces of necessary information are removed to fit the definition. De-identified information is not subject to the privacy regulations because it does not specifically identify an individual.

Privileged and Nonprivileged Information

When working with health records, all health care staff members are responsible for maintaining the confidentiality of patients' health information. The purpose of the Privacy Rule is to ensure that patients who receive medical treatment can control the manner in which specific information is used and to whom it is disclosed.

Confidential communication is a privileged communication that may be disclosed only with the patient's permission. Everything a health care worker sees, hears, or reads about patients remains confidential and does not leave the office. Never talk about patients or data contained in health records where others may overhear. Some employers require employees to sign a confidentiality agreement (Fig. 2.1). Such agreements should be updated periodically to address issues raised by the use of new technologies.

EMPLOYEE CONFIDENTIALITY STATEMENT

As an employee of _____ABC Clinic, Inc._____ (employer), having been trained as an insurance billing specialist with employee responsibilities and authorization to access personal medical and health information, and as a condition of my employment, I agree to the following:

A. I recognize that I am responsible for complying with the Health Insurance Portability and Accountability Act (HIPAA) of 1996 policies regarding confidentiality of patients' information, which, if I violate, may lead to immediate dismissal from employment and, depending on state laws, criminal prosecution.

B. I will treat all information received during the course of my employment, which relates to the patients, as confidential and privileged information.

C. I will not access patient information unless I must obtain the information to perform my job duties.

D. I will not disclose information regarding my employer's patients to any person or entity, other than that necessary to perform my job duties, and as permitted under the employer's HIPAA policies.

E. I will not access any of my employer's computer systems that currently exist or may exist in the future using a password other than my own.

F. I will safeguard my computer password and will not show it in public.

G. I will not allow anyone, including other employees, to use my password to access computer files.

H. I will log off of the computer immediately after I finish using it.

I. I will not use e-mail to transmit patient information unless instructed to do so by my employer's HIPAA privacy officer.

J. I will not take patient information from my employer's premises in hard copy or electronic form without permission from my employer's HIPAA privacy officer.

K. Upon termination of my employment, I agree to continue to maintain the confidentiality of any information learned while an employee and agree to relinquish office keys, access cards, or any other device that provides access to the provider or its information.

Mary Doe
Signature

September 14, 20XX
Date

Mary Doe
Print name

Brenda Shield
Witness

Fig. 2.1 An example of an employee confidentiality agreement that may be used by an employer when hiring an insurance billing specialist.

Privileged information is related to the treatment and progress of the patient. The patient must sign an authorization to release this information or selected facts from the health record. Some states have passed laws allowing certain test results (e.g, the presence of the human immunodeficiency virus [HIV] or alcohol or substance abuse) and other information to be maintained separate from the patient's health record. Some states require a special authorization form be used to release this information.

Example 2.2 lists some of the privileged communications that a health care organization might use that fall under HIPAA compliance regulations.

EXAMPLE 2.2 Privileged Communications in a Health Care Organization

- Intake forms
- Laboratory work requests
- Provider–patient conversations
- Conversations that refer to patients by name
- Provider dictation tapes
- Telephone conversations with patients
- Encounter sheets
- Provider notes
- Prescriptions
- Insurance claim forms
- X-ray films
- E-mail messages

Nonprivileged information consists of ordinary facts unrelated to treatment of the patient, including the patient's name, city of residence, and dates of admission or discharge. This information must be protected from unauthorized disclosure under the privacy section of HIPAA. The patient's authorization is not necessary for the purposes of treatment, payment, or health care operations, unless the record is in a specialty health care facility such as an alcohol treatment center or a special service unit of a general hospital such as a psychiatric unit. Professional judgment is required. The information is disclosed on a legitimate need-to-know basis. For example, an attending physician may require complete access to the health record because the information may have some effect on the treatment of the patient, but an x-ray technician would not necessarily need to know everything in the record.

! COMPLIANCE ALERT

Confidentiality Statement

Most information in patients' health records and the health care organization's financial records is considered confidential and sensitive. Employees who have access to such computer data should have integrity and be well chosen because they have a high degree of responsibility and accountability. It is wise to have those handling sensitive computer documents sign an annual confidentiality statement (see Fig. 2.1). This way the statement can be updated when an individual's responsibilities increase or decrease. The statement should contain the following:

- Written or oral disclosure of information pertaining to patients is prohibited.
- Disclosure of information without consent of the patient results in serious penalty or immediate dismissal.

Designated Record Set

HIPAA gives an individual the right to access their health information in a designated record set maintained by each covered entity and its business associates. Designated record sets include health records, billing and claims records, and health plan enrollment records. A patient is not guaranteed access to information that is not part of a designated record set. Some examples of information that a covered entity is not required to release to a patient are peer reviews, patient safety control records, and business planning records. Other information not included in a designated record set are appointment schedules, requests for diagnostic testing, and birth and death records.

Psychotherapy Notes

Psychotherapy notes have special protection under HIPAA. Disclosure of a patient's mental health records requires specific patient permission. This means that when an insurance payer requests the health records to review the claim, a patient authorization is required.

In general, psychotherapy notes are defined as the information that is the recorded (in any manner) documentation and/or analysis of conversation with the patient. This information should be kept separate from the medical section of the patient health record to be distinguished as psychotherapy notes. For example, Jane Doe tells her psychologist the details of her childhood trauma. The documented conversation specific to her trauma (e.g, what occurred and how she felt) is considered the psychotherapy notes and cannot be released without Jane Doe's specific permission.

Certain clinical data are excluded from the definition of psychotherapy notes. When an individual is using the services of a mental health professional, not all information gathered and recorded in the health record of the mental health provider is considered part of the psychotherapy notes. The law lists the following specific items that are excluded from such notes:

- Medication prescription and monitoring
- Counseling session start and stop times
- Modalities and frequencies of treatment furnished
- Results of clinical tests
- Any summary of the following items: diagnosis, functional status, treatment plan, symptoms, prognosis, and progress to date

It is also important to understand that patients do not have the right to obtain a copy of psychotherapy notes under HIPAA. However, the treating mental health provider can decide when a patient may obtain access to this health information. State law must always be considered. Some states allow patients access to their psychotherapy notes. In these cases, state law would take precedence over HIPAA as a result of the state preemption allowance as described later in this chapter.

Consent and Authorizations

HIPAA imposes requirements to protect not only disclosure of PHI outside of the organization but also internal uses of health information. PHI may not be used or disclosed without permission from the patient or someone authorized to act on behalf of the patient. However, the rule does allow the use or disclosure of PHI if it is specifically for the purposes of treatment, payment, or health care operations (TPO).

Consent is the verbal or written agreement that gives approval to some action, situation, or statement. With regards to HIPAA, a consent is a document that gives health care organizations permission to use or disclose PHI for TPO. Although many health care organizations obtain signed consents from their patients, the Privacy Rule does not require a covered entity to obtain consent for routine uses and disclosures. See Fig. 2.2 for an example of a consent for release of information for TPO.

Treatment includes coordination or management of health care between providers or referral of a patient to another provider. PHI can also be disclosed to obtain reimbursement or payment for services. Other health care operations include performance reviews, audits, and training programs.

In contrast to a consent, the HIPAA Privacy Rule requires a signed authorization for any uses and disclosures that are not routine and are not otherwise allowed by the Privacy Rule. Authorization is an individual's formal, written permission to use or disclose their personally identifiable health information for purposes other than TPO. The authorization must specify the information to be disclosed and the purpose of the disclosure. It must specify who is disclosing the information and who is receiving it. For example, if a patient changes primary care providers, they will need to sign an authorization to have their

---

COLLEGE CLINIC
4567 Broad Avenue
Woodland Hills, XY 12345-0001
Phone: 555/486-9002
Fax: 555/487-8976

CONSENT TO THE USE AND DISCLOSURE OF HEALTH INFORMATION

I understand that this organization originates and maintains health records which describe my health history, symptoms, examination, test results, diagnoses, treatment, and any plans for future care or treatment. I understand that this information is used to:

- plan my care and treatment.
- communicate among health professionals who contribute to my care.
- apply my diagnosis and services, procedures, and surgical information to my bill.
- verify services billed by third-party payers.
- assess quality of care and review the competence of health care professionals in routine health care operations.

I further understand that:

- a complete description of information uses and disclosures is included in a *Notice of Information Practices* which has been provided to me.
- I have a right to review the notice prior to signing this consent.
- the organization reserves the right to change their notice and practices.
- any revised notice will be mailed to the address I have provided prior to implementation.
- I have the right to object to the use of my health information for directory purposes.
- I have the right to request restrictions as to how my health information may be used or disclosed to carry out treatment, payment, or health care operations.
- the organization is not required to agree to the restrictions requested.
- I may revoke this consent in writing, except to the extent that the organization has already taken action in reliance thereon.

☐ I request the following restrictions to the use or disclosure of my health information.

_____

_____   _____
Date   Notice Effective Date

_____   _____
Signature of Patient or Legal Representative Witness

_____   _____
Signature   Title

Date _____   __ Accepted __ Rejected

Fig. 2.2 An example of a consent form used to disclose and use health information for treatment, payment, or health care operations (TPO). This is not required under Health Insurance Portability and Accountability Act (HIPAA), some health care organizations use it. (From Fordney, M. T., & French, L. (2003). *Medical insurance billing and coding: A worktext*. Philadelphia: Elsevier.)

health records sent to the new provider. Health care organizations must be careful when obtaining authorizations for marketing, research, and psychotherapy notes. The authorization form must state if a health care organization receives remuneration for specific marketing or research activities. See Fig. 2.3 for an example of an authorization for release of information.

**REQUIRED ELEMENTS
OF HIPAA AUTHORIZATION**

Identification of person (or class) authorized to request

Identification of person (or class) to whom covered entity is to use/disclose

Description of information to be released with specificity to allow entity to know which information the authorization references

Description of each purpose of the requested use or disclosure

Expiration date, time period, or event

Statement that is revocable by written request

Individual's (patient's) signature and date

Statement of representative's authority

Authorization for Release of Information

PATIENT NAME: Levy   Chloe   E.
             LAST   FIRST   MI   MAIDEN OR OTHER NAME
DATE OF BIRTH: 02 - 12 - 1950 SS# 320 - 21 - 3408 MEDICAL RECORD #: 3075
             MO DAY YR
ADDRESS: 3298 East Main Street   CITY: Woodland Hills   STATE: XY ZIP: 12345-0001

DAY PHONE: 013-340-9800   EVENING PHONE: 013-549-8708

I hereby authorize Gerald Practon, MD   (Print Name of Provider) to release information from my medical record as indicated below to:
NAME: Margaret L. Lee, MD
ADDRESS: 328 Seward Street   CITY: Anytown   STATE: XY ZIP: 45601-0731

PHONE: 013-219-7698   FAX: 013-290-9877

INFORMATION TO BE RELEASED:
                  DATES:
☒ History and physical exam   6-8-20XX
☐ Progress notes
☐ Lab reports
☐ X-ray reports
☐ Other:

I specifically authorize the release of information relating to:
☐ Substance abuse (including alcohol/drug abuse)
☐ Mental health (including psychotherapy notes)
☐ HIV related information (AIDS related testing)
X
SIGNATURE OF PATIENT OR LEGAL GUARDIAN   DATE

PURPOSE OF DISCLOSURE: ☐ Changing physicians   ☒ Consultation/second opinion   ☐ Continuing care
☐ Legal   ☐ School   ☐ Insurance   ☐ Workers Compensation
☐ Other (please specify):

1. I understand that this authorization will expire on 09/01/20XX (Print the Date this Form Expires) days after I have signed the form.

2. I understand that I may revoke this authorization at any time by notifying the providing organization in writing, and it will be effective on the date notified except to the extent action has already been taken in reliance upon it.

3. I understand that information used or disclosed pursuant to this authorization may be subject to redisclosure by the recipient and no longer be protected by Federal privacy regulations.

4. I understand that if I am being requested to release this information by Gerald Practon, MD (Print Name of Provider) for the purpose of:

   a. By authorizing this release of information, my health care and payment for my health care will not be affected if I do not sign this form.
   b. I understand I may see and copy the information described on this form if I ask for it, and that I will get a copy of this form after I sign it.
   c. I have been informed that Gerald Practon, MD (Print Name of Provider) will/will not receive financial or in-kind compensation in exchange for using or disclosing the health information described above.

5. I understand that in compliance with XY (Print the State Whose Laws Govern the Provider) statute, I will pay a fee of $ 5.00 (Print the Fee Charged). There is no charge for medical records if copies are sent to facilities for ongoing care or follow up treatment.

Chloe E. Levy   6/1/XX OR
SIGNATURE OF PATIENT   DATE   PARENT/LEGAL GUARDIAN/AUTHORIZED PERSON   DATE

                                            ☐
RECORDS RECEIVED BY   DATE   RELATIONSHIP TO PATIENT

FOR OFFICE USE ONLY
DATE REQUEST FILLED _____ BY: _____
IDENTIFICATION PRESENTED_____ FEE COLLECTED $_____

Fig. 2.3 Completed authorization for release of information form for a patient who is seeking a consult or second opinion. The required elements for Health Insurance Portability and Accountability Act (HIPAA) authorization are indicated. Note: This form is used on a one-time basis for reasons other than treatment, payment, or health care operations (TPO). When the patient arrives at the new provider's office, a consent for TPO form will need to be signed. (From *Federal Register* 64[212]: Appendix to Subpart E of Part 164: Model Authorization Form, November 3, 1999.)

Verification of Identity and Authority

Before any disclosure, a health care worker must verify the identity of persons requesting PHI if they are unknown to them. They may request identifying information, such as date of birth, Social Security number, or even a code word stored in the health care organization's medical billing system that is unique to each patient. Public officials may present badges, credentials, official letterheads, and other legal documents of authority for identification purposes. Patients and patient representatives should be prepared to show a valid picture ID such as a driver's license.

Health care workers must also verify that the requestor has the right to receive the PHI and identify the need for the PHI. Exercising professional judgment fulfills the verification requirements for most disclosures because the health care worker is acting on "good faith" in believing the identity of the individual requesting PHI. It is good practice when making any disclosure to note the authority of the person receiving the PHI and how this was determined. This shows due diligence with respect to HIPAA.

Any conflicts among various permissions the organization may have on file for a given patient must be resolved before information can be released. For example, if a covered entity has agreed to a patient's request to limit how much of the PHI is sent to a consulting physician for treatment but then receives the patient's authorization to disclose the entire health record to that provider, this would be a conflict. In general, the more restrictive permission would take precedence. Privacy regulations allow resolving conflicting permissions either by obtaining a new permission from the patient or by communicating orally or in writing with the patient to determine the patient's preference. Be sure to document any form of communication in writing.

Minimum Necessary Rule

Another way that HIPAA restricts access to PHI within an organization is through the Minimum Necessary Rule. This requires that the amount of PHI accessed be limited to the minimum amount necessary for a medical staff member to do their job. It should only be shared on a need-to-know basis. Minimum Necessary determinations for *uses of PHI* must be made within each organization and reasonable efforts must be made to limit access to only the minimum amount of information needed by staff members.

In smaller offices, employees may have multiple job functions. If a medical assistant helps with the patient examination, documents vital signs, and then collects the patient's copayment at the reception area, the assistant will likely access both clinical and billing records. Similarly, a coding specialist will need access to the patient's entire health record to code an encounter. However, the receptionist for a health care organization will most likely not need to see the entire record to schedule an appointment for a patient.

Larger organizations may have specific restrictions regarding who should have access to different types of PHI, because staff members tend to have more targeted job roles.

Simple procedure and policy (P&P) about appropriate access to PHI may be sufficient to satisfy the Minimum Necessary requirement.

The Minimum Necessary Rule applies to business associates as well. If a provider is referring a patient to a prosthetic manufacturer, he would be violating the minimum necessary rule if he sent the patient's entire health record. The prosthetic manufacturer does not need to know everything the patient was treated for in the past.

Minimum Necessary determinations for *disclosures of PHI* are distinguished by two categories within the Privacy Rule:

1. For disclosures made on a routine and recurring basis, policies and procedures, or standard protocols, may be implemented for what will be disclosed. These disclosures would be common in the organization. Examples may include disclosures for workers' compensation claims or school physical forms.
2. For other disclosures that would be considered nonroutine, criteria for determining the Minimum Necessary amount of PHI should be established and each request for disclosure should be reviewed on an individual basis. A staff member such as the privacy officer (PO) will likely be assigned to determine this situation when the need arises.

Incidental Uses and Disclosures

Reasonable safeguards must be in place to demonstrate that a health care organization is following the HIPAA Privacy Rule. The safeguards are measurable solutions based on accepted standards that are implemented and periodically monitored to show that the office is in compliance. Reasonable efforts must be made to limit the use or disclosure of PHI. For example, if the front desk receptionist closes the privacy glass between their desk and the waiting area when making a call to a patient, this is a reasonable safeguard to prevent others in the waiting room from overhearing.

Incidental uses and disclosures are permissible under HIPAA only when reasonable safeguards or precautions have been implemented to prevent misuse or inappropriate disclosure of PHI. When incidental uses and disclosures result from failure to apply reasonable safeguards or adhere to the minimum necessary standard, the Privacy Rule has been violated. If the receptionist closes the privacy glass before having a confidential conversation but is still overheard by an individual in the waiting room, this would be incidental. They have applied a reasonable safeguard to prevent their conversation from being overheard.

The OCR has addressed what is permissible with regard to incidental disclosures. Examples follow.

- A provider may discuss a patient's condition or plan of care in the patient's treatment area or hospital room.
- A pharmacist may discuss a prescription with a patient over the pharmacy counter or with a provider or the patient by telephone.

- A patient's name may be called out in the reception room; however, some offices prefer to use first names and not call out last names.

State Preemption

HIPAA's federal privacy regulations apply unless the state laws are more stringent regarding privacy, a situation referred to as state preemption. A state law is considered to be more stringent if it does the following:

- Gives an individual greater access to their health information
- Prohibits disclosure that would be allowed under HIPAA
- Narrows the duration of an authorization to release information

State preemption is a complex technical issue. It refers to instances when state law takes precedence over federal law. The PO determines when the need for preemption arises.

For example, under HIPAA, a covered entity is required to provide an individual access to their health records in a timely manner (30 or 60 days with a possible extension) from the time they are requested. Under New York State law, a provider must permit visual inspection within 10 days and furnish a copy within a reasonable time. In this situation, New York State law would preempt HIPAA and a provider will have to provide visual inspection within a shorter time frame.

Exceptions to HIPAA

There are exceptions to HIPAA. Confidentiality between the provider and patient is automatically waived in the following situations:

- When the patient is a member of a managed care organization (MCO) and the health care organization has signed a contract with the MCO, the MCO has a right to access the health records of their patients, and, for utilization management purposes, the MCO has a right to audit the patient's financial records.
- When patients have certain communicable diseases that are highly contagious, state health agencies require providers to report them. This is true even if the patient does not want the information reported.
- When a medical device breaks or malfunctions, the Food and Drug Administration (FDA) requires health care organizations to report information that will allow it to be advised of the break or malfunction.
- When a patient is a suspect in a criminal investigation or to assist in locating a missing person, material witness, or suspect, police have the right to request certain information.
- When the patient's records are subpoenaed or there is a search warrant, the courts have the right to order health care organizations to release patient information.
- When there is a suspicious death or suspected crime victim, health care organizations must report cases to proper law enforcement authorities.
- When the provider examines a patient at the request of a third party who is paying the bill, the payer has the right to request information. An example of this would be a workers' compensation carrier requesting an independent medical examination on a patient.

- When state law requires the release of information to police that is for the good of society, proper authorities are allowed to access certain information. Examples of this would be cases of child abuse, elder abuse, domestic violence, or gunshot wounds.

 2.4   QUICK REVIEW
Question: What are the objectives of the HIPAA Privacy Rule?

 2.5   QUICK REVIEW
Question: What is a covered entity?

 2.6   QUICK REVIEW
Question: What is PHI? Give some examples.

 2.7   QUICK REVIEW
Question: What is TPO?

 2.8   QUICK REVIEW
Question: What is the Minimum Necessary Rule?

PATIENT'S RIGHTS UNDER HIPAA

All patients have a right to privacy. It is important never to discuss patient information other than with the provider, an insurance company, or an individual who has been authorized by the patient. Under HIPAA, patients are granted the following six federal rights that allow them to be informed about PHI and to control how their PHI is used and disclosed (Box 2.1).

> ### BOX 2.1   Health Insurance Portability and Accountability Act Help
>
> In summary, patients have the right to the following:
> - Be informed of the organization's privacy practices by receiving a Notice of Privacy Practices (NPP)
> - Have their information kept confidential and secure
> - Obtain a copy of their health records
> - Request to have their health records amended
> - Request special considerations in communication
> - Restrict unauthorized access to their confidential health information
>
> Patients cannot prevent their confidential health information from being used for treatment, payment, or routine health care operations (TPO), nor may they force amendments to their health record. As a billing specialist become acclimated to their organization's policies and procedures regarding the handling of protected health information (PHI), they will be better able to recognize that their position plays an important part in Health Insurance Portability and Accountability Act compliance.

Required Notice of Privacy Practices

Under HIPAA, a patient has the right to see a health care organization's Notice of Privacy Practices. A Notice of Privacy Practices (NPP) is a document that is usually given to the patient at the first encounter with a provider or at enrollment with a health plan. The staff must make a reasonable best effort to obtain a signature from the patient acknowledging receipt, and also have it signed by a witness. If the patient cannot or will not sign, this should be documented in the patient's record. The NPP must be posted at every service site and be available in paper form for those who request it. A health care organization's website must have the NPP placed on the site and must deliver a copy electronically on request.

A NPP must be in plain language and contain the following information:
- How the covered entity may use or disclose PHI
- The patient's rights regarding PHI and how to file a complaint
- The covered entity's legal duties including how it is required by law to maintain the privacy of the PHI
- Who the patient may contact for further information about the covered entity's privacy policies

To better understand the requirements of the NPP, refer to Procedure 2.1 at the end of the chapter.

! COMPLIANCE ALERT

Health care organizations are expected to handle requests made by patients to exercise their rights. Health care workers must know their organization's process for dealing with each specific request. Understanding HIPAA and the organization's policy manual will guide the worker to follow the appropriate protocol.

Billing specialists should be familiar with the general forms used within the health care organization. Be aware of the following:
- **Written acknowledgment.** After providing the patient with the Notice of Privacy Practices (NPP), a "good faith" effort must be made to obtain written acknowledgment from the patient receiving the document. If the patient refuses to sign or is unable to sign, this must be documented in the patient record.
- **Authorization forms.** Use and disclosure of protected health information (PHI) is permissible for treatment, payment, or routine health care operations (TPO) because the NPP describes how PHI is used for these purposes. The health care organization is required to obtain signed authorization to use or disclose health information for situations beyond TPO. This functions as protection for the organization. Health care staff must learn about the particular authorization forms used in their office.

Restrictions on Certain Uses and Disclosures of Protected Health Information

Patients have the right to request restrictions on certain uses and disclosures of their PHI. For example, a patient who had a successfully treated sexually transmitted infection many years ago can request that, whenever possible, this material not be disclosed. A health care organization is not required to agree to these requests but must have a process to review the requests, accept and review any appeal, and give a sound reason for not agreeing to a request. Restrictions must be documented and followed. Patients also have the right to revoke any authorization they have given for use and disclosure.

Confidential Communications

Patients have the right to request confidential communications by alternative means or at an alternative location. For example, patients may request a provider call them at work rather than at their home. Patients do not need to explain the reason for the request. The health care office must have a process in place both to evaluate requests and appeals and to respond to the patient. Patients may be required by the office to make their requests in writing. A written document protects the health care organization's compliance endeavors.

Access to Protected Health Information

Patients have the right to access and obtain a copy of their health record. Privacy regulations allow the health care organization to require that the patient make the request for access in writing. Generally, a request must be acted on within 30 days. If the covered entity is unable to respond to the request within 30 days, a one-time 30-day extension may be permitted. If an extension is taken, the health care organization must notify the patient within the initial 30-day period and provide the date that the information will be available.

A health care organization may charge a reasonable, cost-based fee for copies of PHI. This may include only the costs for supplies and labor for copying, postage when mailed, and preparing a summary of the PHI if the patient has agreed to this instead of complete access. If a patient requests an electronic copy of their information or requests that it be transmitted to another person, the covered entity generally must produce it in the form requested if readily producible.

Under HIPAA Privacy Rule, patients do not have the right to access the following:
- Psychotherapy notes
- Information compiled in reasonable anticipation of, or for use in, legal proceedings
- Information exempted from disclosure under the Clinical Laboratory Improvements Act (CLIA) (CLIA will be discussed in Chapter 3)

The office may deny patient access for the previously mentioned reasons without giving the patient the right to review the denial. If the health care provider denies access because the patient would be a danger to themselves or someone else as a result of accessing the confidential health information, the patient has the right to have the denial reviewed by another licensed professional who did not participate in the initial denial decision.

Amendment of Protected Health Information

Patients have the right to request that their PHI be amended. As with other requests, the health care organization may require the request to be in writing. There must be a process to accept and review both the request and any appeal in a timely fashion. The request may be denied for the following circumstances:
- The provider who is being requested to change the PHI is not the creator of the information. For example, a health care provider cannot amend a record sent by a referring provider.
- The PHI is believed to be accurate and complete as it stands in the health care organization's health records.

- The information is not required to be accessible to the patient such as a psychotherapy note.

Generally, the health care organization must respond to a patient's request for amendment within 60 days. If a request is denied, the patient must be informed in writing of the reason for the denial. The patient must also be given the opportunity to file a statement of disagreement.

Accounting of Disclosure of Protected Health Information

Patients have the right to receive an accounting of PHI disclosures. Health care organizations should maintain a log of all disclosures of PHI, either on paper or within the organization's computer system. The process for providing an accounting should be outlined in the health care organization's policy manual. Patients may request an accounting or tracking of disclosures of their confidential information and are granted the right to receive this accounting once a year without charge. Items to be documented must include the following:

- Date of disclosure
- Name of the entity or person who received the PHI, including their address, if known
- Brief description of the PHI disclosed
- Brief statement of the purpose of the disclosure

Disclosures made for TPO, facility directories, and some national security and law enforcement agencies are not required to be recorded.

Facility directories are listings of patients within the facility. Under HIPAA, facilities such as hospitals and nursing homes must be careful about releasing information about the patients in their care. Patient directories may list a patient's name, general condition, and location in the hospital. A patient must be given the opportunity to opt out of the directory. Information may only be released to visitors who ask for a patient by name. Clergy may be given directory information without having to ask for the patient by name.

Information pertaining to infectious disease outbreaks may be released to public health officials. Law enforcement may be given information pertaining to the whereabouts of a fugitive, as well as in cases of suspected abuse or violence. Media must be directed to the facility spokesperson. Public figures such as elected officials and celebrities must be given the same privacy standards as other patients.

Box 2.2 reviews some guidelines for maintaining patient confidentiality.

2.9   QUICK REVIEW

Question: True or False?

_____ A reasonable effort should be made to obtain a signed acknowledgment after a patient is given an NPP.

_____ A patient cannot revoke their authorization to release PHI.

_____ A patient has the right to obtain a copy of their psychotherapy notes in their entirety.

_____ A patient has the right to request a provider change information in their health record.

BOX 2.2   Do's and Don'ts of Confidentiality

Don't: Discuss a patient with acquaintances, yours or the patient's.

Don't: Leave patients' records or appointment books exposed on your desk.

Don't: Leave a computer screen with patient information visible, even for a moment, if another patient may see the data.

Do: Make sure the person making a telephone inquiry is who they say they are. Use one of the following methods of verification:

- Ask for one or more of the following items: patient's full name, home address, date of birth, Social Security number, mother's maiden name, dates of service.
- Ask for a callback number and compare it with the number on file.
- Ask the patient to fax a sheet with their signature on it so that you can compare it with the one on file.
- Some health care facilities may assign a code word or number such as a middle name or date that is easy for patients to remember. If a patient does not know the code word, then ask for personal identifying information as mentioned.

Do: Obtain proper authorization from the patient to release information to another person.

Do: Use care when leaving messages for patients on answering machines or with another person. Leave your name, the office name, and the return telephone number. Never attempt to interpret a report or provide information about the outcome of laboratory or other diagnostic tests to the patient. Let the provider handle it.

Do: Properly dispose of notes, papers, and memos by using a shredding device.

Do: Be careful when using the copying machine, because it is easy to forget to remove the original insurance claim or health record from the document glass.

Do: Use common sense and follow the guidelines mentioned in this chapter to help you maintain your professional credibility and integrity.

Do: Access only the minimum amount of privileged information necessary to complete your job.

Don't: Use PHI (including names and addresses) for marketing purposes without the specific authorization of the patient without the specific authorization of the patient. Sending appointment reminders and general news updates about a health care organization and the services it provides is not considered marketing and does not require patient authorization.

THE SECURITY RULE: ADMINISTRATIVE, TECHNICAL AND PHYSICAL SAFEGAURDS

The Security Rule comprises regulations related to the security of electronic protected health information (ePHI). This refers to any PHI that is produced, saved, transferred, or received in an electronic form. The Security Rule provides regulations related to electronic transactions and code sets, privacy, and enforcement. The Security Rule addresses only ePHI, but the concept of preserving PHI that will become ePHI makes attention to security for the entire organization important. The P&P required by the Security Rule must be maintained for 6 years after they are no longer in use. The Security Rule is divided into three main sections: administrative safeguards, technical safeguards, and physical safeguards. These safeguards reasonably protect PHI from any use or disclosure that violates HIPAA, whether intentional or unintentional (Box 2.3).

BOX 2.3 Examples of Safeguards

Administrative	Technical	Physical
Verifying the identity of an individual picking up health records	Create username and password required to access patient records from computer	Locked, fireproof filing cabinets for storing paper records
Apply sanctions against workforce members who fail to comply with security policies and procedures	Establish procedures to obtain necessary ePHI during an emergency	Establish procedures that allow facility access in support of restoration of lost data under the disaster recovery plan
Perform regular records review of information system activity, such as audit logs, access reports, and security incident tracking reports	Implement procedures that terminate an electronic session after a predetermined time of inactivity	Implement physical safeguards for all workstations that access ePHI, to restrict access to authorized users
Identify a security official who will be responsible for the development of policies and procedures	Implement a mechanism to encrypt and decrypt ePHI	Implement policies and procedures to limit physical access to electronic information systems by identifying authorized individuals by title and/or job function

ePHI, Electronic protected health information.

Administrative Safeguards

Administrative safeguards prevent unauthorized use or disclosure of ePHI through information management controls. Policy and procedures to manage this include the selection, development, implementation, and maintenance of security measures to protect ePHI. These measures guard data integrity, confidentiality, and availability and include the following:

- Information access controls, such as passwords, authorize each employee's physical access to ePHI. These restrict access to records in accordance with the employee's responsibility in the health care organization. For example, usually the health information management (HIM) clerk who has authorization to retrieve health records will not have access to billing records. Each user should have a unique username and an unshared, undisclosed password to log in to any computer with access to PHI. Identifying each unique user allows an organization to audit access and ensure proper access controls are implemented. Passwords for all users should be changed on a regular basis and should never be common names or words.
- Internal audits review who has had access to PHI to ensure that there is no intentional or accidental inappropriate access. This applies to both the medical billing systems as well as the paper records.
- Risk analysis and management is a process that assesses the privacy and security risks of various safeguards and the cost in losses if those safeguards are not in place. Each organization must evaluate its vulnerabilities and the associated risks and decide how to lessen those risks. Reasonable safeguards must be implemented to protect against known risks.
- Termination procedures should be formally documented in the P&P manual and include terminating an employee's access to PHI. Other procedures include changing office security pass codes, deleting user access to computer systems, deleting terminated employees' e-mail accounts, and collecting any access cards or keys.

Technical Safeguards

Technical safeguards are security controls that are put in place to protect and track access to information on computers within the health care organization. These include the following:

- Access controls through limitations created for each staff member based on job category. For example, a receptionist, administrative medical assistant, clinical medical assistant, bookkeeper, or insurance billing specialist will have different levels of access depending on their assigned tasks.
- Audit controls keep track of logins to the computer system, administrative activity, and changes to data. This includes changing passwords, deleting user accounts, and creating new user accounts.
- Automatic logoffs prevent unauthorized users from accessing a computer when it is left unattended. The computer system or software program should automatically log off after a predetermined period of inactivity.

Physical Safeguards

Physical safeguards also prevent unauthorized access to PHI. These physical measures and P&P protect a covered entity's electronic information systems and related buildings and equipment from natural and environmental hazards as well as unauthorized intrusion by a hacker or employee who should not have access. Appropriate and reasonable physical safeguards should include the following:

- Media and equipment controls are documented in the P&P manual regarding management of the PHI. Typical safeguard policies include how the office handles the retention, removal, and disposal of paper records as well as recycling computers and destroying obsolete data drives or software programs containing PHI.
- Physical access controls limit unauthorized access to areas in which equipment and medical charts are stored. Locks on doors are the most common type of control.
- Secure workstation locations minimize the possibility of unauthorized viewing of PHI. This includes ensuring

that password-protected screen savers are in use on computers when unattended and that desk drawers are locked.

⚠ COMPLIANCE ALERT

Organizations and their employees can take a number of preventive measures to maintain computer security.

1. Obtain a software program that stores files in coded form.
2. Never leave electronic storage devices unguarded on desks or anywhere else in sight.
3. Use a privacy filter over the computer monitor so that data may be read only when the user is directly in front of the computer.
4. Log off the computer terminal before leaving a workstation.
5. Read the manuals for the equipment, especially the sections titled "Security Controls," and follow all directions.
6. Store confidential data on external media rather than only on the computer's hard drive. External media should be stored in a locked, secure location, preferably one that is fireproof and away from magnetic fields.
7. Make sure the computer system has a firewall and proper antivirus/antispyware software installed. Hackers can also access digital copiers, laser printers, fax machines, and other electronic equipment with internal memories.
8. Send only an account number when e-mailing a colleague with specific questions. Never send the patient's name or other identifying information over unsecured e-mail.
9. Develop passwords for each user and access codes to protect the data. A password is a combination of letters, numbers, or symbols that an individual is assigned to access the system. Passwords should be changed at regular intervals and never written down. A good password is composed of more than eight characters and is case sensitive. *Case sensitive* means that the password must be entered exactly as stored using upper- or lower-case characters. Delete obsolete passwords from the system. Change any passwords known by an employee who is fired or resigns. Individuals with their own passwords allow the employer to distinguish work done by each employee. If errors or problems occur, focus may then be directed toward correcting the individual user.

A strong password:
- Is at least eight characters long.
- Does not contain the username, real name, or company name.
- Does not contain a complete word.
- Is significantly different from a previous password.
- Contains characters from these four categories: uppercase, lowercase, numbers, symbols. For example: Iluv2pla2BA4$

 2.10   QUICK REVIEW

Question: Give an example of each type of safeguard: administrative, technical, and physical

---

HEALTH INFORMATION TECHNOLOGY FOR ECONOMIC AND CLINICAL HEALTH ACT

The Health Information Technology for Economic and Clinical Health Act (HITECH Act) was a provision of the American Recovery and Reinvestment Act (ARRA) of 2009. ARRA contained incentives for adopting health care IT that are designed to speed up the adoption of electronic health record systems for

many health care organizations. The HITECH Act updated and enhanced the privacy and security responsibilities of covered entities that were established under HIPAA. The HITECH Act brought significant compliance changes to three specific areas:

1. Business associates
2. Notification of breach
3. Civil penalties for noncompliance with the provisions of HIPAA

Business Associates

Under HIPAA, the covered entity is responsible and liable for all activities related to their business associates. If a covered entity becomes aware of a breach involving a business associate, the covered entity is expected to terminate the contract if the breach was not corrected. The HITECH Act also brought greater responsibility to the business associate. It required all business associates to comply with the HIPAA Security Rule in the same manner that a covered entity would. Business associates are expected to implement physical and technical safeguards as outlined in the Security Rule. They are expected to conduct a risk analysis, to develop and implement related policies and procedures, and to comply with written documentation and workforce training requirements. The business associate is now subject to the application of civil and criminal penalties, just as a covered entity is.

Notification of Breach

The HITECH Act defines a breach as the unauthorized acquisition, access, use, or disclosure of PHI, in a manner not permitted by HIPAA, which poses a significant risk of financial, reputational, or other harm to the affected individual.

Mitigation means to "alleviate the severity" or "make mild." In reference to HIPAA, the covered entity has a duty to take appropriate steps in response to a breach of confidential communication. Breaches are considered to be HIPAA violations and may lead to substantial fines. If a breach is discovered, the health care organization is required to mitigate, to the extent possible, any harmful effects of the breach. For example, if a billing specialist learns that they have sent health records by fax to an incorrect party, steps should be taken to have the recipient destroy the PHI. Mitigation procedures also apply to activities of the health care organization's business associates. Being proactive and responsible by mitigating reduces the potential for a more disastrous outcome from the breach or violation.

Under the HITECH Act, if a breach were to occur, the HITECH Act requires a covered entity to notify the affected party directly within 60 days. Any breach is presumed reportable unless the covered entity or business associated can demonstrate that there is a low probability that the information has been compromised.

Breach notification is not required when any of the following occur:

1. The breach was unintentional access or use by someone who acquired the PHI in good faith through the normal scope of their job. For example, if a billing specialist receives and opens an e-mail from a nurse, and then notifies the nurse of

the misdirected e-mail and deletes it, a breach notification is not required.

2. There is a good faith belief that the unauthorized person could not have retained the PHI. For example, if a laptop is lost and recovered and analysis shows that information on the laptop had not been accessed or altered, a breach notification is not required.

3. A health care organization may be asked by law enforcement to delay breach notification if such notification would impede an investigation.

If an organization has used an appropriate method to encrypt and destroy files, it is relieved of the breach notification rule as it applies to that PHI.

Breach notification must be sent in writing via first class mail to each individual affected. If the patient is deceased, the next of kin must be notified. If an address is unknown, an effort must be made to reach the individual through other means. If the breach affects 500 or more individuals, the notice must also be provided to local media outlets such as newspaper and television news.

DHHS must also be notified within 60 days of the breach for breaches affecting 500 or more people. For smaller breaches, DHHS can be notified annually or within 60 days of the end of the year the breach was discovered. A list of covered entities that have had breaches is maintained by DHHS. Organizations on this list must submit logs of breaches to the DHHS on an ongoing annual basis.

HIPAA Omnibus Rule

The final HIPAA Omnibus Rule is an update to the 1996 HIPAA law and 2009 HITECH Act that modified both privacy and security rules for covered entities and their business associates. The new rule, effective March 26, 2013, did the following:

- enhanced patients' privacy rights and protections, especially regarding genetic information
- strengthened the OCR's ability to enforce the HIPAA privacy and security protections in the face of the expanded use of electronic health records
- held business associates who receive PHI and their subcontractors to the same standards of covered entities
- clarified when breaches of unsecured health information must be reported to DHHS
- increased the restrictions on use of PHI in research and marketing
- raised the penalties for negligent disclosures

HIPAA Compliance Audits

The HITECH Act further requires DHHS to provide periodic audits to ensure that covered entities and business associates are complying with HIPAA Privacy and Security Rules and Breach Notification standards. The OCR has developed an audit program that is used to assess HIPAA privacy and security programs and compliance efforts. It examines mechanisms for compliance, identifies best practices, and discovers risks and vulnerabilities that may not be identified through other means. All covered entities, including health plans, health care clearinghouses, health care providers, and business associates, are eligible for an audit. Over the past decade, OCR audits have

focused on how covered entities have implemented controls and processes to meet HIPAA Privacy and Security and Breach Notification Rules.

2.11 QUICK REVIEW

Question: Name three specific areas addressed in HITECH.

CONSEQUENCES OF NONCOMPLIANCE WITH HIPAA AND HITECH

Different governing bodies handle the prosecution of HIPAA violations. DHHS handles issues regarding transaction code sets and security. Complaints can be filed against a covered entity for not complying with these rules. The OCR oversees privacy issues and complaints and refers criminal issues to the Office of the Inspector General (OIG). The OIG provides the workup for referral cases, which may involve the Federal Bureau of Investigation (FBI) and other agencies. Health care organizations are expected to have an active HIPAA compliance plan in place.

Since the 2003 HIPAA Privacy Rule compliance date, the OCR has investigated more than 231,968 complaints.[1] Sometimes the investigation finds that no violation occurred. When a violation has occurred, the OCR attempts to resolve the situation with one of the following:

- Voluntary compliance where the OCR may provide training and technical assistance to bring an entity into compliance;
- Corrective action where the OCR outlines a step-by-step process to correct the violation and ensure it does not happen again; and/or
- Resolution agreement where the covered entity is obligated to perform certain tasks and report to the OCR for 3 years. It often includes a monetary penalty.

Penalties for Noncompliance With the Provisions of HIPAA

There are both civil and criminal penalties for failure to comply with HIPAA regulations. The HITECH Act significantly increased the penalty amounts that may be imposed for violations related to failure to comply with HIPAA rules. These were initially established as follows:

- $100 to $50,000 if the covered entity did not know about the violation
- $1000 to $50,000 if the violation was due to reasonable cause
- $10,000 to $50,000 if the violation was due to willful neglect and was corrected
- $50,000 or more if the violation was due to willful neglect and was not corrected

All penalties have increased due to inflation each year.

The HITECH Act set a maximum penalty of $1.5 million for all violations of an identical provision in a calendar year. Penalties may also be applied on a daily basis if the OCR sees fit to do so. An example of when this may occur would be if a health

---

[1]Department of Health and Human Services. (2020, March 31). Enforcement Highlights. https://www.hhs.gov/hipaa/for-professionals/compliance-enforcement/data/enforcement-highlights/index.html.

care organization refuses to give patients copies of their records when requested. In this case, OCR may apply the penalty per day that the organization was in violation.

Individuals also can be held personally responsible for HIPAA violations with criminal actions as follows:

- Knowing violations: up to $50,000 and/or 1 year in prison
- Misrepresentation or offenses under false pretenses: up to $100,000 and/or 5 years in prison
- Intent to sell, distribute, etc.: up to $250,000 and/or 10 years in prison

Refraining From Intimidating or Retaliatory Acts

HIPAA privacy regulations prohibit a covered entity from intimidating, threatening, coercing, discriminating against, or otherwise taking retaliatory action against individuals for any of the following:

- for exercising HIPAA privacy rights
- for filing a complaint with DHHS
- for testifying, assisting, or participating in an investigation, or
- for reasonably opposing any practice prohibited by the regulation.

Examples of Recent HIPAA Violations

In 2018, Anthem, Inc. was found to have had a breach exposing 78.8 million records. They agreed to a settlement of $16 million to settle the breach. This was the largest HIPAA settlement to date. They were found not only to have insufficient controls in place to prevent such a breach, but they also failed to respond adequately once the breach was detected.

Fresenius Medical Care North America had multiple recent HIPAA violations regarding stolen computers and unencrypted thumb drives. The company settled the case for $3.5 million. In addition to the monetary penalties, the company and all of its entities must conduct comprehensive risk analyses to address further areas of risk. P&P must be developed to address devices, media, and access controls.

The University of Texas MD Anderson Cancer Center was ordered to pay a civil monetary penalty of $4,348,000 to settle a case. The center had lost a laptop and two unencrypted thumb drives thereby exposing 34,883 patients' ePHI. Despite having P&P in place requiring all devices to be encrypted, the health center had failed to implement these policies until after the theft.

Massachusetts General Hospital was fined $515,000 for allowing film crews to record patients without consent for the TV series, Boston Med. The corrective action plan included additional staff training on allowable uses and disclosures of PHI to film and media.

In 2017, Memorial Healthcare System paid HHS $5.5 million and agreed to a corrective action plan to settle HIPAA violations. They self-reported to HHS a potential breach of PHI for over 115,000 patients. A former employee's login credentials had been used for a year to access patient records. HHS found that the organization had failed to review activity or terminate the former employee's access despite having identified this risk several years before the breach.

In January 2017, HHS announced the first settlement based on untimely breach notification. Presence Health in Illinois agreed to pay $475,000 and complete a corrective action plan when it failed to notify affected individuals within 60 days of discovering a breach. Though the notification was otherwise handled correctly, the OCR sent a clear message to other organizations. Every aspect of the HIPAA rules and Breach Notification Rules must be followed to the letter.

These and other OCR Resolution Agreements can be reviewed on the DHHS website (https://www.hhs.gov/hipaa/for-professionals/compliance-enforcement/agreements/index.html).

2.12   QUICK REVIEW

Question: Name four governing bodies that oversee or prosecute HIPAA violations.

ORGANIZATION AND STAFF RESPONSIBILITIES IN PROTECTING PATIENT RIGHTS

HIPAA affects all areas of the health care office, from the reception area to the provider (see Fig. 2.4). In addition to being educated and trained in job responsibilities, every staff member must be educated about HIPAA and trained in the P&P pertinent to the organization.

Obligations of the Health Care Organization

The covered entity must implement written P&P that comply with HIPAA standards. P&P are tailored guidelines established to inform each employee of their role within the organization. It is important that PHI is addressed in these guidelines. HIPAA requires each organization to implement P&P that comply with privacy and security rules. The organization should have a P&P manual to train providers and staff and to serve as a resource for situations that need clarification. Revisions to P&P must be made as needed and appropriate to comply with laws as they change. Documentation must be maintained in written or electronic form and retained for 6 years after its creation or when it was last in effect, whichever is later.

Fig. 2.4 Health Insurance Portability and Accountability Act (HIPAA), privacy, and security affect every level of the health care organization. (From iStock photo.com.)

HIPAA and Social Media

In 2020, there were approximately 3.8 billion social media users worldwide.[2] These social media users were spending almost two and a half hours per day on an average of eight social networking sites.[3] In addition to individual health care workers socializing on various sites, many health care organizations and providers use social media channels as a method of connecting with their patients and attracting new ones. As such, health care organizations must have a social media policy in place to ensure patient privacy is maintained. Training should be given to new employees as part of their orientation, and a refresher should be done annually to make sure the social media rules are not forgotten.

Under HIPAA's privacy rule, sharing protected health information on social media is prohibited. This includes any text, video or pictures that can potentially identify a patient. PHI can only be posted on social media with the patient's written consent outlining both the specific information that can be shared and specific purpose for using it.

Posting images or videos of patients without their consent is a HIPAA violation. This holds true if the patient is not the specific subject of the picture or video, but is simply in the frame, or if their PHI is visible. It is also a HIPAA violation if a health care worker posts gossip about a patient. Remember violations occur even if the patient is not listed by name but can be identified by the information shared.

Having conversations with patients on a health care organization's social media page can be an effective way of engaging them. Regardless of what a patient may share about themselves, it is important to protect their PHI. Violations can still occur even if the patient initiates the conversation. It is best to ask the patient to private message, email or call to continue the conversation.

Best Practices to Avoid Common HIPAA Violations

An insurance billing specialist will likely answer the telephone and speak during the course of their job, and there may be uncertainties about what questions they can and cannot answer. Reasonable and appropriate safeguards must be taken to ensure that all confidential health information is protected from unauthorized and inappropriate access, in both verbal and written forms (Fig. 2.5).

- Consider that conversations occurring throughout the office may be overheard. The reception area and waiting room are often linked and it is easy to hear the scheduling of appointments and exchange of confidential information. It is necessary to observe work areas and maximize efforts to avoid unauthorized disclosures. Simple and affordable precautions include using privacy glass at the front desk and having conversations away from settings where other patients or visitors are present. Health care providers can move their dictation

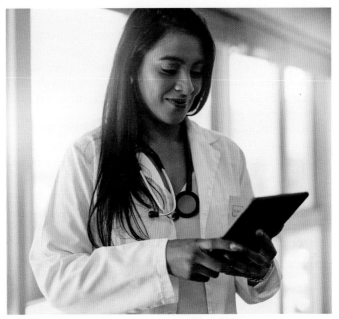

Fig. 2.5 Privacy and security must be considered in every aspect of a health care worker's job, from phone conversations to computer use to physical surroundings. (From iStock photo.com.)

stations away from patient areas or wait until no patients are present before dictating. Telephone conversations made by providers in front of patients, even in emergency situations, should be avoided. Providers and staff must use their best professional judgment.

- Be sure to check in both the patient's health record and the medical billing systems to determine whether there are any special instructions for contacting the patient regarding scheduling or reporting test results. Follow these requests as agreed by the office.
- Patient sign-in sheets are permissible but limit the information a patient is required to list when they sign in and change the sheet periodically during the day. A sign-in sheet must not contain information such as a reason for the encounter or the patient's medical condition. Because some providers specialize in treating patients with sensitive issues, simply showing that a particular individual has an appointment with the provider may pose a breach of patient confidentiality.
- Formal policies for transferring and accepting outside PHI must address how the health care organization keeps this information confidential. When using courier services, billing services, transcription services, or e-mail, transferring PHI must be done in a secure and compliant manner.
- Computers are used for a variety of administrative functions, including scheduling, billing, and managing health records. Computers are typically present at the reception area. Keep the computer screen turned so that viewing is restricted to authorized staff. Screen savers should be used to prevent unauthorized viewing or access. The computer should automatically log off the user after a period of being idle, requiring the staff member to reenter their password.

[2]Market.US. (2020, April 17). Social Media Statistics and Facts. https://market.us/statistics/social-media/.

[3]Smart Insights. (2020, April 17). Global Social Media Research Summary 2020. https://www.smartinsights.com/social-media-marketing/social-media-strategy/new-global-social-media-research/.

- Keep usernames and passwords confidential and change them often. Do not share this information. An authorized staff member, such as the PO, will have administrative access to reset a lost or compromised password. Also, medical billing systems can track users and follow their activity. Safeguards include password protection for electronic data and storing paper records securely.
- Safeguard work areas; do not place notes with confidential information in areas that are easy to view by nonstaff. Cleaning services will access the building, usually after business hours; ensure that PHI is properly safeguarded.
- Place patient health records face down at reception areas so that the patient's name is not exposed to other patients or visitors. When placing health records on the door of an examination room, turn the chart so that identifying information faces the door. If medical charts are kept on countertops or in receptacles, it is important to ensure that nonstaff persons will not access the records.
- Do not post the health care provider's schedule in areas viewable by nonstaff individuals. Schedules are often posted for the convenience of the professional staff, but this may be a breach of patient confidentiality.
- Fax machines should not be placed in patient examination rooms or in any reception area where nonstaff persons may view incoming or sent documents. Only staff members should have access to the faxes.
- Health care workers who open office mail or take telephone calls pertaining to health record requests should direct these requests to the appropriate staff member.
- Exercise good judgment in writing and wording e-mails because they do not give security against confidentiality.
- Send all privacy-related questions or concerns to the appropriate staff member.
- Immediately report any suspected or known improper behavior to the supervisor or the PO so that the issue may be documented and investigated. Any questions about policies and procedures should be directed to the PO (Fig. 2.6).
- Never discuss patients casually with co-workers, friends, or family. Be mindful of the surroundings. Avoid sharing any patient information on social media. Even if a patient is not mentioned by name, someone may recognize the patient.
- Do not respond to inquiries about a patient no matter how well meaning they may seem. Many people who do not work within the health care system are unaware that this is a HIPAA violation.
- Electronic files can be accessed on stolen or misplaced computers and smartphones. Home computers that do not have appropriate security may be easily hacked. Even texting can be hacked so it is important to only use phones to transmit patient data over secure applications that use encryption.
- Do not access health records for patients out of curiosity or as a favor to a family member or friend. Health care workers are allowed the minimum amount of access necessary to do their job. This is a common HIPAA violation that costs health care organizations every year.

Fig. 2.6 Insurance billing specialist consulting with the supervisor or office manager about office policies regarding release of a patient's health record.

Under HIPAA, health care providers and their employees are required to protect PHI and limit the use of it to the minimum amount necessary. Applying HIPAA requirements can be a challenge and penalties for violating HIPAA are high. Health care workers have an obligation to their employer and to the patients they serve.

Compliance is an ongoing effort involving teamwork. Health care workers should monitor their own activities to ensure that they are following the required protocols. Shortcuts cannot be taken when patient privacy and security are involved.

? DISCUSSION POINT

Discuss various ways an insurance billing specialist can prevent HIPAA violations.

PROCEDURE 2.1   Understanding the Notice of Privacy Practices

Go to the following websites and answer the questions below.

https://www.hhs.gov/hipaa/for-professionals/privacy/guidance/privacy-practices-for-protected-health-information/index.html

https://www.hhs.gov/hipaa/for-professionals/privacy/guidance/model-notices-privacy-practices/index.html.

https://www.hhs.gov/sites/default/files/ocr/privacy/hipaa/npp_fullpage_hc_provider.pdf

1. Name three types of covered entities that are not required to develop an NPP.
2. Describe the four main areas of content that must be provided in the NPP.
3. When must a health plan provide an NPP?
4. When must a health care provider give notice?
5. If a patient requests a change to their health record, is the provider obligated to change it?
6. How long does a health care provider have to provide a copy of a patient's health information if it is requested?
7. If a patient requests a list of times their information was shared, how far back must the list go?
8. Name three ways a patient may file a complaint if they feel their rights have been violated?

KEY POINTS

This is a brief chapter review of the key issues presented. To further enhance your knowledge of the technical subject matter, review the key terms and key abbreviations for this chapter by locating the meaning for each in the Glossary at the end of this text, which appears in a section before the Index.

1. The Health Insurance Portability and Accountability Act (HIPAA) has affected confidentiality and disclosure of protected health information (PHI) and completion and electronic transactions in health care. It has also affected how health care organizations address fraud and abuse in claims submission and implementation of compliance and practice standards.
2. While employed by a health care organization, the insurance billing specialist's duty is to have complete knowledge and understanding of HIPAA mandates. Always carry out policies and procedures that comply with federal regulations, and keep up to date with these statutes. This will assist both the provider and the patients.
3. The primary purpose of HIPAA *Title I: Health Insurance Reform* is to provide continuous insurance coverage for workers and their insured dependents when they change or lose jobs. *Title II: Administrative Simplification* focuses on the health care organization setting and aims to reduce administrative costs and burdens.
4. Serious civil and criminal penalties, such as fines and imprisonment, apply for HIPAA noncompliance.
5. *PHI* refers to data that identify an individual and describe their health status, age, sex, ethnicity, or other demographic characteristics, whether that information is or is not stored or transmitted electronically.
6. Under HIPAA, PHI may not be used or disclosed without permission from the patient or someone authorized to act on behalf of the patient. Use or disclosure is permitted if it is specifically required for treatment, payment, or routine health care operations (TPO). The two types of disclosure required by the HIPAA Privacy Rule are to the individual who is the subject of the PHI and to the Secretary of the DHHS to investigate compliance with the rule.
7. *Disclosure* means the release, transfer, provision of access to, or divulging information to a person or entity outside the health care organization. *Use* means the sharing, employment, application, utilization, examination, or analysis of IIHI within an organization that holds such information. When a patient's billing record is accessed to review the claim submission history, the individual's health information is in use.
8. When comparing privileged and nonprivileged information, privileged information is related to the treatment and progress of the patient. The patient must sign an authorization to release this information or selected facts from the health record. Nonprivileged information consists of ordinary facts unrelated to treatment of the patient, including the patient's name, city of residence, and dates of admission or discharge.
9. Under HIPAA, a Notice of Privacy Practices (NPP) document must be given to the patient at the first encounter or at enrollment. The NPP explains the individual's rights and the health care organization's legal duties regarding PHI. Use and disclosure of PHI is permissible for TPO because the NPP describes how PHI is used for these purposes. Thus, a consent form is not required. The health care organization is required to obtain a signed authorization form to use or disclose health information for situations beyond the TPO. This is a protection for the health care organization. Psychotherapy notes are handled separately under HIPAA. Such notes have additional protection, specifically that an authorization for any disclosure of psychotherapy notes must be obtained.
10. The three major categories of security safeguards are administrative, technical, and physical measures that will reasonably protect PHI from any use or disclosure that is in violation of HIPAA.
11. DHHS and the OCR perform HIPAA audits and place substantial fines on covered entities that do not follow HIPAA regulations.

Strongly consider the lessons learned from the privacy, transaction, and security rules in conjunction with OIG compliance recommendations. The most important points are to read the health care organization's P&P manual and to ask questions about the general operations of the organization. Always use the best practice approach to be an informed and effective employee.

INTERNET RESOURCES

OIG HIPAA for Professionals Compliance Enforcement
- https://www.hhs.gov/hipaa/for-professionals/compliance enforcement/agreements/index.html.

OIG HIPAA for Professionals NPP Guidance
- https://www.hhs.gov/hipaa/for-professionals/privacy /guidance/privacy-practices-for-protected-health -information/index.html.

OIG HIPAA for Professionals Model NPP
- https://www.hhs.gov/hipaa/for-professionals/privacy /guidance/model-notices-privacy-practices/index.html.

OIG HIPAA for Professionals Sample NPP for Health Care Providers
- https://www.hhs.gov/sites/default/files/ocr/privacy/hipaa /npp_fullpage_hc_provider.pdf.

STUDENT ASSIGNMENTS

- Study Chapter 2.
- Complete all exercises all in the *Workbook* to reinforce the theory learned in this chapter.
- Turn to the Glossary at the end of this text for a further understanding of the key terms and key abbreviations used in this chapter.

Compliance, Fraud, and Abuse

Cheryl Fassett

OBJECTIVES

After reading this chapter, you should be able to:
1. Define compliance.
2. Discuss the difference between fraud and abuse.
3. List examples of fraud and abuse in the health care setting.
4. Identify the federal and state laws that regulate health care fraud and abuse.
5. Understand the penalties for fraud and abuse.
6. Identify the various fraud and abuse audit programs.
7. Discuss the basic components of an effective compliance program.
8. Discuss potential risk areas for provider groups, billing companies, and hospitals.

KEY TERMS

abuse
Anti-Kickback Law
assumption coding
auditing
Civil False Claims Act
Civil Monetary Penalty
Clinical Laboratory Improvement Amendments
clustering
compliance
compliance plan
Comprehensive Error Rate Testing
corrective action plan
cost reports
Criminal False Claims Act
DRG upcoding/DRG creep

embezzlement
Emergency Medical Treatment and Labor Act
Exclusion Statute
Federal Deposit Insurance Corporation
fraud
Fraud Enforcement and Recovery Act
Health Care Fraud and Abuse Control
Health Care Fraud Prevention and Enforcement Action Team
kickback
medical necessity
Medicare Administrative Contractor
Medicare Integrity Program
monitoring

Occupational Safety and Health Administration
Office of Inspector General
OIG Work Plan
Operation Restore Trust
patient dumping
phantom bills
Physician Self-Referral Law
qui tam
Recovery Audit Contractor
safe harbor
Self-Disclosure Protocol
Stark Law
undercoding
upcoding
Zone Program Integrity Contractor

KEY ABBREVIATIONS

CERT	EMTALA	MAC	PPACA
CLIA	FCA	MIP	RAC
CMP	FDIC	OIG	SDP
CMS	FERA	ORT	ZPIC
DHHS	HCFAC	OSHA	
DOJ	HEAT	P&P	

INSIGHTS FROM THE FIELD

Lisa N.: Certified Professional Coder (CPC), Certified Professional Compliance Officer (CPCO), Certified Documentation Expert - Outpatient (CDEO), Certified Professional Mediacl Auditor (CPMA), Certified Risk Adjustment Coder (CRC), Certified Professional Coding - Instructor (CPC-I)

I have worked in health care for 40 years! I started as a medical assistant, but have been a biller, coder, reimbursement specialist, physician educator, and held various department and practice management positions over the years. I am currently a corporate compliance advisor. I educate providers and perform annual reviews to ensure correct coding and documentation. When I started in medicine, you were able to learn on the job—you didn't have to have any degrees or certifications to get a job in a medical office. Along the way, I was able to get certifications to make me more valuable to my employers. Learning all the guidelines, rules, codes, and so on is challenging enough, but that really doesn't prepare you to be able to interact with providers. Providers can have strong personalities, and I advise you to have a thick skin and hold your ground. Look them in the eye, be professional, and ALWAYS get back to them with an answer to their question. I never have a problem telling a provider that I don't know the answer, but you can bet I'll follow up and let them know. It's okay to admit we don't know it all, but they need to have confidence that you will find out.

COMPLIANCE DEFINED

Health care is one of the most highly regulated industries, holding the health care worker to the highest levels of scrutiny. Any individual working in health care and any business that is involved with the health care industry must conform to the principles and practices identified by state and federal agencies.

Compliance in the health care industry is the ongoing process of meeting regulations, recommendations, and expectations of federal and state agencies that pay for health care services and regulate the industry (Fig. 3.1). Health care compliance involves the following:

- The claims reimbursement processes
- Managed care procedures
- Protection of patients' privacy
- Various guidelines and statutes
- Licensure
- Patient safety
- Attention to the law

A compliance plan outlines the organization's standardized process for handling business functions, much like a user's man-

Fig. 3.1 Compliance involves many players, laws, and standards. A compliance plan is a set of policies, procedures, and guidelines to ensure an organization conducts its business in accordance with applicable laws and regulations.

ual. This will enable consistent and effective management and staff performance.

The first step toward achieving compliance is understanding the laws that regulate the industry. Failure to comply with the associated mandates can lead to criminal penalties and/or civil fines.

3.1 QUICK REVIEW
Question: What is compliance?

FRAUD AND ABUSE LAWS

The US Department of Justice (DOJ), tasked with prosecuting health care fraud and abuse cases, announced that it recovered $2.6 billion in health care fraud in 2019 alone, up from both preceding years.[1] With many regulations and laws in place, there are very tight controls on medical billing. All individuals involved in the provision of health care services and in billing for those services are held to very high standards. Considering complex government regulations and constant scrutiny, it is important for those involved in the reimbursement process to clearly understand fraud and abuse. Both fraud and abuse can expose providers, health care organizations, and heath care workers to criminal and civil liability.

Fraud can occur when deception is used in claim submission to obtain payment from the payer. Individuals who knowingly, willfully, and intentionally submit false information to benefit themselves or others commit fraud. Fraud can also be seen in mistakes that result in excessive reimbursement. It is not necessary to prove intent to defraud. Liability can occur when a person knowingly presents or makes a false record that creates a false claim.

As you will learn later in this textbook, insurance claims require codes that describe what was wrong with the patient (diagnosis codes) and what service was provided to the patient (procedural codes). Codes must be reported accurately on claim forms. A fraudulent claim may be one that has been coded to maximize payment by reflecting a higher service level. An inaccurate diagnosis may be billed to justify a service that was not medically necessary. A claim may also be filed for services that never took place, or for a patient who was never seen. Patients can also commit fraud by stealing a person's identity and using their insurance coverage, or providing false information on their health insurance applications. Further examples of health care fraud are listed in Box 3.1.

Abuse describes incidents or practices by health care organizations, not usually considered fraudulent, that conflict with accepted sound medical business or fiscal practices. An example of abuse in billing practices may be to submit excessive charges for services or supplies, or duplicate billing. Additional examples of health care abuse are listed in Box 3.2.

---

[1]Office of Public Affairs, Department of Justice. (2020, January 9) Justice Department Recovers over $3 Billion from False Claims Act Cases in Fiscal Year 2019. https://www.justice.gov/opa/pr/justice-department-recovers-over-3-billion-false-claims-act-cases-fiscal-year-2019.

BOX 3.1   Examples of Fraud

- Billing for services or supplies not provided (**phantom bills** or invoice ghosts)
- Altering fees on a claim form to obtain higher payment
- Forgiving the deductible or copayment
- Altering health records to generate fraudulent payments
- Omitting relevant information from a claim (for example, failing to reveal whether a spouse has health insurance coverage through an employer)
- Upcoding (for example, submit a code for a complex fracture when the patient had a simple fracture)
- Dispensing less medication than billed for
- Split billing schemes (for example, billing procedures over a period of days when all treatment occurred during one encounter)
- Using another person's insurance card to obtain medical care
- Changing a date of service
- Soliciting offering, or receiving a kickback, bribe, or rebate in return for referring a patient to another provider or facility
- Restating the diagnosis to obtain insurance benefits or better payment
- Deliberately applying for duplicate payment (for example, billing the insurance twice, billing Medicare and the beneficiary for the same service, or billing Medicare and another insurer in an attempt to be paid twice)
- Unbundling or exploding charges (for example, billing a multichannel laboratory test as if individual tests were performed)
- Collusion between a health care organization and an employee of a third-party payer when the claim is assigned (if the health care organization deliberately overbilled for services, overpayments could be generated with little awareness on the part of the Medicare beneficiary)
- Billing based on "gang visits" (for example, a provider visits a nursing home and bills for 20 patient encounter without furnishing any specific services to individual patients)
- Knowingly billing for the same item or service more than once or another party billing the federal health care program for an item or service also billed by the health care organization

⚠ COMPLIANCE ALERT

Anyone in the health care field, even patients, can face charges of fraud and abuse! Billing specialists and other employees can protect themselves by understanding what actions are considered fraudulent and approaching their tasks with integrity.

False Claims Act (1863)

The False Claims Act (FCA) of 1863 is still the US government's main recourse against fraud and abuse. Originally written to protect the government from being sold shoddy equipment in the Civil War, it now extends that protection from military supplies to health care.

A false claim is one for services or supplies that were not provided specifically as presented or for which the health care organization is otherwise not entitled to payment. Presenting a claim for an item or service based on a procedure code known to result in greater payment or to submit a claim for services not medically necessary is also a violation of the FCA. The government uses the FCA in conjunction with other fraud and abuse laws as a primary enforcement tool. There are both civil and criminal aspects to the FCA.

BOX 3.2   Examples of Medical Billing Abuse

- Regularly referring to other providers for unnecessary services
- Charging excessively for services or supplies
- Performing a battery of diagnostic tests when only a few tests are required for services
- Violating Medicare's participating provider agreement
- Calling patients for repeated and unnecessary follow-up encounters
- Billing Medicare beneficiaries at a higher rate than other patients
- Submitting bills to Medicare and not to third-party payers (e.g., claims for injury from an automobile accident, in a store, or at the workplace)
- Breaching an assignment agreement
- Failing to make required refunds when services are not reasonable and necessary
- Requiring Medicare patients to pay full charges, in excess of the Medicare charge limits
- Requiring patients to sign a global waiver agreeing to pay privately for all services that Medicare will not cover and using these waivers to obligate patients to pay separately for a service that Medicare covers as part of a package or related procedures
- Failing to submit claims for covered services to Medicare and requiring the patient to pay for them privately.

Criminal False Claims Act (18 US Code §287)

The Criminal False Claims Act stated that anyone who knowingly makes or presents a false or fraudulent claim to any department or agency of the United States shall be imprisoned up to 5 years and shall be subject to a fine. Though the law did not apply specifically to the health care industry, Health Insurance Portability and Accountability (HIPAA) amendments officially linked the FCA to health care (Fig. 3.2). HIPAA updated the criminal code to include the following:

- *Theft or Embezzlement Statute (18 US Code §669).* This law brings fines and imprisonment against any person who embezzles, steals, or intentionally misapplies any of the moneys, funds, property, or other assets of any public or private health care benefit program. In addition to health care organizations that deal with the Medicare and Medicaid programs, this law applies to financial service industries, bookkeeping and accounting firms, and all business types and industries.

  Embezzlement means stealing money that has been entrusted to one's care. The insurance billing specialist has been entrusted to process and manage health care finances in an

Fig. 3.2 It is crucial that an insurance billing specialist understands fraud and abuse laws. (From iStock photo.com.)

organization. They should take extreme precautions to protect themselves and the organization who employs them. If an undiscovered embezzler leaves an employer, the person's replacement could be accused some months later of doing something they did not do. Be aware of what constitutes fraudulent activity and bring any potential issues to management upon discovery.

Other statutes that reflect fraud investigations targeting health care are as follows:

- *False Statement Relating to Health Care Matters Statute (19 US Code §1035).* Any person who conceals facts, makes fraudulent statements, or falsifies documentation relating to health care services is committing fraud. This holds true for both the delivery of and payment for these services. In doing this, a person is subject to fines and imprisonment.
- *Health Care Fraud Statute (18 US Code §1347).* Any individual who knowingly attempts or carries out a scheme to defraud any health care benefit program is committing fraud and is subject to fines and imprisonment. If a serious body injury or death occurs, the person may face life imprisonment.
- *Obstruction of Criminal Investigations of Health Care Offenses Statute (18 US Code §1518).* A person is subject to fines and imprisonment when he or she prevents, obstructs, or misleads a federal health care criminal investigator.

Civil False Claims Act (31 US Code §§3729-3733)

The Civil False Claims Act authorizes the United States to recover monetary damages from people who file fraudulent claims for payment by the federal government.

A coding or billing specialist who has knowledge of fraud or abuse should take the following measures:

- Notify the provider, both personally and in writings.
- Document the false statement.
- Notify the health care organization's manager.
- Maintain a written audit trail with dated memoranda.
- Do not discuss the problem with anyone who is not immediately involved.

The American Academy of Professional Coders (AAPC) and the American Health Information Management Association (AHIMA), as well as most other professional organizations, have established a code of ethics for their certified members. Health care workers who follow these guidelines will be on the right path to avoid fraud and abuse (Box 3.3).

Qui Tam Provision

A writ of qui tam (pronounced kwee tam) is a provision under the FCA whereby a private individual who assists a prosecution can receive all or part of any penalty imposed. The qui tam provision in the FCA offers financial incentives to private citizens who act as informants and report suspected fraud on behalf of the federal government. This involves fraud by government contractors and other entities that receive or use government funds.

The informant or individual who files a qui tam suit is known as a "relator" or a "whistleblower." A whistleblower can be anyone—an employee, a patient, another provider, or someone who works for a billing company or third-party payer. The lawsuits are filed under seal, so only the federal government knows about

---

BOX 3.3 Key Components in the AAPC and AHIMA Codes of Ethics

Integrity
Respect
Commitment
Competence
Fairness
Responsibility
Professionalism

Both organizations require their members to adhere to legal and ethical principles in coding, health information management, and every aspect of their jobs. They require members to avoid circumstances that may go against the laws and regulations of the health care industry.

For detailed discussion of each of these components, please refer to the AAPC Code of Ethics page (https://www.aapc.com/aboutus/code-of-ethics.aspx) and the AHIMA Code of Ethics page (https://bok.ahima.org/doc?oid=105098#.Xqm77CN_OUk).

AAPC, American Academy of Professional Coders; *AHIMA,* American Health Information Management Association.

---

the allegations. This gives the government time to investigate and decide if it is valid and will intervene.

Qui tam cases for health care fraud and abuse are big business. These lawsuits help recover billions of dollars for the US Treasury and taxpayers every year. In case the government chooses to join, the whistleblower who assists in the qui tam action shares in 15-20% of any money recovered from penalties imposed. If the government does not join the case and the whistleblower pursues it without them, the whistleblower is entitled to 25-30% of the monies collected.

Penalties for Violating the False Claims Act

As originally written, civil penalties for violations of the FCA can result in fines of up to three times the programs' loss plus $11,000 per claim filed. However, with inflation, the amount has increased to a maximum of $23,331 per claim plus triple the damages in 2020.[2] Criminal penalties for submitting false claims may include fines, imprisonment, or both (Box 3.4). Updated penalties for the different health care fraud laws are published in the OIG *Federal Register* annually and vary depending on the alleged violation.[3]

! COMPLIANCE ALERT

Health care organizations and staff are not likely to read the *Federal Register* from cover to cover. However, it is important that you are familiar with it. The *Federal Register* is a newspaper published by the National Archives and Records Administration. It contains federal regulations, proposed rules, and other important documents. New legislation that affects the health care world will always appear in this publication.

---

[2]Kohn, Kohn & Colapinto, National Law Review. (2020, January 17) DOJ Publishes New Fine Rates for False Claims Act Whistleblower Cases. https://www.natlawreview.com/article/doj-publishes-new-fine-rates-false-claims-act-whistleblower-cases
[3]Department of Health and Human Services, *Federal Register.* (2020, January 17) Annual Civil Monetary Penalties Inflation Adjustment. https://www.govinfo.gov/content/pkg/FR-2020-01-17/pdf/2020-00738.pdf.

Civil penalties:
    Up to $22,927[4] per false claim plus triple the damages (money the government lost because of the claim)
Criminal penalties:
    Up to 10 years in jail and $100,000
Administrative sanctions:
    Up to $20,000 per line item per false claim and exclusion from participation in government programs

The FCA was amended in 2009 and 2010 under the Fraud Enforcement and Recovery Act of 2009 (FERA) and the Patient Protection and Affordable Care Act (PPACA). One significant change to the FCA under PPACA was clarification that overpayments under Medicare and Medicaid must be reported and returned within 60 days of discovery. Failure to report and return an overpayment exposes a health care organization to liability under the FCA.

Exclusion Statute (42 US Code §1320a-7)

Under the Exclusion Statute, the OIG is required to exclude individuals, health care providers, and health care organizations who commit criminal offenses from participation in any federal health care programs. Offenses that can earn exclusion from these programs range from Medicare fraud to patient abuse to financial misconduct.

According to OIG, no payment will be made to an excluded individual for anything he or she furnishes, orders, or prescribes. This payment exclusion extends to anyone who employs or contracts with the excluded individual as well as any hospital or provider who allows the excluded individual to provide services.

Health care organizations are required to screen all prospective providers, employees, and contractors against the OIG's List of Excluded Individuals and Entities before hire. Organizations that hire or contract with excluded individuals may be subject to civil monetary penalties. Be sure to check the updated exclusion listings at the OIG website (https://oig.hhs.gov/faqs/exclusions-faq.asp).

! COMPLIANCE ALERT

A health care organization that employees an individual on the OIG List of Excluded Individuals can face the same type of penalties as the excluded individual.

Stark Laws (42 US Code §1395nn)

The Stark Law is commonly referred to as the Physician Self-Referral Law. The original Stark Law pertained only to referrals to clinical laboratories. It was later expanded the service list to include the following:
- Clinical laboratory services
- Radiology services

[4]Medicare Learning Network, Centers for Medicaid and Medicare. (2019, February). Medicare Fraud and Abuse: Prevent, Detect, Report. https://www.cms.gov/Outreach-and-Education/Medicare-Learning-NetworkMLN/MLNProducts/Downloads/Fraud-Abuse-MLN4649244.pdf.

- Physical and occupational therapy services
- Durable medical equipment and supplies, including prosthetics and orthotics
- Radiation therapy services and supplies
- Outpatient speech-language pathology services
- Parenteral and enteral equipment and supplies
- Inpatient and outpatient hospital services
- Home health services
- Outpatient prescription drugs

The Stark Law prohibits the submission of claims for services or referral of patients if the referring provider has a financial relationship with the entity that provides the services. The Stark Law carries exceptions, so it is important to understand the referral processes and in-office ancillary services used by each health care organization. Penalties for violations of the Stark Law include fines and exclusion from participation in the federal health care programs.

Anti-Kickback Statute (42 US Code §1320a-7b[b])

Under the Anti-Kickback Statute (1972), paying for referrals is a crime. A kickback may include any type of gift, reward, or inducement for facilitating a transaction or appointment. Kickbacks can distort health care professionals' decision making, promote overutilization of services and products, and result in unfair competition. Accepting discounts, rebates, or other reductions in price may violate this statute if it involves services payable under a federal program such as Medicare or Medicaid. For example, if a hospital furnishes providers with free office space or tickets to a golf tournament in exchange for their patient referrals, they would both be guilty of paying and receiving kickbacks.

Penalties for paying or accepting kickbacks can include fines, jail terms, and exclusion from participating in federal health care programs. Penalties up to $50,000 per kickback plus three times the amount of the remuneration can be imposed. The PPACA strengthened this statute by clarifying that to prove a fraud, the government needs to only prove intent to break the law, not to violate this statute specifically.

Safe Harbors

A safe harbor is a provision of a statute or a regulation that specifies certain business arrangements that will be deemed not to violate a given rule. There are safe harbors that protect individuals from prosecution under the Anti-Kickback Statue. Certain arrangements are not violations of the Anti-Kickback Statute and are clearly allowed if they fall within a "safe harbor."

For example, in 2013, a safe harbor that allows hospitals to furnish provider groups with electronic health record systems and training to operate them was extended by the Centers for Medicare and Medicaid Services (CMS) and the OIG through 2021. Before this, it could have been viewed as a kickback arrangement for referrals if a hospital gave provider groups this type of resource. However, this safe harbor was essential in CMS's effort to assist smaller provider groups or health care organizations in the health care community to adopt electronic health records technology.

Civil Monetary Penalties Law (41 US Code §1320a-7a)

The Social Security Act allows the DHHS to impose monetary penalties and program exclusions for violations of the Anti-Kickback Statute and other various violations. The US Congress enacted this Civil Monetary Penalty (CMP) statute to help combat health care fraud and abuse. CMP imposes civil monetary penalties and assessments against a person or organization for making false or improper claims against any federal health care program. Penalties can range from $2000 to $100,000 per violation and may also include an assessment of up to three times the amount claimed for each item or service. CMP also allows a health care organization or provider to be excluded from government programs. CMP does not require that intent to defraud is proven.

Operation Restore Trust

Launched in 1995, Operation Restore Trust (ORT) was a program designed to combine the efforts of federal and state agencies to combat fraud, waste, and abuse in the Medicare and Medicaid programs. It was a joint effort overseen by the OIG and CMS allowing the public to report issues that might indicate fraud, abuse, or waste. ORT identified problems and weaknesses within the federally funded programs, recovering more than $25 million in its first year. It also trained state and local organizations to detect fraud and abuse and implemented statistical methods to identify health care organizations for audits and investigations.

Additional Laws and Compliance

Other laws pertaining to fraud and abuse include the Federal Deposit Insurance Corporation (FDIC) mail and wire fraud provisions, as follows:

- §1341: *Frauds and swindles.* An individual is subject to both fines and imprisonment when devising a scheme to defraud or obtain money or property by means of false pretenses by use of the US Postal Service. When an individual submits false paper claims via mail, he or she is also committing mail fraud.
- §1343: *Fraud by wire, radio, or television.* An individual will be fined and/or imprisoned for devising a scheme to defraud or obtain money or property by means of false pretenses, representations, or promises by wire, radio, or television. A health care organization that is committing billing fraud through electronic claim submission may also be found guilty of wire fraud.

Though these laws may not initially seem to fit with health care fraud, if bills are sent through the US Mail, mail fraud can be added to other fraud charges. In this electronic age, most claims for health care services are submitted electronically to insurance companies and government payers. Fraudulent billing can result in wire or mail fraud charges for both providers and patients, with the added benefit of allowing the government to freeze the accused's assets until after the investigation and trial. This is done to preserve funds that could have been obtained by fraud.

Examples of Recent Fraud and Abuse Cases

The year 2019 saw the largest recovery to date for health care fraud under the FCA. A combined effort by the Medicare Fraud

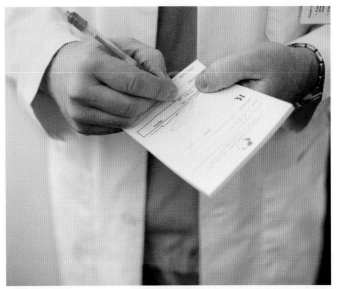

Fig. 3.3 Many fraud cases in the last 10 years have centered around pharmaceuticals and kickbacks. (From iStock photo.com.)

Strike Force, various state Medicaid Fraud Control units, the Federal Bureau of Investigation (FBI), and the OIG resulted in a recovery of $2.6 billion. It involved 505 cases involving health care organizations, providers, and health care workers[5] (Fig. 3.3).

Many of the fraud cases over the last 10 years have involved pharmaceuticals and kickbacks. The DOJ and whistleblowers have filed suits under the FCA and various other fraud laws against drug companies, physicians, hospitals, device manufacturers, health organizations, and health care workers. Some recent cases include the following:

- Insys Therapeutics paid $195 million in civil penalties for paying kickbacks in the form of lavish meals and entertainment to providers who prescribed their products to patients.
- Avanir Pharmaceuticals was fined $95 million for providing kickbacks to providers in long-term care facilities to prescribe one of their drugs to dementia patients, which was not an approved use of the medication.
- Seven pharmaceutical manufacturers paid a combined total of $624 million for illegally paying patient copays on their drugs.
- Encompass Health Corporation, an inpatient rehabilitation facility operator, paid $48 million for submitting inaccurate information to Medicare to receive higher reimbursement, and for admissions that were not medically necessary.
- An Orlando, Florida dermatologist agreed to pay more than $1.7 million to settle a false claims act liability for inflating Medicare claims related to a specific type of wound repair, referred to as Moh's surgery.
- A physician group in Houston, Texas paid over $1.2 million to resolve claims that they improperly billed Medicare for sleep studies.

[5]Shelby Livingston, Modern Healthcare (2020, January 9) Feds Amass $2.6 Billion from 2019 Healthcare Fraud Cases. https://www.modernhealthcare.com/legal/feds-amassed-26-billion-2019-healthcare-fraud-cases.

- A billing specialist in Tampa, Florida was sentenced to 5 years' probation and 4 months home detention for her role in falsifying medical claims submitted to various government payers.
- A urologist in Los Angeles, California was sentenced to 6 years in prison for fraudulent billings of nonexistent patient visits and unnecessary tests.

In many of these cases, found on the DOJ (https://www.justice.gov/briefing-room) and OIG fraud enforcement (https://oig.hhs.gov/fraud/enforcement/criminal/) websites, a whistleblower shared in the recovered monies. The US government is clearly committed to the investigation and prosecution of health care fraud and abuse. It is imperative that health care entities develop their own compliance program to identify and prevent fraud.

It is important to realize health care organization employees can commit fraud and abuse at the coding and billing level. Any questions or concerns should be brought to the compliance office for further investigation. Fraudulent or abusive billing patterns that may draw attention to a health care organization for possible audit are as follows:

- Billing intentionally for unnecessary services
- Billing incorrectly for services of physician extenders, such as nurse practitioner, midwife, physician assistant
- Billing for diagnostic tests without a separate report in the health record
- Changing dates of service on insurance claims to comply with policy coverage dates
- Waiving copayments or deductibles or allowing other illegal discounts
- Ordering excessive diagnostic tests, such as laboratory tests or x-ray studies
- Using two different provider numbers to bill the same services for the same patient
- Misusing provider identification numbers, resulting in incorrect billing
- Using improper modifiers for financial gain
- Failing to return overpayments made by the Medicare program

Many of these errors can be avoided if the coding and billing specialist ensures that documentation of patient care in the health record corresponds with billing information submitted on the insurance claims.

COMPLIANCE AUDITS AND OVERSIGHT

One of the greatest challenges for health care providers, workers, and organizations is the growing number of government and third-party fraud and abuse audit programs that scrutinize payment of health care services (Fig. 3.4).

CMS is the federal agency that administers and oversees the Medicare program and monitors the Medicaid program run by each state. CMS is committed to providing health care services to Medicare and Medicaid beneficiaries while also partnering with various entities and law enforcement agencies to prevent and detect health care fraud and abuse.

Since its establishment in 1976, the Office of Inspector General's (OIG) mission has been to protect the health and welfare

Fig. 3.4 Many types of audits actively search for wrongdoers who commit health care fraud. Fraud and abuse can result in large fines and even jail time. (From iStock photo.com.)

of the beneficiaries of Department of Health and Human Services (DHHS) programs and to safeguard the integrity of the Medicare and Medicaid programs. The OIG was established to find and eliminate fraud, abuse, and waste. The OIG undertakes nationwide audits as well as investigations to review the claim submission processes of health care organizations and reimbursement patterns within the program. The OIG makes recommendations to the DHHS Secretary and the US Congress on correcting problematic areas addressed in the federal programs. The OIG publishes the *Federal Register* which contains various items pertaining to compliance including penalties for fraud and abuse and compliance plan guidance. (See Procedure 3.1 at the end of the chapter.)

Efforts to combat fraud were consolidated and strengthened under the Health Insurance Portability and Accountability Act (HIPAA) of 1996. The Act established a comprehensive program to combat fraud committed against all health plans, both public and private. The legislation required the creation of a national Health Care Fraud and Abuse Control (HCFAC) Program, under the joint direction of the Attorney General and the Secretary of the DHHS acting through the department's Inspector General (DHHS/OIG). The HCFAC Program coordinates federal, state, and local law enforcement activities to combat health care fraud and abuse.

HIPAA legislation has radically changed the focus and mission within the OIG. HIPAA pushed the OIG into a new era, guaranteeing funds for the OIG programs and mandating initiatives to protect the integrity of all health care programs.

HIPAA requires DHHS and the Department of Justice (DOJ) to detail the amounts deposited to the Medicare Trust Fund as well as the source of such deposits in an annual report. The Affordable Care Act (ACA) provides additional tools and resources to help fight fraud that will help to boost HCFAC Program activities. These resources include the following:

- Enhanced screenings and enrollment requirements
- Increased data sharing across government
- Expanded overpayment recovery efforts
- Greater oversight of private insurance abuses

Recovery Audit Program

CMS's Recovery Audit Program is tasked with identifying and correcting improper Medicare payments. Recovery Audit Contractors (RACs) are companies that contract with Medicare to recoup money from inappropriately paid claims. An improper payment may be an overpayment on a claim that did not meet Medicare's rules and guidelines or a provider was paid based on an incorrect fee schedule. It may also be an underpayment in a claims review will show that the procedure should have been coded for a higher level of service.

RACs receive information from Medicare about paid claims and look for potential claim payment errors using computer programs. They look for facilities, suppliers, and individual providers whose billings are higher than the majority of other suppliers or providers in their area. If a RAC finds a provider has received an overpayment, the provider is given the opportunity to discuss the determination before having to return the monies. This differs from the standard CMS appeal process which will be discussed in Chapter 6. RACs are paid a percentage of the money they recover and are highly motivated to find claim errors.

Medicare and Medicaid Integrity Programs

HIPAA includes a provision establishing the Medicare Integrity Program (MIP). This provision gives CMS specific authority to enter into contracts with entities to combat fraud, waste and abuse in the Medicare program.

The goals of the MIP are to identify and reduce Medicare overpayments through a series of audits and reviews of health care organizations' claims and cost report data. Objectives of MIP include identifying plan beneficiaries with additional insurance and educating health care organizations. Program integrity contractors help expand the scope of the MIP. This effort has recovered several billions of dollars in the fight against fraud, waste, and abuse. Similar programs have recently extended into state Medicaid programs and are referred to as Medicaid Integrity Programs. These work to identify and recover inappropriate Medicaid payments.

Zone Program Integrity Contractors

Zone Program Integrity Contractors (ZPICs) continue the efforts of various integrity auditors that were established in HIPAA. A ZPIC is a fraud-investigating contractor hired by CMS to audit and review on their behalf. ZPICs focus on reviewing claims for health care organizations that have suspicious billing patterns. A ZPIC audit is typically done based on a high frequency of specific services, data analysis, or a call to a tip line. It compares a health care organization's services to those of similar organizations. If fraud and abuse are detected, ZPICs report this to the OIG for further investigation.

Comprehensive Error Rate Testing

Medicare claims are processed by Medicare Administrative Contractors (MAC). CMS implemented the Comprehensive Error Rate Testing (CERT) program to measure the accuracy of payments in the Medicare program at both national and regional levels. CERT audits are performed to determine if a MAC is paying claims correctly. Claims are randomly selected for CERT review. The health care organization receives a letter from CMS requesting medical documentation to substantiate services that have been paid. Instructions for returning the documentation are provided and all documentation related to the services in question must be sent to the CERT Documentation Contractor within 75 days of the request. If a health care organization fails to submit the required documentation, the CERT audit will be denied and the organization will be required to return the payment to Medicare. CERT error rates are calculated based on review of records and are then used to form future target areas the OIG will focus on. CERT errors are also used by CMS to measure performance of Medicare contractors.

Health Care Fraud Prevention and Enforcement Action Team

In 2009 the DOJ and DHHS established the Health Care Fraud Prevention and Enforcement Action Team (HEAT) to build and strengthen existing programs to combat Medicare and Medicaid fraud and to crack down on fraud perpetrators. HEAT efforts have included expansion of the DOJ-DHHS Medicare Fraud Strike Force that has been successful in fighting fraud. The Medicare Fraud Strike Force continues its efforts, which are outlined in annual reports issued by the DOJ and DHHS Press Offices.

Special Alerts, Bulletins, and Guidance Documents

Health care organizations and their staff should follow all special fraud alerts published by the OIG to alert the industry of specific patterns or trends related to fraudulent or abusive activities regarding the Medicare and Medicaid programs. Special advisory bulletins report industry practices and arrangements that may indicate fraud and abuse. Other guidance documents include updates, response letters, and alerts important to more specifically targeted matters. All notices are available at the OIG website and on their mailing list.

The OIG Work Plan outlines areas where the OIG will prioritize audit efforts in the next year. It is updated monthly to reflect emerging issues. Examples of recent OIG focus are opioid prescriptions, production of COVID-19 lab test kits and payments to hospitals for lab services. Providers and organizations should refer to the Work Plan to determine areas to focus their own compliance efforts. The Work Plan can be found on the OIG's website https://oig.hhs.gov/reports-and-publications/workplan/index.asp.

The OIG's Self-Disclosure Protocol (SDP) was originally established in 2006. It has been refined many times over the years, most recently in the PPACA (2010). The SDP is a vehicle for providers and health care organizations to voluntarily disclose self-discovered evidence of potential fraud and work together with the OIG in resolving issues efficiently and fairly. The latest revision of this protocol streamlined the disclosure process and made the potential sanctions more proportionate with the disclosed violations.

⚑ 3.5   QUICK REVIEW
Question: What are some of the audits used by CMS to ensure proper payments?

COMPLIANCE PROGRAMS

A compliance plan is a comprehensive set of policies, procedures, and guidelines designed to ensure that an organization conducts its business in accordance with applicable laws and regulations. The OIG offers compliance guidelines for various types of health care organizations such as provider groups, hospitals, and billing companies. These guidelines provide acceptable principles for business operations.

The OIG started publishing various compliance program guidelines in 1998. At that time the guidance recommended by the OIG was voluntary. It was provided as a way for health care organizations to effectively reduce the risk of legal action and create a good faith effort in combating fraud, waste, and abuse. Under the PPACA, mandatory compliance program requirements were implemented and became effective January 1, 2011, for Medicare Advantage (MA) and Medicare Part D programs. Under this legislation, the DHHS Secretary has the authority to define providers, suppliers, and health care organizations that must adopt a compliance plan. Health care providers and organizations are not allowed to enroll in the Medicare or Medicaid programs without certification of a compliance plan.

The goal of a compliance plan is to prevent and reduce improper conduct. An effective program ensures proper billing practices and decreases the chance for fraud and abuse within a health care organization. The organization's governing authority should be knowledgeable about the contents of the plan and exercise reasonable oversight of its implementation and effectiveness, and high-level management should be assigned overall responsibility for the program (Box 3.5).

A well-designed compliance program can do the following:
- Speed the claims processing cycle
- Optimize proper payment or claims
- Minimize billing mistakes
- Reduce the likelihood of a government audit
- Avoid conflict with Stark laws and the Anti-Kickback Statute
- Show a good faith effort to submit claims appropriately
- Relay to staff that there is a duty to report mistakes and suspected or known misconduct

The health care organization's claims processing supervisor should research industry sector program guidance to help with specific concerns regarding the specialty or facility setting. Check the OIG website (https://oig.hhs.gov/compliance/compliance-guidance/index.asp) to view addenda, comments, and drafts of additional compliance guidance subjects.

BOX 3.5 Benefits of a Compliance Program

- Speed the claims processing cycle
- Optimize proper payment on claims
- Minimize billing mistakes
- Reduce the likelihood of a government audit
- Avoid conflict with various federal laws and statutes
- A good faith effort in maintaining compliance
- Create a culture of integrity

! COMPLIANCE ALERT

All employees in a provider group or health care organization are responsible for following the established compliance plan. If something does not seem right, ask the compliance officer or manager for clarification.

Purpose of a Compliance Program

The presence of an OIG compliance strengthens the health care organizations efforts to conduct compliant billing practices. It may also lessen imposed penalties in the event of an OIG audit or other discovery of fraudulent billing activities. Compliance policies and procedures can be found in the health care organization's policy and procedure (P&P) manual. Employees at every level of a health care organization can benefit from knowledge of P&P as they pertain to both HIPAA and OIG compliance guidelines.

Because health care organizations rely on the expertise of their billing and coding staff to process claims accurately and promptly, they also look to these staff members for advice and guidance. An insurance billing specialist will be expected to understand the complexities of the various laws and regulations governing the medical claims process.

Compliance plans effectively become a consensus among the players; providers, claims processing staff, and payers all agree to process claims in accordance with shared values. Consider the organization's OIG compliance program as a way to integrate regulatory requirements directly into claims processing procedures. OIG views the experienced billing specialists as the critical screen for the health care organization's claims. The common denominators in the key benefits identified by OIG are efficiency, consistency, and integrity.

Basic Components of a Compliance Plan

OIG outlines the following seven components of an effective program guidance plan:
- Conducting internal monitoring and auditing
- Implementing compliance and practice standards
- Designating a compliance officer or contact
- Conducting appropriate training and education
- Responding appropriately to detected offenses and developing corrective action
- Developing open lines of communication
- Enforcing disciplinary standards through well-publicized guidelines

Under the PPACA, these elements were adjusted as follows:
- Written policies, procedures and standards of conduct
- Compliance program oversight
- Training and education
- Open lines of communication
- Auditing, monitoring, and disclosure
- Consistent discipline
- Corrective actions

Written Policies, Procedures, and Standards of Conduct

Policies and procedures should be explained to new employees within the first 90 days of employment and then reviewed annually with the entire organization. They should be clearly written and outline expectation for all staff members. They should detail the organization's commitment to ethical behavior and create an atmosphere of integrity from management down. Policies and procedures should be reviewed and updated at regular intervals.

Written standards and procedures address risk areas that a health care organization needs to monitor and follow. In addition to these risk areas, policies should be developed that address the following:

1. Definition of reasonable and necessary
2. Proper medical documentation
3. Corporate integrity (Stark Laws, Anti-Kickback Statute)
4. Federal sentencing guidelines
5. Record retention
6. Overpayments

A health care organization's P&P manual should be easily accessible to review the standards and protocol for these issues.

Compliance Program Oversight

All health care organizations should have a compliance officer. The compliance officer is the key individual who oversees the organization's compliance program monitoring. In smaller health care organizations, compliance may be directed solely by the compliance officer. However, in larger organizations, there may be an officer and a compliance team or committee. The number of members on the compliance committee is not important; it is important to have a well-rounded committee drawing on staff members from many departments including human resources, claims auditing, billing, legal, and medicine. All compliance officers should have access to a health care attorney who is well-versed in all matters of compliance.

The compliance committee acts as a review board. Committees may consist of provider-client staff and billing company staff or a combination of the provider-client, their practice manager, and the billing company staff. The committee, empowered by management, legitimizes the compliance program within the organization. In addition to possessing professional experience in claims processing and auditing, committee members are expected to use good judgment and high integrity to fulfill committee obligations. The compliance committee is tasked with developing and reviewing policies and procedures, training staff, and auditing and enforcing disciplinary standards.

Training and Education

Significant elements of an effective compliance program involve proper education and training of staff. Every employee and individual who interacts with the health care organization may be accountable for potential misconduct and should be considered in the organization's training sessions.

General compliance training sessions should be required at least annually. For staff members involved in coding and billing, a separate training session should be held to cover internal procedures, federal and state laws regarding fraud and abuse, and specific government and other payer reimbursement policies. Periodic professional courses in continuing education should be available to staff members as well as health care providers. Coding and billing personnel should receive continual

training to remain updated on diagnostic and procedural codes for each year.

Effective training can reduce potential errors, penalties, and fines. An educated staff makes fewer errors and reduces the organization's risks.

Open Lines of Communication

Effective lines of communication provide a channel for employees to report suspected or known misconduct without immediately reporting to an external agency. In this way, the health care organization can resolve issues internally. Open door policies ensure an environment in which staff members feel secure to ask about the organization's existing P&P and to report questionable activities. Each employee should know the steps to take in reporting any suspicious business activity.

All health care employees should understand the organization's procedure for reporting misconduct. It is important that employees follow these guidelines to protect their reputation and credibility within the workplace. Depending on the size of the practice, the methods for contacting managerial staff may include anonymous telephone calls through a hotline or written report forms.

Auditing, Monitoring, and Disclosure

A comprehensive auditing and monitoring program will not eliminate misconduct within an organization. It will, however, minimize the risk of fraud and abuse by identifying the risk areas. The compliance officer, with the committee's assistance, should identify problem areas and have established auditing priorities and procedures as part of the organization's compliance program.

Auditing provides a systematic and objective review of a transaction. Auditing is best handled by an objective party and should provide details of errors and recommendations for improvement. Monitoring is not as structured as an audit. It is more of a spot check for quality control. It is a continuous process and should be done on a regular basis to ensure the recommendations of auditors are being followed. Monitoring is also helpful in identifying areas that may require a more thorough formal audit. To determine areas that should be audited and monitored, a compliance committee should consider issues that have been reported to them. The OIG *Work Plan* is also a good place to start.

Special attention should be paid to the risk areas associated with submission and processing claims. Also, a thorough review of the organization's standards and written P&P should be conducted to ensure proper guidelines for complying with state and federal laws and insurance payer requirements.

A compliance program should yield an internal reporting of audit results. These are key to continued education within a health care organization. An audit will not necessarily yield errors. Positive feedback is equally important to staff and providers.

If compliance issues are uncovered during an audit, the health care organization should consider self-disclosure. The FCA allows for reduced damages should the violating person or organization furnish information on the violation within

30 days of discovery. To qualify under the self-disclosure guidelines, an organization needs to conduct a thorough investigation and take corrective action to terminate any improper conduct.

Consistent Discipline

Every health care organization is made up of people, and people make mistakes. For this reason, health care organizations must have established disciplinary guidelines. These must be made well known to employees and other agents who contract with the organization. Employees all want to know what will happen if mistakes are made and what progressive forms of discipline await in situations involving misconduct. Disciplinary standards include the following:

- Verbal warning
- Written warning
- Written reprimand
- Suspension or probation
- Demotion
- Termination of employment
- Restitution of any damages
- Referral to federal agencies for criminal prosecution

Whether the misconduct was intentional or negligent, all levels of employees need to know what is expected of them. The health care organization must publish this information and distribute it to all employees.

When faced with the discovery of an offense or an error, inaction may be interpreted as indifference. This could jeopardize the reputation of the health care organization. The health care organization should have a process for investigating problems and taking necessary corrective action.

Corrective Action

A corrective action plan is a method to address detected offenses. Corrective action plans may include any of the above disciplinary actions as well as appropriate education and training to ensure the errors do not occur again.

Some issues that raise concern include the following:
- Significant changes in claims that are rejected
- Software edits that show a pattern of misuse of codes or fees
- An unusually high volume of charges, payments, or rejections
- Notices from insurance payers regarding claims submitted by the organization

Health care staff members should be encouraged to report concerns for any suspected or known misconduct, with an established chain of command to do so. Some incidences of misconduct may violate criminal, civil, or administrative law. If the situation warrants it, the compliance officer should report the misconduct promptly to the appropriate government authority.

Fraud and abuse should be reported. Contact the DHHS OIG as follows:
- Telephone hotline: 1-800-HHS-TIPS (1-800-447-8477)
- TTY: 1-800-377-4950
- Website: https://oig.hhs.gov/fraud/report-fraud/index.asp

Please note: Suspected fraud and abuse can no longer report fraud to the OIG via e-mail.

3.6 QUICK REVIEW
Question: What are the seven basic components of a compliance plan?

OIG COMPLIANCE PROGRAM GUIDELINES

The Office of the Inspector General has issued compliance program guidelines for various types of health care organizations. These are published in the *Federal Register*. Each outlines steps for creating an effective program, as well as addressing specific risk areas that each type of health care organization will want to focus on.

Individual and Small Group Physician Practices

All providers have a responsibility to make sure that claims submitted for their services are accurate. An effective compliance program will assist a physician practice in achieving this goal. A compliance program should complement patient care. The OIG outlines four specific areas of potential risk for providers and small group practices. The guidelines can be read in their entirety in the *Federal Register*, Vol. 65, No. 194, October 5, 2000.

Coding and Billing

Coding and billing are some of the main areas of fraud investigations for small groups. Attention should be paid to proper health record documentation requirements and using appropriate diagnosis codes to reflect the need for services.

Specific risk areas identified by OIG include the following:
- Billing for items or services not rendered or not provided as claimed
- Submitting claims for equipment, medical supplies, and services that are not reasonable and necessary
- Double billing resulting in duplicate payment
- Billing for noncovered services as though covered
- Known misuse of provider identification numbers, which results in improper billing
- Unbundling, as in billing for each component of the service instead of billing or using an all-inclusive code
- Failure to use coding modifiers properly
- Clustering: reporting one level of service for all patient encounters, regardless of the patient's presenting problem or the amount of work or time spent with the patient
- Upcoding the level of service provided: reporting a higher level of service for patient encounters, regardless of the patient's presenting problem or the amount of work or time spent with the patient
- Undercoding a service provided: reporting a lower level of service for patient encounters or submitting false representation of service provided

Reasonable and Necessary Services

Although the OIG does not want to dictate proper patient care, it does look at medical necessity in determining if treatment is appropriate. Medical necessity refers to the activities that are reasonable and appropriate based on the accepted clinical standard of care. Most insurance carriers will deny payment if they feel the service is not reasonable for the given medical condition. Documentation in the health record should support all clinical decisions.

Payment for services may be delayed, downcoded, or denied if the medical necessity of a treatment is questioned. As a rule, medical necessity is a criterion used by insurance companies, as well as federal programs such as Medicare, when making decisions to limit or deny payment. Some health care organizations use electronic medical necessity software that verifies that the medical services or procedures are justified by the patient's symptoms and diagnosis. Medical treatment must be done in accordance with standards of good medical practice and the proper level of care provided in the most appropriate setting. However, insurers differ on this definition and may or may not cover the services depending on the benefits of the plan.

Documentation

The OIG expects every provider to have timely, accurate, and complete documentation for each patient. The health record may be used to validate the appropriateness of treatment among other things. It must be legible and complete. If an encounter or treatment is not documented, it did not happen in the eyes of the insurance carrier.

Improper Inducements, Kickbacks, and Self-Referrals

All providers should be aware of the federal and state laws that govern ethical practice. It is illegal to give or receive any type of remuneration for a referral. Remuneration can influence medical decision making, cause overuse of services and supplies, and increase the costs billed to government payers like Medicaid and Medicare. Specific attention should be given to the health care provider or group practice's relationship with hospitals, laboratories, pharmacies, suppliers, and vendors. Providers should also be careful not to offer any inducements to patients. They should not routinely waive copays or deductibles.

Third-Party Medical Billing Companies

The OIG recognizes that health care organizations are increasingly relying on third-party billing companies. Some billing companies also provide coding services and other practice management services. Billing companies should familiarize themselves with the compliance guidelines for the type of health care entity they service, as well as those outlined specifically for third party billing companies. It is important that they promote a culture of compliance with regard to the prevention, detection, and resolution of any questionable practices. Risk areas include coding and billing, claims submission, credit balances, and integrity of data systems. The guidelines created for third party billing companies can be read in their entirety in the *Federal Register,* Vol. 63, No. 243, December 18, 1998.

Coding

As discussed earlier in this chapter, insurance claims require reporting of codes to describe what was wrong with the patient (diagnosis codes) and what services were provided to the patient (procedural codes). This will require someone who is involved in the health care organization to assign those codes, based on what the service provider has documented. Assignment of the codes may be done by the service provider, a certified coder, or another individual working for the health care organization. In some cases, coding may be performed by the third-party medical billing company. Regardless of who is doing the coding, they should be knowledgeable and continually hone their skills in this area. In addition to the coding and billing items listed in the individual and small group practices risk section, billing companies that offer coding services should also be aware of the following issues:

- Internal coding practices, including software and coding edits, should be reviewed to ensure they follow federal guidelines.
- Assumption coding should be avoided. A service or diagnosis should not be coded if the documentation does not support it.
- Documentation may be the service provider's responsibility, but coders should be aware of what is required for proper documentation and assist in educating the provider when needed. If documentation is not clear, the coder should query the provider.
- Claims should never be submitted for services provided by unqualified or unlicensed clinical personnel.
- All documentation must be available at the time of coding so that codes may be assigned as accurately as possible.
- Billing companies should be sure not to employ sanctioned individuals.
- Billing companies should promote the confidentiality of all medical, financial, and personal information in their possession.

> **! COMPLIANCE ALERT**
>
> Documentation is not just the responsibility of the provider. Billing specialists need to be aware of the documentation requirements as they relate to medical necessity and supporting the claims sent in for payment.

Claims Submission

Policies and procedures should ensure the following:

- Proper and timely documentation is obtained before billing.
- Claims are only submitted when documentation supports the services.
- Diagnosis coding is based solely on documentation.
- Confusing or lacking documentation is verified with the provider.
- Compensation to coding and billing specialists should not provide incentive to up-code.
- Claims will undergo a pre- and post-submission review.

Credit Balances

Credit balances occur when payments and allowances posted to a claim exceed the amount of the claim. This typically occurs when too much money has been paid by the insurance, the patient, or a combination of the two. It is the responsibility of both the health care organization and the billing company to have a system in place to accurately identify such overpayments in a timely manner. Refunds must be issued on a regular and timely basis.

Integrity of Data Systems

The health care industry relies on computer systems to transmit medical and billing information. Billing companies must have systems in place to not only back up data but also to prevent data corruption by outside sources such as hackers. The system should be checked regularly for viruses and monitored for unauthorized access and disclosures.

Hospitals

Over the last few decades, the ways in which hospitals provide and are reimbursed for services has changed. As a result, the OIG has published multiple guidelines for hospitals. The first publication was in the *Federal Register,* Vol. 63, No. 35, February 23, 1998. A supplemental guidance was published in the *Federal Register,* Vol. 70, No. 19, January 31, 2005. The OIG feels that compliance programs should lead the governing bodies of hospitals. These programs provide guidance to help them adhere to the regulatory laws of health care.

Hospitals have the same risks as those identified for other entities. They must ensure proper documentation, coding, and billing practices. They must adhere to all regulations pertaining to anti-kickbacks and self-referrals. They must be sure to properly refund credit balances. In addition to these, however, they face other risks.

DRG Upcoding

Hospitals are paid by Medicare for inpatient services through reporting of Medicare Severity Diagnosis-Related Groups (MS-DRGs), which will be discussed later in this textbook. DRG upcoding, sometimes referred to as "DRG creep," occurs when an inappropriate diagnosis and/or procedure code causes a patient's case to group to a higher-paying diagnosis-related group. This is similar to upcoding in the individual and small group physician practices.

Patient Dumping

Hospitals must avoid patient dumping. The phrase *patient dumping* was coined through the occurrence of private hospitals refusing to examine or treat the poor or uninsured in the emergency department and transferring them to public hospitals. The Emergency Medical Treatment and Labor Act (EMTALA) requires that anyone that comes to an emergency room be evaluated and stabilized regardless of their ability to pay. Uninsured patients with emergency medical conditions or in active labor cannot be turned away.

Relationships

Excessive payments for medical directorships, low rent for office space, interest-free loans, and high payments in health care organization acquisitions can all spell kickback in an OIG investigation. Health care organizations and individual providers and provider groups need to be particularly careful with contract language to avoid these illegal inducements. Joint ventures and other business arrangements with suppliers, providers, or health care organizations who are in a position to refer business to the hospital should be entered with care.

Cost Reports

CMS requires institutional health care providers, such as hospitals, to submit annual cost reports. These contain information facility utilization data, costs and charges by cost center, and financial settlement data. False cost reports can be submitted to reflect higher operating costs. This also occurs when an institution shifts data from one area to another to show falsely inflated costs related to patient care.

Billing

When outpatient services are incorrectly billed as inpatient services, a duplicate billing can be created in the hospital's system. These types of services are reimbursed under two separate payment systems that will be discussed in detail in Chapters 18 and 19.

When a hospital bills for a discharge instead of a transfer, it commits fraud. Under Medicare guidelines, only the discharging hospital may report the full DRG. A transferring hospital must submit per diem charges instead. A per diem charge would be a "per day" charge. When hospitals discharge a patient, the patient's freedom of choice must be considered when referring them for rehabilitation, long-term care, home health care, or durable medical equipment.

Clinical Laboratory Improvement Amendments

Hospital laboratories must also comply with laboratory guidelines and other legislation such as the Clinical Laboratory Improvement Amendments (CLIA). Every diagnostic test is categorized by its level of complexity. Under CLIA every laboratory is certified to be able to run a certain level of test. The goal of CLIA is to ensure quality laboratory tests regardless of the laboratory that runs them. CLIA is overseen by the Occupational Safety and Health Administration (OSHA). There are additional OIG compliance guidelines for home health care agencies, Medicare Part C carriers, clinical laboratories, nursing facilities, research programs, ambulance suppliers, and pharmaceutical manufacturers. These can be found on the OIG site at https://oig.hhs.gov/compliance/compliance-guidance/.

 3.7   QUICK REVIEW
Question: What are some of the ways a small group practice can be noncompliant with regards to coding and billing?

 3.8   QUICK REVIEW
Question: What is patient dumping?

WHAT TO EXPECT FROM THE HEALTH CARE ORGANIZATION

Health care workers must be aware of the potential liabilities when submitting claims for payment that are deemed to be fraudulent or inappropriate by the federal or state government. The government may impose significant financial and administrative penalties when health care claims are not submitted appropriately, including criminal prosecution against the offending party. According to the OIG, fraud can result from deliberate unethical behavior or simply from mistakes and miscues that cause excessive reimbursement.

Billing specialists involved in the claims processing procedures in the health care organization should understand the importance and urgency in following the legal and ethical path when performing their duties. An honest mistake could lead to a situation that puts the health care organization at risk for investigation of fraud, waste, or abuse if it continues and is not corrected.

Although every health care organization has different policies and procedures, each should have the following:

- An expectation that all employees will adhere to all laws and guidelines that regulate and pay for health care services
- Privacy/security/compliance officer (even if one person)
- A P&P manual
- Employee training and education (at least annually and whenever there are changes in business operations that affect staff members directly)

❓ DISCUSSION POINT

Discuss how compliance plans can help deter fraud and abuse in the health care setting.

PROCEDURE 3.1 Research Items on the OIG website and in the *Federal Register*

Follow these steps and answer the accompanying questions.
1. Go to the OIG website (https://oig.hhs.gov/).
2. Go to the "About Us" tab.
   - How many different offices are part of the OIG?
   - Which office do you think would be responsible for investigating fraud in health care?
3. Go to the "Reports" tab.
   - How often is the Work Plan updated?
   - What are some of the focuses of the most recent Work Plan?
4. Go to the "Fraud" tab.
   - Find and read some of the more recent cases of Medicare fraud.
5. Go to the "Compliance" tab.
   - Find the guidelines for compliance programs for Nursing Facilities.
   - What are some of the areas of concern regarding quality of care?
6. Go to the "Exclusions" tab.
   - Under "Background Information," what is the difference between mandatory and permissive exclusions.
   - Under FAQs, how does an excluded individual get reinstated?
7. Go back to the "Reports" tab and go to the *Federal Register*.
   - Click on the most recent report.
   - Click the search function at the top of the page and search "civil monetary penalties inflation."
   - Go to the most recent document about CMP inflation adjustments.
   - What are some of the examples of health care fraud listed in this document?
   - What are the monetary penalties for committing these acts of fraud?
8. Be prepared to share your findings in a class discussion.

KEY POINTS

This is a brief chapter review of the key issues presented. To further enhance your knowledge of the technical subject matter, review the key terms and key abbreviations for this chapter by locating the meaning for each in the Glossary at the end of this text, which appears in a section before the Index.

1. The difference between fraud and abuse is that fraud occurs when deception is used in a claim submission to obtain payment from the payer. Individuals who knowingly, willfully, and intentionally submit false information to benefit themselves or others commit fraud. Abuse means incidents or practices by health care organizations, not usually considered fraudulent, that are inconsistent with accepted sound medical business or fiscal practices.
2. The Centers for Medicare and Medicaid Services, the Office of the Inspector General, and various other regulatory agencies oversee and investigate health care fraud and abuse.
3. The False Claims Act (1863) is the baseline legislation for health care fraud today.
4. Qui tam or whistleblower lawsuits are those in which an individual files a claim on behalf of the federal government. The whistleblower shares in any recovered funds.
5. Stark laws prohibit the submission of claims for services or referral of patients if the referring provider has a financial relationship with the entity who provides the service.
6. The Anti-Kickback Statute prohibits any type of gift, reward, or inducement for referrals.
7. RACs, ZPICs, MIPs, CERT, and HEAT are various types of audits aimed at recovering monies for government payers who have been fraudulently billed.
8. A compliance program is a set of policies, procedures, and guidelines designed to ensure that an organization conducts business in accordance with laws and regulations.
9. An effective compliance program has seven steps: written policies and procedures; program oversight; training and education; open lines of communication; auditing, monitoring and disclosure; consistent discipline; and corrective actions.
10. The OIG has published several compliance program guidelines for various types of health care organizations.

INTERNET RESOURCES

Office of the Inspector General
- https://oig.hhs.gov/

OIG Exclusion Program
- https://oig.hhs.gov/faqs/exclusions-faq.asp

OIG Enforcement
- https://oig.hhs.gov/fraud/enforcement/criminal/

OIG Workplan
- https://oig.hhs.gov/reports-and-publications/workplan/index.asp

OIG Compliance Guidance
- https://oig.hhs.gov/compliance/compliance-guidance/index.asp

OIG Fraud Reporting
- https://oig.hhs.gov/fraud/report-fraud/index.asp

Federal Register Civil Monetary Penalties
- https://www.govinfo.gov/content/pkg/FR-2020-01-17/pdf/2020-00738.pdf

Department of Justice
- https://www.justice.gov/briefing-room

AAPC Code of Ethics
- https://www.aapc.com/aboutus/code-of-ethics.aspx

AHIMA Code of Ethics
- https://bok.ahima.org/doc?oid=105098#.Xqm77CN_OUk

STUDENT ASSIGNMENT

- Study Chapter 3.
- Complete all exercises *Workbook* to reinforce the theory learned in this chapter.
- Turn to the Glossary at the end of this text for a further understanding of the key terms and key abbreviations used in this chapter.

PART 2

Introduction to Health Insurance

4

Basics of Health Insurance

Cheryl Fassett

OBJECTIVES

After reading this chapter, you should be able to:

1. Describe the history of insurance in the United States.
2. Explain the reasons for the rising cost of health care.
3. Discuss how the Affordable Care Act reforms health care.
4. Discuss the legal principles of insurance and state the four concepts of a valid insurance contract.
5. Explain the difference between an implied and an expressed health care organization patient contract and discuss different types of patients.
6. Discuss how insurance works and define common insurance terms.
7. List and describe the choices a person has when it comes to choosing and obtaining health insurance.
8. Describe the types of health insurance coverage, including federal, state, and private health insurance plans.
9. Explain the life cycle of an insurance claim from date of service to third-party payer processing and payment.
10. List the types of computerized signatures for documents and insurance claims.
11. Describe the proper information to post to the patient's financial account after claims submission and payment received.

KEY TERMS

accounts receivable management
Affordable Care Act
assignment
birthday rule
blanket contract
cancelable
capitation
claim
coinsurance
conditionally renewable
consumer directed health plan
contract
conversion privilege
coordination of benefits
copayment
cost share/cost sharing
daysheet
deductible
dependent
disability income insurance
electronic signature
emancipated minor
encounter form
exclusions
exclusive provider organization
expressed contract
fee-for-service

flexible spending account
group health insurance plan
guaranteed renewable
guarantor
Health Benefit Exchanges
Health Care and Education
    Reconciliation Act
health insurance
health maintenance organization
health reimbursement account
health savings account
implied contract
indemnity health insurance
independent or individual practice
    association
institutional provider
insured
life cycle of a claim
major medical
mandated benefits
Maternal and Child Health Program
Medicaid
medical savings account
medically necessary
Medicare
Medicare/Medicaid
noncancelable policy

noncovered services
nonparticipating provider
optionally renewable
participating physician or provider
Patient Protection and Affordable
    Care Act
physician's representative
point-of-service plan
preauthorization
precertification
predetermination
preexisting conditions
preferred provider organization
premium
revenue cycle
self-funded health plans
self-pay
State Children's Health Insurance
    Program
state disability insurance
third-party payers
TRICARE
Unemployment Compensation
    Disability
Veterans Health Administration
    (CHAMPVA)
workers' compensation insurance

KEY ABBREVIATIONS

ACA	FSA	Medi-Medi	SCHIP
A/R	HCERA	MSA nonpar	SDHP
CDHP	HDHP	NPP par	SDI
CHAMPVA	HMO	PMS	SHOP
COB	HRA	POS plan	SOF
COBRA copay	HSA	PPACA	UCD
DOS	IPA	PPO	VA
EPO	MCHP	ROA	WC

👤 INSIGHTS FROM THE FIELD

Christina S.: Certified Professional Coder (CPC) and Certified Professional Medical Auditor (CPMCA)

I have worked in the health care field for about 19 years. I started in health information management and then moved into medical billing and coding. I am currently a coding compliance educator. I provide education to coders and providers in an effort to improve documentation. I also assist with coding and billing inquiries and developing educational materials. I think one of the most important skills a billing specialist can have is to understand how to navigate around the insurance carrier websites, such as Medicare and Medicaid. It's important to know which providers participate with which carriers and to stay current with their policies.

HISTORY OF HEALTH INSURANCE IN THE UNITED STATES

Health insurance is an agreement between a policyholder and a third-party payer or government program. It reimburses the policyholder for all or a portion of the cost of medical and/or preventive care based on the insurance policy purchased. Its main purpose is to help offset some of the high costs accrued during illness or when an injury occurs. A third-party payer is an entity, such as an insurance company, governmental agency, or employer, that reimburses health care expenses.

To understand the current health care system, a billing specialist needs to understand the history of health care in the United States. The current health care system did not always exist.

Health care insurance originated in the mid-1800s in the United States with the Franklin Health Assurance Company of Massachusetts. It offered coverage for nonfatal injuries in railroad and steamboat accidents. About 10 years later, the Travelers Insurance Company of Hartford marketed a plan that was similar to today's health insurance. In 1911, Montgomery Ward and Company offered benefits to its ill or injured employees. These commercial plans paid only for lost wages when an individual was sick or received an injury. This was the first group plan.

Only large employers offered health insurance to their employees before 1920. As doctors learned more about diseases and effective treatments and more people took advantage of new medical technology, the cost for health care increased.

To help ease the burden of health care costs, Baylor Hospital in Dallas created a system, which eventually became known as Blue Cross, to help people pay their hospital bills. Its counterpart, Blue Shield, started gaining recognition in the late 1930s as a way for doctors to secure payment for health care services. By the 1960s, the success of the Blue Cross and Blue Shield models encouraged other insurers to enter the health care market.

The shortage of labor during World War II also had an impact on the health care market. Employers began to offer health insurance as an added benefit to the employment package. Soon, it was commonplace for employers to provide health insurance. Most private insurance companies sold policies that included hospital care, surgical fees, and health care organizations' services. In addition to those benefits, many plans began offering catastrophic coverage, preventive care, dental insurance, disability income insurance, and long-term or home health care insurance for the chronically ill, physically disabled, and developmentally disabled.

In 1965, federal legislation was passed to assist the elderly and the poor with their health insurance expenses. This led to the government health care programs known as Medicare and Medicaid. Although both programs started small, expenditures in these programs grew dramatically. They currently make up a large percentage of all health care expenses in the United States.

As additional benefits were offered by insurance carriers and the public used more health care services, medical costs and premium rates that were paid for the coverage increased. Developing technologies also played a role. An increase in the aging population with more advanced health care needs has pushed health care spending even higher.

To deal with the rising costs of health care, the federal government adopted cost-containment legislation for government programs such as Medicare and Medicaid. The concept of managed care began in the 1930s, when Kaiser Industries developed a prepaid, integrated health care insurance model for its employees. In the 1980s, insurance carriers began to see the benefits of managed care. Managed care insurance carriers are more involved in health care decisions, such as how much care a patient will receive and who will provide it. This was recognized as a method to help control rising health care expenditures. As a result, many new types of insurance plans arose to control the cost of medical care and to help those who could not afford insurance.

HEALTH CARE REFORM

Over the past 75 years, leaders of the United States, from President Franklin D. Roosevelt to President Donald Trump, have announced reforms of the health care system. A major restructuring of the United States health care system was necessary during the 1990s for the following reasons:

- A growing percentage of Americans were not covered by private or government insurance.
- Employers had to pay rising health care premiums and did not want to cut wages to cover these costs.
- Government needed to reduce the deficit by controlling increases in the Medicare and Medicaid programs.
- Health care providers and hospital costs soared due to inflation, high-tech equipment, expensive medications, and so on.
- The health care system was riddled with inefficiency and fraud.
- Patients overused health care services.

On March 23, 2010, under President Barack Obama, the Patient Protection and Affordable Care Act (PPACA) was signed into law. The related Health Care and Education Reconciliation Act (HCERA), which modifies certain provisions of PPACA, was signed into law on March 30, 2010. These two laws together are commonly referred to as the Affordable Care Act (ACA) or Obamacare. The ACA brought sweeping health insurance reforms. It holds insurance companies accountable, lowers costs, guarantees choice, and enhances the quality of health care for all Americans. Implementation of the ACA began in 2010 and was to be concluded by 2020 (Table 4.1).

The goal of the ACA was to make health care available and affordable for the 32 million Americans who did not have health insurance. The plan expects to provide coverage to 94% of Americans. The ACA provides tax cuts for the middle class and aims to reduce premiums for families and small businesses.

Individual Mandate

The ACA included an individual mandate, which required most Americans to have health insurance coverage or face a penalty. Because of this, the constitutionality of the Act was challenged in March 2012. On June 28, 2012, the Supreme Court of the United States upheld the PPACA in its entirety.

As a result of this mandate, if an individual did not have health insurance, they paid a tax penalty of $95 per individual or 1% of taxable income, whichever is greater, for 2014. In 2015, the fine rose to $325 per individual or 2% of taxable income, and 2016 saw an increase to $695 per individual or 2.5% of income. For every year after 2016, the government refigured the fine based on a cost-of-living adjustment.

This federal mandate was later eliminated in 2019 under President Trump. However, some state penalties continued to remain in effect. For example, by 2020, New Jersey, Massachusetts, Vermont, and the District of Columbia had instituted state penalties for failing to have health insurance.

Health Benefit Exchanges

A primary goal of the ACA was to make health care cheaper and easier to access for the uninsured population. To address this, a key provision of the ACA insurance reform was the creation of Health Benefit Exchanges (or Exchanges). An Exchange is an organized marketplace where uninsured individuals and small business owners can find all the qualified private health plans available in their area. Exchanges were created to lower health care costs by creating a competitive regional private insurance market. Exchanges are administered by the Department of Health and Human Services (DHHS) and Centers for Medicaid and Medicare Services (CMS), along with nonprofit organizations. Small Business Health Options Program (SHOP) Exchanges serve a similar function for small employers and the self-employed. The Exchanges first opened on January 1, 2014.

The Exchanges offer a central site for researching, comparing, and purchasing health insurance coverage. They make the process of finding a health insurance policy easier and more efficient. Exchanges create larger individual and small employer insurance pools. In doing this, they provide individuals and small employers with access to the policies that were written using the ACA's uniform set of national rules.

Individuals and small businesses of up to 100 employees can purchase qualified coverage through exchanges and take advantage of federal subsidies. States allowed businesses with more than 100 employees to purchase coverage in the SHOP Exchange beginning in 2017. Through establishment of the Exchanges, millions of Americans and small businesses have access to more choices of affordable coverage. By holding insurance companies accountable to keep premiums down and prevent insurance industry abuses, the ACA will end discrimination against Americans with preexisting conditions.

The Future of the Affordable Care Act

As discussed, the ACA has affected health care in many positive ways. However, as with any act of legislation, there have been people who opposed the ACA from the start. Some have argued that the government should not be allowed to force people to buy insurance. Some feel that the health plans that are offered on the Exchanges and through employers are not actually "affordable." Since being passed, there have been efforts to repeal or replace the ACA. Currently, the future of it is unclear.

 4.1 QUICK REVIEW

Question: What were some of the reasons the ACA was passed? What were the intended goals?

LEGAL PRINCIPLES OF INSURANCE

The role of a medical insurance billing specialist is to complete the insurance claim accurately, assist in claims submission, and obtain accurate and timely reimbursement. An insurance claim, also called an encounter record, is a bill sent to an insurance carrier requesting payment for services rendered. However, before developing the skill of coding and completing insurance claim forms, it is necessary to understand how insurance works.

Legal situations occur daily in the performance of these job duties. They involve confidentiality of health records, accurate insurance claim transmission, fraud and abuse issues, credit and collection laws, and so on. A billing specialist cannot escape

TABLE 4.1 Timeline for Implementation of the Affordable Care Act From 2010 to 2020

YEAR	TIMELINE
2010	• Implementation of rules to prevent insurance companies from denying coverage to children with preexisting conditions. • Prohibits insurance companies from dropping coverage because of technical errors in insurance contracts when patients get sick. • Prohibits insurance companies from imposing lifetime dollar limits on essential benefits. • Regulates annual limits on insurance coverage. • Provides consumers with an easy way to appeal to their insurance company and to an outside board if the company denies coverage of a claim. • Creates an easy-to-use website where consumers can compare health insurance coverage options. • Tax credits to small businesses that provide insurance benefits to their workers. • Relief for seniors who hit the Medicare prescription drug "doughnut hole." • New insurance plans must cover certain preventive services without cost sharing (i.e., deductibles, copays, or coinsurance). • A prevention and public health fund to invest in proven prevention public health programs. • Further crackdown on health care fraud through new resources and screening procedures for health care organizations. • Access to insurance for uninsured Americans with preexisting conditions. • Extends coverage for young adults. • Provided coverage for early retirees. • Rebuilds the primary care workforce. • Holds insurance companies accountable for unreasonable rate hikes. • Allows states to cover more people on Medicaid through additional federal funding. • Provides payments for rural health care organizations.
2011	• Provides prescription drug discounts. • Covers free preventive care for seniors through annual wellness visits and personalized prevention plans. • Improves health care quality and efficiency. • Improves care for seniors after they leave the hospital. • Provides for new innovations to bring down costs. • Increased access to services at home and in the community. • Strengthens community health centers. • Brings down health care premiums. • Addresses overpayments to big insurance companies and strengthens Medicare Advantage.
2012	• Links payment to quality outcomes. • Encourages integrated health systems through Accountable Care Organizations. • Reduces paperwork and administrative costs by implementation of electronic health records. • Helps understand and fight health disparities through collection of racial, ethnic, and language data. • Provides new voluntary options for long-term care insurance.
2013	• Improves preventive health coverage through additional funding to state Medicaid programs. • Expands authority to bundle payments and pay health care organizations at a flat rate for an episode of care. • Increases Medicaid payments for primary care doctors. • Provides additional funding for the State Children's Health Insurance Program.
2014	• Eliminates discrimination as a result of preexisting conditions or gender. • Eliminates annual limits on insurance coverage. • Ensures coverage for individuals participating in clinical trials. • Makes care more affordable. • Establishes Health Insurance Exchanges. • Creates small business tax credits. • Increases access to Medicaid. • Promotes individual responsibility. • Ensures free choice through establishment of health insurance exchanges.
2015	• Pays health care organizations based on value, not volume. Health care organizations receive higher payments based on the quality of care they provide. • Annual health insurance industry fees will be imposed on health insurance companies to fund some of the provisions of the Affordable Care Act. The fees continue to increase yearly until 2018.
2016	• States will be permitted to form health care choice compacts and allow insurers to sell policies in any state participating in the compact. • Reduces Medicare payments to certain hospitals for hospital-acquired conditions by 1%.
2018	• Provides for a 40% excise tax to be imposed on high-cost group health plans.
2020	• Eliminates Medicare Part D (doughnut hole) coverage gap.

Data from https://obamacarefacts.com/health-care-reform-timeline.

liability by pleading ignorance. It cannot be overemphasized that keeping up to date on health care plan policies and procedures is essential. Most legal issues pertaining to private health insurance claims fall under state or civil law, whereas issues with government programs fall under federal laws.

Insurance Contracts

The first concept with which a billing specialist needs to be familiar is the insurance contract or policy. A contract is a legal and binding written document that exists between two or more parties. Essentially, any agreement between two or more persons that is enforceable by law is considered a contract. There is no standard health insurance contract. Individuals who take out a policy receive an original document composed by the insurance company.

The following four items are part of a valid insurance contract:
1. The person must be a mentally competent adult and not under the influence of drugs or alcohol when signing the contract.
2. The insurance company must offer an individual health insurance coverage and the individual must accept the offer.
3. An exchange of value (the first premium payment) submitted with the application, known as a *consideration,* must be present.
4. A legal purpose, which is an insurable interest in the case of a health insurance policy, must exist.. This means that the policyholder expects to continue in good health, but the insurance policy will provide something of value if an accident or illness strikes.

A policy can be challenged and coverage may not be in effect if the purchaser of the insurance policy or subscriber makes a fraudulent statement. After a policy has been in force for 2 years (3 years in some states), it may not be challenged.

Implied or Expressed Contracts

A health care organization and its staff must be aware of the health care organization's obligations to each patient and liabilities regarding service, as well as the patient's responsibilities to the health care organization. The health care organization patient contract begins when the health care organization accepts the patient and agrees to treat him or her. An implied contract is created by the actions of the parties involved. It is not written or spoken. For example, if Mary Johnson goes to Dr. Doe's office and Dr. Doe provides a medical service to her, this is an implied contract. If the patient is unconscious when treatment is rendered, treatment is based on an implied-in-fact contract. An expressed contract can be verbal or written.

Self-Pay Patients

For patients who do not have health insurance, the contract for treatment is between the health care organization and the patient. The patient is liable for the entire bill and is considered a self-pay patient.

Guarantor

A guarantor is a person who accepts treatment or signs a form agreeing to pay. When a patient presents to a health care facility or provider for care, it is an implied contract. However, most

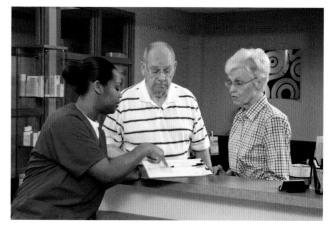

Fig. 4.1 Receptionist explaining where a guarantor's signature goes on a patient registration form for the medical services.

health care organizations have the guarantor sign a form to help in their collection strategies. This creates an expressed contract (Fig. 4.1). Usually, a patient of legal age (18 or 21, depending on state law) is their own guarantor. In the case of a minor child, the parent who presents the child for care at the time of the initial visit is considered the guarantor. If the patient is a child of a divorced parent, the custodial parent bears the responsibility of the child's medical expenses unless the divorce decree states otherwise. An adoptive parent may be the custodial parent or guarantor and therefore solely liable for the child's bill.

Emancipated Minor

An emancipated minor is a person younger than 18 years of age who:
- Lives independently,
- Is totally self-supporting,
- Is married or divorced,
- Is a parent even if not married,
- Is in the military and possesses decision-making rights, or
- Is a college student living away from home, even when financially dependent on parents.

Parents are not liable for the medical expenses incurred by an emancipated minor. The patient record should contain the minor's signed statement that he or she is emancipated.

Employment and Disability Examinations

When an employer requests an examination for employment or an insurance company requests an examination for a disability claim, the health care organization's contract is with the insurance carrier or employer that requests the exam, not the patient. An employer may request a medical exam for a new employee to show they are physically able to perform a job duty or for an existing employee who is requesting some sort of work accommodation for a disability.

Workers' Compensation Patients

Workers' compensation (WC) cases involve a person being injured on the job. These cases may be referred to as industrial accidents or illnesses. In these types of cases, the contract exists between the health care organization and the insurance company. When there is a dispute as to whether the injured party was hurt at work, a Patient Agreement form must be signed by the patient, who agrees to pay the health care organization's fees if the case is declared to be non–work related.

🖋 4.2 QUICK REVIEW

Question: If there is no insurance policy, who is responsible for paying medical services?

THE INSURANCE POLICY

Insurance policies are complex and contain a great deal of language that is difficult to understand. Most health insurance coverage includes benefits for hospital, surgical, and other medical expenses such as preventive services, physical therapy, prescriptions, and lab tests.

Major medical benefits contracts are designed to offset large medical expenses caused by prolonged illness or serious injury. Some of these policies include coverage for extended care or skilled nursing health care organization benefits. While premiums are cheaper than other forms of health insurance, these plans do not cover any preventive or minor health issues.

In a health insurance policy, the insured is known as a subscriber, member, policyholder, or recipient and may not necessarily be the patient seen for the medical service. The insured is the individual or organization protected in case of loss under the terms of an insurance policy.

A policy might also include dependents of the insured. Generally, this term refers to the spouse and children of the insured, but under some contracts, parents, other family members, and domestic partners may be covered as dependents. Under the ACA, health plans must allow employees to keep their children on their plans until age 26.

Policy Application

Before a policy is issued, the insurance company decides whether it will enter into a contract with the applicant. Information is obtained about the applicant so that the company can decide whether to accept the risk. Generally, the application form has two sections: The first part contains basic information about the application, and the second part concerns the health of the individual.

An insurance policy is a legally enforceable agreement. If a policy is issued, the applicant becomes part of the insurance plan. The policy becomes effective only after the insurance company offers the policy and the person accepts it and then pays the initial premium. If a premium is paid at the time the application is submitted, the insurance coverage can be put into force before the policy is delivered. Depending on the laws in some states, the applicant also can have temporary conditional insurance if the agent issues a specific type of receipt.

Policy Renewal Provisions

Health insurance policies may have renewal provisions that state the circumstances under which the company may refuse to renew, may cancel coverage, or may increase the premium. It is important for the insurance billing specialist to understand that a patient's coverage may change from appointment to appointment. It is always a good routine to verify insurance information each time the patient comes in for an appointment. A billing specialist may check eligibility verification to see if the patient is a member of the insurance plan and that the member identification number is correct. This may seem redundant, but it avoids a delay in payment.

In private health insurance, there are five classifications of renewal provisions:

1. A cancelable policy grants the insurer the right to cancel the policy at any time and for any reason. The insurance company notifies the insured that the policy is canceled and refunds any advance premium the policyholder has paid. In some states, this type of policy is illegal.
2. In an optionally renewable policy, the insurer has the right to terminate coverage on the premium or anniversary date. The insurer may not cancel the policy at any time in between.
3. Conditionally renewable policies grant the insurance company a limited right to refuse to renew a health insurance policy at the end of a premium payment period. Reasons stated in the policy may relate to age, employment status, or both, but may not relate to the insured's health status.
4. The guaranteed renewable classification is desirable because the insurer is required to renew the policy as long as premium payments are made. However, these policies often have age limits.
5. In a noncancelable policy, the insurer cannot increase premium rates and must renew the policy until the insured reaches the age specified in the contract. Some disability income policies have noncancelable terms.

Policy Terms

To keep the insurance in force, a person must pay a monthly, quarterly, or annual fee called a premium. If the premium is not paid, a grace period of 10 to 30 days is usually given before insurance coverage ceases.

Most policies have a deductible, which is a specific amount of money that must be paid each year before the policy benefits begin. Generally, the higher the deductible, the lower the cost of the policy. Most policies also have a cost-sharing requirement. This means that the insured will assume a percentage of the fee, called coinsurance (e.g., 20%), or pay a specific dollar amount, called a copayment or copay (e.g., $5 or $10), for covered services.

Routinely waiving deductibles and copayments is fraudulent because, by agreeing to participate with an insurance, the health care organization has agreed to accept a patient portion. Generally, deductibles, coinsurance, and copayments should be collected at the time of service. The Medicare program is an exception to this rule. It does not recommend collecting the deductible in advance from the beneficiary.

A provider may consider writing off a portion of the amount owed by the patient in cases of financial hardship. It is good practice to get a patient's request for this consideration in writing. Additional documentation should be kept on file to prove the patient's financial status.

Generally, it is the patient's responsibility to give a written notice of a claim to the insurance company within a certain time limit. However, some insurance carriers require that the provider of service be obligated to submit the claim. Usually as a courtesy, the claim is filed for the patient by the health care organization.

The insurance billing specialist must be able to abstract proper information from the patient record, which is used to code the diagnoses and services rendered, to complete an insurance claim form, to make entries to a patient's financial accounting record, and to follow up on unpaid claims. If any one of these procedures is not done properly, the third-party payer may not pay the claim correctly. Following up on unpaid claims is done by contacting the claims representative, called a claims adjudicator or an adjuster.

Coordination of Benefits

A coordination of benefits (COB) statement is included in most policies and contracts with health care organizations. When the patient has more than one insurance policy, insurance companies must coordinate the reimbursement of benefits to determine which carrier is going to be the primary payer and which carrier is the secondary payer. This prevents the duplication or overlapping of payments for the same medical expense. The combination of payments from the primary and secondary carriers cannot be more than the amount of the health care organization's charges (Example 4.1).

Carriers may pend or delay a claim, stating that they are attempting to coordinate benefits with the other carrier. This process can be time-consuming and may take 90 days or more to resolve. A billing specialist should be diligent in following up on this situation so that the stalled cash flow issue can be resolved. In some situations, the patient ultimately may be responsible for the bill. If the patient understands this, they will pay sooner and resolve the account balance quicker.

Birthday Rule

The birthday rule is an informal rule that the health insurance industry has widely adopted for the COBs when children are listed as dependents on two parents' health plans. Under the birthday rule, the health plan of the parent whose birthday comes first in the calendar year is designated as the primary plan. This applies to the month and day only, not the year of birth. If both mother and father have the same birthday, the plan of the person who has had coverage longer is the primary payer.

EXAMPLE 4.1   Coordination of Benefits for Dual Coverage Case

Mr. Smith has Insurance A and Insurance B. The claim is for $100. The claim is sent to Insurance A. Insurance A allows $80 for the procedure and pays $80. The claim is then sent to Insurance B. Insurance B also allows $80 for the procedure. The claim that was sent to Insurance B was not for $100 but for the remaining $20. The $20 is within the amount allowed by Insurance B, therefore, Insurance B pays the $20. Some carriers try to play by their own rules by stating that because Insurance A paid $80 and the $80 equals the amount Insurance B pays, Insurance B will pay no more for the claim. These rules were established by the National Association of Insurance Commissioners and approved by every state insurance commissioner. Be observant of insurance claims like this.

According to the National Association of Insurance Commissioners, the birthday rule is not insurance law. Some insurance plans do not follow these customs, and it may be necessary to contact the plan for confirmation.

In cases of divorce, remember it is not the health care organization's responsibility to enforce family court laws. The divorce decree is between the parents of the child. Have the parent accompanying the child pay the bill at the time of service. The responsible party can reimburse them. If a copy of the court decision is presented, bill the insurance of the parent deemed responsible.

General Policy Limitations

Health insurance policies may contain exclusions or limitations of the policy. Exclusions are services that are never covered by the health insurance policy. These noncovered services are outlined in the insurance policy. A noncovered service is one that is not considered medically reasonable for the patient's diagnosed condition. For example, if a patient has a straightforward case of bronchitis, a magnetic resonance imaging scan (MRI) may not be considered medically necessary when a simple chest x-ray would be sufficient to diagnose the condition and rule out pneumonia. A noncovered service may also refer to any benefits that are not covered within the guidelines of the patient's insurance policy. For example, a patient may need eyeglasses, but it may not be a covered benefit on their policy. Examples of noncovered services may include items such as acupuncture, eyeglasses, contact lenses, dental treatment surgery, services related to sex transformations, and cosmetic and aesthetic treatments. Most insurance policies also have limitations for covered services that are not deemed medically necessary.

"Medically necessary" is defined as accepted health care services and supplies that are appropriate for the evaluation and treatment of an injury, illness, or disease and its symptoms. The concept of medical necessity is based on the accepted standards of care. For example, a patient may request to have a test for a vitamin deficiency performed because they read an article and think they may have it. However, the insurance may not pay for the service unless the patient presents with bone pain, muscle weakness, mood changes, or other signs or symptoms that may indicate medical necessity for the procedure to be performed.

In the past, insurance companies issued policies that did not provide benefits for conditions that existed and were treated before the policy was issued. These are called preexisting conditions. The ACA prohibited insurers from denying coverage or charging higher premiums to any person with preexisting conditions.

Mandated benefits are state and/or federal laws that require coverage for treatment of specific health conditions for some categories of dependents, such as children placed for adoption. Health care benefits may be mandated by state law, federal law, or, in some cases, both. For example, under the Newborns' and Mothers' Health Protection Act (NMHPA) of 1996, health plans may not limit benefits for any length of hospital stay related to childbirth for the mother or newborn child. Additionally, there is a federal mandate that requires health plans to provide someone who is receiving benefits related to a mastectomy with coverage for reconstruction of the breast. The Americans with

Disabilities Act (ADA) requires insurance companies to provide the same benefits to disabled and nondisabled individuals regarding premiums, deductibles, and limits on coverage.

Case Management Requirements

Many private third-party payers have certain requirements that must be met before they approve hospital admissions, inpatient or outpatient surgeries, and elective procedures. First, eligibility requirements must be obtained. These are conditions that must be met before the patient receives benefits under a specific insurance plan or government program. The carrier can refuse to pay part of or the entire fee if these requirements are not met.

Precertification refers to discovering whether treatments such as surgeries, hospitalizations, or tests are covered under a patient's contract. Preauthorization relates not only to whether a service or procedure is covered but also to finding out whether it is medically necessary. Predetermination means discovering the maximum dollar amount that the carrier will pay for surgery, consulting services, radiology procedures, and so on.

A health care organization should obtain precertification or predetermination when a procedure is tentatively scheduled. The information that may be required to obtain precertification approval by fax, telephone, or online is shown in Fig. 4.2. A form similar to the one shown in Fig. 4.3 can be used

COLLEGE CLINIC
4567 Broad Avenue
Woodland Hills, XY 12345-0000

Phone: 555/486-9002   Fax: 555/590-2189

Insurance Precertification Form

Date: __5/4/XX__
To: Insurance Carrier __Cal-Net Care__   From: __Janet__ Office Mgr.
    Address __9900 Baker Street__
    __Los Angeles, CA 90067__

Check those that apply: Admission certification ✔   Outpatient ___ Inpatient ✔
                           Surgery certification ✔   Emergency situation ✔

Patient's name __Ronald Stranton__   Date of Birth: __4-14-49__
Patient's address __639 Cedar Street__   Sex: Male ✔ Female ___
__Woodland Hills, XY 12345__   Social Security No. __527-XX-7250__
Insured's Name __Same__   Policy Group ID No. __A59__
Insured's Address _____   Employer: __Aerostar Aviation__

Treating physician __Clarence Cutler, M.D.__   NPI #: __430 500 47XX__
Primary Care Physician __Gerald Practon, M.D.__ NPI #: __462 7889 7XX__

Name of Hospital __College Hospital__   Admission Date: __5/4/XX__
                                                Estimated Length of Stay: __3-5 d__
Admitting Diagnosis __Volvulus__   Diagnosis Code: __K56.2__
Complicating conditions to substantiate need for inpatient hospitalization_____
__Complete bowel obstruction__
Date current illness or injury began __5/2/XX__
Procedure/surgery to be done __Reduction of Volvulus__   Procedure code __44050__

Second opinion needed   Yes ___ No ✔ Date performed _____

Telephone precertification: __Emergency Cert. 5/4/XX__
Name of representative certifying __McKenzie Kwan__
Direct-dial telephone number of representative __1-800-463-9000 ext. 227__

Reason(s) for denial _____
Certification approved   Yes ✔ No ___ Certification approval No. __69874__
Authorization for services Yes ✔ No ___ Authorization No. __69874E__

Note: The information contained in this facsimile message is confidential and privileged information intended only for the use of the individual or entity named above. If the reader of this message is not the intended recipient, you are hereby notified that any dissemination, distribution, or copying of this communication is strictly prohibited. If you have received this communication in error, please immediately notify me by telephone and return the original facsimile to me via the U.S. Postal Service. Thank you.

Fig. 4.2 Insurance precertification form. This form can be faxed to the insurance company or used when telephoning to obtain approval for hospitalization under a patient's insurance policy or managed care plan.

COLLEGE CLINIC
4567 Broad Avenue
Woodland Hills, XY 12345-0001

Phone: 555/486-9002   Fax: 555/487-8976

INSURANCE PREDETERMINATION FORM

Perry Cardi, MD
_____Physician_____

Patient: __Leslee Austin__   Telephone # __(555) 486-8452__
Address: __209 Refugio Road__   Date of Birth __04-07-44__
City __Woodland Hills__   State __XY__   ZIP __12345-0001__
Social Security # __629-XX-9260__   Accident Yes_____ No __X__
Insurance Company __American Insurance__   Member # __Am 45692__
Insurance Co. Address __4040 Broadway Ave__   Group # ____123P____
__Valley Vista, XY 12345__   Telephone # __(555) 238-5000__
Policy holder __Leslee Austin__
Relationship to insured: Self __X__ Spouse____ Child____ Other____
Type of coverage: HMO __X__ PPO___ 80/20___ 70/30___ Other____
Procedure/Service __Cardioversion (CPT 92960)__
Diagnosis __Atrial fibrillation (ICD–10–CM 48.91)__

- -

BENEFITS:
Coverage effective date: From __02/01/XX__ To __01/31/XX__
Preexisting exclusions: __Lupus erythematosus__   Second opinion requirements: Yes ____ No __X__
Major medical   Yes __X__ No ____   Precertification/Preauthorization Yes __X__ No ____
Deductible   Yes ____ No __X__ Amount $_____   Reference # __432786__
 Per family: Yes ____ No __X__ Amount $_____   Authorized by: __Lucille Vasquez__
 Deductible paid to date: Amount $_____
Out of pocket expense limit: Amount $_____
                                       Per: _____

- -

COVERAGE: COVERAGE DETAILS AND LIMITS
 Procedures/Services
  Office visits   YES __X__   NO _____   __Physical exam; one per year__
  Consultations   YES __X__   NO _____   _____
  ER visits   YES __X__   NO _____   _____
  X-ray   YES __X__   NO _____   _____
  Laboratory   YES __X__   NO _____   __Need authorization__
  Office surgery   YES __X__   NO _____   __Need authorization__
  Hospital surgery   YES __X__   NO _____   _____
  Anesthesia   YES __X__   NO _____   __Need authorization__
  DME   YES __X__   NO _____   _____
 Physician payment schedule: RVS____ RBRVS____ UCR____ Other __X__

- -

 Payment sent to: Provider __X__ Patient ____ Time limit after submission? __30 days__
 Verification by: ____Karen Reynolds____   Date: __07-14-XX__

Fig. 4.3 Insurance predetermination form. This form can be sent to the insurance company to find out the maximum dollar amount that will be paid for primary surgery, consulting services, postoperative care, and so on.

to obtain predetermination. Preauthorization forms can also be used to document the information received when verifying the patient's insurance coverage. It should become part of the patient's record and be used for reference when billing future insurance claims.

After the information is received from the third-party payer, give the patient an estimate of fees for the proposed surgery; state how much the insurance is expected to pay, and make the patient aware of any balance amounts that may be due by them. It is further recommended that the patient sign a statement that

they are aware of their responsibility and agree to pay it on receipt of the bill. An example of suggested wording for a letter is given in Fig. 4.4. This written estimate makes collection quicker and easier.

4.3   QUICK REVIEW

Question: Under the birthday rule, under which insurance would Little Johnny Junior be covered if his mom has Blue Shield and a date of birth of 1/5/1978, while his dad has Aetna and a date of birth of 9/16/76?

COLLEGE CLINIC
4567 Broad Avenue
Woodland Hills, XY 12345-0000

Phone: 555/486-9002   Fax: 555/487-8976

Current date

Patient's name
Address
City, State, ZIP code

Dear

This letter gives you an estimate of the fees for your proposed surgery. Verification of coverage and benefit information has been obtained from your insurance company. Listed are your benefits for the proposed surgical expenses and the estimated balance after your insurance carrier pays.

Surgical procedure	Craniotomy		
Date of surgery	February 21, 20XX		
Name of hospital	College Hospital		
Hospital address	4500 Broad Ave., Woodland Hills, XY 12345		

		Insurance pays	Estimated balance
Surgeon's fee	1930.00	1420.50	509.50
Preoperative visit			
Preoperative tests			

You have a policy deductible of $1000   which   has ✓ has not been met.

The surgery requires the use of an anesthesiologist, assistant surgeon, and a pathologist. These physicians will bill you separately for their services. The hospital will also bill you separately.

This office will file your insurance claim for the surgical procedure, so the insurance payment should come directly to us. If the insurance carrier sends you the payment, then you are responsible to get the payment to this office within five days. Your balance after surgery should be approximately $1203.85. You are responsible for any remaining balance after our office receives the insurance payment.

This notice gives our estimation of the balance for which you will be responsible. Please sign below to indicate you have received and understand this notification.

_____   _____

Signature   Date

Thank you for choosing our medical practice. If you have any questions, please call me.

Sincerely,

Karen Martinez, CMA
Administrative Medical Assistant

Fig. 4.4 Sample letter to a patient supplying an estimate of the fees for proposed surgery.

CHOICE OF HEALTH INSURANCE

A person can obtain health insurance through a group plan or an individual contract. Any insurance plan issued directly to an individual and their dependents is called an individual contract, or personal insurance. Usually, this type of policy has a higher premium and, often, the benefits are less than those obtainable under a group health insurance plan.

A group contract is any insurance plan that covers a group of employees or other group and their eligible dependents. They are insured under a single policy issued to their employer or leader. Individual certificates are given to each insured individual or family unit. A group policy usually provides better benefits and offers lower premiums than individual contracts. The coverage for each person in the group is the same. A new employee must sign a waiver if they decline enrollment. Under the PPACA, employers may change the kind of medical benefits they offer their employees. For example, an employer may choose to increase copayments and deductibles or choose a plan that offers fewer benefits.

Some individuals can obtain comprehensive group coverage through plans sponsored by the professional organizations to which they belong. This is called a blanket contract.

Conversion Privilege

If the person leaves the employer or organization or the group contract is terminated, the insured may continue coverage under an individual policy if the group contract has a conversion privilege. Usually, conversion from a group policy to an individual policy increases the premium and could reduce the benefits.

COBRA

The Consolidated Omnibus Budget Reconciliation Act (COBRA) of 1985 requires employers with 20 or more workers to extend group health insurance coverage in light of certain events. Coverage is extended to the employee and their dependents at group rates for up to 18 months. Qualifying events include being laid off, reduction in hours, or voluntary or involuntary termination. In the event of the death of a covered employee, a divorce from a covered employee, or an employee becoming entitled to Medicare, the extension of coverage for the spouse or dependents may be extended to 36 months. In all these situations, the former employee, the spouse, or the dependent is responsible for paying the premiums for the coverage.

Medical Savings Accounts

A medical savings account (MSA) is a type of tax-free savings account that allows individuals and their employers to set aside money to pay for health care expenses. An employer can set up an MSA for their employees and make an annual contribution to the MSA, which is tax deductible for both employer and employee. MSA balances can be carried over from year to year. MSAs are portable, allowing individuals to take their MSA with them when they retire, change jobs, or relocate. When health care services are provided, the patient files a claim with the MSA to receive reimbursement and uses the explanation of benefits (EOB) from the insurance company as documentation. Medicare beneficiaries are eligible to enroll in a similar tax-advantaged savings account, which may be referred to as a Medicare medical savings account.

Health Savings Accounts

The Medicare Reform Act was signed into law in December 2003, giving Americans a tool for defraying medical costs called health savings accounts (HSAs). HSAs are open to anyone younger than 65 years of age who enrolls in a high-deductible health plan. Employers and/or employees may fund an HSA up to a set Internal Revenue Service (IRS)-mandated dollar amount each year. In 2020, this amount was $3,550 for a single insured plan and $7,100 for a family plan. The IRS also sets annual out-of-pocket expenses, including deductibles and copayments. In 2020, for example, these could not exceed $6,900 for single coverage and $13,800 for family coverage. If a high-deductible

health plan has a higher out-of-pocket maximum, it may not be an HSA-eligible plan. These accounts are a tax-favored savings plan in which a working person can deposit money in an HSA and deduct the amount of the deposits from taxable income. Withdrawals from HSAs are tax-free when used for qualifying medical expenses. Money left unspent in an HSA may be rolled over year after year.

Health Reimbursement Arrangements

An alternative plan is a health reimbursement account (HRA). HRAs are typically offered in tandem with high-deductible plans. The employer owns the account and only the employer is eligible to make contributions. The employer is allowed to determine contribution limits and define covered expense. Employers can determine whether the balance can be rolled over from one year to the next. If the employee leaves, the money remains with the employer.

High-Deductible Health Plans

High-deductible health plans (HDHPs) give tax advantages that assist in saving for future medical expenses. They have annual out-of-pocket limits and higher annual deductibles than traditional health insurance plans. They are typically combined with an HSA or HRA.

Flexible Spending Accounts

Another option is a health care flexible spending account (FSA). FSAs are employer sponsored. They allow a specific amount of wages to be put aside for qualified medical expenses and dependent care. In 2020, an individual could put up to $2750 in an FSA each year, with the cap increasing by the annual inflation rate in subsequent years. Money deducted from an employee's paycheck and deposited into an FSA is not subject to payroll taxes, resulting in substantial payroll tax savings. Before implementation of the ACA, one disadvantage of using an FSA was that funds not used by the end of the plan year were lost to the employee, known as the "use it or lose it" rule. Under the terms of the ACA and effective in plans from 2013 and later, the employee is allowed to carry over up to $500 per year to the following year without losing the funds.

 4.4   QUICK REVIEW
Question: What is the difference between an HSA and an HRA?

TYPES OF HEALTH INSURANCE

Many forms of health insurance coverage are currently in effect in the United States. Types of third-party payers include private insurance, government plans, managed care contracts, and workers' compensation. A brief explanation of the programs discussed in this text is given here, but for an in-depth study, refer to the appropriate chapters that follow.

There are various options available to employers and individuals when purchasing health insurance alone or as a group. Some are traditional insurance plans, such as indemnity plans, while others are managed care plans, such as health maintenance organizations (HMOs), exclusive provider organizations (EPOs), and independent practice associations (IPAs).

Federal and state governments oversee many types of insurance plans for elderly or indigent people. There are also several plans for military personnel and their families. While workers' compensation insurance plans are not funded by the government, they are regulated by state governments.

PRIVATE INSURANCE

Indemnity Health Insurance

Indemnity health insurance plans are referred to as traditional or fee-for-service health plans. They are designed to allow patients maximum flexibility and choice when it comes to health care organizations. Subscribers pay a fixed monthly premium and services are paid at a percentage of covered benefits after an annual deductible is met. Health care organizations are paid each time a service is rendered on a fee-for-service basis.

Self-Funded Health Plans

Some employers choose to be self-insured. In these self-funded health plans, the employer pays for all of the employees' health care costs directly without using a third-party payer. This is different from a traditional insurance coverage where the employer pays premiums to the health insurance company who then pays for the health care costs. In this type of plan, the employer will set aside monies in a trust to cover these expenses.

Consumer Directed Health Plans

These plans are a rapidly emerging approach to health care services that are also referred to as self-directed health plans (SDHPs). Consumer directed health plans (CDHPs) allow the consumer to design and customize their own health plan, based on their specific needs and circumstances. Typically, the CDHP involves the pairing of a high-deductible preferred provider organization plan with a tax-advantaged account, such as an HSA.

MANAGED CARE PLANS

Exclusive Provider Organization

An exclusive provider organization (EPO) is a type of managed health care plan in which subscriber members are eligible for benefits only when they use the services of a limited network of health care organizations. EPOs combine features of both health maintenance organizations (HMOs) and preferred provider organizations (PPOs). Employers agree not to enter into an agreement with any other plan for coverage of eligible employees. EPOs are regulated under state health insurance laws.

Health Maintenance Organization

A health maintenance organization (HMO) is an organization that provides a wide range of comprehensive health care services for a specified group at a fixed periodic payment. The emphasis is on preventive care. Health care organizations are prepaid by capitation, which is a payment system based on a flat rate per patient in the plan. Health care organizations are prepaid based on the number of HMO members. An HMO can be sponsored by the government, medical schools, hospitals, employers, labor unions, consumer groups, insurance companies, or hospital medical plans.

Independent or Individual Practice Association

An independent or individual practice association (IPA) is a type of managed care plan in which a program administrator contracts with a number of health care organizations. These organizations agree to provide treatment to subscribers in their own offices or clinics for a fixed capitation payment per month. Subscribers to IPA plans have limited or no choice of health care organization. IPA health care organizations continue to see their fee-for-service patients.

Point-of-Service Plan

A point-of-service (POS) plan is a managed care plan consisting of a network of health care organizations and hospitals that provides an insurance company or employer with discounts on its services. Patients can refer themselves to a specialist or see an out-of-network health care organization for a higher copayment.

Preferred Provider Organization

A variation of a managed care plan is a preferred provider organization (PPO). This is a form of contract medicine by which a large employer, or any organization that can produce a large number of patients, contracts with a hospital or a group of health care organizations to offer medical care at a reduced rate.

MEDICARE

Medicare is a national four-part program. It consists of a hospital insurance system (Part A), supplementary medical insurance (Part B), Medicare Plus Choice Program (Part C), and the Medicare Prescription Drug benefits (Part D). It is for individuals who are at least 65 years of age. It was created by the 1965 Amendments to the Social Security Act and is operated under the provisions of the Act. Benefits are also extended to permanently disabled people and those with end-stage renal disease. Refer to Chapter 6 for further discussion on Medicare.

MEDICAID

Medicaid is a program sponsored jointly by federal, state, and local governments to provide health care benefits to medically indigent persons on public assistance, aged individuals who meet certain financial requirements, and the disabled. Some states have expanded coverage for other medically needy individuals who meet special state-determined criteria. Coverage and benefits vary widely from state to state. Refer to Chapter 7 for further discussion on Medicaid and other state programs.

MILITARY PLANS

Tricare

A government-sponsored program called TRICARE provides military and non-military hospital and medical services. It covers spouses and dependents of active service personnel, retired service personnel and their dependents, and dependents of members who died on active duty. Active duty service members are not eligible for TRICARE but have benefits like TRICARE Prime, in which the Department of Defense covers all allowable charges for medically necessary care. Refer to Chapter 8 for further discussion on TRICARE.

Veterans Health Administration

The Veterans Health Administration or Civilian Health and Medical Program of the Department of Veterans Affairs (CHAMPVA) is administered by the Department of Veterans Affairs (VA). This federal program covers medical bills for veterans with total, permanent, service-connected disabilities, as well as their spouses and dependents. It also covers the surviving spouses and children of veterans who died as a result of service-connected disabilities. Refer to Chapter 8 for further discussion on CHAMPVA.

⚡ WORKERS' COMPENSATION INSURANCE

Workers' compensation insurance (WC) is a contract that insures a person against on-the-job injury or illness. The employer pays the premium for the employees. Refer to Chapter 9 for further discussion on WC.

Examples of Insurance Billing

Sometimes, it is difficult to comprehend the full scale of insurance billing. A patient's care is often overseen by various providers and departments. As an example of total medical billing, six cases are presented in Box 4.1 to explain the entire billing picture, from simple to complex.

In these scenarios, an insurance billing specialist in the offices of the attending health care provider, assistant surgeon, anesthesiologist, radiologic group, and private clinical laboratory submits an insurance claim form called the CMS-1500 for reimbursement to the insurance payer (Fig. 4.5A). If the health care organization does not participate, it gives the patient the necessary information to submit his or her own claim to the insurance company. Chapter 14 discusses how to complete this form.

In the hospital and hospital emergency department, a member of the hospital staff inputs services into a central computer system. This produces an itemized statement and completed insurance claim form via computer to be submitted to the third-party payer. The term institutional provider refers to hospitals, skilled nursing facilities, hospice, home health agencies, or any other health-related service facilities. These use a CMS-1450, also known as the UB-04 claim form, for billing medical services. Some types of services, such as speech pathology and physical therapy, are also billed on this form. Chapter 19 discusses how to complete this form (Fig. 4.5B).

⚖ | 4.5   QUICK REVIEW

Question: Who is covered by the following types of insurance?
1. Medicare
2. Medicaid
3. TRICARE
4. Indemnity
5. Workers' Compensation

HANDLING AND PROCESSING INSURANCE CLAIMS

Most offices today are computerized and use practice management software (PMS) for scheduling, electronic health records, coding, billing, accounts receivable management, and other administrative functions. However, some smaller offices thrive in the paper environment and will continue to do so. A computerized office may still generate paper insurance claim forms and send them to the insurance payer.

Different methods exist for processing insurance claims for the health care organization. The most common ones follow.
1. Posting charges and submitting to the insurance payer on the CMS-1500 or CMS-1450 claim form. These forms can be completed and transmitted electronically or prepared manually under certain circumstances.
2. Contracting with an outside billing service company to prepare and electronically transmit claims on behalf of the health care organization's office.

BOX 4.1   Examples of Medical Billing

CASE 1

A new patient comes in with complaints of a sore throat and an infected nail. The provider's office bills for:
- Office visit, penicillin injection
- Office surgery for infected nail
- Sterile surgical tray (may or may not be billed, depending on third-party payer)

CASE 2

A patient comes in because of an accident and has complaints that require evaluation and management services, x-ray films, and laboratory studies (urinalysis) performed in the provider's office.
The provider's office bills for:
- Office visit
- Office visit x-ray studies (including interpretation)
- Laboratory tests (urinalysis, including interpretation)

CASE 3

A patient is seen by the primary care provider after office hours in the hospital emergency department.
- The provider's office bills for the hospital visit in the emergency department.
- The hospital bills for hospital outpatient emergency department services (use and supplies).

CASE 4

A provider sends a patient's Papanicolaou (Pap) test to a private clinical laboratory.
- The provider's office bills for the office visit and handling of the specimen.
- The laboratory bills for the Pap test.

CASE 5

A patient is sent to a local hospital for an upper gastrointestinal radiographic series. An x-ray technician obtains the films in the hospital and a privately owned radiologic group does the interpretation.
- The hospital bills for the technical component of the upper gastrointestinal x-ray series (use of equipment).
- The radiologic group bills for the professional component of the upper gastrointestinal x-ray series (the interpretation).

CASE 6

A patient is seen in the office and is immediately hospitalized for a hysterectomy.
- The surgeon's office bills for initial hospital admission and surgical procedure.
- The assistant surgeon bills for assisting the surgeon during hysterectomy.
- The anesthesiologist bills for anesthesia administered during hysterectomy.
- The hospital bills for hospital room, operating room, anesthesia supplies, medications, x-ray films, laboratory tests, and medical and surgical supplies (dressings, intravenous lines). The hospital might also bill for blood for transfusions, electrocardiogram, radiation therapy, and respiratory therapy.

---

3. Direct data entry (DDE) in the payer's system. The billing specialist logs into the insurance company's system and keys in the data required to process the claim. Keep in mind that Health Insurance Portability and Accountability (HIPAA) regulations will determine whether a health care organization is a covered entity and whether it is required to submit claims electronically.

HEALTH INSURANCE CLAIM FORM

APPROVED BY NATIONAL UNIFORM CLAIM COMMITTEE (NUCC) 02/12

1. MEDICARE MEDICAID TRICARE CHAMPVA GROUP HEALTH PLAN FECA BLK LUNG OTHER (Medicare#) (Medicaid#) (ID#DoD#) (Member ID#) (ID#) (ID#) (ID#)	1a. INSURED'S I.D. NUMBER (For Program in Item 1)

2. PATIENT'S NAME (Last Name, First Name, Middle Initial)
3. PATIENT'S BIRTH DATE MM DD YY SEX M F
4. INSURED'S NAME (Last Name, First Name, Middle Initial)
5. PATIENT'S ADDRESS (No., Street)
6. PATIENT RELATIONSHIP TO INSURED Self Spouse Child Other
7. INSURED'S ADDRESS (No., Street)
CITY STATE
8. RESERVED FOR NUCC USE
CITY STATE
ZIP CODE TELEPHONE (Include Area Code) ( )
ZIP CODE TELEPHONE (Include Area Code) ( )
9. OTHER INSURED'S NAME (Last Name, First Name, Middle Initial)
10. IS PATIENT'S CONDITION RELATED TO:
11. INSURED'S POLICY GROUP OR FECA NUMBER
a. OTHER INSURED'S POLICY OR GROUP NUMBER
a. EMPLOYMENT? (Current or Previous) YES NO
a. INSURED'S DATE OF BIRTH MM DD YY SEX M F
b. RESERVED FOR NUCC USE
b. AUTO ACCIDENT? YES NO PLACE (State)
b. OTHER CLAIM ID (Designated by NUCC)
c. RESERVED FOR NUCC USE
c. OTHER ACCIDENT? YES NO
c. INSURANCE PLAN NAME OR PROGRAM NAME
d. INSURANCE PLAN NAME OR PROGRAM NAME
10d. CLAIM CODES (Designated by NUCC)
d. IS THERE ANOTHER HEALTH BENEFIT PLAN? YES NO If yes, complete items 9, 9a, and 9d.

READ BACK OF FORM BEFORE COMPLETING & SIGNING THIS FORM.
12. PATIENT'S OR AUTHORIZED PERSON'S SIGNATURE I authorize the release of any medical or other information necessary to process this claim. I also request payment of government benefits either to myself or to the party who accepts assignment below. SIGNED _____ DATE _____
13. INSURED'S OR AUTHORIZED PERSON'S SIGNATURE I authorize payment of medical benefits to the undersigned physician or supplier for services described below. SIGNED _____

14. DATE OF CURRENT ILLNESS, INJURY, or PREGNANCY(LMP) MM DD YY QUAL.
15. OTHER DATE QUAL. MM DD YY
16. DATES PATIENT UNABLE TO WORK IN CURRENT OCCUPATION FROM MM DD YY TO MM DD YY
17. NAME OF REFERRING PROVIDER OR OTHER SOURCE 17a. 17b. NPI
18. HOSPITALIZATION DATES RELATED TO CURRENT SERVICES FROM MM DD YY TO MM DD YY
19. ADDITIONAL CLAIM INFORMATION (Designated by NUCC)
20. OUTSIDE LAB? YES NO $ CHARGES
21. DIAGNOSIS OR NATURE OF ILLNESS OR INJURY Relate A-L to service line below (24E) ICD Ind. A. B. C. D. E. F. G. H. I. J. K. L.
22. RESUBMISSION CODE ORIGINAL REF. NO.
23. PRIOR AUTHORIZATION NUMBER

24. A. DATE(S) OF SERVICE From To	B. PLACE OF SERVICE	C. EMG	D. PROCEDURES, SERVICES, OR SUPPLIES CPT/HCPCS MODIFIER	E. DIAGNOSIS POINTER	F. $ CHARGES	G. DAYS OR UNITS	H. EPSDT Family Plan	I. ID. QUAL.	J. RENDERING PROVIDER ID. #
1									NPI
2									NPI
3									NPI
4									NPI
5									NPI
6									NPI

25. FEDERAL TAX I.D. NUMBER SSN EIN
26. PATIENT'S ACCOUNT NO.
27. ACCEPT ASSIGNMENT? (For govt. claims, see back) YES NO
28. TOTAL CHARGE $
29. AMOUNT PAID $
30. Rsvd for NUCC Use $
31. SIGNATURE OF PHYSICIAN OR SUPPLIER INCLUDING DEGREES OR CREDENTIALS (I certify that the statements on the reverse apply to this bill and are made a part thereof.) SIGNED DATE
32. SERVICE FACILITY LOCATION INFORMATION a. NPI b.
33. BILLING PROVIDER INFO & PH # ( ) a. NPI b.

NUCC Instruction Manual available at: www.nucc.org   PLEASE PRINT OR TYPE   APPROVED OMB-0938-1197 FORM 1500 (02-12)

Fig. 4.5A CMS-1500 form is used by health care providers for submitting claims for medical services.

Fig. 4.5B CMS-1450 (also known as the UB-04 form) is used by facilities such as hospitals and skilled nursing facilities for submitting claims.

LIFE CYCLE OF AN INSURANCE CLAIM

The **life cycle** or **revenue cycle** of an insurance claim includes the administrative and clinical functions that are required to capture and collect payment for services provided by a health care organization.

The revenue cycle of an insurance claim outlines the basic steps (Fig. 4.6) in handling and processing insurance claims in a health care organization's office. The cycle begins when the patient makes an appointment and continues until payment is received.

Step 1: Preregistration

Some health care organizations preregister a new patient during the initial telephone call. Some have a designated staff member contact the patient before the appointment time. Some send a letter confirming the appointment with an informative brochure about the health care organization and a patient registration form. This form may be printed off the organization's website, completed online, or completed when the patient arrives for his or her appointment.

It is a good idea to have new patients arrive 15 to 20 minutes before the scheduled appointment. This allows time to collect vital statistics and insurance information and to discuss the patient's responsibility with respect to payment policies. A patient registration form also may be called a patient information form or intake sheet (Fig. 4.7).

Instruct the patient to fill in all spaces and indicate not applicable (N/A) if an item does not apply. If the patient has a medical problem that makes it difficult to complete the form, such as rheumatoid arthritis of the hands or limited vision, then the insurance billing specialist should interview the patient and fill in the necessary data.

Read the form carefully after completion to ensure that complete and accurate personal and financial information has been obtained from the patient. The patient registration form should contain the following facts:

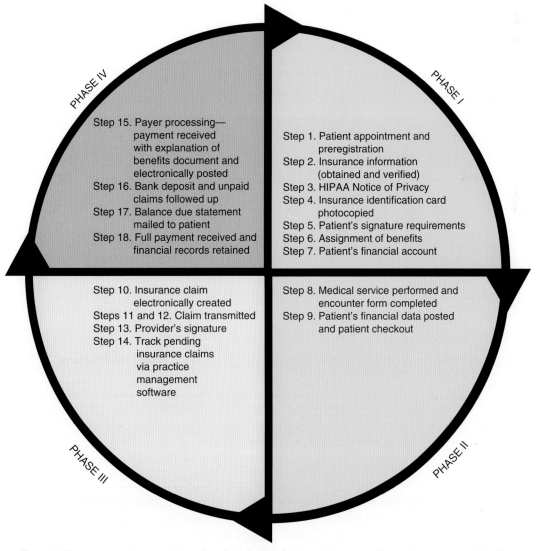

Fig. 4.6 Revenue cycle overview showing the basic steps in processing an insurance claim in a health care organization's office, to the third-party payer, and after payment is received.

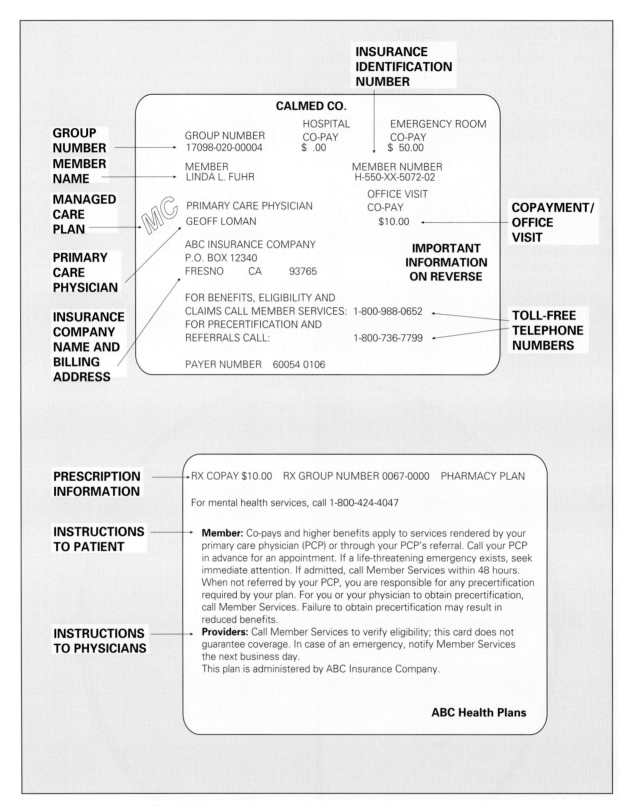

Fig. 4.7 Front *(top)* and back *(bottom)* sides of an insurance card.

- *Name: First, middle initial, and last.* The name must match that shown on the insurance identification card. Some pediatric patients do not have the same last name as their parents or stepparents. Insurance payments show the policyholder's name, and it is time consuming to find and give credit to the patient's account without this information. Medical billing systems allow a cross-reference of the patient, subscriber, and guarantor's names, as well as Social Security numbers, so that, when the policyholder's name is searched, the patient's name also appears.

- *Street address*, including apartment number, zip code, and *telephone numbers* with area code (cell and landline)
- *Business address, telephone number with extension, and occupation*
- *E-mail address*
- *Date of birth*. HIPAA requires eight digits (year/month/day) to be submitted to payers; for example, the eight-digit format of January 2, 1936, is 19360102. A medical billing system may collect these data in a different format but transmit them in the required eight-digit format.
- *Person responsible for account*, either guarantor or insured's name
- *Social Security number*
- *Spouse's name and occupation*
- *Referring provider's name* or another referral source
- *Driver's license number*
- *Emergency contact*, such as a close relative or friend, with name, address, and telephone number
- *Insurance billing information*: all insurance company names, addresses, policy numbers, and group numbers. This is important for the COBs. Medicare and Medicaid patients are given the option of joining managed care programs and are allowed to switch every 30 days. Always ask each older patient whether he or she is covered by traditional Medicare or a Medicare HMO. A good patient information sheet has space where this information can be written in by the patient.

Fig. 4.8 Patient presenting an insurance identification card to the receptionist for photocopying.

write the date on the copy, using this as the basis for revising data on file.

> **! COMPLIANCE ALERT**
>
> If the health care organization is submitting an insurance claim for the patient, the patient is not required to sign a release-of-information form for obtaining payment for services. However, some health care organizations prefer to operate at a higher level of privacy and continue to obtain patients' signatures on release-of-information forms.

Step 2: Verification of Insurance

Verify insurance and all other information that may have changed since the last encounter. This may be done by giving the patient a copy of the previously completed patient registration form and asking him or her to correct any incorrect data in red.

Step 3: Notice of Privacy Practices

Each patient is given a Notice of Privacy Practices (NPP) that explains how his or her health information is used. Have the patient sign a form stating that he or she has received the NPP. If the patient refuses or is unable to sign, document this in the patient's health record. An NPP is mandatory under federal law through HIPAA.

Step 4: Insurance Identification Card

Photocopy or scan both sides of all of the patient's insurance identification cards (see Fig. 4.7). A copy produces error-free insurance data and can be used in lieu of completing the insurance section of the patient registration form. Ask for photo identification, such as a driver's license, to verify that the person has not used someone else's card. Call the insurance company to verify coverage and applicable deductible or copayment, and whether the insurance plan requires precertification for any services. On a return visit, ask to see the card and check it with the data on file (Fig. 4.8). If it differs, photocopy both sides and

Step 5: Patient's Signature Requirements

Under HIPAA regulations, a patient's signed authorization is not required for treatment, payment, or routine health care operations (TPO). However, many organizations continue to have patients sign an authorization allowing the release of any medical or other information necessary to process the claim. If the patient is physically or mentally unable to sign, the person representing the patient may sign for the patient. Most patient registration forms include a statement to sign regarding these two authorizations (see bottom of Fig. 4.9).

Electronic billers are permitted to obtain a lifetime authorization from the beneficiary to release health or other information necessary to process a claim. The signature should be retained in a file for future use on all electronic claims. This authorization allows the office to submit claims on the beneficiary's behalf. To do this, the patient signs a brief statement that reads as follows:

(Name of Beneficiary) (Health Insurance Claim Number)
"I request that payment of authorized benefits be made either to me or on my behalf to (name of health care organization or supplier) for any services furnished me by health care organization or supplier. I authorize any holder of medical information about me to release to my insurance carrier and its agents any information needed to determine these benefits or the benefits payable for related services."

Patient Registration

I was referred to this office by: Margaret Taylor   City: Oxnard   Date: 01/20/13

PATIENT INFORMATION			PRIMARY INSURED INFORMATION		
Name (Last) Fuhr	(First) Linda	(Middle) L	Name of insured (Last) Fuhr	(First) Gerald	(Middle) T
Name you like to be called Linda			Address (If different)		
Address 3070 Tipper street			City	State	Zip
City Oxnard	State CA	Zip 93030	Policyholder's birthdate 06-15-64	Sex ☒ M ☐ F	Home phone number 555-276-0101
Patient's birthdate 11-05-65	Sex ☐ M ☒ F	Home phone number 555-276-0101	SSN 545-XX-2771		Work phone number 555-921-0075
SSN 550-XX-5172		Work phone number 555-372-1151	Email address GFUHR64@AOL.COM		Cell phone number 555-243-2736
Email address LFUHR65@AOL.COM		Cell phone number 555-243-1777	Insurance name ABC Insurance Company		
Employer or school name Macys	Title Sales associate		Insurance address P.O. Box 12340, Fresno, CA 93765		
Patient status ☒ Employed		☐ Full time student	ID number H-550-XX-5172-02		Group number 17098
☐ Single	☒ Married	☐ Other	Primary insured's relationship to patient Spouse		
Ethnicity ☐ Hispanic	☐ Non-Hispanic	☒ Not specified	Employer Electronic Data Systems		
Race ☐ African American ☒ Caucasian or European American ☐ Native American	☐ Asian American ☐ Pacific Islander		Employer address 2700 West 5th Street Oxnard, CA 93030		
Preferred language English			Comments None		

EMERGENCY CONTACT INFORMATION		SECONDARY INSURANCE INFORMATION		
Name Hannah Gildea	Relationship Aunt	Name of insured (Last)	(First)	(Middle)
Address 4621 Lucretia St., Oxnard, CA 93030		Policy holder's birthdate	Sex ☐ M ☐ F	
Home phone number 555-274-0132	Cell phone number 555-243-1388	Insurance name None		
Email address GILDEAH@YAHOO.COM		Insurance address		
Does your emergency contact have power of attorney? ☐ Yes ☒ No	Advance health directive? ☒ Yes ☐ No	ID number	Group number	

FOR WORK-RELATED PROBLEMS, PLEASE FILL OUT BELOW

Workers' comp insurance	Policy number	Address	City	State	Zip
Claim number	Date of injury	Employer at time of injury			
Has this injury been reported to the employer? ☐ Yes ☐ No		Employer address			

INSURANCE SIGNATURE AUTHORIZATION

I authorize any holder of medical or other information about me to release to the insurance company any information needed for this or a related claim. I permit a copy of this authorization to be used in place of the original, and newest payment of medical insurance benefits to, (PHYSICIAN NAME OR PRACTICE NAME): _____

X *Linda Fuhr*   Jan. 20, 20XX

ORDER # 58-8429 • © 2012 BIBBERO SYSTEMS, INC. • PETALUMA, CALIFORNIA
TO REORDER CALL TOLL FREE: (800) 242-2376 OR FAX (800) 242-9330 MFG IN U.S.A.

Fig. 4.9 Patient registration information form showing a comprehensive listing of personal and financial information requested from the patient on his or her first visit to the office. (Courtesy Bibbero Systems, Inc., Petaluma, Calif. Telephone: 800-242-2376; fax: 800-242-9330; website: www.bibbero.com.)

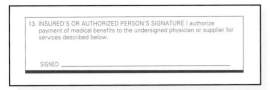

13. INSURED'S OR AUTHORIZED PERSON'S SIGNATURE I authorize payment of medical benefits to the undersigned physician or supplier for services described below.

SIGNED _____

Fig. 4.10 Section 13 from the health insurance claim form CMS-1500, illustrating authorization for assignment of benefits.

Step 6: Assignment of Benefits

The signature requirement for the assignment of benefits is included in Block 13 of the CMS-1500 insurance claim form (Fig. 4.10). For the health care organization to receive payment directly from the insurance payer, the patient must sign an assignment of benefits statement for each insurance company. However, before explaining an assignment, it is important to define the difference between participating (par) and nonparticipating (nonpar) providers.

A par health care organization has a contractual agreement with an insurance plan to render care to eligible beneficiaries and bill the third-party payer directly (Example 4.2). The third-party payer pays its portion of the allowed amount, and the health care organization bills the patient for the balance after the disallowed portion is adjusted off of the account. Managed care plans also refer to par providers as member health care organizations. If the amount of the patient's responsibility can be determined, it is collected at the time of the encounter.

EXAMPLE 4.2 Participating Provider

Dr. Gomez accepts assignment and is a par provider for the Liberty Health Insurance Plan. Pedro Nunez, a new patient, is seen in the office with complaints of a sore throat and infected nail, for which a $150 fee is charged for the office visit, office surgery, and penicillin injection. The patient has met his deductible for the year.

Provider fee (total billed amount)	$150
Provider contracted rate (allowable charge)	$140
Patient coinsurance or copayment amount	$10
Insurance claims payment	$130
Provider's adjusted (write-off) amount	$10

Dr. Gomez collects $10 from the patient and is paid a total of $140.

A nonpar provider is a health care organization without a contractual agreement with an insurance plan. It is not required to accept a contracted amount for care to eligible beneficiaries (Example 4.3). The health care organization may or may not file

EXAMPLE 4.3 Nonparticipating Provider

Dr. Warner does not accept assignment and is a nonpar provider for the XYZ Health Insurance Plan. Estelle Cutter, an established patient, is seen in the office complaining that her ears are full of earwax that needs to be removed. A $60 fee is charged.

Provider fee (total billed amount)	$60
Usual, customary, and reasonable (UCR)	$55
Patient coinsurance or copayment amount	$10
Insurance claims payment	$44
Provider may bill patient over UCR	$6

Dr. Warner collects $16 from the patient and is paid a total of $60 because he can collect the difference between his fee and the patient's copayment, plus the insurance payment.

an insurance claim as a courtesy to the patient and may require full payment at the time of service. The patient should be made aware that their insurance plan will cover a considerable amount less on the claim when receiving services from a nonpar provider.

If a health care organization accepts assignment, the insurance carrier sends the payment directly to them. An agreement is obtained by having the patient sign an assignment of insurance benefits document that directs payment to the health care organization. The CMS-1500 claim form contains this provision, as well. An assignment of benefits becomes a legally enforceable document, but must refer to specific hospitalization, course of treatment, or office visits. Each course of treatment needs to have an assignment document signed by the patient, unless an annual or lifetime signature authorization is maintained in the patient's file.

Accepting assignment, participating, and nonparticipating can mean different things for different carriers.

ASSIGNMENT OF BENEFITS FOR PRIVATE CARRIERS

For private insurance companies with whom the health care organization does not have a contractual agreement, accepting assignment means that the claim will be paid to the health care organization's office instead of the patient. Because there is no signed agreement between the health care organization and the carrier, the difference between the billed amount and the carrier's allowed amount is not written off, but collected from the patient in the same way as any copayment or deductible.

ASSIGNMENT OF BENEFITS FOR MANAGED CARE

In managed care plans, a par or preferred provider is a health care organization that has contracted with a plan to provide medical services to plan members. A nonpar provider refers to a health care organization that has not contracted with a managed care plan to provide medical services to plan members. The assignment is automatic for individuals who have signed with managed care contracts.

ASSIGNMENT OF BENEFITS FOR MEDICAID

For Medicaid cases, there is no assignment unless the patient has other insurance in addition to Medicaid. The Medicaid fiscal intermediary pays all providers directly.

ASSIGNMENT OF BENEFITS FOR MEDICARE

The words *participating*, *nonparticipating*, and *assignment* have slightly different meanings in the Medicare program. A health care organization that accepts assignment on Medicare claims is called a participating (par) health care organization. It may not bill or accept payment for the difference between the submitted charge and the Medicare allowed amount. However, an attempt must be made to collect the 20% coinsurance and any amount applied to the deductible.

A health care organization that does not participate is called a nonparticipating health care organization and has an option regarding assignment. The health care organization either may not accept assignment for all services or may exercise the option of accepting assignment for some services and collecting from the patient for other services performed at the same time and place. The health care organization collects the fee from the patient but may bill no more than the Medicare-limiting charge. The check is sent to the patient.

STATE LIC.# C1503X
SOC. SEC. # 000-11-0000
PIN # _____

College Clinic
4567 Broad Avenue
Woodland Hills, XY 12345-4700

Phone: 555-486-9002

☐ Private   ☒ Bluecross   ☐ Ind.   ☐ Medicare   ☐ Medi-cal   ☐ Hmo   ☐ Ppo

Patient's last name Smith	First Lydia		Account #: 13845	Birthdate 09/ 13 / 92	Sex ☐ Male ☒ Female	Today's date 09/ 17 / 20XX
Insurance company Blue Shield of CA	Subscriber Lydia Smith			Plan # 0473	Sub. # 186-72-10XX	Group 849-37000

ASSIGNMENT: I hereby assign my insurance benefits to be paid directly to the undersigned physician, I am financially responsible for non-covered services.
SIGNED: Patient,
or parent, if minor *Lydia Smith*   Today's date   09 / 17 / 20XX

RELEASE: I hereby authorize the physician to release to my insurance carriers any information required to process this claim.
SIGNED: Patient,
or parent, if minor *Lydia Smith*   Today's date   09 / 17 / 20XX

✓	DESCRIPTION	CODE	FEE	✓	DESCRIPTION	CODE	FEE	✓	DESCRIPTION	CODE	FEE
	OFFICE VISITS	NEW EST.			Venipuncture	36415			OFFICE PROCEDURES		
	Blood pressure check	99211			TB skin test	86580			Anoscopy	46600	
	Level II	99202 99212			Hematocrit	85013			Ear lavage	69210	
	Level III	99203 99213			Glucose finger stick	82948			Spirometry	94010	
X	Level IV	(99204) 99214	180.00		IMMUNIZATIONS				Nebulizer Rx	94664	
	Level V	99205 99215			Allergy inj. X1	95115			EKG	93000	
	PREVENTIVE EXAMS	NEW EST.			Allergy inj. X2	95117			SURGERY		
	Age 65 and older	99387 99397			Trigger pt. inj.	20552			Mole removal (1st)	17110	
	Age 40 - 64	99386 99396			Therapeutic inj.	96372			(2nd to 14th)	17003	
	Age 18 - 39	99385 99395			VACCINATION PRODUCTS				Flat warts (1st - 14th)	07110	
	Age 12 - 17	99384 99394			DPT	90701			15 or more	17111	
	Age 5 - 11	99383 99393			DT	90702			Biopsy, 1 lesion	11100	
	Age 1 - 4	99382 99392			Tetanus	90703			Addt'l. lesions	11101	
	Infant	99381 99391			MMR	90707			Endometrial Bx	58100	
	Newborn ofc	99432			OPV	90712			Skin tags to 15	11200	
	OB/NEWBORN CARE				Polio inj.	90713			Each addt'l. 10	11201	
	OB package	59400			Flu	90662			I & D abscess	10060	
	Post-partum visit N/C				Hemophilus B	90645			SUPPLIES/MISCELLANEOUS		
	LAB PROCEDURES				Hepatitis B vac.	90746			Surgical tray	99070	
	Urine dip	81000			Pneumovax	90670			Handling charge	99000	
	UA qualitative	81005			VACCINE ADMINISTRATION				Special report	99080	
X	Pregnancey urine	81025	20.00		Age: Through 18 yrs. (1st inj.)	90460			DOCTOR'S NOTES:		
	Wet mount	87210			Age: Through 18 yrs. (ea. addt'l. inj.)	90461					
	kOH prip	87220			Adult (1st inj.)	90471					
	Occult blood	82270			Adult (ea. addt'l. inj.)	90472					

DIAGNOSES	**ICD-10-CM**				
Abdominal pain/unspec.	R10.9	Colitis/unspec.	K51.90	FUO	R50.9
Absess	L02._	Confusion	R41.0	Gastritis	K29.70
Allergic reaction	T78.40_	CHF	I50.9	Gastroenteritis (colitis)	K52.9
Alzheimer's disease	G30	Constipation	K59.00	G.I. bleed	K92.2
Anemia/unspec.	D64.9	COPD	J44.9	Gout/unspec.	M10.9
Angina/unspec.	I20.9	Cough	R05	Headache	R51
Anorexia	R63.0	Crohn's disease/unspec.	K50.90	Health exam	200._
Anxiety/unspec.	F41.9	CVA	I63.9	Hematuria/unspec.	R31.9
Apnea, sleep	G47.30	Decubitus ulcer	L89._	Herpes simplex	B00.9
Arrhythmia, cardiac	I49.9	Dehydration	E86.0	Herpes zoster	B02.9
Arthritis, rheumatoid	M06.9	Dementia/unspec.	F03	Hiatal hernia	K44.9
Asthma/unspec.	J45.909	Depression, major/unsp.	F32.9	HTN (HBP)	I10
Atrial fibrillation.	I48.0	Diab I, no complications	E10.0	Hyperlipidemia/unspec.	E78.5
B-12 deficiency.	E53.8	Diab II, no complications	E11.9	Hypothyroidism/unspec.	E03.9
Back pain, low	M54.5	w/kidney complic.	E11.2_	Impotence	N52._
BPH	N40	w/ophthalmic compl.	E11.3_	Influenza, respiratory	J10.1
Bradycardia/unspec.	R00.1	w/neurolog compl.	E11.4_	Insomnia	G47.0
Bronchitis, acute	J20._	w/circulatory crmpl.	E11.5_	IBS, diarrhea	K58.
Bronchitis, chronic.	J42	Insulin use.	Z79.4	Lupus, systemic erythim.	M32.9
Bursitis/unspec.	M71.9	Diarrhea/unspec.	R19.7	MI, acute.	I21._
CA, breast	C50._	Diverticulitis.	K57.92	MI, old.	I25.2
CA, lung	C34._	Diverticulosis.	K57.90	Migraine	G43.9
CA, prostate	C61	Dizziness	R42	Myalgia	M79.1
Cellulitis	L03._	Dysuria	R30.0	Neck pain	M54.2
Chest pain/unspec.	R07.9	Edema/unspec.	R60.9	Neuropathy	G62.9
Cirrhosis, liver/unspec.	K74.60	Endocarditis	I38	Nausea	R11.1
Cold, common	J00	Esophageal reflux	K21.0	X Nausea/vomiting	R11.0
		Fatigue (lethargy)	R53.83	Obesity/unspec.	E66.9

Osteoarthritis (site).	M19._
Otitis media	H66.9_
Parkinson's disease	G20
Pharyngitis, acute.	J02.9
Pleurisy	R09.1
Pneumonia.	J18.9
Pneumonia, viral	J12.9
Prostatitis/unspec.	N41.9
PVD	I73.9
Radiculopathy	M54.1_
Rectal bleeding	K62.5
Renal failure	N19
Sciatica.	M54.3_
Shortness of breath	R03.02
Sinusitis, chr./unspec.	J32.9
Syncope	R55
Tachycardia/unspec.	R00.0
Tachy., supraventric	I47.1
Tendinitis/unspec.	M77.9
TIA	G45.9
Ulcer, duodenal/unspec.	K26.9
Ulcer, gastric/unspec.	K25.9
Ulcer, peptic/unspec.	K27.9
URI/unspec.	J06.9
UTI	N39.0
Vertigo	R42
Weight gain	R63.5
Weight loss	R63.4

Diagnosis/additional description:
Pregnancy

Doctor's signature/date
Dr. B. Caesar
09-17-20XX

Return appointment information:	-with whom	(Self) other
Days Wks. (Mos.) 1 month		

PLEASE RMEMBER THAT PAYMENT IS YOUR OBLIGATION, REGARDLESS OF INSURANCE OR OTHER THIRD PARTY INVOLVEMENT.

Rec'd. by:
☐ Cash
☐ Check
_____

Total today's fee   200.00

Amount rec'd. today

INSUR-A-BILL ® BIBBERO SYSTEMS, INC. • PETULUMA, CA • © 7/90 (BM1092)   (REV. 7/11)

Fig. 4.11 Encounter form: Procedural codes for professional services are taken from the Current Procedural Terminology (CPT) book and diagnostic codes are taken from the *International Classification of Diseases, Tenth Revision, Clinical Modification (ICD-10-CM)* book. (Courtesy Bibbero Systems, Inc., Petaluma, Calif. Telephone: 800-242-2376; fax: 800-242-9330; website: www.bibbero.com.)

✚ ASSIGNMENT OF BENEFITS FOR TRICARE

A health care organization that participates in TRICARE agrees to accept the allowable charge as the full fee and cannot charge the patient the difference between the health care organization's charge and the allowable charge. The exception to this is when the health care organization does not accept assignment on the claim.

A par or nonpar health care organization can submit a claim and choose to not accept assignment on a claim-by-claim basis. In the event the health care organization does not accept assignment, TRICARE sends the patient all payments. TRICARE does not communicate with the health care organization if the provider has questions about the claim. It is up to the health care organization to bill the sponsor for payment. The health care organization can collect 115% of the TRICARE allowable from the patient when a CMS-1500 claim form is marked "no" in the accepting assignment block.

⚡ ASSIGNMENT OF BENEFITS FOR WORKERS' COMPENSATION

There is no assignment for industrial cases. The WC carrier pays the fee for services rendered according to its fee schedule, and the check automatically goes to the health care organization. The patient is not responsible for payment of services for any work-related injury or illness.

Step 7: Patient's Financial Account

Patient information is entered into the PMS program. Accuracy is crucial because the data will be used to construct the claim for transmission to the insurance company. If the health care organization is not computerized, a manual system includes paper daysheets and patient ledger cards.

Step 8: Encounter Form

An encounter form (also called a charge slip, multipurpose billing form, patient service slip, routing form, superbill, or transaction slip) is attached to the patient's health record during the encounter (Fig. 4.11). This contains the patient's name, the date, and, in some instances, the previous balance due. It also contains the procedural and diagnostic codes and the date the patient should return for a follow-up appointment. This two- or three-part form is a combination bill, insurance form, and routing document used in both computer- and paper-based systems. This also can be a computerized multipurpose billing form that may be scanned to input charges and diagnoses into the patient's computerized account. Time is saved and fewer errors occur because no keystrokes are involved.

Health care organizations use the encounter form as a communications tool or routing sheet and as an invoice to the patient. When used as a routing sheet, it becomes a source document for insurance claim data. The encounter form is completed by the health care organization. Both a procedural code for services performed and a diagnostic code are chosen by the provider of services. In some situations, a certified coder may review the patient's health record to assign a proper code on the basis of the documentation.

The encounter form's procedure and diagnostic code sections should be updated and reprinted biannually with correct descriptions because changes, additions, and deletions occur that may

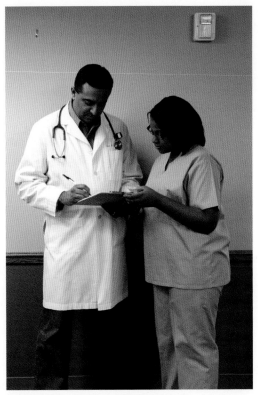

Fig. 4.12 Provider checking off procedures on the encounter form at the conclusion of a patient's office visit.

affect the organization. Remove all codes not used or seldom used and revise and add current, valid, commonly used codes for the organization. Because there is no grace period, update encounter forms twice a year: by October 1 for changes in diagnostic codes and by January 1 for changes in procedural codes.

Some health care organizations develop encounter forms for different services (e.g., surgical services, office services, and out-of-office services such as hospital visits, emergency, outpatient health care organization, nursing home, or house calls). The provider signs the encounter form and indicates whether the patient needs another appointment (Fig. 4.12).

Some health care organizations may have patients carry the encounter form to the reception desk, where fees are determined and input for billing. The patient is given the opportunity to pay and make a future appointment.

Step 9: Financial Accounting Record and Accounts Receivable Management

The value of maintaining careful records of all insurance matters cannot be overemphasized. Accounts receivable (**A/R**) management breathes life into the organization's cash flow. *A/R management* refers to establishing the patient financial accounting record and carrying out the claims process. For compilation of claim data, services are entered into the computer by either front desk personnel or the in-office billing department. If the organization outsources this function, an off-site billing company retrieves the data and processes the claims. All charges and patient payments are posted to their respective accounts.

A financial account is set up in the medical billing system. Data obtained from the patient registration process are keyed into the program and a patient account is established. Usually, an account number is automatically assigned by the program and used for tracking and reporting. All items posted to each patient account are housed in the computer database for accurate and easy retrieval.

Using the encounter form, daily transactions are recorded by the billing staff. Professional fees, payments, adjustments, and balances due are also posted in the practice management software program. Accuracy is especially important when keying data into the computer because this is where the data begins to build an insurance claim.

In the paper environment, a ledger card or financial accounting record is maintained for each patient who receives professional services (Fig. 4.13). An established patient who is injured on the job requires two ledgers, one for private care and one for WC services. At the end of each day, a daysheet is generated and

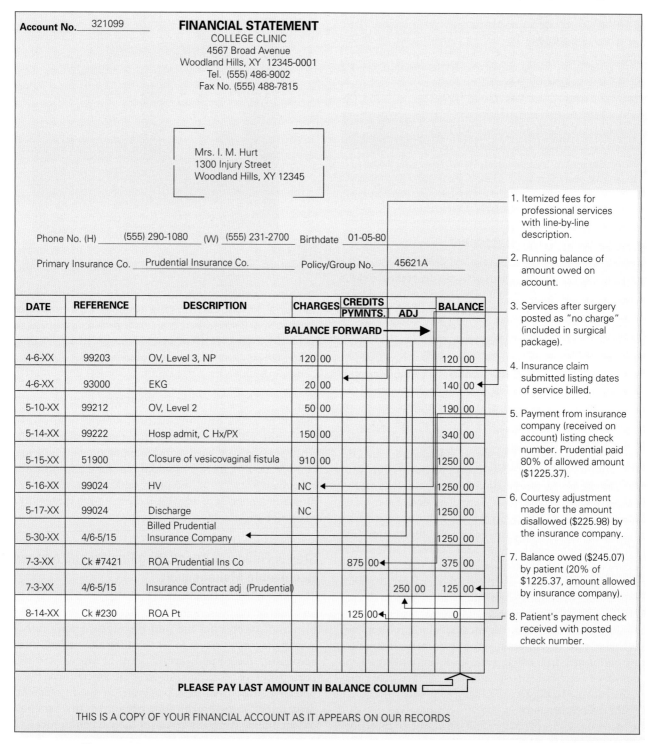

Fig. 4.13 Financial accounting record illustrating posting of professional service descriptions, fees, payments, adjustments, and balance due.

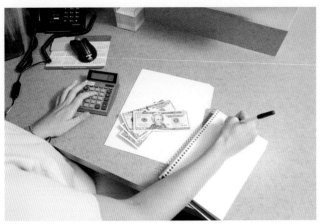

Fig. 4.14 Health care organization employee posting to a patient's financial accounting record or daysheet.

printed. A daysheet, or daily record sheet, is a register for recording daily business transactions. The totals from this can be compared with the encounter forms to ensure that all charges, payments, and adjustments have been properly posted. Also, the daysheet is a useful tool for checks and balances when assessing the bank deposit slip for accuracy.

The paper environment allows transactions to be recorded on the patient ledger cards. All patients seen on one day have their charges (debits) recorded on the daysheet, along with all payments and adjustments (credits). Each day, the totals are carried forward and a new daysheet is set up to receive posting for that day (Fig. 4.14). The patient's ledger card should show an entry of the date an insurance claim is sent, including the date of services that were billed. Each service must be posted on its own line, and a running balance is calculated in the right column. When the ledger is filled, the account balance is carried over to a new card. Step-by-step instructions for completing a ledger card are given in Procedure 4.1, at the end of the chapter.

Step 10: Insurance Claim

Under HIPAA guidelines, health care organizations with more than 25 full-time employees or providers with more than 10 full-time employees must send all claims electronically in the approved format. An insurance billing specialist completes the claim information for all services provided. A claim is submitted by using exact procedural and diagnostic codes, including the use of any appropriate documents such as operative reports or invoices. The claim is then mailed or sent electronically to the correct third-party payer.

The minimum information required by third-party payers is as follows:

- What was done? Services and procedures, using procedure codes and appropriate modifiers
- Why was it done? Diagnoses
- When was it performed? Date of service (DOS)
- Where was it received? Place of service (POS)
- Who did it? Provider name and identifying number

A helpful hint is to group together, or batch, all outstanding charges to the same type of insurance at one time. This cuts down on errors, makes claims easier to track, and, in the

paper environment, makes manual completion of the forms less tedious.

It is preferable to electronically transmit claims as soon as possible after services are rendered. Time limits for filing claims range from 30 days to 1½ years from the DOS. This can vary depending on the commercial carrier, federal or state program, or whether the claim is for an illness or accident. Claims filed after the time limit will be denied and a detailed appeals process may be required to have the claim reconsidered.

Financial losses from delays in processing can occur in some instances. If a patient has had a long-term illness, insurance benefits can expire before a claim is processed. If several providers treat the same patient, some insurance companies pay only one of them. Typically, whoever files the claim first is paid first. In this scenario, the other health care organizations may have to wait for disbursement by the health care organization that received the check. Submit hospitalized patients' insurance claim forms promptly on discharge or on a regular schedule. A good practice is to do this weekly or twice a month, depending on the office protocol and regardless of the discharge date for long-term inpatients.

Patients who pay at time of service and who wish to submit their own insurance claims are given two copies of the encounter form. The patient retains one copy for personal records, attaches the second copy to the insurance claim form, and forwards it to the insurance company.

Step 11: Submitting the Paper Claim

If a paper claim is submitted, a copy of the claim form is placed in the office's pending file or the patient's health record chart, depending on office protocol. The date the claim is mailed is noted on the patient's ledger card and recorded on the insurance claims register. Mail claims in batches to each carrier to save on postage.

Step 12: Transmitting the Electronic Claim

When filing claims electronically, a batch is created and a digital file is stored in a predetermined directory. These files are either transmitted directly to the insurance payer or through a clearinghouse.

Claims are transmitted either electronically as required by HIPAA or, in cases of exemption, on a paper form. When sending paper claims, make a copy for office records and create an insurance claims register or spreadsheet to track and follow up claims. Refer to Fig. 4.15 for the phases of adjudication by the third-party payer for payment, partial payment, denial, or rejection.

Step 13: Provider's Signature

Providers rarely sign the insurance claim form. However, when a signature is required, it can be accepted in several formats—handwritten, facsimile stamp, or electronic signature. An electronic signature is digital data attached to a computerized document as verification of the provider's intent to sign the document. State and government programs require a signature. In the Medicare program, certificates of medical necessity require an original signature.

Electronic claim for services is received by the insurance payer via transmission.	1. Claim for services is received by the insurance payer. If a paper form is submitted, an image is captured (scanned or microfilmed) and/or data is keyed into payer system. Electronic claims are transmitted into administrative system.
Data content checked with common data file procedure code numbers matched to policy benefits.	2. Claim data is electronically checked against payer database to assess common files. Identification and demographics of the patient is cross checked with subscriber identification number and benefits are confirmed. If the patient is not identified, the claim is rejected and a denial is sent to the health care provider.
Procedure and diagnostic codes matched.	3. Procedure code numbers are electronically matched with the policy's master benefits list. A claims processor compares the claim with the policy benefits. Procedure codes are cross-matched with diagnostic code numbers and again compared with policy benefits.
Claim form checked with common data file.	4. The claim form is checked against the common data file.
Allowed or approved amount determined.	5. Determination is made of "allowed or approved" charges. Claims are rejected for a variety of reasons, including that the patient's condition is not covered under the policy benefits, that the number of visits exceeds the allowed amount under the policy, or that the policy has expired.
Deductible amount determined.	6. The patient's deductible amount is determined. This amount is due from the patient and varies according to his or her policy requirements. Most payers require a yearly deductible, e.g., Mary Jones has a $500 yearly deductible. Every January 1, the out-of-pocket expense due from Ms. Jones for the given calendar year must be met in the amount of $500 before the insurance payer will pay the full benefits under the conditions of Mrs. Jones' policy. Medicare's Part B annual deductible is $110.
Copayment determined.	7. Copayment or coinsurance requirement determined. This amount varies (e.g., depending on the subscriber's policy, the insurance payer may require a predetermined copayment at every visit or a percentage due for services after the payer processes and pays on the claim). Patients are usually billed for the balance by a statement sent from the health care provider after insurance reimbursement is received, called balance billing.
Explanation of benefits form generated when adjudication process completed.	8. Explanation of benefits (EOB) or remittance advice form is generated by the software program.
Explanation of benefits and insurance check sent to provider.	9. Explanation of benefits and insurance payment check are mailed to provider by insurance carrier.

Fig. 4.15 Adjudication: Insurance payer life cycle of an insurance claim shows the basic steps of a third-party payer to pay an insurance claim and the documents generated.

Sometimes, a provider gives signature authorization to one person on the staff to sign insurance claims. That person is known as the physician's representative or attorney-in-fact (Fig. 4.16). For an authorization of this type, a document should be signed before a notary public. If the health care organization is ever audited and fraud or embezzlement is discovered, the person who had signature authorization, as well as the provider, can be brought into the case. The federal government will prosecute if this involves a Medicare patient; the state government will prosecute if a Medicaid patient is involved.

There are three levels of computerized or electronic signatures, listed in order of their strength.
- Level 1—digitized signature
- Level 2—button, personal identification number (PIN), biometric, or token
- Level 3—digital signature

An electronic signature looks like the signer's handwritten signature (Fig. 4.17). The signer authenticates the document by key entry or with a pen pad using a stylus to capture the live signature. It also can be defined as an individualized computer access and identification system. Examples are a unique PIN, series of letters, electronic writing, voice, computer key, token, or fingerprint transmission (biometric system).

A digital signature may be lines of text or a text box stating the signer's name, date, and time, as well as a statement indicating that a signature has been attached from within the software application (Fig. 4.18). Level 3 is the strongest signature because it protects the signature by a type of tamper-proof seal that breaks if the message content is altered.

Use of a signature stamp is not recommended. Most insurance carriers have updated signature policies advising

PROVIDER'S NOTARIZED SIGNATURE AUTHORIZATION

State of _____Iowa_____)
)ss
County of _Des Moines_)

Know all persons by these presents:

That I _John Doe, MD_ have made, constituted, and appointed and by these presents do make, constitute and appoint _Mary Coleman_ my true and lawful attorney-in-fact for me and in my name place and stead to sign my name on claims, for payment for services provided by me submitted to the _Blue Cross and Blue Shield of Iowa_, My signature by my said attorney-in-fact includes my agreement to abide by the full payment concept and the remainder of the certification appearing on all _CMS-1500_ claim forms. I hereby ratify and confirm all that my said attorney-in-fact shall lawfully do or cause to be done by virtue of the power generated herein.

In witness whereof I have hereunto set my hand this _20th_ day of _January_ 20 _XX_.

_____John Doe, MD_____
(Signature)

Subscribed and sworn to before me this _20th_ day of _January_ 20 XX _____

_____
Notary Public

My commission expires _____ .

Fig. 4.16 Example of a provider's signature authorization form that can be completed, notarized, and sent to the third-party payer after a copy is retained for the health care organization's records.

Fig. 4.17 Example of a provider's electronic signature.

Electronically signed:
David Smith, MD
07/12/2008 10:30:08

Fig. 4.18 Example of a provider's digital signature. This is an example of the strongest signature authentication.

providers that stamp signatures are no longer acceptable because of misuse or abuse. State laws may require that insurance claims or other related documents have an original signature. Billing specialists must follow state laws regardless of any carrier manual regulations. For information on state laws, contact the state legislature.

! COMPLIANCE ALERT

Use of a signature stamp is not recommended. Most insurance carriers have updated signature policies advising providers that stamp signatures are no longer acceptable because of misuse or abuse.

Step 14: Track Pending Insurance Claims

In the computerized medical billing system, a date is noted each time a claim is generated for submission, whether it is sent electronically or is printed on a paper claim form from the computer. An aging A/R report is used to determine outstanding balances. This can be generated using the date the claim was filed as a point to assess how many days old the claim is. The aging report is used to obtain the total A/R amount. This shows a snapshot of how much money is due to the organization from each patient or insurance carrier.

When submitting paper claims, keep a duplicate of the claim on file. If payment is not received within a predetermined amount of time, the claim must be followed up. This file also may be referred to as a suspense, follow-up, or tickler file. The term *tickler* came into existence because it tickles or jogs the memory at certain dates in the future.

Whether claims are billed electronically or in paper format, a billing specialist should check with the insurance carrier to determine if the company features an online claim-tracking service on its website. This will allow a health care organization to follow up on unpaid claims and to check the status of a claim quickly using the insurance company's website.

Step 15: Insurance Payments

After the claim is processed by the insurance payer, an EOB or remittance advice (RA) is generated and either sent on paper or transmitted electronically to the health care organization. Record of payment or denial of the claim is posted to the patient's financial account.

The payment is posted or credited to the patient's account and current daysheet indicating the date posted, name of insurance company, check or voucher number, amount received, contracted adjustment, and outstanding balance.

In both the electronic and paper environment, there may be claims that are not processed in a timely manner by the insurance payer. To follow up on these, a monthly review of outstanding claims, also known as an unpaid claims report or aged receivables, should be generated to determine further collection activity needed (Fig 4.19).

Step 16: Bank Deposit

The health care organization should receive a payment from the third-party payer within 2 to 8 weeks from claim submission. The payment should accompany the RA sent by the insurance payer. Electronic funds transfer (EFT) may be used in place of a mailed paper check. EFT allows the automatic deposit of funds from the payer to the health care organization's bank account. In either electronic or paper office environments, all checks and cash are entered on the bank deposit slip and deposited at the bank.

Step 17: Monthly Statement

The claim transaction is completed when the claim generated for each date of service has been processed by all responsible parties and the patient's financial account is at zero. For the patient who has insurance, a monthly statement for any outstanding balance should be sent indicating that insurance has been billed and the amount due is the patient's responsibility. The patient statement should always reflect the same fee as that submitted to the insurance company, minus the amount paid by the patient copayment and/or the insurance amount paid or adjusted off. Patients who do not have insurance should receive a monthly statement indicating all outstanding balances due, minus any payments or adjustments applied since the last billing statement.

Some companies offer services to enable patients to pay their bills online securely through the health care organization's website. They also have electronic or eStatements that reduce processing and mailing costs by delivering patient statements securely or leaving balance due reminders. Online bill payment may be set up to automatically draft patients' debit/credit cards. This eliminates checks and postage and speeds up payments.

Step 18: Financial Records Retained

Whether an office is computerized or still operates in a paper-based environment, a health care organization cannot escape the volumes of paperwork that business produces. Financial records must be retained and may include the following (not an all-inclusive list):

Outstanding Claims
Primary Insurance
August 10, 20XX

Billing No.	Patient Name	Primary Insurance	Claim Sent	Bill Balance
1002	Simpson, Teri E	United Western Benefit		47.50
1003	Lee, Michael	United Western Benefit		83.55
1005	Bortolussi, Jabe	ABC Insurance Company	05/25/20XX	465.00
1006	Blackwood, Crystal L	TRICARE	05/25/20XX	16.07
1007	Helms, Clinton A	Medicare Health Systems Corporation	05/25/20XX	33.25
1008	Jameson, Richard D	Royal Pacific Insurance Company	05/25/20XX	41.07
1010	Kelsey, Ron	XYZ Insurance	06/09/20XX	66.23
1011	Simpson, Teri E	United Western Benefit		16.07
1012	Simpson, Teri E	United Western Benefit		40.20
1013	Simpson, Teri E	United Western Benefit		16.07
1014	Simpson, Teri E	United Western Benefit		8.00
1015	Lee, Michael	United Western Benefit		16.07
1016	Lee, Michael	United Western Benefit		28.55
1017	Lee, Michael	United Western Benefit		40.20
1018	Martin, John R	Medicare Health Systems Corporation		149.86
1019	Jameson, Richard D	Royal Pacific Insurance Company		86.42
1020	Nunez, Margaret A	Aetna Health Plan		18.25
Report Count: 17				1172.36

Fig. 4.19 Practice management software screen showing outstanding claims, patients' balances due, and names of insurance companies to follow up on claims.

- Copy of the completed patient information form, patient authorization or signature-on-file for assignment of benefits form, copies of insurance identification cards, responsible-party authorization, and insurance correspondence
- Explanation of benefits or RA documents sent from insurance payers
- Logs of all telephone conversations and actions taken regarding insurance disputes or collection activities. If these notes are not stored in the corresponding patient health record, the health care organization will likely have a master file set up where all logs are kept.
- Encounter forms and referral and authorization slips
- Daysheets and deposit slips

4.6 QUICK REVIEW
Question: What is assignment of benefits?

4.7 QUICK REVIEW
Question: What is the difference between a par and nonpar provider?

4.8 QUICK REVIEW
Question: What are acceptable formats for provider signatures?

KEEPING UP TO DATE

- Make a folder or binder of pertinent insurance information. Obtain information booklets and policy manuals from the local offices of the various insurance companies. Obtain sample copies of all forms required for the insurance plans used most in the health care organization's office. Keep samples of completed claim forms.
- Changes occur daily and monthly, so keep well informed by reading Medicaid, Medicare, TRICARE, and local medical society bulletins. Maintain a chronologic file on each of these bulletins for easy reference, always keeping the latest bulletin on top.
- Attend any workshops on insurance in the health care industry offered in the area. Network with other insurance specialists to compare policies and discuss common problems. The American Association of Medical Assistants (AAMA) and other professional organizations have chapters in many states that feature educational workshops and lectures.
- Become a member of one of the following professional organizations. On a monthly basis, each of these associations distributes journals or newsletters featuring current information.
  - American Academy of Professional Coders (AAPC)
  - American Medical Billing Association (AMBA)
  - Medical Association of Billers (MAB)
  - Medical Group Management Association (MGMA)
  - Healthcare Financial Management Association (HFMA)
  - Healthcare Billing and Management Association (HBMA)
  - Professional Association of Health Care Office Management (PAHCOM)
  - American Health Information Management Association (AHIMA)
- Make good use of the internet.

DISCUSSION POINT
Discuss: What do you feel some of the pros and cons may be of working in an office that does electronic billing over paper billing?

PROCEDURE 4.1 Prepare and Post to a Patient's Financial Accounting Report

Follow these steps to post charges, payments, adjustments, and balances to a patient's ledger/account (see Fig. 4.13).

1. **Personal Data:** Insert the patient's name and address to prepare the ledger card. Some ledgers may require additional information (attending provider's name; type of insurance; insurance company's name with policy and group numbers; patient's home and work telephone numbers; birth date; Social Security number; driver's license number; spouse's and/or dependents' names; and name, address, and telephone number of nearest relative), depending on the style of card chosen for a health care organization.

2. **Date:** Post the date of service (DOS) in the date column, description of the services in the professional service description column, and charge amount in the charge column. The posting date is the actual date that the transaction is recorded. If the DOS differs from the posting date, reference the DOS in the description column. This date column should never be left blank.

3. **Reference:** List a current procedural terminology (CPT) procedure code number in the reference column.

4. **Description:** Write a brief description of the transaction that is being posted, such as *OV* for office visit or *HV* for hospital visit. Indicate the evaluation and management (E/M) service levels (1 through 5) using the last digit of the E/M code (e.g., 9920**5** = Level **5**). List the name of other services or surgical procedures (e.g., electrocardiogram, vaccination, tonsillectomy).

5. **Charges:** Add the charge to the running current balance and enter the current balance in the right column.

6. **Payments:** Post the date the payment is received and indicate received on account (**ROA**) and who made the payment (e.g., patient [pt] or name of insurance company) in the description column. List the type of payment (cash, check, debit card, money order, or credit card) and voucher or check number (e.g., ck #430) in the reference column.

7. **Adjustments:** Post the date the adjustment is being made and indicate the type of adjustment (e.g., insurance plan adj., contract adj., courtesy adj.).

8. **Billing Comments:** Indicate when the insurance company was billed by posting the current date and name of the insurance company. Include the dates of services being billed in the reference column (e.g., 4/20/XX through 5/1/XX). Indicate when the patient statement was sent and amount due if different from the current balance (e.g., patient billed $45.00 balance after insurance payment).

9. **Other Comments:** Indicate other comments that pertain directly to the account (e.g., account sent to ABC Collection Agency, account scheduled for small claims court).

10. **Charges:** Refer to the fee schedule and post each fee (charge) on a separate line in the "Charge" column. Charges are debited (subtracted) from the account balance.

Continued

PROCEDURE 4.1   Prepare and Post to a Patient's Financial Accounting Report—cont'd

11. **Payments:** Enter the amount paid in the "Payment" column, credit (subtract) the payment received from the amount in the running current balance column, and enter the current balance.
12. **Adjustments:** Post the contracted insurance plan discount in the "Adjustment" column by referencing the DOS, insurance company name, and type of contract discount (e.g., HealthNet PPO discount or Medicare courtesy adjustment). Adjustments are credited to the account balance.
13. **Current Balance:** Line by line, credit and debit by adding and subtracting postings to the running balance to determine the amount for the current balance column as shown in Fig. 4.14. If a line is used to indicate a date an action was taken (e.g., insurance company or patient

billed, account sent to collection), bring down the running balance from the previous line. This column must always contain an amount and should never be left blank. *Optional:* Post the adjustment on the same line as the payment.
14. Submit an itemized billing statement to the patient for the balance due.

Date	Description	Charge	Payment	Adjustment	Balance
					1250.00
7-3-XX	ROA Prudential Ins #7421		875.00	250.00	375.00

KEY POINTS

This is a brief chapter review of the key issues presented. To further enhance your knowledge of the technical subject matter, review the key terms and key abbreviations for this chapter by locating the meaning for each in the Glossary at the end of this text, which appears in a section before the Index.

1. An insurance contract is a legal document in which the insured receives coverage that helps offset the cost of medical services. The four concepts of a valid insurance contract follow:
   a. The person must be a mentally competent adult and not under the influence of drugs or alcohol when signing the contract.
   b. The insurance company must make an offer (the signed application) and the person must accept the offer (issuance of the policy) without concealment or misrepresentation of facts on the application.
   c. An exchange of value (the first premium payment) submitted with the application, known as a *consideration,* must be present.
   d. A legal purpose must exist, which is an insurable interest in the case of a health insurance policy. This means that the policyholder expects to continue in good health, but that the insurance policy will provide something of value if an accident or illness strikes.

2. The insurance billing specialist must understand insurance terminology and policy provisions as they relate to billing and claims submission. An implied contract is created by the actions of the persons involved. On the other hand, an expressed contract can be verbal or written. However, most health care organization patient contracts are implied.

3. There are many types of private and federal insurance programs, such as managed care, workers' compensation, Medicare, Medicaid, and TRICARE.

4. An aging accounts receivable report to determine outstanding balances can be generated using the date that the claim was filed as a point to assess how many days old the claim is. This report is used to understand how much money is due to the organization from each patient account.

5. Each type of insurance has different time limits for claims submission; if submitted after the designated time, claims will be denied.

6. Because federal program regulations have ongoing changes and new diagnostic and procedural codes are adopted annually, it is imperative that the insurance billing specialist keep up to date on technical information and have access to current reference books.

INTERNET RESOURCES

Timeline for Health Care Reform
- https://obamacarefacts.com/health-care-reform-timeline

STUDENT ASSIGNMENT

- Study Chapter 4.
- Complete all of the exercises in the *Workbook* to reinforce the theory learned in this chapter.
- Turn to the Glossary at the end of this text for a further understanding of the key terms and key abbreviations used in this chapter.

5

The Blue Plans, Private Insurance, and Managed Care Plans

Linda M. Smith

OBJECTIVES

After reading this chapter, you should be able to:

1. Discuss the difference between a private indemnity insurance plan and a managed care plan.
2. State the provisions of the Health Maintenance Organization Act of 1973.
3. Explain the different types of health maintenance organizations.
4. List features of an exclusive provider organization.
5. Define and discuss provider sponsored organizations.
6. Name the features of preferred provider organizations.
7. Explain the features of a point-of-service plan.
8. Define and discuss consumer directed health plans.
9. Discuss triple-option health plans.
10. State the purpose of utilization management and the techniques used.
11. Define a *carve out* and provide an example.
12. Discuss the patient information letter and its contents.
13. Identify four types of referrals for medical services, tests, and procedures.
14. State the purpose of creating an insurance plan reference guide.
15. Describe types of payment mechanisms used by insurance plans.

KEY TERMS

ancillary services
Blue Cross/Blue Shield Association
capitation
carve-out plans
Chapter 11
coinsurance
collection rate
concurrent review
consumer directed health plan
copayment
deductible
direct contract model HMO
direct referral
disenrollment
exclusive provider organization
fee-for-service
formal referral

gatekeeper
group model HMO
health maintenance organization
indemnity insurance plan
Individual Practice Association (IPA) HMO
managed care
managed care organizations
National Committee for Quality Assurance
network model HMO
out-of-pocket
per capita
per member per month
point-of-service plan
preferred provider organization
prepaid group practice model

primary care provider
private health insurance
provider networks
provider sponsored organization
Retrospective reviews
self-referral
staff model HMO
stop-loss
tertiary care
traditional insurance plan
triple option health plan
usual, customary and reasonable
utilization management
utilization review
verbal referral
withhold

KEY ABBREVIATIONS

BCBSA	FFS	NCQA	PPO
CDHP	HMO	PCP	PSO
copay	IPA	PMPM	UCR
EPO	MCO	POS	UR

INSIGHTS FROM THE FIELD

Nancy T.: Certifed Professional Coder (CPC) and Certified Professional Coding Instructor (CPC-I)

I started working in a physician's office as a teenager. My job was to help with the billing. We used ledger cards which we photocopied to bill to the patient. I worked every high school and college break in various health care positions. During a college fellowship with the New York Senate, I met the Vice President of Blue Shield. Because of my medical billing experience, I was offered a job with Blue Cross Blue Shield where I spent the next 29 years as an insurance specialist and a fraud examiner.

The most valuable skill an insurance billing specialist can have is the willingness to learn.

Every time my employer asked me to take on a new task, I always said yes, as long as they provided me with the training, the books, or material that I needed to learn the job. I learned quickly that once you learn a concept, it is yours. And although the health care environment is ever-changing, the concepts never go away. I worked with great people. Co-workers shared their knowledge with me. I built spreadsheets and kept information organized in notebooks.

You have to be a good technician today. It's not enough to complete a form. You have to be able to get into computer networks and get the information you need. Go to insurance plans' websites and work your way through them. It takes time. Take the time to dig through and to get the most facts.

And even when you think you have learned it all, and you've been doing the job for 20 years, things are going to change.

PRIVATE HEALTH INSURANCE

Private health insurance plans are marketed by the private health insurance industry rather than through government-sponsored programs. Although there are many types of private health insurance plans, they are classified as either traditional fee-for-service plans or managed care plans. We will explore both of these types of private health plans in this chapter.

Most private health insurance companies are publicly traded companies that operate to generate a profit for shareholders, although a smaller percentage operate as nonprofit organizations. Private insurance companies must meet the requirements of the state insurance agency in which they conduct business. Each state has different laws that dictate what services are mandated for coverage by private insurance companies and their obligations to beneficiaries. Private health insurance is generally offered through employers or other organizations. There are numerous private insurance companies across the United States

who typically offer a variety of traditional fee-for-service and managed care plans.

Blue Cross/Blue Shield Plans

Blue Cross/Blue Shield (BCBS) is the oldest private insurance company in the United States. The organization is also one of the largest private insurance companies providing health care coverage to nearly one in three Americans.[1] It was founded in the 1930s as a not-for-profit organization. In 1994 the Blue Cross/Blue Shield Association (BCBSA) petitioned and was allowed to convert their status to for-profit corporations. Often referred to as the "Blues," the Blue Cross plans were developed to cover hospital expenses and the Blue Shield plans were established primarily to cover physician services.

The BCBSA developed into what is now a national association of approximately 36 independent, community-based, and locally operated BCBS companies. Each company is an independent franchise of the BCBSA and they often differ in corporate structure and policies. Each independent company offers local and national programs with several types of plans, including traditional indemnity plans and a broad range of managed care plans. Blue Cross/Blue Shield Companies also offer coverage through federal employee programs (FEPs) and Medicare managed care plans. The BCBSA provides some form of health insurance in every state within the United States, the District of Columbia, and Puerto Rico.

Blue Shield Identification Card

The patient's BCBS identification card provides important information needed for billing purposes. The first step in obtaining the correct information is to identify the BCBSA trademark on the card and then locate the name and address of the BCBS home company that the patient is a member of. The address for claims submission should be identified on the back of the identification card. The BCBS card will also provide the type of plan the patient is enrolled in (for example, traditional, health maintenance organization, preferred provider organization, point-of-service plan; see Fig. 5.1)

Health care organizations should have available for reference the current provider manual for its state's BCBS plans, which should provide the details needed for claim processing. In Fig. 5.2, an example of a completed Blue Shield claim form is

---

[1]Source: https://www.bcbs.com/about-us.

Fig. 5.1 Blue Cross Blue Shield identification card. (A) front of card. (B) Back of card. (Courtesy of Blue Cross and Blue Shield Association.)

DRAFT - NOT FOR OFFICIAL USE

BLUE SHIELD
NO SECONDARY COVERAGE

CARRIER

HEALTH INSURANCE CLAIM FORM

APPROVED BY NATIONAL UNIFOR MCLAIM COMMITTEE (NUCC) 02/12

| | PICA | | | | | | | | PICA | | |

1. MEDICARE (Medicare#) MEDICAID (Medicaid#) TRICARE (ID#DoD#) CHAMPVA (Member ID#) GROUP HEALTH PLAN [X] (ID#) FECA BLK LUNG (ID#) OTHER (ID#)	1a. INSURED'S I.D. NUMBER (For Program in Item 1) 142768100
2. PATIENT'S NAME (Last Name, First Name, Middle Initial) Jones, Ivan, R	3. PATIENT'S BIRTH DATE 07 01 1945 SEX M [X] F	4. INSURED'S NAME (Last Name, First Name, Middle Initial) Jones, Ivan, R
5. PATIENT'S ADDRESS (No., Street) 27 Hill Avenue	6. PATIENT RELATIONSHIP TO INSURED Self [X] Spouse Child Other	7. INSURED'S ADDRESS (No., Street)
CITY Woodland Hills STATE XY	8. RESERVED FOR NUCC USE	CITY STATE
ZIP CODE 123450000 TELEPHONE (Include Area Code) ( )		ZIP CODE TELEPHONE (Include Area Code) ( )

PATIENT AND INSURED INFORMATION

9. OTHER INSURED'S NAME (Last Name, First Name, Middle Initial)	10. IS PATIENT'S CONDITION RELATED TO:	11. INSURED'S POLICY GROUP OR FECA NUMBER A563
a. OTHER INSURED'S POLICY OR GROUP NUMBER	a. EMPLOYMENT? (Current or Previous) YES [X] NO	a. INSURED'S DATE OF BIRTH MM DD YY SEX M F
b. RESERVED FOR NUCC USE	b. AUTO ACCIDENT? YES [X] NO PLACE (State)	b. OTHER CLAIM ID (Designated by NUCC)
c. RESERVED FOR NUCC USE	c. OTHER ACCIDENT? YES [X] NO	c. INSURANCE PLAN NAME OR PROGRAM NAME Blue Shield
d. INSURANCE PLAN NAME OR PROGRAM NAME	10d. CLAIM CODES (Designated by NUCC)	d. IS THERE ANOTHER HEALTH BENEFIT PLAN? YES [X] NO If yes, complete items 9, 9a, and 9d.

READ BACK OF FORM BEFORE COMPLETING & SIGNING THIS FORM.

12. PATIENT'S OR AUTHORIZED PERSON'S SIGNATURE I authorize the release of any medical or other information necessary to process this claim. I also request payment of government benefits either to myself or to the party who accepts assignment below.

SIGNED Signature on file   DATE

13. INSURED'S OR AUTHORIZED PERSON'S SIGNATURE I authorize payment of medical benefits to the undersigned physician or supplier for services described below.

SIGNED Signature on file

14. DATE OF CURRENT: ILLNESS, INJURY, or PREGNANCY(LMP) 08 04 20XX QUAL. 431	15. OTHER DATE QUAL. MM DD YY	16. DATES PATIENT UNABLE TO WORK IN CURRENT OCCUPATION FROM MM DD YY TO MM DD YY
17. NAME OF REFERRING PROVIDER OR OTHER SOURCE DN Perry Cardi MD	17a. 17b. NPI 67805027XX	18. HOSPITALIZATION DATES RELATED TO CURRENT SERVICES FROM MM DD YY TO MM DD YY
19. ADDITIONAL CLAIM INFORMATION (Designated by NUCC)		20. OUTSIDE LAB? YES [X] NO $ CHARGES

21. DIAGNOSIS OR NATURE OF ILLNESS OR INJURY Relate A-L to service line below (24E)   ICD Ind. 0

A. N401   B.   C.   D.
E.   F.   G.   H.
I.   J.   K.   L.

22. RESUBMISSION CODE   ORIGINAL REF. NO.

23. PRIOR AUTHORIZATION NUMBER

24. A. DATE(S) OF SERVICE From MM DD YY To MM DD YY	B. PLACE OF SERVICE	C. EMG	D. PROCEDURES, SERVICES, OR SUPPLIES (Explain Unusual Circumstances) CPT/HCPCS MODIFIER	E. DIAGNOSIS POINTER	F. $ CHARGES	G. DAYS OR UNITS	H. EPSDT Family Plan	I. ID. QUAL.	J. RENDERING PROVIDER ID. #
1	08 07 XX	11		99213	A	90 00	1		NPI	1245897700
2									NPI	
3									NPI	
4									NPI	
5									NPI	
6									NPI	

PHYSICIAN OR SUPPLIER INFORMATION

25. FEDERAL TAX I.D. NUMBER SSN EIN XX12210XX [X]	26. PATIENT'S ACCOUNT NO. 0721	27. ACCEPT ASSIGNMENT? (For govt. claims, see back) [X] YES NO	28. TOTAL CHARGE $ 90 00	29. AMOUNT PAID $	30. Rsvd for NUCC Use
31. SIGNATURE OF PHYSICIAN OR SUPPLIER INCLUDING DEGREES OR CREDENTIALS (I certify that the statements on the reverse apply to this bill and are made a part thereof.) Concha Antrum MD 030320XX SIGNED Concha Antrum MD DATE	32. SERVICE FACILITY LOCATION INFORMATION a. NPI b.	33. BILLING PROVIDER INFO & PH # (555) 4869002 College Clinic 4567 Broad Avenue Woodland Hills XY 123450001 a. 3664021CC b.

NUCC Instruction Manual available at: www.nucc.org   PLEASE PRINT OR TYPE   OMB APPROVAL PENDING

Fig. 5.2 A completed Blue Shield claim form.

provided. Further guidance for completion of a CMS 1500 claim form for a Blue Shield patient will be explained in Chapter 14 of this textbook. Note the following information included on the claim form:

- The name of the insurance carrier the claim is being prepared for is identified in the top right-hand corner of the form.
- In box #1, Group Health Plan has been checked to identify this patient has Blue Shield (a private insurance).
- In box #1a., the patient's Blue Shield identification number has been entered.
- In box #11, the patient's group policy number has been entered.
- In box #27, the accept assignment box has been checked "yes" to indicate that the provider accepts assignment.

Fee-for-Service Plans

Until the early 1970s, most private health insurance companies offered only fee-for-service (FFS) plans. These are also referred to as traditional insurance plans or indemnity insurance plans. In an FFS plan, the insured pays a fixed monthly premium. The insured may obtain care from any health care organization and the organization is paid each time a service is rendered. The insured must meet an annual deductible. A deductible is a specific dollar amount that the patient must pay before an insurance plan begins covering health care costs. Once the annual deductible has been met, the insurance company will pay a percentage of the covered benefits. The remaining percentage is then paid by the insured; this is referred to as the coinsurance amount.

Generally speaking, fee-for-service plans offer more flexibility. However, patients usually pay higher premiums and there are usually more out-of-pocket expenses to the patient. Out-of-pocket expenses are those that the patient is responsible for paying. Payments to health care providers are usually based on usual, customary, and reasonable (UCR) rates that are set by the insurance carrier. The UCR is the amount that the insurance company will pay for a specific disease, illness, or medical problem.

5.1   QUICK REVIEW

Question: What types of insurance plans does the BCBSA offer?

MANAGED CARE

Through the 1960s and into the early 1970s, the financing and delivery of health care began to gain governmental attention. In an attempt to restrain the growth of health care costs for US citizens, legislators started to take notice of a model of health care coverage that used a managed care approach. Managed care refers to a group of techniques intended to reduce the cost of providing health care while improving the access to care and the quality of care. Managed care plans are a type of health insurance in which the plan contracts with health care providers and medical facilities to offer services to patients in their plan at a reduced cost. The contracted providers make up

the plans' network and the plans' rules determine how much of the patients' care the plan will pay for. Plans with the greatest restrictions, such as which providers the patient can see, usually cost less. Plans that offer greater flexibility to the patient typically cost more.

One of the earliest forms of managed care were prepaid group practice models. In these plans, the insurance carrier contracts with a network of providers to offer services to patients in advance for a full range of health services the patients in their plan are entitled to. US legislators noticed this type of plan initiated in 1929 by two Los Angeles physicians, Donald Ross and Clifford Loos, who entered into a prepaid contract to provide comprehensive health services to 2000 employees of a local water company. Ross-Loos is now known as the *CIGNA Health Insurance Corporation.*

Another pioneer of the prepaid model of health care is the Kaiser Foundation Health Plans, which were started in 1937. The Kaiser construction company requested that Dr. Sidney R. Garfield and a few physicians working for him provide medical care for workers who were building a fresh-water aqueduct across the California desert to Los Angeles. Dr. Garfield charged the insurance carriers $1.50 per worker per month and the workers 5 cents per day. In return, he provided comprehensive health care. Then, in 1938, Henry J. Kaiser and his son, Edgar, started a joint venture to complete the Grand Coulee Dam in Washington and invited Dr. Garfield to form a medical group to furnish care to the workers for 7 cents per day prepaid by the employer. The group expanded to include the workers' wives and children. Currently, Kaiser Permanente is one of the nation's largest not-for-profit private health plans.[2]

Health Maintenance Organization Act of 1973

A health maintenance organization (HMO) is a type of managed care plan that provides coverage of health services for a prepaid, fixed annual fee. In an HMO, enrollees of the plan must seek services through a panel of providers who are members of the HMO network. The term "health maintenance organization" originated in the 1970s by a policy advisor to the federal government on medical care whose name was Paul Ellwood. The term became institutionalized when Congress passed the Health Maintenance Organization Act of 1973 (Public Law 93-222), which began the movement to managed care in the United States. The emphasis of the movement was to do away with the FFS system, which rewarded health care providers for providing more services rather than for providing the appropriate services.

The Health Maintenance Organization Act gave the federal government authority to assist HMO development in several ways, including (1) providing grants, loans, and loan guarantees to offset the initial operating deficits of new HMOs that meet federal standards and (2) requiring most employers to offer an HMO to their employees as an alternative to traditional health insurance. Benefits under the HMO Act fall under two categories, basic and supplemental health service, and are listed in Box 5.1.

Over the past 20 years, managed care has evolved from the early prepaid models and HMOs into many different types of

---

[2]Source: https://about.kaiserpermanente.org/who-we-are/fast-facts.

BOX 5.1   Health Maintenance Organization Act Benefits of 1973

Basic Health Services

- Alcohol, drug abuse, and addiction medical treatment
- Dental services (preventive) for children younger than age 12 years
- Diagnostic laboratory, x-ray, and therapeutic radiology services
- Emergency health services in or out of the health maintenance organization (HMO) service area
- Family planning and infertility services
- Health education and medical social services
- Home health services
- Hospital services (inpatient and outpatient)
- Mental health services on an outpatient basis, short-term (not to exceed 20 encounters) ambulatory, evaluative, and crisis intervention
- Health care services and consultant or referral services without time or cost limits
- Preventive health services (for example, physical examinations for adults, vision and hearing tests for children through age 17 years, well-baby care, immunizations, health education)

Supplemental Health Services

- Dental care not included in basic benefits
- Extended mental health services not included in basic benefits
- Eye examinations for adults
- Intermediate and long-term care (nursing facilities and nursing homes)
- Prescription drugs
- Rehabilitative services and long-term physical medicine (for example, physical therapy)

plans. Managed care has become the predominant form of health care in most parts of the United States.[3] **Managed care organization (MCO)** is a generic term applied to various types of managed care plans. Although often criticized by disgruntled patients and consumer-advocacy groups, MCOs are credited with keeping down medical costs by reducing unnecessary hospitalizations, forcing providers to discount their rates, and causing the health care industry to become more efficient and competitive. Critics of managed care claim that managed care plans control costs by denying medically necessary services to patients, even in life-threatening situations, or by providing low-quality care. The criticism has led many states to pass laws mandating managed care standards.

Accreditation

The **National Committee for Quality Assurance (NCQA)** is a not-for-profit organization that accredits managed care health plans. NCQA has built a rigorous set of standards to which health plans must attest and adhere. Health plans are evaluated on the quality of care patients receive, how happy patients are with their care, and health plans' efforts to keep improving. Receiving a seal of approval means that the health plan has met all key elements required by state and federal laws allowing them to participate in managed care programs. NCQA is the most comprehensive evaluation in the industry and the only assessment that bases results of clinical performance and consumer experience.

[3]Source: https://www.ncsl.org/.

Participating Providers

In managed care plans, a **preferred provider** is a participating health care provider or organization that has contracted with the plan to provide medical services to plan members. The managed care will reimburse participating providers at a negotiated fee. When plan members see participating providers, they typically have lower out-of-pocket expenses. A non-participating provider refers to a health care organization that has not contracted with a managed care plan to provide medical services to plan members.

Participating hospitals, physicians, and other health care providers come together in various types of structures to form an organized and comprehensive system of care that managed care plans can offer to their members. These groups are referred to as *provider networks*.

Primary Care Provider

Most managed care plans use a **primary care provider (PCP)** as a gatekeeper. A **gatekeeper** is a health care practitioner who controls patient access to specialists and diagnostic testing services. PCPs are most often doctors; however, some managed care plans allow physician assistants or nurse practitioners to serve as PCPs. PCPs generally practice in the fields of internal medicine, family practice, general practice, or pediatrics.

Identification Card

Each enrollee of a managed care plan is given an identification card. To see an example of a card from this type of plan, refer to Fig. 5.3. The card usually lists the patient's name, member

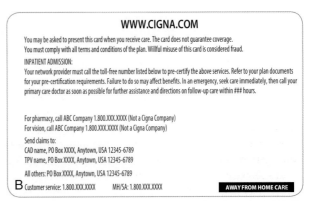

Fig. 5.3 Managed Care insurance identification card. (A) Front of card. (B) Back of card.

number, group number, and primary care provider's name. The name of the MCO and type of plan with the amount of copayment for various outpatient services (for example, office encounter, emergency department, urgent care center, and pharmacy) may be included by some plans.

Both sides of the patient's card should be photocopied because they contain important information such as the insurance companies' address and telephone numbers used for inquiries and authorizations.

 5.2   QUICK REVIEW
Question: What is a managed care plan?

MANAGED CARE SYSTEMS

Managed care systems all have a network of physicians, hospitals, and other health care providers they contract with to provide services to their plan members at the lowest possible cost. However, not all managed care plans are alike. Some of the main differences in managed care plans are typically related to:

- **Contractual structures**. Managed care plans often operate differently, based on how they have contracted with health care professionals and health care organizations to offer services. In some cases, the health care providers are employed by the MCO, and in others they are private health care organizations in contract with the MCO.
- **Premium costs to the patient**. Some plans offer affordable, low-cost premiums with limited flexibility and limited coverage. Higher premium plans offer greater flexibility to health care services with fewer restrictions to the patient and expanded coverage.
- **Choice of health care providers**. Some plans will allow patients to only see providers in their network. Other plans allow patients to see out-of-network providers with more out-of-pocket costs to the patient.
- **Gatekeepers**: Some plans require patients to use gatekeepers for all referrals while others allow the patient to bypass gatekeepers to see specialists.
- **Cost containment measures**. Some plans may incorporate cost containment measures such as precertification for diagnostic testing, hospital admissions, hospital stays, and second surgical opinion, whereas others may not.
- **Out-of-pocket expense to patients**. Expense to patients in the form of copayments and coinsurance varies from plan to plan. The amount of out-of-pocket expense is typically dependent upon premium cost and choice of health care providers.
- **Method of reimbursement**. Although all plans contract with health care organizations and negotiate fees, the methods of reimbursement may differ. Some will reimburse using a prepaid method of reimbursement, while others will reimburse on an FFS basis. Some plans also offer different types of incentive payments to participating health care organizations. The various methods of reimbursement are outlined later in the chapter.

Some of the most common types of managed care plans are defined in this section.

Health Maintenance Organizations

A HMO is a managed care plan or program that offers comprehensive medical services to its members in a particular geographic area, usually in return for a fixed or prepaid fee. There are five different HMO models. How the HMO is structured influences the way health care organizations deliver services. The five models of HMOs are listed in the Table 5.1.

Preferred Provider Organizations

A preferred provider organization (PPO) is another common type of managed care plan. A PPO contracts with a group of providers (designated as "preferred") to deliver care to members. PPO members have the freedom to choose any health care provider or hospital for services, but they receive a higher level of benefits if the preferred providers are used. There are usually coinsurance requirements and deductibles. Occasionally the PPOs pay 100% of the cost of care but most do not. As with major medical policies, coinsurance requires the patient to pay 20% to 25% of the allowed amount up to a certain point and then the PPO pays 80% to 100% of the balance. Predetermination of benefits may be required, as well as fee limits, quality control, and utilization review (UR).

Exclusive Provider Organizations

An exclusive provider organization (EPO) is a type of managed care plan that combines features of HMOs (e.g, enrolled population, limited provider panel, gatekeepers, utilization management, capitated provider reimbursement, and authorization system) and PPOs (for example, flexible benefit design, negotiated fees, and FFS payments). It is referred to as exclusive because employers agree not to contract with any other plan. The member must choose medical care from network providers with certain exceptions for emergency or out-of-area services. If a patient decides to seek care outside the network, generally he or she is not reimbursed for the cost of the treatment. Technically, many HMOs can be considered EPOs. However, EPOs are regulated under insurance statutes rather than federal and state HMO regulations.

Point-of-Service Plans

The typical point-of-service (POS) plan combines elements of an HMO and a PPO while offering some unique features. It is basically an HMO consisting of a network of health care professionals and hospitals that provides an insurance company or an employer with discounts on its services. In a POS program, members choose a PCP who manages specialty care and referrals. A POS plan allows the covered individual to choose services from a participating or nonparticipating provider with different benefit levels. The POS program pays members a higher level of benefits when they use network providers. The member may use providers outside the network, but higher deductibles and coinsurance percentages for out-of-network services act as incentives for members to stay within the network.

TABLE 5.1   Health Maintenance Organization Models

Model	Contractual Structure	Reimbursement Structure
Group Model HMO	The HMO contracts with a multi-specialty medical group practice to provide all types of health care services to its members. The group practice may work exclusively with the HMO, or it may provide services to non-HMO patients as well. The health care providers are employed by the group practice and not by the HMO.	The HMO pays the medical group a negotiated, per capita (per person) amount for each patient enrolled over a stated period. It is up to the group to then distribute payment among its health care providers.
Staff Model HMO	The HMO employs the health care providers to furnish services to its members. Health care providers see patients in their own facilities. The HMO must employ health care providers of various specialties to meet the needs of their members.	Health care providers are usually paid on a salary basis and may also receive bonus or incentive payments based on their productivity and performance.
Network Model HMO	The HMO contracts with two or more health care organizations to provide health services. These health care organizations may be broad-based, multispecialty groups or several small groups of primary care and specialty providers.	Health care providers in the network are usually paid using a capitation method of payment. Capitation is a payment system used by managed care plans in which health care providers and hospitals are paid a fixed per capita (per person) amount for each patient enrolled over a stated period. The provider of services is paid a capitation amount for each HMO patient, regardless of whether the patient is actually seen by the service provider in any given month.
Individual Practice Association (IPA) HMO	The HMO contracts with a group of independent practicing health care providers, referred to as an Individual Practice Association (IPA). The IPA is a separate legal entity. The IPA contract allows health care providers to remain independent and in their own separate offices. The health care providers are allowed to treat both HMO and non-HMO patients. Health care providers are not employees of the IPA and are not paid salaries.	Health care providers are paid for their services on a capitation or FFS basis. Services are paid out of a fund drawn from the premiums collected from the subscriber, union, or corporation by an organization that markets the health plan. The IPA usually withholds a portion of the capitation to cover operating costs for risk sharing and incentive purposes.
Direct Contract Model HMO	The HMO contacts directly with private health care providers in the community to furnish services to their members. A broad panel of service providers, including primary care and specialty providers are recruited.	Service providers are generally compensated on either an FFS basis or a capitation basis.

The POS plan may also provide nonparticipating benefits through a supplemental major medical policy. The key advantage of POS programs is the combination of HMO-style cost management and PPO-style freedom of choice.

Triple-Option Health Plans

Triple-option health plans allow members to select from three choices: HMOs, PPOs, or "traditional" indemnity insurance. Some of these plans allow the employee to change plans more often than traditional arrangements. They incorporate cost containment measures, such as precertification for hospital admission, hospital stays, and second surgical opinions.

Provider-Sponsored Organization

A provider-sponsored organization (PSO) is a managed care plan that is owned and operated by a health system, physicians group, or hospital instead of an insurance company. PSOs are gaining in popularity and growing in number. Many health systems are developing strategies to establish or expand their own health plans. They represent a move away from traditional FFS care to value-based care.

Consumer Directed Health Plans

Consumer directed health plans (CDHPs), also known as high-deductible plans (HDPs), are becoming more common as employers and individuals look for more economical health

insurance options. CDHPs shift more of the payment responsibility to the plan member by requiring a large deductible that the family or patient is financially responsible for. Once the deductible is met, the insurance benefits will kick in.

Claim Forms

MCOs will provide health care organizations with provider manuals that will outline their specific requirements for claims processing. An example of a managed care claim form is provided in Fig. 5.4 Further guidance for completion of a CMS 1500 claim form for a managed care patient will be explained in Chapter 14 of this textbook. Note the following information included on the claim form:

- The name of the insurance carrier the claim is being prepared for is identified in the top right-hand corner of the form.
- In box #1, Group Health Plan has been checked to identify this patient has a managed care plan (a private insurance).
- In box #1a., the insured's managed care identification number has been entered.
- In box #4, the name of the insured is entered. Note that it is the spouse of the patient who received services.
- In box #11, the insured's group policy number has been entered.
- In box #27, the accept assignment box has been checked "yes" to indicate that the provider accepts assignment.

ABC Managed Care
NO SECONDARY COVERAGE

DRAFT - NOT FOR OFFICIAL USE

HEALTH INSURANCE CLAIM FORM

APPROVED BY NATIONAL UNIFOR MCLAIM COMMITTEE (NUCC) 02/12

| | | PICA | | | | | | | PICA | | |

1. MEDICARE	MEDICAID	TRICARE	CHAMPVA	GROUP HEALTH PLAN	FECA BLK LUNG	OTHER	1a. INSURED'S I.D. NUMBER (For Program in Item 1)
☐ (Medicare#)	☐ (Medicaid#)	☐ (ID#DoD#)	☐ (Member ID#)	☒ (ID#)	☐ (ID#)	☐ (ID#)	142867

2. PATIENT'S NAME (Last Name, First Name, Middle Initial)	3. PATIENT'S BIRTH DATE	SEX	4. INSURED'S NAME (Last Name, First Name, Middle Initial)
Short, Mary, S	MM 06 DD 26 YY 1953	M ☐ F ☒	Short, Thomas, A

5. PATIENT'S ADDRESS (No., Street)	6. PATIENT RELATIONSHIP TO INSURED	7. INSURED'S ADDRESS (No., Street)
16 Apple Lane	Self ☐ Spouse ☒ Child ☐ Other ☐	16 Apple Lane

CITY	STATE	8. RESERVED FOR NUCC USE	CITY	STATE
Woodland Hills	XY		Woodland Hills	XY

ZIP CODE	TELEPHONE (Include Area Code)		ZIP CODE	TELEPHONE (Include Area Code)
123450000	( )		123450000	( )

9. OTHER INSURED'S NAME (Last Name, First Name, Middle Initial)	10. IS PATIENT'S CONDITION RELATED TO:	11. INSURED'S POLICY GROUP OR FECA NUMBER
		781000

a. OTHER INSURED'S POLICY OR GROUP NUMBER	a. EMPLOYMENT? (Current or Previous)	a. INSURED'S DATE OF BIRTH	SEX
	☐ YES ☒ NO	MM 11 DD 10 YY 1952	M ☒ F ☐

b. RESERVED FOR NUCC USE	b. AUTO ACCIDENT? PLACE (State)	b. OTHER CLAIM ID (Designated by NUCC)
	☐ YES ☒ NO	

c. RESERVED FOR NUCC USE	c. OTHER ACCIDENT?	c. INSURANCE PLAN NAME OR PROGRAM NAME
	☐ YES ☒ NO	ABC Managed Care

d. INSURANCE PLAN NAME OR PROGRAM NAME	10d. CLAIM CODES (Designated by NUCC)	d. IS THERE ANOTHER HEALTH BENEFIT PLAN?
		☐ YES ☒ NO If yes, complete items 9, 9a, and 9d.

READ BACK OF FORM BEFORE COMPLETING & SIGNING THIS FORM.

12. PATIENT'S OR AUTHORIZED PERSON'S SIGNATURE I authorize the release of any medical or other information necessary to process this claim. I also request payment of government benefits either to myself or to the party who accepts assignment below.

SIGNED Signature on file   DATE _____

13. INSURED'S OR AUTHORIZED PERSON'S SIGNATURE I authorize payment of medical benefits to the undersigned physician or supplier for services described below.

SIGNED Signature on file

14. DATE OF CURRENT: ILLNESS, INJURY, or PREGNANCY(LMP)	15. OTHER DATE	16. DATES PATIENT UNABLE TO WORK IN CURRENT OCCUPATION
MM 01 DD 07 YY 20XX QUAL. 431	QUAL.	MM DD YY FROM TO MM DD YY

17. NAME OF REFERRING PROVIDER OR OTHER SOURCE	17a.	18. HOSPITALIZATION DATES RELATED TO CURRENT SERVICES
DN Perry Cardi MD	17b. NPI 67805027XX	MM DD YY FROM TO MM DD YY

19. ADDITIONAL CLAIM INFORMATION (Designated by NUCC)

20. OUTSIDE LAB?	$ CHARGES
☐ YES ☒ NO	

21. DIAGNOSIS OR NATURE OF ILLNESS OR INJURY Relate A-L to service line below (24E)   ICD Ind. 0

A. J180   B. _____   C. _____   D. _____
E. _____   F. _____   G. _____   H. _____
I. _____   J. _____   K. _____   L. _____

22. RESUBMISSION CODE	ORIGINAL REF. NO.

23. PRIOR AUTHORIZATION NUMBER

24. A. DATE(S) OF SERVICE From MM DD YY To MM DD YY	B. PLACE OF SERVICE	C. EMG	D. PROCEDURES, SERVICES, OR SUPPLIES (Explain Unusual Circumstances) CPT/HCPCS MODIFIER	E. DIAGNOSIS POINTER	F. $ CHARGES	G. DAYS OR UNITS	H. EPSDT Family Plan	I. ID. QUAL.	J. RENDERING PROVIDER ID. #
1	01 09 XX		11		99203	A	120 00	1		NPI	1245897700
2										NPI	
3										NPI	
4										NPI	
5										NPI	
6										NPI	

25. FEDERAL TAX I.D. NUMBER	SSN EIN	26. PATIENT'S ACCOUNT NO.	27. ACCEPT ASSIGNMENT? (For govt. claims, see back)	28. TOTAL CHARGE	29. AMOUNT PAID	30. Rsvd for NUCC Use
XX12210XX	☐ ☒		☒ YES ☐ NO	$ 120 00	$	$

31. SIGNATURE OF PHYSICIAN OR SUPPLIER INCLUDING DEGREES OR CREDENTIALS (I certify that the statements on the reverse apply to this bill and are made a part thereof.)

Concha Antrum MD   030320XX

SIGNED Concha Antrum MD DATE

32. SERVICE FACILITY LOCATION INFORMATION	33. BILLING PROVIDER INFO & PH # (555) 4869002
	8461 College Clinic
	4567 Broad Avenue
	Woodland Hills XY 123450001
a. NPI b.	a. 3664021CC b.

NUCC Instruction Manual available at: www.nucc.org   PLEASE PRINT OR TYPE   OMB APPROVAL PENDING

Fig. 5.4 A completed managed care claim form.

UTILIZATION MANAGEMENT

Utilization management, also referred to as utilization review (UR), is a set of techniques used by managed care plans to control health care costs. Utilization management is performed thorough case-by-case assessments of the appropriateness of care and medical necessity of health care services according to evidence-based criteria or guidelines. The managed care plans' UR committee watches over how health care organizations use medical care resources. Ideally, utilization management should help the patient get the best care at the best price in the best setting.

Preauthorization

One utilization management technique used by MCOs is a preauthorization process to review a request for medical treatment. The MCO will confirm that the patient's plan provides coverage for the services prior to treatment. The MCO uses their predetermined guidelines of care for any given condition to determine if the patient's condition qualifies for the service requested. For example, an MCO might require preauthorization for a patient to have a magnetic resonance image (MRI) of the brain for a particular condition. This is an expensive diagnostic testing that is only performed when it is medically necessary. If preauthorization of the medical care, tests, or procedures is denied, the patient must be informed of the denial, the cost for the service, and their obligation to pay before obtaining the service. If the patient decides they cannot afford the cost for the service, they should also be counseled on their rights to receive the service and the risks associated with not having it.

Concurrent Reviews

Concurrent reviews are another technique used to approve treatment or services during *active* management of the condition. The purpose of the review is to ensure the patient is getting the appropriate care timely and cost-effectively. Hospital systems may use concurrent reviews to assess hospital length of stay and keep patients in the hospital no longer than necessary. It would be further utilized to manage the patient who is discharged from a hospital stay and setting up an appropriate rehabilitation plan, home health, or transfer to another type of health care facility.

Retrospective Reviews

Retrospective reviews are another UR technique. Retrospective reviews look at services that were already provided and compare them with treatment guidelines. Review of past cases by various health care providers oftentimes results in revisions to treatment guidelines to ensure care is adequate and medically current for the condition. Retrospective reviews are also

performed when a treatment that is normally preauthorized was done without approval. For example, the patient may have been unresponsive, and the provider was unable to obtain preauthorization of the service.

> **! COMPLIANCE ALERT**
>
> **Right to Audit Records**
> Many insurance contracts contain a clause stating "for quality care purposes, the insurance carrier or MCO has a right to access the health records of their patients and for utilization management purposes." They have the right to audit those patients' financial records that relate only to the medical services provided to the member by the health care provider.

MANAGEMENT OF INSURANCE PLANS

Contracts

An insurance billing specialist may be involved in negotiating contracts with private insurance and managed care companies. The health care organization must consider the financial implications that a contract with a private insurance company or an MCO will have on the organization's total revenue stream. Negotiated contracts should also have provisions that will lead to a positive working relationship with the payer, provide quality improvement strategies within the organization, and result in a higher level of patient satisfaction.

Although reimbursement is the key to finalizing most contracts, there are requirements in the billing process that should not be overlooked. The contract should identify the following:

- Authorization process for treatment
- Time limit for submitting claims and appealing denied claims
- How responsive the payer will be for processing claims and interest paid for overdue payment
- Process for adding new service lines
- Credentialing process for new health care providers
- Access to payer policies for all procedures
- How new policies and procedures imposed by the carrier will be communicated
- Noncovered services, excluded benefits, and carve-out plans

Carve-out plans refer to health insurance contracts that exclude specific diseases or injuries from coverage. For example, mental health services and chiropractic care are commonly carved out from coverage provided by an insurance plan. In those situations, mental health or chiropractic services are provided through a separately purchased contract at a higher premium. The insurance carrier may require that a specific group of health care providers be seen for related conditions and services that are usually reimbursed according to a different arrangement or rate formula than those services specified under the primary insurance contract.

Patient Information Letter

Patients should be informed of what is expected from them and in turn, what they can expect from the health care organization or provider. The patient information letter should outline the names of the insurance plans that the health care organization is currently participating in and outline any possible restrictions, noncovered items, and expectations for collection of deductibles, copayment, or coinsurance amounts. Note that if the patient neglects to notify the office of any change in eligibility status in the plan, such as **disenrollment**, the patient is then held personally responsible for the bill. It is also important to post a sign in the waiting room advising patients to check with the receptionist about participating plans. Fig. 5.5 shows a sample letter of appropriate wording and content. File a copy of the letter given to the patient in the patient's medical record. If the patient refuses to agree with private insurance or managed care policy, document this in the medical record. Reimbursement may depend on the documentation.

Scheduling Appointments

Screen patients when they call for appointments to determine whether they belong to a health plan that the health care organization is participating with. Keep on hand an alphabetic list and profile of all plans with which the health care organization has a signed contract. If the patient is not in a participating plan, let the patient know and suggest that he or she locate a participating health care provider. If the patient still wishes to schedule services, advise them of the organization's policy for billing of nonparticipating insurances. Most organizations will require payment at time of service if the provider of services does not participate with their insurance.

Verification of Benefits

Verification of the patient's plan and coverage is an important step in managing all types of insurance plans. Verifying benefits and claim submissions requirements can eliminate confusion between the health care provider and the patient. It can also reduce the number of delayed or unpaid claims.

Verification should be done prior to the patient being treated. The most important step in the insurance verification process is to look at the patient's insurance card and confirm the insurance carriers' name and the type of plan (PPO, EPO, FFS) the patient is enrolled in. Insurance cards should always be copied on both sides and maintained in the patient's financial records.

Contact the insurance plan to confirm eligibility and plan benefits. Typically, insurance carrier phone numbers are located on the back side of the card. Payers also have websites that enrolled providers can use to verify benefits and eligibility. Verification should include:

COLLEGE CLINIC
1400 Avon Road, Suite 200
Woodland Hills, XY 12345

January 1, 20XX

TO: OUR PATIENTS

RE: PREFERRED PROVIDER ORGANIZATIONS

The following is a list of the PPOs and health insurance plans that we are members of and, therefore, will bill for you:

1. Georgia County Foundation
2. VIP Health Plan
3. Blue Cross Prudent Buyer Plan
4. Georgia County PPO
5. Northwest PPO
6. Blue Shield PPO

We are participating providers in several different PPOs. In order that we may maintain proper records for referrals and/or hospitalization, we request that each patient who is enrolled in a specific PPO keep our office currently informed regarding his or her eligibility status in that plan. Each time you are in the office for a visit, please verify with the receptionist that we have the correct coverage information.

If you have not informed us of changes in the status of your eligibility within the plan, you will be held responsible for any outstanding balance on your account due to that change.

Additionally, when your physician feels it is necessary to either hospitalize you or refer you to another physician outside this group, it is your responsibility to inform your physician that you belong to a specific PPO, as there may be restrictions imposed by that PPO regarding admission and referrals. If you fail to inform your physician at the time of referral or admission, our group may not be held responsible for noncoverage charges due to these restrictions.

If you have any questions regarding the above, please ask to speak to our insurance specialist.

I have read and understand the above text.

Signed: _____ Date: _____
          Patient (subscriber)

Fig. 5.5 Letter to preferred provider organization *(PPO)* subscribers outlining restrictions and noncovered services.

- Insurance name, phone number, and claims address
- Insurance ID and group number
- Name of insured
- Relationship of the insured to the patient
- Effective date for the policy
- Confirm active coverage in the plan for the date services will be provided.
- Confirm whether the insurance covers the procedure, diagnosis, or services to be provided.
- Confirm that your health care organization participates with the plan.
- Identify any limitations of the policy, including exclusions or documentation requirements for bills.
- Determine whether a referral or prior approval is necessary for the services to be provided.

- Confirm any remaining deductibles, coinsurance responsibility, and applicable copays.

Having a solid insurance verification process in place will make medical billing practices for all insurance plans more efficient and more successful.

Referrals and Prior Approval

Many insurance plans require prior approval or preauthorization for certain services or referral of a patient to see a specialist. The following are several types of referrals that a plan may use.

- **Formal referral.** An authorization request is required by the MCO contract to determine if referral is medically necessary. This may be obtained via telephone or a completed authorization form (Fig. 5.6) mailed or transmitted by fax or e-mail.

College Clinic
4567 Broad Avenue
Woodland Hills, XY 12345-0001
Telephone: (555) 486-9002
Fax: (555) 487-8976

MANAGED CARE PLAN AUTHORIZATION REQUEST

☐ Health Net   ☐ Met Life
☒ Pacificare   ☐ Travelers
☐ Secure Horizons   ☐ Pru Care
☐ Other

Member/Group No.: 54098XX

TO BE COMPLETED BY PRIMARY CARE PHYSICIAN OR OUTSIDE PROVIDER

Patient Name: Louann Campbell   Date: 7-14-20XX

☐ Male   ☐ Female   Birthdate: 4-7-1952   Home Telephone Number: (555) 450-1666

Address: 2516 Encina Avenue, Woodland Hills, XY 12345-0439

Primary Care Physician: Gerald Practon, MD   Provider ID #: TC 14021

Referring Physician: Gerald Practon, MD   Provider ID #: TC 14021

Referred to: Raymond Skeleton, MD   Office Telephone number: (555) 486-9002

Address: 4567 Broad Avenue, Woodland Hills, XY 12345

Diagnosis Code: M54.40   Diagnosis: Low back pain with Sciatica

Diagnosis Code: Diagnosis:

Treatment Plan: Orthopedic consultation and evaluation of lumbar spine; R/O herniated disc L4-5

Authorization requested for: ☐ Consult only ☐ Treatment only ☐ Consult/Treatment
                              ☐ Consult/Procedure/Surgery ☐ Diagnostic Tests

Procedure Code: 99244   Description: New patient consultation

Procedure Code: Description:

Place of service: ☒ Office ☐ Outpatient ☐ Inpatient ☐ Other   Number of Visits: 1

Facility: Length of Stay:

List of potential future consultants (i.e., anesthetists, surgical assistants, or medical/surgical):

Physician's Signature: Gerald Practon, MD

TO BE COMPLETED BY PRIMARY CARE PHYSICIAN

PCP Recommendations: See above   PCP Initials: GP

Date eligibility checked: 7-14-20XX   Effective Date: 1-15-20XX

TO BE COMPLETED BY UTILIZATION MANAGEMENT

Authorized: Auth. No.   Not Authorized

Deferred: Modified:

Effective date: Expiration date: Number of visits:

Fig. 5.6 A managed care plan treatment authorization request form completed by a primary care provider *(PCP)* for preauthorization of a professional service.

- Direct referral. An authorization request form is completed and signed by the PCP and handed to the patient. Certain services may not require completion of a form and may be directly referred (for example, obstetric care, dermatology).
- Verbal referral. The PCP informs the patient and telephones the referring service provider for an appointment.
- Self-referral. The patient refers himself or herself to a specialist. The patient may be required to inform the PCP.

Patients may be unaware of preapproval requirements. A good precaution is to ask the patient about insurance coverage at the time the appointment is made. If the patient is a member of a managed care plan, carefully review the patient's preauthorization requirements. If approval is necessary for certain situations, inform the patient of this before he or she sees the service provider. If a patient has obtained the written authorization approval, ask the patient to fax or mail a copy because it may have an expiration date noted on it. Even if preapproved, the treatment must be medically necessary, or payment may be denied after submission of a claim. If an authorization is delayed and the patient comes in for the scheduled services, the plan should be called to obtain a verbal authorization. The date, time, and name of the authorizing person should be documented; otherwise, the patient's appointment for services should be rescheduled. A referral recommendation must be documented in the patient's record and, if applicable, sent to the referring service provider.

A tracking system, such as a referral tracking log, should be in place for pending referrals so that care may be rendered in a timely manner and patients do not get "lost" in the system (Fig. 5.7). This log should include the date on which the authorization is requested, the patient's name, procedure or consultant requested, insurance plan, effective and expiration dates, dates of follow-up, name of person who approved or denied the request, and appointment date for consult or procedure. Sometimes authorization approvals are sent to the PCP and not to the referring

or ordering provider. In these cases, follow-up must be made with the PCP. A maximum 2-week turnaround time should be allowed, and all authorization requests should be tracked.

If a managed care plan refuses to authorize payment for recommended treatment, tests, or procedures, have the PCP send a letter to the plan that is worded similarly to that shown in Fig. 5.8. Include medical documentation, such as office and hospital encounter notes, laboratory reports, and x-ray reports, to support the insurance claim. Then, after all efforts have been exhausted, send a letter such as the one shown in Fig. 5.9 to the patient informing them of this fact and asking the patient to appeal the denial of benefits.

In capitated managed care plans, when a PCP sends a patient for consultation to a specialist who is not in the managed care plan, the specialist bills the PCP. This is done because the PCP receives a monthly capitation check from the plan and any care for the patient must come from the capitation pool. This type of plan encourages PCPs not to refer patients so that they can retain profits.

If a specialist recommends referral to another specialist (tertiary care), ensure that the recommendation is provided in writing. Call the specialist at a later date to determine whether the recommendation was acted on. If the patient refuses to be referred, ensure that this is documented. If a referral form is necessary, do not telephone or write a letter. The managed care plan may refuse payment if the proper form is not completed.

When a referral authorization form is received, make a copy of the form for each approved office encounter, laboratory test, or series of treatments. Then use the form as a reference to bill for the service. All copies being used indicates that all services that the patient's plan has approved are completed. Ask the PCP or the managed care plan for a new authorization to continue treatment on the patient. The request should be generated in a timely manner so that treatment is not delayed.

AUTHORIZATION REQUEST LOG								
Date requested	Patient name	Procedure/ consult	Insurance plan	1st F/U	2nd F/U	3rd F/U	Approved	Scheduled date
2/8/XX	Juan Percy	Bone scan-full body	Health Net	2/20			J. Smith	2/23/XX
2/8/XX	Nathan Takai	MRI-L-knee	Pru-Care	2/20	3/3			
2/9/XX	Lori Smythe	Consult Neuro G. Frankel MD	FHP	2/22			T. Hope	2/26/XX
2/10/XX	Bob Mason	Cervical collar	Secure Horizons	2/22	3/5	3/19		

Fig. 5.7 An authorization request log to be used as a system for tracing referral of patients for diagnostic testing, procedures, and consultations.

Ms. Jane Smith
Chairperson
Utilization Review Committee
ABC Managed Care Plan
111 Main Street
Anytown, XY 12345-0122

Dear Ms. Smith:

On _____ I prescribed_____ for_____ .
　　　Date　　　　　　　　　List treatment, test, procedure　Patient's name

On _____ you refused to authorize for that treatment. I find that I
　　　Date
must take issue with your determination for the following reasons:

In my medical judgment, the treatment is a very important part of my overall care of_____
_____ . This patient suffers from_____ . The treatment is
Patient's name　　　　　　　　　　　　　　　Describe condition
necessary to _____ . Failure to perform the treatment could
　　　　　　Describe why necessary
result in the following problem(s):

Enclosed are copies of the laboratory and radiological reports. For these reasons, I urge you
to reconsider your refusal to authorize payment for the procedure I have prescribed.

By copy of this letter to_____ I am reiterating my suggestion that
　　　　　　　　　　Patient's name
he/she obtain the treatment despite your refusal to authorize payment, for the reasons I
have set forth in this letter and in prior discussions with _____ .
　　　　　　　　　　　　　　　　　　　　　　　Patient's name

Yours truly,

John Doe, MD
Enclosures
cc: (Name of patient)

Fig. 5.8 A letter to a managed care plan when there is a refusal to authorize payment for a recommended treatment, test, or procedure.

Mr. Avery Johnson
130 Sylvia Street
Anytown, XY 12345-0022

Dear Mr. Johnson:

On _____ I prescribed_____ for you. On _____ ,
　　　Date　　　　　　　　Treatment, test, procedure　　　　　　Date

_____refused to authorize for same. On that basis,
　Name of Managed Care Plan
you have informed me of your decision to forego the treatment I have prescribed. I
expressed my concerns regarding your decision during our discussion on_____ about
　　　　　　　　　　　　　　　　　　　　　　　　　　　Date
the potential ramifications of your refusal to undergo the treatment.

The purpose of this letter is to recommend that you appeal_____
　　　　　　　　　　　　　　　　　　　　　　　Name of Managed Care Plan's
denial of benefits and reconsider your decision to forego the treatment in light of the
potential consequences of your refusal.

Should you wish to discuss this further, please do not hesitate to contact me.

Sincerely yours,

John Doe, MD

Fig. 5.9 A letter sent by the provider to inform the patient about refusal of payment for treatment, test, or procedure by the managed care plan.

INSURANCE PLAN REFERENCE GUIDE

Plan name/address	Telephone eligibility	Copay	Preauthorization requirements	Test restrictions	Contracted lab(s) radiology	Contracted hospital(s)	Promised payment
Aetna PPO POB 43 WH XY 12345	555-239-0067	$20	hosp/surg/all dx tests	PE 1/yr	ABC Labs	College Hosp	30 days
Blue PPO POB 24335 WH XY 12345	555-245-0899	$30	referral specialist	PE 1/yr	Main St. Lab	St. John MC	30 days
Health Net POB 54000 WH XY 12345	555-408-5466	$10	hosp/surg see check list referrals	Mammo-gram 1/yr	Valley Lab	St. Joseph MC	45 days
Travelers MCO POB 1200 WH XY 12345	555-435-9877	$10	surg/hosp admit referrals	Pap >50 q3yr <50 q1yr	College Hosp Metro Lab	College Hosp	30 days

Fig. 5.10 Insurance plan quick reference guide to help keep track of specifics for each Insurance plan in which the health care organization participates.

Diagnostic Tests

Many insurance plans require that patients have laboratory and radiology tests performed at plan-specified facilities. These are referred to as *network facilities*. Obtain the necessary authorizations for such services and allow sufficient time to receive the test or x-ray examination results before the patient's return appointment. When verifying benefits, ask if the deductible applies; that is, if a provider orders a radiology service that is on site, the deductible may not apply, but if the patient is sent to an outside facility, the deductible applies.

Inform the patient ahead of time when there is doubt about coverage for a test or if the insurance plan indicates that a test is not covered. Disclose the cost and have the patient sign a waiver agreement to pay for the service, thus enabling the billing of the patient for the service. If an authorization is denied because a test is deemed "medically unnecessary" and the health care provider wishes to appeal, the provider can present clinical reasons to the insurance carrier's medical director to receive approval and bring attention to possible expansion of benefits for future patients.

Insurance Plan Guide

Creating a grid or matrix of all private insurance companies and MCOs with which the health care organizations has contracts can help keep up with the many complexities of dealing with the various plans. Use a sheet of paper and list each plan with the billing address vertically in a column to the left. Then list significant data horizontally across the top. Suggested titles for column categories are as follows: eligibility telephone numbers, copayment amounts, preauthorization requirements, restrictions on tests frequently ordered, participating laboratories, participating hospitals, and the contract's

time limit for promised payment. Referring to this grid can provide specifics about each plan's coverage and copayment amounts at a glance (Fig. 5.10). A good procedure is to include this information on each patient's data sheet when benefits are verified.

 5.5   QUICK REVIEW

Question: Identify items included in a contract with an MCO that are key requirements in ensuring the insurance billing specialist obtains payment for services provided by the health care organization.

REVENUE CYCLE MANAGEMENT

Private insurance companies, as well as federal and state programs, typically reimburse using an FFS payment schedule, whereas MCOs have a multitude of payment methodologies.

Deductibles

Deductibles are generally associated with traditional or FFS insurance plans. Usually there is no deductible for a managed care plan. If the patient has a plan with a deductible, be sure to verify the amount of the deductible with the insurance company, ask patients if they have met their deductibles, and collect them in the early months of the year (January through April). Deductibles are applied to claims as they are received and processed by the plan.

Copayments

In a managed care plan, a copayment is a predetermined fee paid by the patient to the provider at the time service is rendered. It is commonly referred to as a copay and is a form of cost sharing because the managed care plan or insurance company pays the remaining cost. Remember to verify the copayment amount when inquiring about insurance plan benefits. Always collect the copay at the time of the patient's office encounter. Billing for small amounts is not cost effective. Copays are commonly made for office encounters, prescription drugs, inpatient mental health services, urgent care encounters, and emergency department encounters. However, the amount may vary according to the type of service. In some plans there may be a separate copayment for x-ray studies and durable medical equipment.

Payment Models and Mechanisms

Concierge medicine. Because insurance companies are paying less for services and there is an increase in documentation and paperwork, some health care organizations have opted to collect a monthly and/or annual retainer fee from patients. This system may be referred to as "concierge medicine" or "direct pay." A monthly fee for the health care providers' services can range from $50 to $150 or an annual fee can range from $1200 to $10,000. Services might include same-day appointments, more time for an office encounter, and contact with the health care professional via telephone, e-mail, and text messaging. If the patient also has an insurance plan, the patient may have to do the paperwork and file the insurance claim.

Cash-only practices. Some health care organizations have decided not to participate with any insurance plans and prefer patients pay cash. If the patient has insurance, some service providers generate a completed claim form so that the patient can submit the claim to the insurance company.

Value-based reimbursement. Value-based reimbursement programs reward health care providers with incentive payments for the quality of care they provide. They are part of a larger quality strategy to reform how health care is delivered and paid for.

The Affordable Care Act instituted the Hospital Value-based Purchasing Program and the Hospital Readmission Reduction Program, which made a positive impact on the US health care system. As a result, there is a greater movement from long-standing volume-based health care models toward value-based care models. For example, the FFS model rewards volume and intensity of service so that more procedures and hospital admissions give more money to the service provider versus value-based health care, which aligns payment and measures objectively the clinical quality of health care. Some of these value-based models are listed here.

Pay for performance. Health care organizations receive FFS payments and receive compensation or bonuses for complying with certain clinical goals. For example, a goal might be to immunize 80% of the organization's patients by age 2 using nationally approved guidelines. If the provider exceeds that goal, reaching a higher percentage, then the health care organization receives a bonus.

Bundled payment/episode of care. Health care organizations agree to accept a single negotiated fee to deliver all medical services for one patient for a specified procedure or condition (for example, hip replacement surgery, pregnancy and birth, certain cardiac procedures). This can reduce costs for payers and increase payment to service providers. The service provider tries to improve efficiency and quality within episodes. However, one must watch that the costs of services for the procedures or conditions do not exceed the agreed-on reimbursement amount.

Patient-centered medical home. The medical home consists of a single team managing with better coordination of medical care that agrees to provide more services. It is paid a negotiated FFS plus a monthly payment based on per-member-per-month (PMPM) and/or a pay-for-performance incentive. The team or group must show certain organizational and structural capabilities (for example, extended office hours, use of electronic medical records, e-prescribing, patient disease registries).

Shared saving (one-sided risk). A combination of payment systems (FFS, pay for performance, bundled payments, global payments, or capitation) that rewards health care organizations that reduce total health care spending on their patients below an expected level set by the payer. The organizations receive a share of the savings.

Shared risk. Health care organizations receive performance-based incentives to share cost savings combined with disincentives to share the excess costs of health care delivery. There is an agreed-upon budget with the payer and the service provider must cover a portion of costs if savings targets are not achieved (for example, a percentage of premium or a set amount [50/50 sharing of excess costs]). If the payer wants the provider to accept more risk, the health care organization can either obtain stop-loss insurance or carve out certain patients or conditions. Another way of limiting risk would be to include a risk corridor arrangement. A corridor protects from high loss but at the same time obstructs opportunities for gains.

Provider-sponsored health plans (PSHPS). A large provider network or hospital system assumes 100% of the financial risk for insuring the patient population. It collects premiums from employers or individuals and directs how care is delivered to patients and how much is spent on giving that care. To set this up, the organization must have an insurance license and obtain approval as a health plan for the state in which it operates commercial, Medicare Advantage, or Medicaid plans. Such systems have responsibilities, such as claims payment, customer service, insurance reporting, and so on.

Full risk: capitation models. These are value-based systems involving managed care plans that can range from FFS and capitation to salaried health care providers. Details about other payment mechanisms follow.

Contact capitation. Contact capitation is based on the concept of paying health care organizations for actual patient encounters or "contacts." A scenario under this payment method occurs when a patient is referred to a specialist for care. A "contact" occurs when the patient receives treatment from a specialist. The patient is assigned to the specialist for a defined period called the *contact period*. The length of the contact period is set in advance for each type of specialty by the panel of participating specialty providers and MCO. The contact period is generally tailored to the demographic and health care needs of the group. Each new patient encounter during a contact period initiates a "contact point." Contact points determine how much to pay each health care provider. The average contact point value is determined by dividing the net specialty capitation pool or total amount of money set aside to be used for a particular specialty by the number of contacts in a certain period. The average contact value is used to determine the amount paid to each specialist during each month in the contact period.

Case rate pricing. For specialists, another payment method is case rate pricing. This means that the specialist contracts with the managed care plan for an entire episode of care. This may be done for certain high-volume, expensive surgical procedures (for example, knee surgery, cataracts, bypass surgery).

Stop-loss limit. Some contracts have a stop-loss section, which means that if the patient's services are more than a certain amount, the health care provider can begin asking the patient to pay (FFS). Monitor each patient's financial accounting record in those instances.

Contract Payment Time Limits

Usually state laws dictate the time limit within which a private insurance or managed care plan must pay. The contract may or may not state the terms of payment, time limits, and late payment penalties, all of which can vary from one plan to another. Prompt payment laws require payment within 30, 45, 55, or 60 days. To diminish late payment of claims, a contract can specify that late claims accrue interest (for example, 5% interest for claims paid after the payment time limit has elapsed). Some states have enacted laws enforcing interest penalties for late payment for either or both private payers, as well as managed care plans. Therefore, the insurance billing specialist should know the laws for the pertinent state. A time limit payment provision is an important factor for the health care organization to consider prior to signing a participation contract.

Monitoring Payment

Monitor payments made from all private insurance and managed care plans and note whether the payment received is less than the agreed amount as stated in the contract. If payment has been reduced, send a letter to the plan citing, "As per contract, see page xx about the fee for the consultation."

Sometimes a procedure (for example, angioplasty with an assistant) may be done and the plan will not pay for an assistant, stating that it is not usual practice. However, perhaps the standard practice in a specific region is to always use an assistant for an angioplasty. When this is emphasized, the plan may remit additional payment.

Some states may have screening fees for emergency services and may or may not require prior approval for such services as defined by the Consolidated Omnibus Budget Reconciliation Act of 1985 (COBRA). Some states have adjudication laws with penalties if the plan does not pay promptly. The following steps should be taken if claims are not paid in a timely manner (30 days):

1. Write to the plan representative and list unpaid claims, claims paid after the payment time limit, and claims paid in error.
2. Send a statement to the director of the plan notifying him or her that if the bill is not paid, the employer's benefits manager or patient will be contacted and alerted to outstand-

ing, slow-paying accounts. Explain that this will prevent the health care organization from renewing the plan's contract and ask the recipient to contact the plan's representative. The consumer has a choice of private and managed care plans; if the present plan does not fulfill his or her expectations, the plan loses members because of dissatisfaction.
3. Take examples and statistics to the next renegotiating session when health care organization's contract is expiring.

Statement of Remittance

Private insurance plans pay based on the services given to the patient (monthly check with a statement of remittance or explanation of benefits [EOB]). Many managed care plans pay using the same FFS basis (Example 5.1 and Example 5.2).

EXAMPLE 5.1   Example of Private Fee-for-Service Insurance Plan Payment

The patient has a private FFS insurance plan and incurs medical expenses of $1000.
- The patient's $200 deductible has not been met.
- The insurance plan pays 80% of the remaining $800.
- The patient is responsible for the deductible ($200) and the 20% coinsurance ($160).
- The total out-of-pocket expense is $360.00.

EXAMPLE 5.2   Example of Managed Care Insurance Plan Payment

The patient has a managed care plan which pays on an FFS basis and incurs medical expenses of $1000.
- The patient's $250 copayment is collected at the time of service.
- The managed care pays the remaining $750 balance.
- There is no further out-of-pocket expense to the patient.

Other managed care plans may pay under a capitation system (monthly check for the number of patients in the plan) (Example 5.3).

EXAMPLE 5.3   Example of Capitation Payment

Example
A primary care provider is under contract with an HMO to pay a capitated payment of $35 per month to provide primary care services to 100 of their plan members. The capitated monthly rate is referred to as **per member per month (PMPM)**. The PCP will receive a capitation payment of $3500 per month to provide care to patients whether they are seen or not and despite how many times they may be seen during that month.

In the capitation system, a monthly check arrives written out for the total amount of monthly capitation. The accompanying paperwork lists all eligible patients being paid for on a PMPM basis divided into two groups: commercial and senior. Patients categorized as commercial are usually younger than age 65 and are paid at a lesser rate because their risk is lower (for example, they do not need to see the doctor frequently). The senior patient category includes those older than 65 years of age; these are paid

STATEMENT OF REMITTANCE

PATIENT NAME (ID NUMBER)	SERVICE DATE MO. DAY YR	P O S	NO SVC	PROCEDURE NUMBER AND DESCRIPTION	AMOUNT BILLED	AMOUNT ALLOWED	RISK WITHHELD	CO PAY	AMOUNT PAID	ADJ. CODE
380224171-01 ALAN E.				CLAIM NO. 62730406 ACCOUNT NO.						
	092620XX	03	1	81000 URINALYSIS-ROUTINE	10.00	10.00	1.00	0	9.00	
	092620XX	03	1	82270 OCCULT BLOOD ANY S	10.00	10.00	1.00	0	9.00	
	092620XX	03	1	99243 LEVEL 3 CONSULT	110.00	110.00	11.00	0	99.00	
	092620XX	03	1	36415 VENIPUNCTURE W/CEN	10.00	10.00	1.00	0	9.00	
				CLAIM TOTALS =	140.00	140.00	14.00	0	126.00	
558700321-01 RONALD B.				CLAIM NO. 62730407 ACCOUNT NO.						
	092520XX	03	1	99213 LEVEL 3 EST VISIT	90.00	90.00	9.00	9.00	72.00	
				CLAIM TOTALS =	90.00	90.00	9.00	9.00	72.00	
473760096-01 DORMA L.				CLAIM NO. 62730408 ACCOUNT NO.						
	092520XX	03	1	99213 LEVEL 3 EST VISIT	90.00	90.00	9.00	9.00	72.00	
				CLAIM TOTALS =	90.00	90.00	9.00	9.00	72.00	

VENDOR SUMMARY: TOTAL AMOUNT PAID $1,600.00   TOTAL WITHHELD $160.00
                 AMOUNT PAID YEAR-TO-DATE: $42,400.00   AMOUNT WITHHELD YEAR-TO-DATE $4,240.00

Fig. 5.11 Statement of remittance or explanation of benefits for noncapitated patients or contracted fee-for-service indicating the amount billed, amount allowed, risk withheld, amount paid, and any copayment to be made by the patient.

at a higher rate because of the increased risk. Always verify the individual capitated amounts listed by each name on the accompanying paperwork against the monthly eligibility list to balance the amount of the check. Contact the MCO if an error appears. If a specialist is capitated, there may be thousands of patients on the capitation plan and a list of patients will not be provided. The capitation amount for a specialist may be only a few cents per month calculated according to the risk of the patient needing specialty services.

In the system where payment is based on services rendered and a statement of remittance or EOB is generated, such statements itemize services that have been rendered to patients and usually indicate the amount billed, amount allowed, amount paid, and any copayment to be made by the patient (Fig. 5.11).

Accounting

Insurance plans vary in their financial reimbursement structure and careful accounting procedures are required. Accounting can become a confusing issue because of a mixture of private and managed care patients with copayment requirements, coinsurance amounts, deductibles, and withholds. Good billing and accounts receivable management software is designed to handle each plan in the computer separately to eliminate mistakes.

Time of Service Payment

Copayments are typically collected at the time of service. And in some cases, the health care organization will require payment of coinsurance at the time of service. In those situations, post first the charge and then the coinsurance prepayment, calculated based on either the percentage of the charge the plan allows or the flat copayment amount (for example, $15 for each office encounter). After receiving the EOB document from the insurance

plan, post an adjustment entry of the disallowed amount, which is calculated on a percentage of the MCO's allowable charge to balance the account (Fig. 5.12). An overpayment should be shown as a refund or credit to the account.

Withhold

Some MCOs may retain a percentage of the allowable charges to the health care organization until the end of the year to cover operating expenses. This is known as withhold. A statement of remittance from the MCO shows the risk amounts withheld for each patient's services in the eighth column of Fig. 5.11. The withhold plus interest is returned to the health care organization at the end of the plan year if the budgeted services for the plan are not overused. However, the withhold or a portion of it is retained by the plan if services are overused. Thus, the health care organizations share in any surplus or pay part of any deficit at year's end. This risk sharing creates an incentive for limiting care by the gatekeeper and limiting referrals to specialists, thereby keeping medical costs down. The withhold can cover all services or be specific to hospital care, ancillary services (laboratory, x-ray use), or specialty referrals.

A managed care plan that withholds a percentage of the allowable charge must be tracked in the health care organization's accounts receivable so that it is not prematurely written off as a bad debt. To do this, develop a capitation accounting worksheet listing the dates of service, patients' names, Current Procedural Terminology (CPT) code for the service rendered, FFS charges, withheld amounts, and disallowed amounts (Fig. 5.13). Then total all columns. The total of the withheld column is a debit entry that indicates what the managed care plan owes to the health care organization pending its year-end reconciliation. When the withheld amount arrives, the accounting worksheet

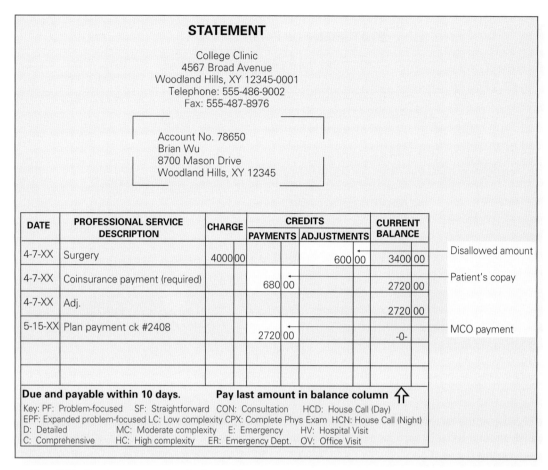

Fig. 5.12 Posting to a patient's financial accounting record (ledger card) showing a charge of $4000. The plan allows $3400; therefore, the patient's prepaid coinsurance amount is $680 (20% of $3400). The managed care plan sent a check for $2720 (80% of $3400) and the disallowed amount ($600) is adjusted off the account, which brings the account balance to zero.

DEBIT

Date	Patient	Service	Charge	Withhold	Disallow	
5/15/20XX	Mason	99204	106.11	5.94	21.22	Disallowed
5/15/20XX	Mason	93000	34.26	1.92	3.43	amounts
5/15/20XX	Mason	81000	8.00	.38	2.40	
5/15/20XX	Self	93501	1500.00	240.00	300.00	
Total			1648.38	248.24	327.05	

Total withheld amount owed by MCO

Fig. 5.13 A managed care plan when payment is on a fee-for-service basis. Note the disallowed portion of the charge, which is based on the plan's allowable charge. A portion of the allowable charge is withheld.

can be compared with the amount withheld during the year. The amount of withholds that are not returned to the health care organization is adjusted once withholds are settled. The total of the column for disallowed amounts shows the amount written off by the health care organization. Combine the withheld returned amount with the managed care payment for the year to determine whether it is worthwhile for the organization to participate in the plan. Some organizations can use the information to renegotiate increased fees when the managed care contract is to be renewed.

Analysis of Insurance Plans

Revenue cycle management reports are generated via computer and are the responsibility of the manager or accountant in most health care organizations. However, it can be an asset for an insurance billing specialist to have some knowledge of the content of these reports. Most health care organizations monitor and analyze plan payments to determine collection rates for each payer. The collection rate is the percentage of money that will be received on each service dollar charged to that insurance carrier. This helps the health care organizations to assess collection activities and to make decisions regarding future contracts.

If the organization has capitation contracts, they will also compare profit or loss of those plans to what would have been received from FFS plans. To do this, one designs a capitation accounting sheet for each capitated plan. This sheet shows a listing of dates of service and professional service descriptions (procedures, injections, and laboratory work) as well as charges and payments (Fig. 5.14). As managed care plan patients receive services, actual service fees are posted in a charge column from the service provider's fee schedule as if the patient were a private payer. In a payment column copayments and the monthly capitation payment are posted. Then all columns are totaled. It is necessary to apply a discount to the total charged amount for a realistic comparison because the health care organization usually paid on an allowed amount rather than an actual charge.

Calculate the difference between the actual charge and the average allowed amount to do this.

Compare the capitated payment amounts plus copayment amounts with the total discounted charges at the end of the year. This gives an accurate idea of whether the capitated payment received is adequate for the services the health care organization provided. Compiling monthly records and reviewing them at the end of the year helps a health care organization to assess the gain or loss of each capitation plan.

Bankruptcy

The U.S. bankruptcy code 11 (referred to as Chapter 11) is a form of bankruptcy that involves reorganization of a debtor's business affairs, debts and assets. If a private insurance plan or an MCO declares a Chapter 11 bankruptcy filing, the plan is obligated to pay all bills incurred before the filing. However, in some situations, another entity may take over the plan and all services incurred after filing are paid by the new payer. If the patient had treatment before the filing, a delay in getting reimbursed may occur because the insurance plan cannot repay debts incurred before its filing until it has worked out a reorganization plan. Health care organizations under contract with the insurance plan are obligated to honor their contractual commitments. If their contracts expire or if they have escape clauses, they may be required to continue accepting patients, depending on the contract provisions.

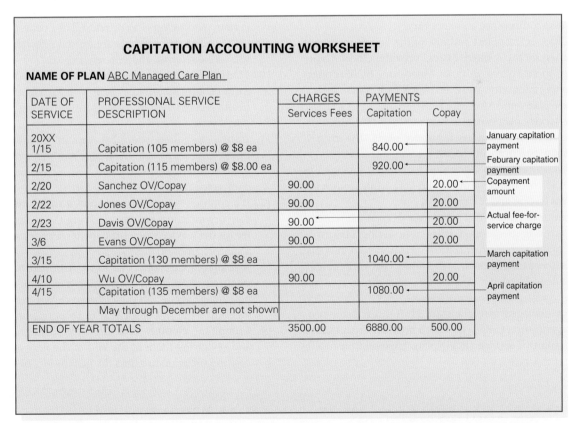

CAPITATION ACCOUNTING WORKSHEET

NAME OF PLAN ABC Managed Care Plan

DATE OF SERVICE	PROFESSIONAL SERVICE DESCRIPTION	CHARGES Services Fees	PAYMENTS Capitation	Copay	
20XX 1/15	Capitation (105 members) @ $8 ea		840.00		January capitation payment
2/15	Capitation (115 members) @ $8.00 ea		920.00		Feburary capitation payment
2/20	Sanchez OV/Copay	90.00		20.00	Copayment amount
2/22	Jones OV/Copay	90.00		20.00	
2/23	Davis OV/Copay	90.00		20.00	Actual fee-for-service charge
3/6	Evans OV/Copay	90.00		20.00	
3/15	Capitation (130 members) @ $8 ea		1040.00		March capitation payment
4/10	Wu OV/Copay	90.00		20.00	
4/15	Capitation (135 members) @ $8 ea		1080.00		April capitation payment
	May through December are not shown				
END OF YEAR TOTALS		3500.00	6880.00	500.00	

Fig. 5.14 An accounting sheet for a capitation plan from January through April showing dates of service, professional service descriptions, members' charges, and capitation payments and copayments received by the health care organization. Charges and payments columns may be totaled at the end of the year to compare capitation with fee-for-service earnings.

Some clauses allow a health care organization to withdraw from seeing patients or leave if the insurance plan is in bankruptcy proceedings for more than 4 months. However, bankruptcy courts have broad powers to prevent health care providers from leaving insurance plans in bankruptcy proceedings if the court deems such actions to be detrimental to the rehabilitation of the debtor.

5.6 QUICK REVIEW

Question: Explain why it would be important for the insurance billing specialist to analyze revenue cycle management reports related to MCO reimbursement?

DISCUSSION POINT

Managed care has become the dominant form of health insurance in the United States. Why do you think this is happening and how does this make the role of the insurance billing specialist more complex?

PROCEDURE 5.1 Interpreting Information From an Insurance Card

Objectives: To accurately interpret information from an insurance card, for the purposes of filing an insurance claim form.

Directions:
1. Examine the Blue Cross Blue Shield insurance card in Figs. 5.1A and B and determine what information is provided from the front and back of it.
2. Identify the insurance carrier's trademark
3. Identify the subscriber's name.
4. Identify the identification number
5. Identify the group number
6. Identify the type of plan
7. Identify the copayment amount for office visits, specialty visits, emergency room visits
8. Identify the annual deductible amount
9. Identify the insurance website where additional resources can be obtained
10. Identify the customer service phone numbers
11. Identify the address where claim forms can be

KEY POINTS

This is a brief chapter review, or summary, of the key issues presented.

1. There are numerous private insurance companies across the United States who typically offer a variety of traditional and managed care plans. Private health insurance is generally offered through employers or other organizations. Plan benefits and coverage, as well as deductibles, copayments, and coinsurance amounts vary.
2. The BCBSA is the oldest and one of the largest insurance companies in the United States, providing health care coverage to nearly one in three Americans. BCBSA offers traditional indemnity plans, managed care plans, federal employee plans, and Medicare plans.
3. Fee-for-service plans are also referred to as traditional insurance plans or indemnity insurance plans. The insured may obtain care from any health care organization.
4. *Managed care* refers to a group of techniques intended to reduce the cost of providing health care while improving the access to care and the quality of care.
5. Primary care providers (PCPs) act as gatekeepers who control patient access to specialists and diagnostic testing services.
6. Health maintenance organizations (HMOs) have models, such as the group model, staff model, network model, Independent Physician Association, and direct contract model.
7. Types of managed care plans are HMOs, exclusive provider organization (EPO), preferred provider organization (PPO), point-of-service (POS) plan, triple-option health plan, provider-sponsored organization (PSO), and consumer directed health plans (CDHP).
8. Utilization management is a set of techniques used by managed care plans to control health care costs. The techniques should help the patient get the best care at the best price in the best setting.
9. Some managed care plans may require prior approval for certain medical services or referral of a patient to a specialist. Four types of referrals are formal referral, direct referral, verbal referral, and self-referral.
10. Many private insurance carrier and managed care organization contracts provide them with the right to access the health records of their patients for utilization management purposes.
11. Insurance billing specialist should monitor payments made from all private insurance and managed care plans to determine if payment received is correct and in line with contracted rates.
12. If a contract has a stop-loss limit, it means that the health care organization can begin asking the patient to pay the fee for the service when the patient's services are more than a specific amount.
13. A managed care plan that has a withhold provision may retain a percentage of the monthly capitation payment or a percentage of the allowable charges to the health care provider until the end of the year to cover operating expenses.
14. Compiling monthly revenue cycle management reports and reviewing them at the end of the year helps a health care organization to assess the gain or loss of each plan.

STUDENT ASSIGNMENT

- Study Chapter 5.
- Complete all exercises in the *Workbook* to reinforce the theory learned in this chapter.
- Turn to the Glossary at the end of this text for a further understanding of the key terms and key abbreviations used in this chapter.

6

Medicare

Linda M. Smith

OBJECTIVES

After reading this chapter, you should be able to:

1. Explain the history of Medicare.
2. Explain the eligibility criteria for Medicare.
3. Abstract important information from a patient's Medicare card.
4. Identify the benefits of Medicare.
5. List five federal laws adopted to increase health benefits for employed elderly individuals.
6. Explain various Medicare programs and other insurance coverage combinations.
7. Name the federal program that relates to utilization and quality control of health services.
8. State the benefits of a participating versus nonparticipating provider.
9. Explain the national and local Medicare coverage policies that must be adhered to.
10. Explain when to obtain a patient's signature on an Advance Beneficiary Notice of Noncoverage.
11. Identify noncovered Medicare services.
12. Define and discuss a Medicare prepayment screen.
13. Discuss the different Medicare payment methodologies.
14. Explain the resource-based relative value scale system that Medicare uses to establish fees.
15. Explain how the Medicare Access and CHIP Reauthorization Act of 2015 have affected Medicare reimbursement.
16. State the Medicare mandatory claim submission guideline.
17. Define a Medicare Administrative Contractor and explain their responsibilities.
18. Determine the time limit requirements for transmitting a Medicare claim.
19. State the components of a Medicare remittance advice.
20. Explain the importance of identifying Medicare overpayments.

KEY TERMS

adjudication
adjustment
Advance Beneficiary Notice of Noncoverage
Advanced Alternative Payment Model
approved charges
assignment
beneficiaries
benefit period
Centers for Medicare and Medicaid Services
Conditional Payment
Correct Coding Initiative
crossover claim
custodial services
disability
donut hole
dual eligible
durable medical equipment
end-stage renal disease
formulary
generic drugs
hospice

hospital insurance
jurisdiction
limiting charge
Local Coverage Determination
medical necessity
Medicaid
Medicare
Medicare Access and CHIP Reauthorization Act of 2015
Medicare administrative contractors
Medicare Advantage Plan
Medicare Beneficiary Identifier
Medicare Claims Processing Manual—Internet Only Manual
Medicare fee schedule
Medicare Improvements for Patients and Providers Act
Medicare Learning Network
Medicare/Medicaid
Medicare Part A
Medicare Part B
Medicare Part C
Medicare Part D
Medicare secondary payer

Medicare Select
Medicare Summary Notice
Medigap
Merit-based Incentive Payment System
National Coverage Determination
national health insurance
national provider identifier
nonparticipating provider
nursing facility
participating provider
premium
prepayment screen
preventive services
prospective payment system
Quality Improvement Organization
Recovery Audit Contractor Initiative
remittance advice
resource-based relative value scale
respite care
United States Preventive Services Task Force (USPSTF).
value-based programs

103

KEY ABBREVIATIONS

ABN	LGHP	MLN	PFFS plan
APM	MAC	MMA	PPS
CCI	MACRA	MSA	PSO
CMS	MA plan	MSN	QIO
DHHS	MBI	MSP	RA
DME	Medi-Medi	NCDs	RAC Initiative
ERA	MFS	NF	RBRVS
ESRD	MG	nonpar	USPSTF
GPCIs	MIPPA	NPI	
LCDs	MIPS	par	

INSIGHTS FROM THE FIELD

Jacqueline G.: Certified Professional Coder (CPC) and Revenue Cycle Billing Specialist

Medicare is complex, and there is no way to know all the Medicare guidelines. You need to start with the basics of Medicare billing and then expand your knowledge into the specific services provided by your health care organization. Know what is covered and what is not covered by Medicare for the specialty you are billing. Pay attention to detail and use all of the tools provided to you to avoid fraudulent billing. Using the Medicare website is important. Understand why a claim may have denied and then learn how to correct it or avoid similar errors in the future.

After 45 years in the field, so much has changed, and I have evolved with all of it. I have learned so much, I have passed advice and knowledge on to others while still learning something new every day. The field has an ever-challenging landscape, which is what I love.

BACKGROUND

National health insurance is a legally enforced system of health insurance that insures a country's population against the costs of health care. It is usually established by national legislation but may be administered by the public sector, the private sector, or a combination of both.

The first move toward a national health insurance system began in Germany when the Sickness Insurance Law of 1883 was passed, and industrial employers were mandated to provide insurance for their low-wage workers. Other countries such as the United Kingdom and most of Western and Central Europe began to follow suit to create other variations of national health insurance. At present, nearly 50 countries have legislation mandating universal or near-universal health coverage. National health insurance programs differ in both how money is collected and how services are provided.

The idea of a national health insurance system for Americans dates back to the presidency of Theodore Roosevelt in 1912. He envisioned a national health plan for the entire populations and individuals of all ages. Although his vision did not become reality during his term, he passed on his effort for a national health care program to President Harry Truman and President John F. Kennedy. Their presidencies also had significant impact in

shaping the health plan. In 1965, Medicare legislation was signed by President Lyndon B. Johnson. It did not provide health coverage for the entire populations; however, it was established to provide national health coverage for Americans 65 years and older. Former President Truman attended the signing of this legislation and was issued the very first Medicare card.

6.1   QUICK REVIEW
Question: Did Theodore Roosevelt's vision of a national health insurance plan for the *entire* US population become a reality?

POLICIES AND REGULATIONS

Medicare is administered by the Centers for Medicare and Medicaid Services (CMS), a federal agency within the US Department of Health and Humans Services (DHHS). The CMS is responsible for implementation of all rules, regulations, and health-related policies governing the Medicare program. The CMS is subdivided into three divisions:

1. The Center for Medicare Management oversees traditional fee-for-service (FFS) Medicare, which is health care coverage provided through the federal government. CMS oversees development of payment policy and management of FFS contractors.
2. The Center for Beneficiary Choices provides information on managed care options for individuals entitled to receive Medicare benefits. A Medicare managed care option is Medicare a health plan that is offered by a private company that contracts with the federal government to provide Medicare-eligible individuals with health care coverage.
3. The Center for Medicaid and State Operations focuses on federal-state programs such as Medicaid, the State Children's Health Insurance Program, and insurance regulations.

The Parts of Medicare

The Medicare program consists of four parts.

- Part A (hospital insurance) covers inpatient care in hospitals, critical access hospital care, and nursing facility care. It also covers hospice care, some home health care, and certain blood services. A hospice is a public agency or private organization that is primarily engaged in providing pain relief, symptom management, and supportive services to terminally ill people and their families.

- Part B (medical insurance) covers physician care, outpatient hospital care, and other related health services that Part A does not cover, such as some of the services of physical and occupational therapists and some home health.
- Part C (Medicare Advantage) provides alternatives for patients entitled to Medicare benefits through managed care plan options.
- Part D provides prescription drug coverage.

Eligibility Requirements

Individuals who may be eligible for Medicare are:

- Those who are age 65 or older
- Those who are under 65 with a disability. A disability is defined by the Social Security Administration (SSA) as the inability to engage in any substantial employment due to physical or mental impairment that can be expected to last for 12 continuous months or result in death.
- Those with end-stage renal disease (ESRD). ESRD occurs when a patient who has chronic kidney disease has a gradual loss of kidney function and reaches an advances stage requiring dialysis or transplant.

Medicare Enrollment

The SSA offices take applications for Social Security, control the Medicare eligibility process, and provide information about the Medicare program.

If an individual receives Social Security or Railroad Retirement benefits, he or she is automatically enrolled in Medicare Parts A and B starting on the first day of the month that the individual turns 65 years of age. Those individuals or their spouse must have worked and paid Medicare taxes for at least 10 years. For those individuals who apply for Social Security benefits early (at age 62 years), they receive reduced Social Security retirement benefits; however, they do not receive Medicare benefits. If an individual is younger than 65 years of age and disabled, he or she will automatically get Medicare Parts A and B after getting Social Security disability or Railroad Retirement benefits for 24 months.

All persons who meet eligibility requirements determined by SSA are eligible for Medicare Part A (hospital coverage) at no charge. Medicare Part B recipients pay an annual fee for coverage, known as a premium to the SSA, and some pay a Medicare surtax on federal income tax payments. This premium may be deducted automatically from the patient's monthly Social Security check if he or she wishes. Premium amounts change from year to year.

To confirm a Medicare patients' enrollment in the Medicare program, verification can be accessed through CMS's HIPAA Eligibility Transaction System (HETS) or through the Medicare Administrative Contractor call center, web portal, or Interactive Voice Response (IVR) unit. An internet link has been provided for HETS at the end of this chapter under *Internet Resources*.

Non-U.S. Citizens

A non-U.S. citizen is an individual who is living in the country without government permission; they are not citizens of the United States. In the Medicare program, a non-U.S. citizen may be eligible for Part A or B coverage. To be eligible, the applicant must have lived in the United States as a permanent resident for 5 consecutive years.

Health Insurance Card

Patients who are entitled to receive Medicare benefits are referred to as beneficiaries. On enrollment into the Medicare program the beneficiary is issued a red, white, and blue Medicare identification card. In the past, Medicare identified the patient by their name and their Social Security number. However, the Medicare Access and CHIP Reauthorization Act of 2015 required removal of Social Security numbers from Medicare insurance cards to fight medical identity theft. The transition period to replace the patient's Social Security number by a Medicare Beneficiary Identifier (MBI) started April 1, 2018 and ended January 1, 2020. Effective January 1, 2020, all Medicare claims must be submitted with the patient's MBI. The MBI is 11 characters in length and is made up only of numbers and uppercase letters. The patient's Medicare card provides the patient's MBI number, hospital and medical coverage status, and coverage start dates (Fig. 6.1).

Benefits

As mentioned earlier, the four parts of the Medicare program are part A, part B, part C, and part D. It is essential for the

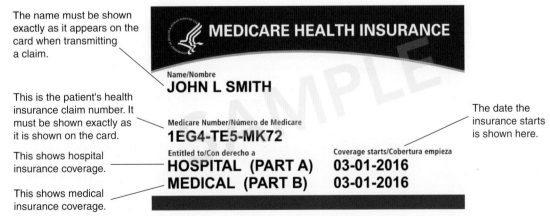

The name must be shown exactly as it appears on the card when transmitting a claim.

This is the patient's health insurance claim number. It must be shown exactly as it is shown on the card.

This shows hospital insurance coverage.

This shows medical insurance coverage.

The date the insurance starts is shown here.

MEDICARE HEALTH INSURANCE

Name/Nombre
JOHN L SMITH

Medicare Number/Número de Medicare
1EG4-TE5-MK72

Entitled to/Con derecho a
HOSPITAL (PART A)
MEDICAL (PART B)

Coverage starts/Cobertura empieza
03-01-2016
03-01-2016

Fig. 6.1 Important information on a patient's Medicare health insurance identification card.

insurance billing specialist to understand the benefits of each of the parts.

Medicare Part A: Hospital Benefits

Part A of Medicare provides hospital insurance benefits to eligible individuals. Funds for this health service come from special contributions from employees and self-employed persons, with employers matching contributions. These contributions are collected along with regular Social Security contributions from wages and self-employment income earned during a person's working years. Individuals over 65 do not pay a premium for Part A as long as they (or their spouse) have worked for 40 or more quarters (10 years). If the individual is not eligible for Social Security benefits, they can enroll in Part A, but they must pay a coverage premium.

Medicare Part A provides benefits to applicants in any of the following situations:

1. A bed-ridden patient in a hospital (up to 90 hospital days for each benefit period). A benefit period begins on the day a patient enters a hospital and ends when the patient has not been a bed patient in any hospital or nursing facility (NF) (formerly called *skilled nursing facility*) for 60 consecutive days. It also ends if a patient has been in an NF but has not received skilled nursing care for 60 consecutive days. Hospital insurance protection is renewed every time the patient begins a new benefit period. There is no limit to the number of benefit periods a patient can have for hospital or NF care.

2. A bed patient in an NF receiving skilled nursing care (up to 100 extended care days for each benefit period). An NF offers nursing or rehabilitation services that are medically necessary to a patient's recovery. To be considered medically necessary, the medical services must be the appropriate care and generally accepted care to be reasonable and adequate for the diagnosis and treatment of the individual's illness or injury. Services would not be considered medically necessary if they are custodial. Custodial services are those that assist the patient with personal needs (e.g., dressing, eating, bathing, and getting in and out of bed).

3. A patient receiving home health care services. Patients must be confined to their homes and require skilled nursing care or therapy. Services must be medically necessary and physician ordered.

4. A patient who needs care in a psychiatric hospital (up to 190 days in a lifetime).

5. A terminally ill patient diagnosed as having 6 months or less to live who needs hospice care.

6. A terminally ill patient who needs respite care. Respite care is a short-term inpatient stay that may be necessary for the terminally ill patient to give temporary relief to the person who regularly assists with home care. Inpatient respite care is limited to stays of no more than 5 consecutive days for each respite period.

Fig. 6.2 contains information on four major classifications of inpatient hospital cost-sharing benefits for Medicare Part A.

MEDICARE (PART A): HOSPITAL INSURANCE–COVERED SERVICES FOR 2020

Services	Benefit	Medicare Pays	Patient Pays
HOSPITALIZATION Semiprivate room and board, general nursing and miscellaneous hospital services and supplies. (Medicare payments based on benefit periods.)	First 60 days	All but $ 1408	$ 1408 deductible
	61st to 90th day	All but $ 352 a day	$ 352 a day
	Days 91 and beyond. Coinsurance per each "lifetime reserve day" after day 90 for each benefit period (up to 60 days over a lifetime).	All but $ 704 a day	$ 704 a day
	Beyond lifetime reserve days	Nothing	All costs
NURSING FACILITY CARE Patient must have been in a hospital for at least 3 days and enter a Medicare-approved facility generally within 30 days after hospital discharge.[2] (Medicare payments based on benefit periods.)	First 20 days	100% of approved amount	Nothing
	21st to 100th day	All but $ 176.00 a day	Up to $ 176.00 a day
	Beyond 100 days	Nothing	All costs
HOME HEALTH CARE Part-time or intermittent skilled care, home health aide services, durable medical equipment and supplies, and other services.	Unlimited as long as Medicare conditions are met and services are declared "medically necessary."	100% of approved amount; 80% of approved amount for durable medical equipment.	Nothing for services; 20% of approved amount for durable medical equipment.
HOSPICE CARE Pain relief, symptom management, and support services for the terminally ill.	If patient elects the hospice option and as long as doctor certifies need.	All but limited costs for outpatient drugs and inpatient respite care.	Limited cost sharing for outpatient drugs and inpatient respite care.

Fig. 6.2 Four major classifications of Medicare Part A benefits. (Updated from *Medicare & You 2020*, US Government Printing Office.)

Miscellaneous hospital services and supplies might consist of intensive care unit (ICU) costs, blood transfusions, drugs, x-ray and laboratory tests, medical supplies (casts, surgical dressings, and splints), use of wheelchair, operating room (OR) and recovery room costs, and therapy (physical, occupational, and speech language). There are no benefits for personal convenience items (television, radio, and telephone), private duty nurses, or a private room unless the private room is determined medically necessary. Similar benefits also relate to nursing facilities.

Benefits for hospice and respite care consist of nursing and physicians' services, drugs, therapy (physical, occupational, and speech-language pathology), home health aid, homemaker services, medical social services, medical supplies and appliances, short-term inpatient care, and counseling.

Medicare Part B: Medical and Preventive Care Benefits

Coverage into Part B Medicare is not automatic, and participation is voluntary. Eligible individuals must enroll in Part B. A medical insurance premium is calculated based on Social Security rates and is automatically deducted from monthly checks for those who receive Social Security benefits, Railroad Retirement benefits, or a Civil Service annuity. Funds for this program come equally from those who sign up for it and the federal government.

Medicare Part B provides benefits for medically necessary physician services, outpatient care, home health services, durable medical equipment, mental health services, ambulance services and rehabilitative services such as physical therapy.

Part B also covers many preventive services at no cost to patients. Preventive services consist of health care services that include check-ups, patient counseling, screenings to prevent illness, and other health-related problems. The following is a list of the preventive services available to Medicare beneficiaries as of March 2020.

- Alcohol Misuse and Counseling
- Annual Wellness Visit
- Bone Mass Measurement
- Cardiovascular Disease Screening Tests
- Colorectal Cancer Screening
- Counseling to Prevent Tobacco Use
- Depression Screening
- Diabetes Screening
- Diabetes Self-Management Training
- Glaucoma Screening
- Hepatitis B Virus Screening
- Hepatitis B Vaccine and Administration
- Hepatitis C Virus Screening
- Human Immunodeficiency Virus Screening
- Influenza Virus Vaccine and Administration
- Initial Preventive Physical Examination
- Intensive Behavioral Therapy for Cardiovascular Disease
- Intensive Behavioral Therapy for Obesity
- Lung Cancer Screening
- Medical Nutrition Therapy
- Pneumococcal Vaccine and Administration
- Prolonged Preventive Services
- Prostate Cancer Screening
- Screening for Cervical Cancer with HPV Tests
- Screening for STIs and HIBC to Prevent STIs
- Screening Mammography
- Screening Pap Tests
- Screening Pelvic Examinations
- Ultrasound Screening for Abdominal Aortic Aneurysm
- Vaccinations

Medicare's preventive service benefits are updated periodically, based on recommendations by the United States Preventive Services Task Force (USPSTF). The USPSTF is an independent panel of national experts in disease prevention who work to improve the health of all Americans by making evidence-based recommendations about preventive services. Medicare's specific coverage requirements and/or limitations for preventive services can be found on the Medicare website. A link to the *Preventive Services Guide* is provided at the end of this chapter under *Internet Resources*.

Medicare Part C: Medicare Advantage Plan

Medicare Part C was created with the passing of the Balanced Budget Act of 1997. Under the Medicare Part C program, patients eligible for Medicare benefits were given the option of choosing between traditional Medicare (described earlier) or a Medicare Advantage Plan (MA plan). Medicare Advantage Plans are offered by private insurance companies approved by Medicare. Medicare pays these companies to cover Medicare beneficiaries. This program was formed to increase the number of health care options, in addition to those that are available under Medicare Parts A and B (a Medicare beneficiary can join an MA plan if he or she has both Parts A and B and lives in the service area of the plan). Individuals who have ESRD must meet special situational requirements to join an MA plan.

Individuals enrolled in a Medicare Advantage Plan will have an identification card issued to them by the private insurance company. The information on that insurance should be used to bill the Medicare Advantage Plan, rather than using the traditional red, white, and blue Medicare card. However, traditional red, white, and blue Medicare cards are not forfeited, and an elderly patient may present with two cards. Special care should be taken when the patient presents for services to identify if the patient has the traditional Medicare or a MA plan and the effective date of the plan (Fig. 6.3).

MA plans receive a fixed amount of money from Medicare to spend on their Medicare members. Some plans may require members to pay a premium similar to the Medicare Part B premium. There are many different types of Medicare Advantage plans. Plans available under this program may include the following: health maintenance organization (HMO), point-of-service (POS) plan, preferred provider organization (PPO), private fee-for-service (PFFS) plan, and provider-sponsored organization (PSO). These different types of managed care plans were outlined in Chapter 5.

A Medicare medical savings account (MSA) plan is another managed care option that may be offered. In an MSA plan, the patient chooses an insurance policy approved by Medicare that has a high annual deductible. Medicare pays the premiums for this policy and deposits the dollar amount difference between

Fig. 6.3 A senior Medicare Advantage plan card.

what it pays for the average beneficiary in the patient's area and the cost of the premium into the patient's MSA. The patient uses the MSA money to pay medical expenses until the high deductible is reached. If the MSA money becomes depleted, the patient pays out of pocket until the deductible is reached. Unused funds roll over for use in the following year. MSA plans vary, and the actual deposit and deductible amounts may be different from Example 6.1.

> **EXAMPLE 6.1   Medicare Savings Accounts**
>
> Mr. Jones joins a Medicare medical savings account (MSA) plan and the plan deposits $2500 into his account. He has a yearly deductible of $4000. If he uses all of the money in his account for Medicare-covered services, he will have to spend $1500 out-of-pocket before he meets his deductible ($4000) and before the Medicare MSA plan will begin paying for his health care. Once Mr. Jones meets his deductible, the MSA plan will pay all his Medicare-covered health care services and he pays nothing. He must continue to pay the monthly Part B premium.

Another type of an MA plan is a special needs plan (SNP), which provides focused and specialized health care for specific groups of people, like those who have both Medicare and Medicaid, live in a nursing home, or have certain chronic medical conditions.

Medicare Advantage plans must cover all the services that traditional Medicare covers except hospice care. Traditional Medicare covers hospice care even if the patient is in a Medicare Advantage plan. In all types of MA plans, the patient is always covered for emergency and urgent care. Many MA plans also offer extra benefits such as dental care, eyeglasses, or wellness programs.

Medicare Part D

Drug benefits started being offered to Medicare beneficiaries on January 1, 2006, under The Medicare Prescription Drug, Improvement, and Modernization Act (MMA). This legislation, known as Medicare Part D, offers Medicare beneficiaries with a prescription drug benefit. It covers prescription drugs used for conditions not already covered by Medicare Parts A and B. It is a standalone prescription drug plan offered by insurance

companies and other private companies providing drug coverage that meet standards established by Medicare. Other names for these plans are *Part D private prescription drug plans (PDPs)* and *Medicare Advantage prescription drug plans (MA-PDs)*.

The two ways to get Medicare prescription drug coverage are as follows:
- Join a Medicare prescription drug plan that adds drug coverage to the original Medicare plan.
- Join an MA plan, that includes prescription drug coverage as part of the plan.

Individuals who enroll pay a monthly premium that varies depending on the plan. Enrollees pay an annual deductible that varies from plan to plan. The patient may also pay a percentage of the drug cost or a flat fee per prescription, referred to as a copayment. The amount of copayment required also varies from plan to plan.

The Medicare Part D program was designed for plans to include a gap in coverage, frequently referred to as a donut hole. The donut hole refers to a temporary limit on what the drug plan will cover for drugs. The donut hole (coverage gap) begins after the patient and the drug plan together have spent a certain amount for covered drugs.

Due to the difficulty many patients experienced in being able to cover the out-of-pocket costs associated with the donut hole, the ACA has been steadily closing the donut hole. The most recent changes to closing the donut hole occurred in 2020. Currently, there are four different periods of Part D coverage (see Table 6.1).

Each Medicare drug plan has its own list of covered drugs, referred to as a formulary. Many Medicare drug plans place drugs into different tiers on their formularies. Drugs in each tier have a different cost.
- Tier one represents generic drugs. Generic drugs are equivalents of brand-name drugs and are the same in dosage form, safety, strength, route of administration, quality, performance characteristics and intended use. Generics are ensured by the Food and Drug Administration to be as safe and effective. Generic drugs typically cost 30% to 70% less than brand-name drugs.
- Tier two covers preferred brand-name drugs and has a higher copayment than tier one. Preferred brand-name drugs do

TABLE 6.1 4 Different Periods of Part D Coverage

Period	Period Defined	2020 Guidelines
Period 1: Deductible Period	Some plans (but not all) have a deductible period. The deductible is the amount of money the patient must pay out-of-pocket before their Medicare drug plan coverage kicks in.	Deductibles vary from plan to plan; some plans have no deductible. However, in 2020, no plan's deductible can be higher than $435.
Period 2: Initial Coverage Period	After the deductible is met, the prescription drug plan will help pay for covered prescription drugs. Some plans will require copayment or coinsurance payment by the patient.	Length of stay in initial coverage period varies based on drug costs and plan benefits. For most plans in 2020, the initial coverage period ends after a total of $4020 in drug costs has been paid by the drug plan and the patient.
Period 3: Coverage gap	After the initial coverage period has passed and the maximum drug cost has been met, the patient enters the coverage gap known as the **donut hole.**	In 2020, the patient is responsible for no more than 25% of the cost of their drugs while they are in the donut hole. They patient remains in the donut hole until they have paid $6350 in out-of-pocket costs for covered drugs.
Period 4: Catastrophic Coverage	After the patient has paid the maximum out-of-pocket costs, they have reached catastrophic coverage. During the catastrophic coverage period, the patient pays significantly lower copays or coinsurance for covered drugs the remainder of the year.	In 2020, patients reach catastrophic coverage after they have paid a maximum of $6350 in out-of-pocket costs for covered drugs.

not have a generic equivalent available. They have been in the market for a time and are widely accepted.

- Tier three drugs are the nonpreferred drugs. Non-preferred drugs are brand-name drugs that are not included on the plan's formulary and are higher-cost medications that have recently come on the market. In most cases an alternative preferred brand-name drug is available. If a brand-name drug is prescribed when a generic equivalent is available, the patient must pay the difference in cost in addition to the copayment. Nonpreferred drugs have higher copayments, or the patient may have to pay a higher percentage of the full drug cost.
- The fourth classification, identified as "S," represents specialty drugs. These are the most expensive drugs on the drug list. They are used to treat complex conditions like cancer and multiple sclerosis. They can be generic or brand name. Specialty drugs require a percentage of total cost of the drug.
- The following are several classes of drugs excluded from coverage under Medicare:
  - Drugs for cosmetic purposes
  - Drugs for symptomatic relief of cough and colds
  - Drugs for weight loss or gain
  - Erectile dysfunction drugs (unless there are medically accepted indications approved by the Food and Drug Administration)
  - Fertility drugs
  - Prescription vitamins or minerals, except prenatal

A provider who prescribes a drug that can be covered by either Part B or Part D must clarify the condition and part coverage on the prescription form (Example 6.2). When a patient has coverage under a Medicare Part D plan, obtain a photocopy of the patient's Medicare supplement or MA plan card. Then check whether the drug that the patient needs is covered by the plan, which generic drugs are available, and whether a drug needs prior authorization.

EXAMPLE 6.2 Prescription Note Clarifying Medical Use of Drug and Coverage Determination

Patient with psoriasis (autoimmune disorder) is prescribed methotrexate. Generally, this immunosuppressive drug is prescribed for transplant patients and is covered under Medicare Part B.

Added prescription note should read: "Psoriasis for Part D."

Medicare for Railroad Workers and Their Families

Patients who are receiving Railroad Retirement benefits or Railroad Disability checks will get Medicare from the Railroad Retirement Board. The Railroad Retirement Board automatically enrolls the patient in Medicare Parts A and B, and medical insurance premiums are automatically deducted from their monthly Railroad Retirement benefit checks. Those who do not receive a monthly check pay their premiums directly or in some cases have premiums paid on their behalf under a state assistance program. Railroad Retirement beneficiaries generally are entitled to benefits for covered services received from a qualified facility in the United States. However, under certain circumstances, a Medicare beneficiary may receive care in Canada or Mexico. Benefits and deductibles under Parts A and B are the same as for other Medicare recipients.

Some railroad retirees are members of a railroad hospital association or a prepayment plan. These members pay regular premiums to the plan and then receive health services that the plan provides without additional charges. In some plans, small charges are made for certain services such as drugs or home visits. Many prepayment plans make arrangements with Medicare to receive direct payments for services they furnish that are covered under Medicare Part B. Claims for services provided should be sent to the address of the Medicare railroad retiree center, listed on the back of the patient's Medicare card. After the claim is processed, a remittance advice (RA) document is generated to the service provider explaining the decision made on the claim and the services for which Medicare paid.

Employed Elderly Benefits

To understand various types of scenarios that may be encountered when transmitting claims for elderly individuals, one must know about several federal laws that regulate health care coverage of those aged 65 and older who are employed. Such individuals may have group insurance or a Medigap policy and may fall under billing categories of Medicare first payer or Medicare secondary payer (MSP) (all are discussed in detail later in this chapter). The federal laws that affect employed elderly individuals are shown in Box 6.1.

6.2   QUICK REVIEW

Question: What are the four parts of Medicare? Can you differentiate the benefits provided under each?

ADDITIONAL INSURANCE PROGRAMS

Many Medicare recipients have Medicare in combination with other insurance plans. This section explains various coverage combinations.

Medicare/Medicaid

Medicaid is a joint federal and state program that helps pay medical costs if the patient has limited income and resources and meet other requirements. Some people qualify for both Medicare and Medicaid and are called dual eligible. Patients designated as Medicare/Medicaid (Medi-Medi) are on both Medicare and Medicaid simultaneously. In these cases, Medicare processes the claims as the primary payer. Generally, the claim to Medicare can be completed in a manner that will allow for a crossover claim or claim transfer directly to the Medicaid program after Medicare payment has been made. Medicaid is always considered to be the payer of last resort and will process the payment as a secondary payer. If the Medicare payment exceeds the Medicaid fee schedule, little or no payment is made by Medicaid. If the beneficiary has not met his or her annual Medicare deductible, the Medicaid claim may result in payment of the Medicaid allowed amount.

Medicare/Medigap

A Medigap (MG) policy is private insurance that helps pay some of the health care costs that traditional Medicare FFS Medicare plans do not cover. Coverage is commonly provided for copayments, coinsurance, and deductibles, all considered to be gaps in Medicare coverage. In some cases, a Medigap policy may also cover health care services that Medicare considers to be noncovered services. Patients pay monthly premiums to private insurance carriers for this supplemental insurance. Beneficiaries can elect not to enroll in a Medigap policy, and beneficiaries with a Medicare Advantage Plan do not need Medigap coverage. Every Medigap policy must follow federal and state laws designed to protect the Medicare patient, and it must be clearly identified as Medicare supplement insurance. All policies offer the same basic benefits, but some offer additional benefits. The

BOX 6.1   Federal Laws Affecting Employed Elderly Individuals

Omnibus Budget Reconciliation Act
The OBRA of 1981 required that in the case of a current or former employee or dependent younger than age 65 years and eligible for Medicare solely because of ESRD, the employer's group coverage is primary for up to 30 months. The Balanced Budget Act of 1997 mandated this change in the length of the coordination period. OBRA applies to all employers regardless of the number of employees. OBRA of 1986, effective in 1987, required that if an employee or dependent younger than age 65 years has Medicare coverage because of a disability other than ESRD, the group coverage is primary, and Medicare is secondary. This Act applies only to large group health plans (**LGHPs**) having at least 100 full- or part-time employees.

Tax Equity and Fiscal Responsibility Act
The TEFRA of 1982 established that an employee or spouse aged 65–69 years is entitled to the same health insurance benefits offered under the same conditions to younger employees and their spouses. The group insurance is primary, and Medicare is secondary. TEFRA applies to employers with at least 20 full- or part-time employees.

Deficit Reduction Act
The DEFRA of 1984, effective in 1985, was an amendment to TEFRA and stated that a spouse age 65–69 years or an employee of any age is entitled to the same group health plan offered to younger employees and their spouses. The group's coverage is primary, and Medicare is secondary. DEFRA applies to employers with at least 20 full- or part-time employees.

Consolidated Omnibus Budget Reconciliation Act
The COBRA of 1985, effective in 1986, is another amendment to TEFRA eliminating the age ceiling of 69 years. An employee or spouse age 65 or older is entitled to the same group health plan offered to younger employees and their spouses. COBRA requires that third-party payers reimburse for certain care rendered in government-run veteran and military hospitals. The group's coverage is primary, and Medicare is secondary. COBRA applies to employers with at least 20 full- or part-time employees.

Tax Reform Act
The Tax Reform Act was passed in 1986 and clarified certain aspects of COBRA. A spouse and dependents may elect to receive continued coverage even if the employee does not wish insurance coverage and terminates the plan. However, the spouse and dependents must have been covered under the plan before the covered employee terminates it. Spouses who are widowed or divorced while receiving continued coverage must report such changes to the benefit plan administrator within 60 days of the employee's death to determine how many additional months of coverage are available.

COBRA, Consolidated Omnibus Budget Reconciliation Act; *DEFRA,* Deficit Reduction Act; *ESRD,* end-stage renal disease; *OBRA,* Omnibus Budget Reconciliation Act; *TEFRA,* Tax Equity and Fiscal Responsibility Act.

patient can choose which one meets their needs. The policies are categorized by alpha letters A through N (Fig. 6.4). All policies are not available in all states, so individuals in some states have fewer options than others.

Some insurance companies offer Medicare Select policies that are slightly different that other supplemental plans. This is a Medigap policy that limits the patient's coverage to a network of doctors and hospitals, except in emergency situations. These health care providers charge less for the services they provide to members.

The chart below shows basic information about the different benefits Medigap policies cover.

100% = the plan covers 100% of this benefit

No benefit = the policy doesn't cover that benefit

% = the plan covers that percentage of this benefit

N/A = not applicable

Medigap Benefits	Medigap Plans									
	A	B	C	D	F*	G	K	L	M	N
Part A coinsurance and hospital costs up to an additional 365 days after Medicare benefits are used up	100%	100%	100%	100%	100%	100%	100%	100%	100%	100%
Part B coinsurance or copayment	100%	100%	100%	100%	100%	100%	50%	75%	100%	100%***
Blood (first 3 pints)	100%	100%	100%	100%	100%	100%	50%	75%	100%	100%
Part A hospice care coinsurance or copayment	100%	100%	100%	100%	100%	100%	50%	75%	100%	100%
Skilled nursing facility care coinsurance	No benefit	No benefit	100%	100%	100%	100%	50%	75%	100%	100%
Part A deductible	No benefit	100%	100%	100%	100%	100%	50%	75%	50%	100%
Part B deductible	No benefit	No benefit	100%	No benefit	100%	No benefit	No benefit	No benefit	No benefit	No benefit
Part B excess charge	No benefit	No benefit	No benefit	No benefit	100%	100%	No benefit	No benefit	No benefit	No benefit
Foreign travel exchange (up to plan limits)	No benefit	No	80%	80%	80%	80%	No benefit	No benefit	80%	80%
Out-of-pocket limit in 2020**	N/A	N/A	N/A	N/A	N/A	N/A	$5880	$2940	N/A	N/A

* Plan F also offers a high-deductible plan. If you choose this option, this means you must pay for Medicare-covered costs up to the deductible amount of $2340 in 2020 before your Medigap plan pays anything.

** After you meet your out-of-pocket yearly limit and your yearly Part B deductible, the Medigap plan pays 100% of covered services for the rest of the calendar year.

*** Plan N pays 100% of the Part B coinsurance, except for a copayment of up to $20 for some office visits and up to a $50 copayment for emergency room visits that don't result in inpatient admission.

Fig. 6.4 Medigap plans effective as of 2020 from a Medicare government publication.

The Medigap insurance carrier is usually billed after Medicare. If the beneficiaries' claim to Medicare has been submitted with the appropriate information, the Medicare contractor will automatically forward a crossover claim to the Medigap contractor for processing. This automation allows for faster claims processing.

Medicare Secondary Payer

Medicare secondary payer guidelines apply in situations when Medicare is not the beneficiary's primary health insurance coverage. In those cases, Medicare is considered the secondary payer. It is important that the billing specialist ensure that Medicare does not pay for services that the primary insurance carrier is responsible for. The MSP rules state that Medicare is the secondary payer when the patient falls into one of the following categories:

- Aged workers under group health plans with more than 20 covered employees
- Disabled individuals aged 64 and younger who are covered under a group health plan with more than 100 covered employees or covered under a family member's current employment

- Medicare beneficiaries under an employer-sponsored group health plan who have ESRD during the first 18 months of the patient's eligibility for Medicare
- Cases of workers' compensation when the injury or illness occurs at work
- Individuals with black lung disease either currently or formerly employed who fall under the Federal Black Lung Program
- Individuals receiving benefits under the Department of Veterans Affairs (VA) and Medicare
- Individuals covered under a federal research grant program
- Automobile accident cases and third-party liability insurance cases.

In the above situations, Medicare is only billed after the primary insurance has processed the initial claim and has issued the health care provider a remittance statement detailing the services that were billed and payment determination. The remittance statement must be forwarded with the claim to Medicare. CMS has developed a questionnaire that can be used to determine if Medicare benefits are primary or secondary. The link for this questionnaire is listed under *Internet Resources* at the end of this chapter.

Managed Care and Medicare

Managed care plans were outlined in Chapter 5. When a patient's primary insurance is a managed care plan that requires fixed copayments at the time service is rendered, it is possible to obtain reimbursement from Medicare for those amounts. A claim must be filed with Medicare after the managed care organization (MCO) has paid. When Medicare's copayment reimbursement has been received, the provider must refund to the patient the copayment amount previously collected.

If the health care organization is paid a capitated amount by the managed care plan, they are paid a fixed per capita amount for each patient enrolled over a state period. There are no RA statements available from the managed care plan to forward to Medicare in these situations. Therefore, the patient must sign a statement that explains the situation. Attach the statement and the copayment receipts to the claim. The statement may read as shown here (Fig. 6.5).

```
Patient Name _____
Medicare Number _____
There is no Explanation of Benefits documentation
available for the attached billed services. I am currently
enrolled with _____ managed care plan
for my health care. My physician, _____ MD,
is paid on a capitated basis, and the copayment that
I pay is $ _____ for each service or visit.
    Patient's signature_____
    Date _____
```

Fig. 6.5 Explanation of Capitated Primary Insurance with Medicare Secondary.

Automobile or Liability Insurance Coverage

If the patient was involved in an automobile accident, the patient's automobile insurance is primary. Or, if it has been deemed that it is the legal responsibility of a person, business, or organization to pay for health care services, liability insurance coverage would be primary to Medicare. A health care professional who treats a Medicare patient who has filed a liability claim must bill the liability insurer first. After 120 days have gone by without a payment from the liability insurer and if the services performed are covered Medicare benefits, the health care professional may seek conditional payment from Medicare. A conditional payment is a payment Medicare makes for services another payer may be responsible for, so the patient does not have to use their own money to pay the bill. However, if a claim is filed with Medicare, the provider must drop the claim against the liability insurer.

- If the payment made by the liability insurer is less than the health care professional's full charge, the service provider may file a claim to Medicare. The provider cannot receive a higher combined reimbursement than what Medicare would have paid if they had been the primary payer (see Examples 6.3 and 6.4).

6.3   QUICK REVIEW
Question: In what cases would Medicare be considered a secondary payer?

EXAMPLE 6.3   Liability Scenario 1
- Patient received services; provider's full charge is $300.
- The liability insurance paid $200.
- The Medicare allowed amount for this service is $150.
- In this case a claim for the $100 balance would not be filed to Medicare because the liability insurance paid more than what Medicare would have allowed.
- The remaining balance of $100 will have to be written off by the service provider.

EXAMPLE 6.4   Liability Scenario 2
- Patient received services; provider's full charge is $300.
- The liability insurance paid $100.
- The Medicare allowed amount for this service is $150.
- In this claim a claim for $50 may be filed to Medicare for the difference between what the liability insurance paid ($100) and what the Medicare allowed amount is ($150)
  The remaining balance of $150 will have be written off by the service provider

UTILIZATION AND QUALITY CONTROL

Quality Improvement Organizations

DHHS has one of the largest federal programs dedicated to improving health quality for Medicare patients, the Quality Improvement Organization (QIO) program. The organization reviews for medical necessity, which CMS defines as the performance of services and procedures that are consistent with the diagnosis in accordance with standards of good medical practice, performed at the proper level, and provided in the most appropriate setting. QIO also reviews for reasonableness, appropriateness, and completeness and adequacy of care given in inpatient, outpatient, and emergency departments of hospitals; nursing facilities; home health agencies; PFFS plans; and ambulatory surgical centers.

It is extremely important that each patient's care be well documented from the treatment standpoint as well as for justifying maximum reimbursement. A health care provider or organization who receives a letter from a QIO about quality of care should consult their attorney before responding by letter or personal appeal. A photocopy of the patient's medical record can be used to substantiate the claim if there is detailed clinical documentation.

Medicare Billing Compliance Issues

Because Medicare is a federal program, there is federal legislation that sets down the policies that must be followed. Therefore, whoever participates in the program must comply with all regulations. General health care compliance has been discussed in Chapter 3; however, it is important to remind any staff member who may be involved in the health care organization of the issues they should be aware of. The following are issues that have been discussed in previous chapters or that will be outlined in later chapters of the textbook. The issues may include but are not limited to the following:
- Release of medical information

PAYMENT EXAMPLES FOR PARTICIPATING PROVIDERS

	Actual charge	Medicare approved amount*	2020 Annual Deductible	Medicare pays	Beneficiary responsible for	Medicare adjustment
Doctor A participates in the Medicare program.	$480	$400	$198 already satisfied	$320 (80% of approved amount)	$80 (20% of approved amount)	$80 (difference between actual charge and approved amount)
Doctor B participates in the Medicare program; however, the patient has not met the deductible amount.	$480	$400	$198 has not been met	$161.60 (80% of approved amount determined after subtracting the deductible)	$238.40 (deductible plus 20% of approved amount)	$80 (difference between actual charge and approved amount)

Fig. 6.6 Payment examples for two physicians who participate with Medicare and the amounts that the patient is responsible for paying with deductible satisfied and not met.

- Reassignment of payment
- Limiting charges for health care service providers
- Correct procedural code assignment and service utilization
- Accurate diagnostic code assignment
- Medical necessity of services performed
- Billing for ancillary employees (physician assistants and nurse practitioners), called "incident-to" billing
- Documentation related to selection of procedural codes for services performed
- Ancillary orders and supervision requirements
- Teaching physician and resident billing
- Routine waiver of copayments, deductibles, or professional courtesy discounts
- Stark I and II anti–referral and compensation regulations
- Overpayment refunds

6.4 QUICK REVIEW
Question: What is the definition of medical necessity and why is it important?

PROGRAM FUNDAMENTALS

Provider

Health care providers are given the option to participate or not participate in the Medicare program. Most providers choose to participate in the Medicare program as there are payment incentives.

Participating Provider

In a **participating (par) provider** agreement, a service provider or health care organization agrees to accept payment from Medicare. Participating providers must accept **assignment** for all claims. Accepting assignment means the patient has signed a statement to have Medicare send payment directly to the provider of services.

The fee that Medicare decides the medical service is worth is referred to as the **approved charge**. Medicare beneficiaries are required to meet their annual deductible, which is based on the calendar year January 1 through December 31 ($198 for calendar year 2020). Medicare will then reimburse 80% of the approved charges. The remaining 20% of the approved charge is paid by the patient (see Fig. 6.6).

Nonparticipating Provider

Although there are few benefits, some health care providers may elect to not participate in the Medicare program. For instance, pediatric specialists rarely provide medical care to Medicare patients, so they do not see a value in participation. A specialist in cosmetic surgery may choose to not participate, as the services they provide would not be a covered benefit under Medicare.

A **nonparticipating (nonpar)** service provider or health care organization does not have a signed agreement with Medicare and has an option about assignment. The service provider may decline assignment for all services or accept assignment for some services and collect from the patient for other services performed at the same time and place. An exception to this policy is mandatory assignment for clinical laboratory tests and services by physician assistants.

Nonpar providers who accept assignment receive only 95% of the Medicare-approved amount. Medicare will pay 80% of the nonpar Medicare approved amount directly to the provider and the provider collects the remaining 20% from the patient.

The nonpar provider can choose *not* to accept assignment for all Medicare patients, or they can decide to *not* accept assignment on a case-by-case basis. If the nonpar provider does not accept assignment, the provider will receive only 95% of the Medicare-approved amount. However, because the provider chose not to accept assignment, Medicare will send payment directly to the patient, and the nonpar provider bills the patient. Medicare sets a limiting charge of 115% of the nonpar rate that can be billed to the patient. A **limiting charge** is a percentage limit on fees, specified by legislation, that nonpar service providers may bill Medicare beneficiaries above the allowed amount. Because Medicare sends the payment to the patient, and service providers must often "chase the money," providers should evaluate whether the ability to balance bill and collect a higher fee from the patient is worth the potential extra billing and collection costs. Furthermore, some hospitals and states prohibit or limit balance billing, so health care organizations and service providers must ascertain whether these restrictions apply before making a Medicare participation or nonparticipation decision (see Example 6.5).

EXAMPLE 6.5 Medicare Nonparticipating and Limiting Charges

Amount	Example
Medicare Fee Schedule (MFS) allowed amount	$200.00
Nonparticipating provider allowed amount	$190.00 ($200.00 × 95% = 5% lower than MFS allowed amount.)
Limiting charge	$218.50 ($190.00 × 115% of MFS allowed amount)
Beneficiary coinsurance and limiting charge portion due to provider	$66.50 ($38.00 plus $28.50) Coinsurance-20% of MFS allowed amount ($190.00 × 20% = $38.00) PLUS $218.50-Limiting charge -190.00-Nonparticipating allowed amount $28.50-Additional amount that can be collected from beneficiary.

Prior Authorization

Prior authorization is a requirement for a health care provider to obtain approval from an insurance carrier to provide a medical service. Generally, traditional Medicare does not require prior authorization.

On the other hand, Medicare Advantage plans often require prior authorization for surgical procedures, diagnostic testing, out-of-network care, nonemergency hospital care, and referrals to specialists. Some of these procedures requiring authorization are on a mandatory list, whereas others are chosen by the regional carrier. The mandatory list is composed of procedures such as the following:

- Bunionectomy
- Carotid endarterectomy
- Cataract extractions
- Cholecystectomy
- Complex peripheral revascularization
- Coronary artery bypass graft surgery
- Hysterectomy
- Inguinal hernia repair
- Joint replacements (hip, shoulder, or knee)
- Transurethral prostatectomy

Each MA plan has different prior authorization requirements. To obtain prior authorization, the MA plans generally have a toll-free line to call for authorization or may require the completion of a preauthorization form. Check with the plan on its policy for preauthorization.

Medicare prescription drug (Part D) plans very often require prior authorization to obtain coverage for certain drugs. In many instances the health care provider must first contact the plan to determine if there is coverage for the drug and if a prior authorization is required. If the prescription is filled without prior authorization, the medical plan will probably not pay for the drug and the patient will be charged full-retail price for the drug.

National and Local Coverage Determinations

Although traditional Medicare does not generally require prior authorization of services to ensure payment, coverage policies have been developed that must be adhered to for assurance of payment.

National Coverage Determinations (NCDs) and Local Coverage Determinations (LCDs) are decisions by Medicare and its administrative contractors. The NCD/LCDs provide coverage information for medical services.

An NCD is mandated by CMS at the federal level, and all Medicare contractors must follow those guidelines. An LCD is mandated at the Medicare contractor level, and those guidelines are only applicable to that carrier's defined area of responsibility referred to as their jurisdiction. Medicare contractors develop LCDs when there is no NCD or when there is a need to further define an NCD.

Both NCDs and LCDs are developed to decide whether to cover a particular service in accordance with CMS's definition of services that are medically necessary. The NCD and LCD are educational and administrative tools to assist physicians, health care providers, and suppliers in transmitting correct claims for payment. Typically, procedural and diagnosis codes describing what is covered and what is not covered can be part of the NCD/LCD. The NCDs/LCDs also specify under what clinical circumstances they consider a service to be reasonable and necessary. Coverage determinations also outline how contractors review claims to determine whether Medicare coverage requirements have been met.

NCD and LCD coverage policies are developed by CMS medical directors and staff with input from the public. CMS requires that local policies be consistent with national guidance. Use of NCDs and LCDs helps avoid situations in which claims are paid or denied without a full understanding of the basis for payment and denial. NCDs are available on the CMS website, whereas LCDs may be obtained from the Medicare contractor.

Advance Beneficiary Notice of Noncoverage

NCDs and LCDs should be reviewed before furnishing services to ensure payment of them.

An advance beneficiary notice is a written notice the insurance billing specialist must issue to an FFS beneficiary before furnishing items or services that are usually covered by Medicare but are not expected to be paid. The Advance Beneficiary Notice of Noncoverage (ABN) allows the beneficiary to make an informed decision about whether to get the item or service that may not be covered and accept financial responsibility if Medicare does not pay.

If it is expected that Medicare will deny payment (entirely or in part), the patient should be instructed to sign an Advance Beneficiary Notice of Noncoverage (ABN), also known as a *waiver of liability agreement,* as shown in Fig. 6.7. This form

A. Notifier:

B. Patient Name: C. Identification Number:

Advance Beneficiary Notice of Non-coverage
(ABN)

NOTE: If Medicare doesn't pay for **D.**_____below, you may have to pay.
Medicare does not pay for everything, even some care that you or your health care provider have good reason to think you need. We expect Medicare may not pay for the **D.**_____below.

D.	E. Reason Medicare May Not Pay:	F. Estimated Cost

WHAT YOU NEED TO DO NOW:
- Read this notice, so you can make an informed decision about your care.
- Ask us any questions that you may have after you finish reading.
- Choose an option below about whether to receive the **D.**_____listed above.
  - **Note:** If you choose Option 1 or 2, we may help you to use any other insurance that you might have, but Medicare cannot require us to do this.

G. OPTIONS: Check only one box. We cannot choose a box for you.
☐ **OPTION 1.** I want the **D.**_____listed above. You may ask to be paid now, but I also want Medicare billed for an official decision on payment, which is sent to me on a Medicare Summary Notice (MSN). I understand that if Medicare doesn't pay, I am responsible for payment, but I can appeal to Medicareby following the directions on the MSN. If Medicare does pay, you will refund any payments I made to you, less co-pays ordeductibles.
☐ **OPTION 2.** I want the **D.**_____listed above, but do not bill Medicare. You may ask to be paid now as I am responsible for payment. I cannot appeal if Medicare is not billed.
☐ **OPTION 3.** I don't want the **D.**_____listed above. I understand with thischoiceI am **not** responsible for payment, and I cannot appeal to see if Medicare wouldpay.

H. Additional Information:

This notice gives our opinion, not an official Medicare decision. If you have other questions on this notice or Medicare billing, call **1-800-MEDICARE** (1-800-633-4227/**TTY:** 1-877-486-2048).
Signing below means that you have received and understand this notice. You also receive a copy.

I. Signature:	J. Date:

CMS does not discriminate in its programs and activities. To request this publication in an alternative format, please call: 1-800-MEDICARE or email: AltFormatRequest@cms.hhs.gov.

According to the Paperwork Reduction Act of 1995, no persons are required to respond to a collection of information unless it displays a valid OMB control number. The valid OMB control number for this information collection is 0938-0566. The time required to complete this information collection is estimated to average 7 minutes per response, including the time to review instructions, search existing data resources, gather the data needed, and complete and review the information collection. If you have comments concerning the accuracy of the time estimate or suggestions for improving this form, please write to: CMS, 7500 Security Boulevard, Attn: PRA Reports Clearance Officer, Baltimore, Maryland 21244-1850.

Form CMS-R-131 (Exp. 06/30/2023)   Form Approved OMB No. 0938-0566

Fig. 6.7 Advance Beneficiary Notice of Noncoverage, Form CMS-R-131, which is also referred to as a *responsibility statement* or *waiver of liability agreement.*

---

should not be given to someone who is in a medical emergency, confused, legally incompetent, or otherwise under great duress. It cannot be signed after a patient has received the service and must specifically state what service or procedure is being waived. Write the specific time frequency limitation for a particular service, such as screening colonoscopy once every 10 years. Each space on the ABN must be completed before providing the ABN to the patient. Blank or partially completed ABNs, even with the patient's signature, are not acceptable. An ABN may be mailed to a patient when presenting it face to face is not possible, but the patient must have an opportunity to ask questions. When the ABN is mailed, it should be sent with a cover letter

explaining that the procedure will be denied by Medicare and include contact information so that the patient can ask questions before the procedure.

To determine which services require an ABN, refer to the NCDs and the LCDs from the insurance carrier. An office policy should be in place for handling patients who refuse to sign an ABN. The Medicare carrier then informs the patient that he or she is responsible for the fee. Keep this signed waiver with other patient financial documents and not with the patient's medical record.

If the service was not reasonable because of Medicare guidelines but the patient thought it was covered and there is no advance notice given with signed waiver of liability agreement, the following apply:

- The provider cannot bill the patient.
- The patient does not have to pay the deductible or coinsurance.
- The patient is refunded any amount paid to the provider on the item or service.

If assignment is accepted and the health care provider patient thought the service was covered under reasonable assumptions, the following apply:

- Medicare is billed to pay for the service.
- The patient must pay the deductible and coinsurance.
- Medicare will not seek a refund of money already paid to the health care provider.

Nonpar providers must refund any amount collected from the beneficiary when services are later found to be not reasonable and necessary.

! COMPLIANCE ALERT

Advance Beneficiary Notice of Noncoverage

Medicare considers the appropriate use of an Advance Beneficiary Notice of Noncoverage (ABN) document as a compliance issue. Ask the patient to sign an ABN document if it is confirmed that the service is not covered or if there is a possibility that a service may be denied for medical necessity or limitation of Medicare benefits. A step-by-step procedure of how to complete an ABN form is presented at the end of this chapter (Procedure 6.2).

Noncovered Services

Noncovered Medicare services are services that are never covered by Medicare. Some of the items or services that Medicare does not cover include the following:

- Long-term care
- Most dental care
- Eye examinations related to prescribing glasses
- Dentures
- Cosmetic surgery
- Acupuncture
- Hearing aids and exams for fitting them
- Routine foot care
- Routine physical examinations
- Services furnished outside the United States, except under certain limited services

Noncovered services are billed to the patient. It is not necessary to give a patient an ABN when a service is never covered by Medicare.

Prepayment Screens

Medicare prepayment screens or prepayment edits are put in place to prevent payment for noncovered and incorrectly coded services. Prepayment screens are also used to target claims for review before payment. The screens may be placed to target specific health care services that have high claim error rates or unusual billing practices that are considered to be a financial risk to Medicare.

The screens or edits are computer triggers that suspend claims processing. These screens are used to identify and review claims

for medical necessity and determine compliance with other appropriate criteria. The suspended claim is held in a pended state until it is checked by a reviewer who decides whether the services are appropriate, medically necessary, or meet other specific criteria.

CMS requires Medicare contractors to implement prepayment screens or edits that include the following:

- *Procedure to procedure,* which screen for multiple services reported on a date of service to ensure they are not inclusive in the primary procedure. For example, an exploratory laparotomy is always inclusive in an open abdominal procedure when performed on the same date of service. Medicare implemented the Correct Coding Initiative (CCI), a methodology used to identify procedures that are usually described by a single code or are inherent to another procedure. The CCI will be discussed further in Chapter 13.
- *Procedure to provider* permits selective screening of services that need review. For example, Medicare may identify a provider who appears to be reporting an usually large amount of endoscopy services in comparison to other in the provider's specialty.
- *Frequency to time* allows screening for a certain number of services provided within a given period. For example, Medicare limits medically necessary routine foot care to one treatment every 60 days.
- *Diagnosis to procedure edits* allows screening for services submitted with a specific diagnosis. For example, vitamin B12 injections are only reimbursed if treatment is related to pernicious anemia, absence of the stomach, or distal ileum.
- *Procedure to specialty code* permits screening of services provided by a certain specialty or type of bill. For example, a physical therapist could not report a code for excision of tonsils.
- *Procedure to place of service* allows selective screening of claims where the service was provided. For example, a nursing home admission must be performed in a nursing home. If it were reported with hospital as the place of service, the claim would be suspended.

6.5 QUICK REVIEW

Question: Explain how an insurance billing specialist can determine coverage information for medical services prior to the service being provided to the patient.

MEDICARE REIMBURSEMENT

Traditional Medicare has different payment methodologies, depending on the type of services provided.

Medicare Fee Schedule

Since January 1992, CMS has reimbursed using a Medicare fee schedule (MFS) to pay doctors and other providers/suppliers. The fee schedule is a comprehensive listing of accepted charges or established allowances for all medical services. CMS has developed fee schedules for health care professionals, physicians, ambulance services, clinical laboratory services, and durable medical equipment.

The resource-based relative value scale (RBRVS) is the system that Medicare uses for establishing fees. This system considers work value, overhead expense, and malpractice values for all Current Procedural Terminology (CPT) codes that are published in the *Federal Register* each November. These are adjusted for each Medicare local carrier by geographic practice cost indices (GPCIs) by using a formula that gives the total value for a code. This payment methodology will be discussed further in Chapter 13.

When using the MFS payment methodology, the approved amount is the amount that the Medicare participating providers agree to accept. It is listed on the RA as an allowed charge for a procedure. This charge is typically lower than the fee the health care provider lists on the claim. When a health care provider accepts assignment, he or she may bill the patient only 20% of the Medicare-allowed charge. If the insurance billing specialist can confirm the amount of annual deductible that has not been met, it is permissible to collect the deductible at the time of service. However, the Medicare copayment should not be collected until Medicare pays.

Prospective Payment System

Since October 1983, CMS has used the prospective payment system (PPS) to reimburse hospitals. PPS is a method of reimbursement in which Medicare payment is made based on predetermined, fixed amounts. For example, an inpatient hospital stay may be reimbursed according to the diagnosis the patient was treated for. If the patient were hospitalized for pneumonia, the PPS would reimburse a predetermined and fixed amount designated for pneumonia inpatient stays. CMS uses separate PPS for reimbursement to acute inpatient hospitals, home health agencies, hospice, hospital outpatient, inpatient psychiatric facilities, inpatient rehabilitation facilities, long-term care hospitals, and skilled nursing facilities. These payment methodologies will be discussed further in Chapter 19.

Value-Based Programs

In an effort to lessen health care cost growth and to identify and encourage high quality of care to patients, legislation was passed in 2008 to change reimbursement methodologies. Since that time, CMS has developed a multitude of programs to transform to more affordable health care through value-based programs. Value-based programs are also known as pay-for-performance programs and are based on value-based purchasing (VBP) principles. Value-based programs reward health care organizations with incentive payments for the quality of care they give to people with Medicare. Payments are linked to the quality and efficiency of care provided with the shift away from paying providers based solely on their volumes of services. A timeline displaying implementation of the various value-based programs is seen in Fig. 6.8.

Medicare Improvements for Patients and Providers Act (MIPPA)

One of the first value-based programs developed by Medicare was the ESRD Quality Incentive Program (QIP). Previously,

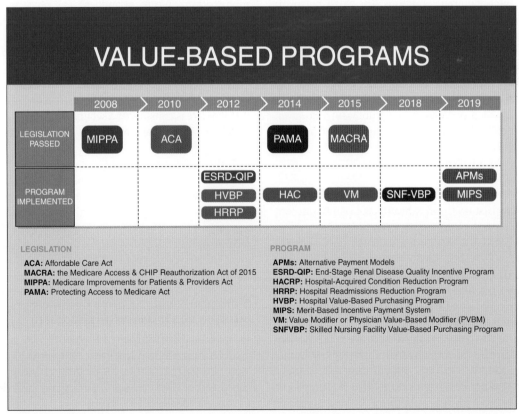

Fig. 6.8 Timeline for implementation of the Center for Medicare and Medicaid's value-based programs that has reformed how health care is delivered and paid for. (https://www.cms.gov/Medicare /Quality-Initiatives-Patient-Assessment-Instruments/Value-Based-Programs/Value-Based-Programs.)

ESRD care was paid through a bundled payment system. Under a bundled payment system, providers and/or health care organizations are paid a single payment for all the delivery of care within a specific period. Under the Medicare Improvements for Patients and Providers Act (MIPPA), CMS was required to implement quality incentives into the ESRD bundled payment system. The ESRD-QIP was established to promote high-quality services to outpatient dialysis facilities treating patients with ESRD. This changed the way CMS pays for treatment of patients with ESRD by linking a portion of payment directly to facilities performance on quality-of-care measures. The ESRD-QIP reduces payments to ESRD facilities that do not meet or exceed certain performance standards. Payment reductions occur when the facility's score on applicable measures does not meet established standards. The ESRD-QIP now operates under a fully bundled, case-mix adjusted PPS and has implemented Medicare's first-ever mandatory pay-for-performance program.

Other programs that follow value-based program values are as follows:

- Hospital Value-Based Purchasing Programs (HVBP): A program to adjust payments to hospitals under the Inpatient Prospective Payment System (IPPS) based on the quality of care they provide.
- Hospital Readmissions Reduction Program (HRRP): A program implemented in 2012 that reduced payment to IPPS hospitals with excess readmissions.
- Hospital-Acquired Condition Reduction Program (HACRP): A program established to provide an incentive for hospitals to reduce hospital-acquired conditions. The worst-performing hospitals are subject to a payment reduction.
- Value Modifier or Physician Value-Based Modifier (PVBM): This program provides for differential payment to a physician or group of physicians under the Medicare fee schedule based on the quality of care furnished compared with the cost of care during a performance period.
- Skilled Nursing Facility Value-Based Purchasing Program (SNFVBP): The SNFVBP program rewards skilled nursing facilities with incentive payments for the quality of care they give to people with Medicare.

Medicare Access and CHIIP Reauthorization Act of 2015

Another piece of legislation to affect health care reimbursement was the Medicare Access and CHIP Reauthorization Act of 2015 (MACRA). MACRA established a quality payment program (QPP), which was a new way to pay providers. Under the QPP, which started on January 1, 2017, providers are rewarded for giving high-quality and high-value care through the Advanced Alternative Payment Model (APM) or the Merit-based Incentive Payment System (MIPS).

APM provides ways to pay health care providers for the care they give to Medicare beneficiaries by sharing the risk. Accountable care organizations (ACOs), patient-centered medical homes (PCMH), and bundled payment models are examples of APMs. Health care providers who qualify for APMs will receive lump-sum incentive payments.

Most Medicare providers will fall under the MIPS payment adjustment option. MIPS defines the financial impact on providers by creating a composite score for each provider. The composite score is based on the following performance categories:

- Quality
- Promoting Interoperability
- Cost
- Improvement Activities

The health care organizations select measures from the categories described that fit their practice and then report on those measures. The health care organization must have a qualified electronic medical record to report the measures.

The final score earned by a clinician for a given performance year then determines the MIPS payment adjustments to be incurred by that provider. Essentially, the composite score will lead to each provider having their own individual fee schedule. Payment adjustments are applied to Medicare Part B payments 2 years after the performance year. For example, providers who report in the performance year 2020 will receive adjustments in 2022, which is referred to as the payment adjustment year.

> **6.6 QUICK REVIEW**
> Question: What is the system used to establish fees for Medicare payment? Under this system, what are the three components that are used to establish the fees?

CLAIM SUBMISSION

The Social Security Act requires that health care providers submit claims for their Medicare patients. This mandatory claims submission requirement applies to all physicians and suppliers who provide covered services to Medicare beneficiaries. Violations to this requirement can lead to civil monetary penalties of up to $2000 per violation. Exceptions to the mandatory filing rule would include:

- If services are provided for free to the beneficiary
- If services are submitted to a primary insurance carrier; Medicare is considered a secondary payer and the health care organization does not possess all information necessary to file the claim.
- If the health care provider opts out of the Medicare program (except in emergency or urgent care situations)

Initial claims for payment under Medicare must be submitted *electronically* unless the health care service provider qualifies for a waiver of exception. The waiver is a provision of the Administrative Simplification Compliance Act (ASCA) requirement for electronic submission of claims and will be discussed further in Chapter 15.

Medicare Administrative Contractors

Claims for traditional FFS Medicare services are sent to a Medicare administrative contractor (MAC). A MAC is a private insurance carrier that has been contracted by CMS to process Medicare Part A and Part B medical claims for Medicare FFS beneficiaries. CMS relies on MACs to do the following:

- Process Medicare FFS claims
- Make and account for Medicare FFS payments
- Enroll providers in the Medicare FFS program
- Handle provider reimbursement services

- Process redetermination requests
- Respond to provider inquiries
- Educate providers about Medicare FFS billing requirements
- Establish local coverage policies
- Review medical records for selected claims
- Coordinate with CMS and other MACs

Currently, there are 12 Part A and Part B MACs contracted with CMS to process Medicare FFS claims (Fig. 6.9). Each MAC processes claims for a defined geographical area or jurisdiction that services institutional providers, physicians, practitioners, and suppliers. Some of those Part A and Part B MACs also process home health and hospice claims. Providers should send the Medicare claim to the MAC covering the jurisdiction where the services were furnished, rather than where the patient resides.

There are an additional four MACs that process claims for durable medical equipment (DME) suppliers (see Fig. 6.10).

A/B MAC Jurisdictions
as of June 2019

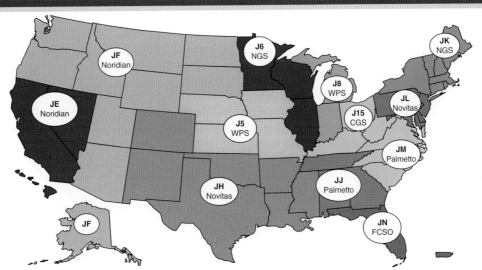

Fig. 6.9 Medicare Administration Contractor (MAC) jurisdiction map for Medicare Part A and Part B Regions map as of June 2019. (https://www.cms.gov/Medicare/Medicare-Contracting/Medicare-Administrative-Contractors/Downloads/AB-Jurisdiction-Map-Jun-2019.pdf.)

DME MAC Jurisdictions
as of June 2019

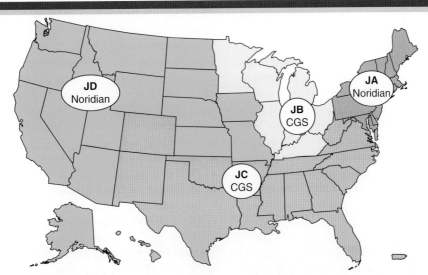

Fig. 6.10 Medicare Administrative Contractor (MAC) jurisdiction map for Durable Medical Equipment suppliers as of June 2019. (https://www.cms.gov/Medicare/Medicare-Contracting/Medicare-Administrative-Contractors/Downloads/DME-Jurisdiction-Map-Jun-2019.pdf.)

DME is any equipment that provides therapeutic benefits to a patient in need because of certain medical conditions and/or illnesses. Medicare covers medically necessary DME if it is prescribed and meets the following criteria:

- Can withstand repeat use (durable)
- Used for a medical reason
- Not usually useful to someone who is not sick or injured
- Used in the patient's home
- Has an expected lifetime of at least 3 years

Examples of DME-covered items include (but are not limited to) blood sugar monitors, canes, commode chairs, crutches, hospital beds, infusion pumps and supplies, nebulizers, patient lifts, traction equipment, and walkers.

Medicare beneficiaries who are enrolled in an MA plan should have claims submitted to the beneficiary's MA plan.

Provider Identification Numbers

Medicare claims must be submitted with the service provider's national provider identifier (NPI). The NPI is a unique 10-digit identification number issued to all covered health care providers. As outlined in the Health Insurance Portability and Accountability Act (HIPAA), service providers must also share their NPI with other providers that may need it for billing purposes. For additional information, refer to Chapter 2.

Time Limit for Claims Submission

The Affordable Care Act (ACA) set the time limit policy for Medicare claims submission. Service providers must submit claims to traditional Medicare and Railroad Retirement within 12 months of the date of service. Medicare will deny claims if they arrive after the deadline date, and they are not subject to appeal.

In limited circumstances, Medicare will allow for exceptions to the one calendar year time limit for filing FFS claims.

- Administrative error: If the deadline was not met because of administrative error, the MAC may extend the timely filing limit through the last day of the sixth month after the month in which the error was corrected.
- Retroactive Medicare entitlement: If the deadline was not met because patient was not entitled to benefits at time of service, and then was notified later that enrollment would be retroactive, the MAC will extend the timely filing limit through the last day of the sixth month after the beneficiary received notification of Medicare entitlement to benefits.
- Retroactive disenrollment from an MA plan: If the beneficiary was enrolled in a MA program but later disenrolled before the service was performed and the MA plan recoups payment from the service provider, Medicare will extend the timely filing limit through the last day of the sixth month after the month in which the MA plan recovered its payment from the service provider.

Instructions for Claims Submissions

MACs are mandated to pay for services deemed medically necessary and reasonable for the diagnosis and treatment of illness and injury. Medicare is not required to pay for noncovered and undocumented services. Claims must be submitted accurately

and in accordance with the current Medicare billing policies. Care must be taken to ensure that all documentation required to support the medical need for the service rendered is submitted when requested by the MAC.

Instructions for claims submissions can be found in the Medicare Claims Processing Manual—Internet Only Manual Publication (IOM Pub.) 100-04. The publication includes general billing requirements for various health care professionals and suppliers, as well as claims submission information specific to a health care professional or supplier type. Another helpful resource is the Medicare Learning Network (MLN). The MLN offers free educational materials for health care professionals on programs, policies, and initiatives. Links to both the IOM and MLN can be found under *Internet Resources* at the end of the chapter.

Further guidance for completion of a CMS 1500 claim form for a Medicare patient will be explained in chapter 14 of this textbook; however, see Fig. 6.11 for an example of a completed Medicare claim form. Note the following information included on the claim form:

- The name of the insurance carrier the claim is being prepared for is identified in the top right-hand corner of the form.
- In box #1, Medicare has been checked to identify this patient has Medicare.
- In box #1a., the patient's Medicare identification number has been entered.
- In box #27, the accept assignment box has been checked "yes" to indicate that the provider accepts assignment.

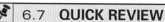

6.7 QUICK REVIEW
Question: Where would the insurance billing specialist send a completed Medicare claim for processing?

AFTER CLAIM SUBMISSION

Remittance Advice

A RA is a notice of payment and explains any adjustments made to a payment during the Medicare adjudication process. Adjudication is the process of paying claims submitted or denying them after comparing the claim to benefit and coverage requirements. RAs provide itemized claims processing decisions regarding the following:

- Payments
- Deductible and copays
- Adjustments
- Denials
- Missing or incorrect data
- Refunds
- Claims withholding because of MSP or penalty situations

Health care service providers who accept assignment receive payment from the MAC for the claims they submitted as well as a RA. And although providers who do not accept assignment must submit a claim for services they provide Medicare beneficiaries, the payment for services will be sent to the patient. The provider of services will receive an informational RA to report

DRAFT - NOT FOR OFFICIAL USE

MEDICARE
NO SECONDARY COVERAGE

HEALTH INSURANCE CLAIM FORM

APPROVED BY NATIONAL UNIFOR MCLAIM COMMITTEE (NUCC) 02/12

| | PICA | | | | | | | | PICA | |

1. MEDICARE	MEDICAID	TRICARE	CHAMPVA	GROUP HEALTH PLAN	FECA BLK LUNG	OTHER	1a. INSURED'S I.D. NUMBER (For Program in Item 1)
[X] (Medicare#)	[ ] (Medicaid#)	[ ] (ID#DoD#)	[ ] (Member ID#)	[ ] (ID#)	[ ] (ID#)	[ ] (ID#)	1EG4-TE5-MK71

2. PATIENT'S NAME (Last Name, First Name, Middle Initial)
Smith, Mary

3. PATIENT'S BIRTH DATE MM 12 DD 30 YY 1910   SEX M [ ] F [X]

4. INSURED'S NAME (Last Name, First Name, Middle Initial)
Smith, Mary

5. PATIENT'S ADDRESS (No., Street)
16 Oregon Street

6. PATIENT RELATIONSHIP TO INSURED
Self [X] Spouse [ ] Child [ ] Other [ ]

7. INSURED'S ADDRESS (No., Street)

CITY: Woodland Hills   STATE: XY

8. RESERVED FOR NUCC USE

CITY   STATE

ZIP CODE: 12345   TELEPHONE (Include Area Code): (555) 7321520

ZIP CODE   TELEPHONE (Include Area Code): ( )

9. OTHER INSURED'S NAME (Last Name, First Name, Middle Initial)

10. IS PATIENT'S CONDITION RELATED TO:

11. INSURED'S POLICY GROUP OR FECA NUMBER

a. OTHER INSURED'S POLICY OR GROUP NUMBER

a. EMPLOYMENT? (Current or Previous) [ ] YES [X] NO

a. INSURED'S DATE OF BIRTH MM DD YY   SEX M [ ] F [ ]

b. RESERVED FOR NUCC USE

b. AUTO ACCIDENT? [ ] YES [X] NO   PLACE (State)

b. OTHER CLAIM ID (Designated by NUCC)

c. RESERVED FOR NUCC USE

c. OTHER ACCIDENT? [ ] YES [X] NO

c. INSURANCE PLAN NAME OR PROGRAM NAME
Medicare

d. INSURANCE PLAN NAME OR PROGRAM NAME

10d. CLAIM CODES (Designated by NUCC)

d. IS THERE ANOTHER HEALTH BENEFIT PLAN?
[ ] YES [X] NO If yes, complete items 9, 9a, and 9d.

READ BACK OF FORM BEFORE COMPLETING & SIGNING THIS FORM.
12. PATIENT'S OR AUTHORIZED PERSON'S SIGNATURE I authorize the release of any medical or other information necessary to process this claim. I also request payment of government benefits either to myself or to the party who accepts assignment below.

SIGNED Signature on file   DATE

13. INSURED'S OR AUTHORIZED PERSON'S SIGNATURE I authorize payment of medical benefits to the undersigned physician or supplier for services described below.

SIGNED

14. DATE OF CURRENT: ILLNESS, INJURY, or PREGNANCY(LMP) MM DD YY QUAL.

15. OTHER DATE QUAL. MM DD YY

16. DATES PATIENT UNABLE TO WORK IN CURRENT OCCUPATION FROM MM DD YY TO MM DD YY

17. NAME OF REFERRING PROVIDER OR OTHER SOURCE
DN Gerald Practon MD

17a.
17b. NPI 46278897XX

18. HOSPITALIZATION DATES RELATED TO CURRENT SERVICES FROM MM DD YY TO MM DD YY

19. ADDITIONAL CLAIM INFORMATION (Designated by NUCC)

20. OUTSIDE LAB? [ ] YES [X] NO $ CHARGES

21. DIAGNOSIS OR NATURE OF ILLNESS OR INJURY Relate A-L to service line below (24E)   ICD Ind. 0

A. I10   B.   C.   D.
E.   F.   G.   H.
I.   J.   K.   L.

22. RESUBMISSION CODE   ORIGINAL REF. NO.

23. PRIOR AUTHORIZATION NUMBER

24. A. DATE(S) OF SERVICE From MM DD YY To MM DD YY	B. PLACE OF SERVICE	C. EMG	D. PROCEDURES, SERVICES, OR SUPPLIES (Explain Unusual Circumstances) CPT/HCPCS | MODIFIER	E. DIAGNOSIS POINTER	F. $ CHARGES	G. DAYS OR UNITS	H. EPSDT Family Plan	I. ID. QUAL.	J. RENDERING PROVIDER ID. #
1	03 10 XX	11		99213	A	90.00	1		NPI	64211067XX
2									NPI	
3									NPI	
4									NPI	
5									NPI	
6									NPI	

25. FEDERAL TAX I.D. NUMBER XX12210XX   SSN [ ] EIN [X]

26. PATIENT'S ACCOUNT NO. 8122

27. ACCEPT ASSIGNMENT? (For govt. claims, see back) [X] YES [ ] NO

28. TOTAL CHARGE $ 90.00

29. AMOUNT PAID $

30. Rsvd for NUCC Use $

31. SIGNATURE OF PHYSICIAN OR SUPPLIER INCLUDING DEGREES OR CREDENTIALS (I certify that the statements on the reverse apply to this bill and are made a part thereof.)
Brady Coccidioides   031020XX
SIGNED Brady Coccidioides MD DATE

32. SERVICE FACILITY LOCATION INFORMATION

a. NPI   b.

33. BILLING PROVIDER INFO & PH # (555) 4869002
College Clinic
4567 Broad Avenue
Woodland Hills XY 123450001

a. 3664021CC   b.

NUCC Instruction Manual available at: www.nucc.org   PLEASE PRINT OR TYPE   OMB APPROVAL PENDING

CARRIER / PATIENT AND INSURED INFORMATION / PHYSICIAN OR SUPPLIER INFORMATION

Fig. 6.11 Example of a completed CMS-1500 claim form for a Medicare patient.

the amount of payment and the adjustments the MAC made during adjudication. RAs can be sent in either electronic format (Electronic Remittance Advice [ERA]) or a paper format (Standard Paper Remittance Advice [SPR]). Both ERA and SPR have the same format; however, the advantage of an ERA is that it electronically posts payments and the billing specialist does not have to post them manually.

The RA provides detailed payment information about a health care claim and helps the billing specialist understand the actions the MAC took while processing the claim. Some RA codes may indicate a need to resubmit a claim with corrected information, whereas others may indicate whether the provider may appeal the payment decision. The RA also identified any adjustment to the claim. An *adjustment* refers to any change that related to how a MAC paid a claim differently than the original billing.

Claim Adjustment Reason Codes (CARCs) provide financial information about claim decision. CARCs communicate adjustments the MAC made and offer explanation when the MAC pays a particular claim or service line differently that what was on the original claim. If there is no adjustment to a claim, then there is no CARC. Several examples of CARCs can be identified in Example 6.6.

Remittance Advice Remark Codes (RARCs) further explain an adjustment or relay informational messages that CARCs cannot express. Additionally, there are some informational RARCs, starting with the work "alert" that MACS use to provide general adjudication information. These RARCs are not always associated with a CARC when there is no adjustment. Examples of RARCS can be noted in Example 6.7.

EXAMPLE 6.6 Claim Adjustment Reason Codes

Code	Financial Information
1	Deductible amount
2	Coinsurance amount
3	Copayment amount
4	The procedure code is inconsistent with the modifier used or a required modifier is missing.
5	The procedure code is inconsistent with the place of service.
6	The procedure code is inconsistent with the patient's age.

EXAMPLE 6.7 Examples of Remittance Advice Remark Codes

Code	Explanation
M51	Missing/incomplete/invalid procedure code.
M53	Missing/incomplete/invalid days or units of service.
M56	Missing/incomplete/invalid payer identifier.

Medicare Summary Notice

A patient is mailed a similar document called a Medicare Summary Notice (MSN) every 3 months. This document notifies the patient of Medicare Part A and Part B covered services that were paid on their behalf. Because many patients do not know what is meant by *amount charged, Medicare approved, deductible,* and

coinsurance, it often becomes necessary for the insurance billing specialist to educate the patient

Posting Payments

The charge submitted by the service provider or health care organization will be higher than the charge approved by the MAC. This does not mean that the provider's charges are unreasonable. However, the difference between the service provider's charge and the amount that is allowed under the Medicare fee schedule must be adjusted. This reduction is known as a contractual adjustment or may be referred to as a write-off. See Example 6.8.

EXAMPLE 6.8 Example of Contractual Adjustment

Service provider's charge is:	$200.00
Medicare approved/allowed amount is:	$150.00
Contractual adjustment is:	$50.00

Because some services may be disallowed or the payments on them may be lower than those charged by the health care provider, know how to post payments to the patient's financial accounting record card or computerized account. Fig. 6.12 illustrates how payments and contractual adjustments are posted.

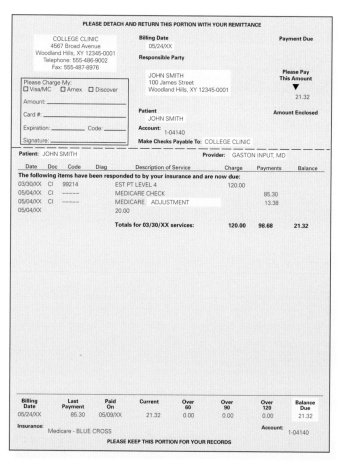

Fig. 6.12 Electronically generated financial accounting record (ledger card) illustrating how payments and contractual adjustments should be posted.

Medicare does not allow for the standardized waiving of copayments. Medicare regulations require that a patient be billed for the copayment at least three times before the balance is adjusted off as uncollectable. Document this as further justification if the patient is suffering financial hardship.

When an RA is received, it may list many patients (Fig. 6.13). Do not post the entire payment made in a lump sum to the daysheet. Individually post each line item paid to the patient's financial accounting record card or computerized account and to the daysheet. To prevent funds from going astray, some offices prefer to post Medicare payments to a separate daysheet and deposit each multiple reimbursement check separately. The daysheet totals will then agree with the deposit slip totals and not get confused with other monies collected.

Fig. 6.14A illustrates an example of a Medicare/Medicaid case after payment by Medicare. Medicare applied the patient's full $147 deductible amount to the Medicare-allowed amount, reducing payment to $26.40. The Medicaid RA (see Fig. 6.14B) shows reimbursement of the coinsurance and deductible amounts dual-billed to Medicaid.

When referring to the Medicaid program, a *cutback* means a reduction, which is reducing Medicare's allowable charges to Medicaid's allowable charges. This would require an adjustment entry on the patient's financial accounting record. Cutbacks are common on Medicaid claims.

Medicare Overpayments

A Medicare overpayment is a payment the health care organization or provider has received in excess of amounts properly payable under Medicare guidelines. Overpayments commonly occur because of insufficient documentation, medical necessity errors, and administrative and processing errors. Medicare overpayments can also occur in the following situations:

- The carrier processes the charge more than once.
- The health care provider receives duplicate payments from Medicare and a secondary payer.
- The health care provider is paid directly on an unassigned claim.
- The item is not covered but is paid.
- The payment is made on erroneous information.

After Medicare identifies an overpayment, it becomes a debt that the health care organization owes the federal government. Federal law requires the CMS to try to recover all identified overpayments. In fact, civil monetary penalties may be imposed if the health care provider knows of an overpayment and does not report and return it.

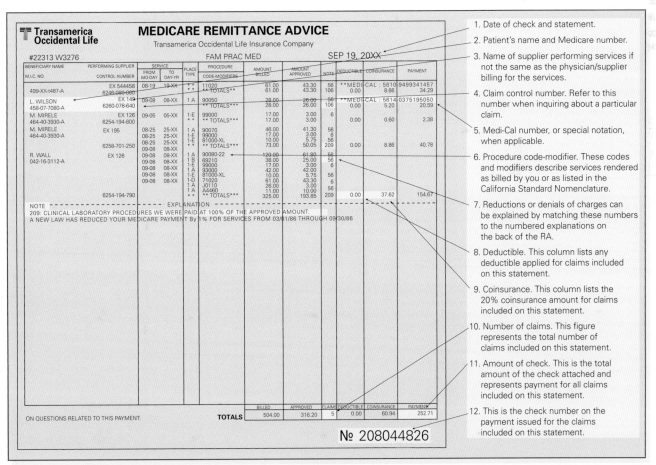

A

Fig. 6.13 Medicare remittance advice (RA) document. (A) Front. Insurance carriers are required to use Centers for Medicare and Medicaid Services messages for Medicare RA, but each carrier has its own code numbers to denote the messages. (B) Back of Medicare RA document. (https://med.noridianmedicare.com/web/jddme/topics/ra/ra-tutorial.)

EXPLANATION OF NOTES   Additional notes may be listed on the front of this form.

1 – See enclosed letter.

2 – Claim was filed after the time limit.

4 – These bills are handled by a special intermediary.

5 – This payment is for an adjustment of a previous claim.

6 – Charges over the maximum Medicare allowance are not covered.

7 – Services before Medicare entitlement are not covered.

8 – Services after Medicare entitlement ended are not covered.

10 – Other charges submitted with this claim may be on a separate statement which you have received or will receive soon.

12 – Routine examinations and related services are not covered.

13 – Immunizations or other routine and preventative services are not covered.

16 – We need an itemization of this charge. Please resubmit your claim with this information.

17 – Prescription drugs are not covered.

18 – Charges for this physician/supplier are not covered.

19 – We need a full description of the service or supply to consider this charge. Please resubmit your claim with this information.

23 – We need a written report for this service. Please resubmit your claim with this information.

26 – More than $312.50 annual psychiatric expense is not covered.

27 – We need from the prescribing physician the specific length of time this medical equipment is needed. Please resubmit your claim with this information.

30 – This charge was previously considered.

37 – Claims for these services will be made by a home health agency or hospital.

39 – Equipment that is not medically necessary is not covered. (See Note 89)

42 – These supplies or services are not covered.

45 – Over 62$\frac{1}{2}$% of psychiatric expenses is not covered.

46 – Routine foot care is not covered.

47 – Routine eye examinations or eye refractions are not covered.

48 – Partial payment of this claim was made to the beneficiary.

49 – This service cannot be considered until the hospital makes the necessary arrangement with the carrier for its processing.

50 – The beneficiary is not responsible for this reduction/denial under the assignment agreement.

54 – Care before and/or after surgery is included in the surgery benefit. (See Note 50)

56 – This is the full charge allowed based upon the prevailing or usual and customary rate.

62 – Payment has been reduced because this test is commonly part of an automated test group. (See Note 50)

66 – This service is not covered when done by this laboratory.

70 – There were no charges or bills with your claim form. Please resubmit your claim with this information.

72 – We need a signed and dated prescription showing medical necessity and specific length of time needed. Please resubmit your claim with this information.

73 – Before another month's payment can be made, we need a new signed and dated prescription showing further necessity of the medical equipment and specific length of time needed.

80 – We need to know the place of service to consider this charge. Please resubmit your claim with this information.

83 – SSA advises us that they are unable to verify the patient's eligibility for Part B Medical Insurance Plan. For this reason, no payment can be made on this claim.

84 – The patient's HIC number shown on this claim was incorrect. Please use the correct HIC number on all future claims.

85 – The patient's name shown on this claim was incorrect. Please use the correct name on all future claims.

86 – Over 62$\frac{1}{2}$% of the allowable charges for psychiatric services is not covered.

89 – If you did not know that Medicare does not pay for this medical service, you may request a review of this decision. See below paragraph entitled "Your right to review of a case."

90 – This service by a chiropractor is not covered.

93 – Over $500.00 annual expense billed by a physical therapist is not covered.

95 – These specific services by this supplier are not covered.

96 – Please verify the date of this service. Resubmit your claim with this information.

99 – We need a complete diagnosis before the claim can be considered. Please resubmit your claim with this information.

106 – The Medicare covered services on this claim have been forwarded for additional processing under Medi-Cal.

107 – This claim was not forwarded for Medi-Cal processing. Please bill Medi-Cal directly and attach a copy of this statement.

108 – The bills for these services have been transferred to Blue Shield of California Medicare Claims, Chico, CA 95976. You will hear from them.

129 – Payment for services prior to July 1 is based on the previous year's payment rate.

131 – Payment for this physician service in a hospital department is reduced since this service is commonly performed in the physician's office. (See Note 50)

138 – This amount is more than Medicare pays for maintenance treatment of renal disease.

147 – This charge is not covered because an allowance for purchase of the same equipment was previously made.

151 – Your claim was transferred to a Health Maintenance Organization for processing.

153 – These are more visits (treatments) for this diagnosis than Medicare covers unless there were unusual circumstances. (See Note 89)

154 – This service is not covered for your patient's reported condition. (See Note 89)

155 – Only one visit per month to a nursing home is covered unless special need is indicated. (See Note 89)

156 – This laboratory test for the reported condition and/or illness is not covered. (See Note 89)

158 – Procedures whose effectiveness has not been proven are not covered. (See Note 89)

161 – The frequency of services for this condition are not covered. (See Note 89)

162 – More than one visit per day for this condition are not covered. (See Note 89)

172 – This type of services billed by a psychologist are not covered.

179 – The amount for this service is included in the approved amount for the consultation/office/hospital visit.

181 – Payment for this service is included in the major surgical fee.

187 – We need the name and address of the individual doctor who performed this service. Please resubmit your claim with this information.

192 – Medicare benefits have been reduced because the patient's employer group health plan has paid some of these expenses.

198 – A claim must be sent to the patient's employer group health plan first. After the claim has been processed by that plan, resubmit this claim with the bills and the notice the other insurance company sent you.

203 – Clinical laboratory services. Blood Gas Studies and Rhythm Strips (1–3 leads) furnished in a hospital setting are reimbursed through the hospital.

205 – The date of this service is after the patient's expiration date provided to us by SSA. If service was rendered to this patient on this date, have the patient's estate contact the local Social Security Office for assistance.

206 – For payment, these services must be billed by the performing laboratory with the assignment accepted.

213 – We did not send this claim to Medicaid. Please send this statement and a copy of the claim to the agency that handles Medicaid in your area.

216 – This service or item cannot be processed until your application for a Medicare provider identification number is received and approved.

218 – Since you are Medicare participating, we have processed this claim as assigned. Future claims must be billed on assignment. If the bill was paid in full, you must immediately refund the amount due to the beneficiary.

219 – We need this charge submitted on your letterhead bill. Please resubmit your claim with this information.

221 – The name and Medicare number submitted on this claim do not match. Please verify for whom these services were rendered and provide the correct name and number on the claim and resubmit.

223 – We did not consider this for payment because you did not send the extra information we asked for. Payment can be requested again by sending us another claim form and all the information.

226 – Medicare will pay rent for the prescribed number of months or until the equipment is no longer needed, whichever occurs first. This is the first monthly rental payment.

227 – You will receive a notice each month when additional rental payments are paid.

231 – Medicare will no longer pay for rental on this item since the purchase price has been paid.

237 – The amount of this payment is the difference between the approved purchase allowance and the rental payments you have received.

YOUR RIGHT TO REVIEW OF A CASE

If you have a problem or question about the way a claim was handled or about the amount paid, please write Transamerica Occidental Life, Box 54905, Terminal Annex, Los Angeles, California 90054, within 6 months of the date of this notice. We will give your request full consideration.

Your Social Security office will help you file a request for review of a claim if it is more convenient for you.

WHERE TO SEND REFUNDS

When refunding a payment you should send a check with a letter of explanation. The letter should include your Transamerica Occidental/Medicare check number, beneficiary name and Medicare identification number (HICNo.), control number to which the payment relates, and any other information which may be pertinent to the refund. Send this information to:

Transamerica Occidental Life
C/O Check and Payment Control
Box 54905, Terminal Annex
Los Angeles, CA 90054-0905

KEY TO CODES FOR PLACE AND TYPE OF SERVICE

Place of service	Type of service
1. Office	A. Medical care
2. Home	B. Surgery (includes treatment of fractures)
3. Inpatient hospital	C. Consultation
4. Skilled nursing facility	D. Diagnostic X-ray
5. Outpatient hospital	E. Diagnostic laboratory
6. Independent laboratory	F. Radiation therapy
7. Other	G. Anesthesia
8. Independent kidney disease treatment center	H. Assistance at surgery
	I. Other medical service
	J. Whole blood or packed red cells

B

Fig. 6.13, cont'd.

MEDICARE REMITTANCE ADVICE

XYZ Insurance Company

Physician or supplier name	Dates of service From To MMDD MMDDYY	See back serv typl	Procedure Code	Billed amount	Amount allowed	See ** act cde	Beneficiary obligation Deductible Co-ins		Medicare payment to Beneficiary provider

BENEFICIARY: BILL HUTCH   HIC NUMBER: 5432-112-34
CONTROL NO.: 92106-30810-00   DE/MI: 2121D52

John Doe MD 0310	0310XX	D 03	49000	245.00	180.00	101	147.00	1.00	0.00	26.40
CLAIM TOTALS:				245.00	180.00	101	147.00	1.00	0.00	26.40

A

MEDICAID REMITTANCE ADVICE

RECIPIENT NAME	RECIPIENT MEDICAID ID NO.	CLAIM CONTROL NUMBER	SERVICE DATE MO DAY YR	PROCEDURE CODE	PATIENT ACCT. NO.	QTY.	MEDICARE ALLOWED	MEDICAID ALLOWED	PATIENT LIABILITY	COMPUTED MCR AMT.	MEDICAID PAID	EOB MESSAGE
BILL HUTCH	521345678	4006984891200	03 10 XX	49000		001	180.00	148.00		26.40	.00	
		4006984891200	00 00 XX			000	180.00	148.00		26.40	148.00	
BLOOD DEDUCT	00 DEDUCTIBLE	147.00 COINSUR	1.00 CUTBACK 32.00									CUTBACK 443

B

Fig. 6.14 (A) A Medicare/Medicaid case after payment by Medicare. (B) The Medicaid remittance advice shows reimbursement of the coinsurance and deductible amounts dual billed to Medicaid.

If an overpayment is identified, the health care organization has 60 days to report and return it. When Medicare identifies an overpayment of $25 or more, the MAC will initiate the overpayment recovery process by sending an initial demand letter requesting repayment. If overpayment is not repaid to the MAC in full within 30 days, interest will be charged. If the health care organization disagrees with an overpayment decision, an appeal can be filed with the MAC.

Recovery Audit Contractor Program

The Recovery Audit Contractor (RAC) Initiative originally created a demonstration program that became permanently implemented when Congress enacted the Tax Relief and Health Care Act of 2006. This extended the RAC Initiative to all 50 states by 2010. Its goals are to identify Medicare underpayments and overpayments and recover overpayments using automated review and complex review. An automated review is done electronically without human review, and a complex review is done using human review of the medical record. A single RAC will serve one of four geographic regions (regions A, B, C, and D) and perform recovery audit services for all Medicare claim types in that region. RACs may identify improper payments from claims they review that may show incorrect payment amounts, noncovered services, incorrectly coded services, miscoding, and duplicate services. RACs are paid a percentage of the incorrect payments they recover. When an underpayment is found, a RAC will communicate this to the MAC. If both underpayments and overpayments are found, the RAC will offset the underpayment from the overpayment. On overpayments, interest accrues from the date of the final determination. Claims identified as overpayments are subject to the Medicare appeals process.

Review and Redetermination Process

Chapter 16 outlines in detail the steps to take to have a claim reviewed and the process of appealing a claim in the Medicare program.

6.8 QUICK REVIEW

Question: What is a Medicare overpayment and why is it important for the insurance billing specialist to promptly report and return it?

DISCUSSION POINT

Medicare is a federal health insurance program specifically for patients 65 years of age and older and for patients who are disabled. What special skills do you think would be critical for the insurance billing specialist to deal effectively with Medicare beneficiaries?

PROCEDURE 6.1 Determine Whether Medicare Is Primary of Secondary and Determine Additional Benefits

1. Go to the CMS website and download the questionnaire that is used to determine if Medicare beneficiaries have other payers that may be primary to Medicare. The questionnaire can be found at: https://www.cms.gov/medicare/coordination-of-benefits-and-recovery/providerservices/downloads/pro_othertool.pdf
2. Work with several classmates to review the questionnaire. Ask each classmate to identify themselves as one of the following.
   - An individual injured or ill because of an automobile accident.
   - An individual with an employer sponsored group health plan. The individual is 66 years of age and still working. His employer has more than 20 employees.
   - An individual who receives Black Lung benefits.
   - An individual who is presenting with an injury that was caused by an accident at the workplace.
3. Review the questionnaire with your classmates to determine if Medicare insurance would be the primary or secondary payer for the scenario they are representing.
4. Make sure than regardless as to whether the patient's Medicare is primary or secondary, that the Medicare card is reviewed, and copy both sides of the card into the patient's record.

PROCEDURE 6.2 Complete an Advance Beneficiary Notice of Noncoverage Form

There are 10 blanks for completion labeled A through J:
- Notifier(s): Enter the name, address, and telephone number of the provider.
- Patient Name: Enter the first and last name and middle initial of the Medicare beneficiary.
- Identification Number: Enter a number for the Medicare beneficiary that helps link the notice with a related claim. However, this field is optional and choosing not to enter a number does not invalidate the ABN. The beneficiary's Medicare health insurance claim number will no longer be used.
- Enter name of item(s), service(s), test(s), or procedure(s). If not enough space, use an attached sheet, noting it in the box.
- Reason Medicare May Not Pay: Explain the reason why you think the service may not be covered by Medicare (e.g., Medicare does not pay for this test for the condition or Medicare does not pay for these tests as often as this [denied as too frequent]).
- Estimated Cost: Enter a cost estimate for any item or service described in field D.
- Options: Patient should choose and check one of the three boxes. If the beneficiary cannot make a choice, the notice should be annotated.
- Additional Information: Insert more comments for clarification (e.g., provide context on Medicare payment policy applicable to a specific benefit or other payer information).
- Signature: Medicare beneficiary should sign the notice.
- Date: Insert the date on which the beneficiary signed the ABN.

ABN, Advance Beneficiary Notice of Noncoverage.

■ KEY POINTS

This is a brief chapter review, or summary, of the key issues presented.

1. Medicare is administered by the Centers for Medicare and Medicaid Services (CMS).
2. Medicare is a health insurance program for people aged 65 or older, people younger than aged 65 with certain disabilities, and people of all ages with end-stage renal disease (ESRD).
3. Medicare Part A is for hospital insurance benefits and Medicare Part B is for medical insurance benefits.
4. Medicare Part C is referred to as *Medicare Advantage plan (MA plan)*. This plan offers a number of health care options in addition to those available under Medicare Part A and Part B.
5. Medicare Part D prescription drug plan is a standalone drug plan, presented by insurance and other private companies, that offers drug coverage that meets the standards established by Medicare.
6. On enrollment into the Medicare program, the Medicare beneficiary is issued an identification card.
7. Patients who received railroad retirement benefits will get Medicare from the Railroad Retirement Board.
8. Medigap is a specialized Medicare supplemental insurance policy whose predefined minimum benefits are regulated by the federal government and devised for the Medicare beneficiary.
9. Medicare secondary payer (MSP) is a primary insurance plan of a Medicare beneficiary who must pay for any medical care or services first before a Medicare fiscal intermediary is sent a claim.
10. The US Department of Health and Human Services' Quality Improvement Organization program is dedicated to improving the quality of services provided to Medicare beneficiaries.
11. Because Medicare is a federal program, providers that transmit claims to Medicare must comply with billing and coding regulations issued by CMS.
12. Participating providers and health care organizations agree to accept assignment on all Medicare claims and may bill the patient only for the Medicare deductible and coinsurance amounts.
13. National Coverage Determinations (NCDs) and Local Coverage Determinations (LCDs) are coverage policies that must be adhered to when determining if services to Medicare beneficiaries will be considered medically necessary and payable.
14. An Advance Beneficiary Notice of Noncoverage (ABN) is an agreement given to the patient to read and sign before

rendering a service if the participating provider thinks that it may be denied for payment because of medical necessity or limitation of liability by Medicare.

15. A Medicare fee schedule (MFS) is a method of reimbursement for services provided by health care providers, ambulance services, clinical laboratory services, and durable medical equipment (DME), agencies, hospice, hospital outpatient, inpatient psychiatric facilities, inpatient rehabilitation facilities, long-term care hospitals, and skilled nursing facilities.

16. The Medicare Access and CHIP Reauthorization Act of 2015 (MACRA) is legislation enacted to establish a new payment methodology to pay providers by rewarding high-quality and high-value care.

17. Medicare requires mandatory claims submission, which applies to all health care providers and suppliers who provide covered services to Medicare beneficiaries.

18. The time limit for sending in Medicare claims is within 12 months from the date of service.

19. Instructions for Medicare claims submission can be found in the Medicare Claims Processing Manual—Internet Only Manual Publication 100.04.

20. Medicare sends a payment check and a nationally standardized document to participating providers called a Medicare remittance advice (RA) and a similar document to the patient called a Medicare Summary Notice (MSN).

INTERNET RESOURCES

HIPAA Eligibility Transaction Systems (HETS)
- https://www.cms.gov/Research-Statistics-Data-and-Systems/CMS-Information-Technology/HETSHelp

Internet Only Manual (IOM):
- https://www.cms.gov/Regulations-and-Guidance/Guidance/Manuals/Internet-Only-Manuals-IOMs

Medicare Learning Network (MLN)
- https://www.cms.gov/Outreach-and-Education/Medicare-Learning-Network-MLN/MLNGenInfo

Medicare Secondary Payer (MSP) Questionnaire
- https://www.cms.gov/medicare/coordination-of-benefits-and-recovery/providerservices/downloads/pro_othertool.pdf

Preventive Services Guide
- https://www.cms.gov/Medicare/Prevention/PrevntionGenInfo/medicare-preventive-services/MPS-QuickReferenceChart-1.html

STUDENT ASSIGNMENT

- Study Chapter 6.
- Complete all exercises in the *Workbook* to reinforce the theory learned in this chapter.

- Turn to the Glossary at the end of this text for a further understanding of the key terms and key abbreviations used in this chapter.

7

Medicaid and Other State Programs

Linda M. Smith

OBJECTIVES

After reading this chapter, you should be able to:

1. Explain what the Medicaid program is.
2. Discuss the history of Medicaid.
3. Describe added benefits for Medicaid recipients afforded by the Patient Protection and Affordable Care Act and the Health Care and Education Reconciliation Act of 2010.
4. Discuss the different types of Medicaid programs.
5. Explain the purpose of the Medicaid Child Health Insurance Program.
6. Identify those eligible for the Medicaid Qualified Medicare Beneficiaries program.
7. Name and describe the two Medicaid eligibility classifications.
8. List valuable information to abstract from the patient's Medicaid card.
9. Describe the Medicaid basic benefits.
10. Explain basic operations of a Medicaid-managed care system.
11. Explain basic Medicaid claim procedure guidelines.
12. Discuss a health care organization's responsibility as a participant in the Medicaid program.
13. Identify the payer of last resort patients who have Medicaid and other coverage.
14. Interpret and post a remittance advice.
15. Describe filing an appeal for a Medicaid case.
16. Explain the purpose of the Medicaid Fraud Control Unit.

KEY TERMS

categorically needy
Children's Health Insurance Program
coinsurance
covered services
Early and Periodic Screening, Diagnosis, and Treatment
federal poverty level
fiscal agent
Medicaid
Medi-Cal

medically needy
Medicare Savings Programs
payer of last resort
prior approval
recipient
share of cost
spousal impoverishment
Supplemental Security Income
Temporary Assistance for Needy Families

KEY ABBREVIATIONS

CHIP	MN	POS machine	SLMB
DEFRA	MSP	QI program	SSI
EPSDT	OBRA	QMB	TANF
FPL	OOY claims	RA	

🔒 INSIGHTS FROM THE FIELD

Ella R.: Insurance Billing Specialist

The most important part of Medicaid billing is to always verify the patient's eligibility. Eligibility can change day-by-day, so it is essential to use the Medicaid Eligibility Verification system. In New York State, there is a web-based application that allows providers to create and submit electronic claims, which is also helpful. Learning to navigate through these programs is a skill that should be learned.

MEDICAID

Medicaid is not so much an insurance program as it is an assistance program. Medicaid is a government program for individuals and families whose income and resources are insufficient to pay for health care. The Medicaid program is jointly funded by the state and federal governments. On a federal level, the Centers for Medicare and Medicaid Services (CMS) monitors the programs and establishes requirements for service delivery, funding, quality, and eligibility standards. The states are required to comply with all federal Medicaid laws.

Each state is allowed to administer and manage its own Medicaid program. This includes establishing eligibility requirements, determining the scope and types of services the state program will cover, and setting the rate of payment. Medicaid eligibility and benefits may vary from state to state.

History

Federal participation in providing medical care to needy persons began between 1933 and 1935 when the Federal Emergency Relief Administration made funds available to pay the medical expenses of the needy unemployed. The Social Security Act of 1935 created the public assistance programs. Although no special provision was made for medical insurance, the federal government paid a share of the monthly income assistance payments, which the individual could use to meet the costs of medical care. Thirty years later, Title XIX of the Social Security Act became federal law, and Medicaid legally came into being in 1965.

Since 1983, the trend in many states has been to expand Medicaid eligibility requirements and services. Changes in Medicaid eligibility allowing more people into the program were made by many states after the passage of the Deficit Reduction Act (**DEFRA**) of 1984 and the Child Health Assurance Program (CHAP) by the federal government. On July 1, 2006, as part of DEFRA, a federal law became effective requiring new applicants and current beneficiaries renewing their benefits to submit birth certificates, passports, or other documents to establish their legal right to benefits as US citizens. If no documentation of citizenship can be found, sworn affidavits from the beneficiary and at least one or two other individuals can be used.

In 2002 and 2003, states across the nation faced steep budget shortfalls. A vast majority of them made cuts of some kind in their Medicaid programs by imposing or boosting copayments, coinsurances, and deductibles or by eliminating some services. States are allowed to develop their own individual cost-sharing strategies such as copayments, coinsurances, and deductible amounts for certain Medicaid-covered benefits. The cost-sharing strategies are based on income, and services cannot be withheld from Medicaid patients for failure to pay out-of-pocket expenses. Additionally, out-of-pocket costs cannot be imposed for emergency services, family-planning services, pregnancy-related services, or preventive services for children. Children, terminally ill individuals, and individuals residing in an institution are also exempt from out-of-pocket expenses.

In 2010, health care reform legislations, known as the *Patient Protection and Affordable Care Act (PPACA)* and the *Health Care and Education Reconciliation Act (HCERA)*, were passed. These Acts affect the Medicaid program by expanding access for childless adults, nonelderly, and nonpregnant individuals, and include preventive services and long-term care benefits. Additional funds were allocated for maternal and child health services.

PPACA created the Community First Choice Option, a plan that allowed state Medicaid plans to provide medical assistance for home- and community-based attendant services and support to eligible individuals. The Community First Choice Option became available in 2011.

TABLE 7.1 Department of Health and Human Services Federal Poverty Guidelines

Year	Annual Income for One Person	Annual Income for a Four-Person Family
2020	$12,760	$26,200
2019	$12,490	$25,750
2018	$12,140	$25,100

Federal poverty levels used to determine eligibility for certain Medicaid programs as outlined by the Department of Health and Human Services. (https://aspe.hhs.gov/poverty-guidelines). FLPs are the same in 48 of the 50 states with the exception of Alaska and Hawaii, which have higher FLPs due to the higher cost of living.

PPACA created the opportunity for states to expand Medicaid to cover nearly all low-income Americans younger than 65, using the federal poverty level (FPL). The FPL is a federally set "poverty line" that indicates the minimum amount of annual income an individual or family needs to pay for essentials such as housing, utilities, clothing, food, and transportation. FPLs are the same in 48 of the 50 states. The two exceptions are Alaska and Hawaii, which have higher FPLs due to the higher cost of living. The FPL is issued every year by the Department of Health and Human Services (HHS). States generally apply a percentage of the FPL to determine eligibility for Medicaid. The limits vary based on the state; however, many states use 138% of the FPL for Medicaid eligibility. In those cases, if the patient's income is below 138% of the FPL, the patient qualifies for Medicaid coverage (Table 7.1).

7.1 QUICK REVIEW
Question: What category of individuals was Medicaid established for to help with medical expenses?

MEDICAID PROGRAMS

As stated earlier, Medicaid programs vary from state to state. Some may have different names. For example, Medi-Cal is California's Medicaid health care program. South Carolina's Medicaid program is called Healthy Connections. The state of Arizona has the Arizona Health Care Cost Containment System (AHCCCS) as their Medicaid agency, which offers health care programs to serve their residents. An internet link has been provided for a complete list of the names of Medicaid programs in all states at the end of this chapter under *Internet Resources*.

Children's Health Insurance Program

The Children's Health Insurance Program (CHIP) is an insurance program that provides low-cost health coverage to children in families that earn too much money to qualify for Medicaid but not enough to buy private insurance. The federal and state government work in partnership to fund this program.

CHIP is administered by states, according to federal requirements. To be eligible for CHIP, a child must be:
- Under 19 years of age
- Uninsured and ineligible for Medicaid
- A citizen of the United States or meet immigration requirements

- A resident of the state
- Eligible within the state's CHIP income range, based on family income, or any other specified rules set by the state

States also have the option to provide coverage to low-income uninsured pregnant women under CHIP.

All states have a CHIP program; program names may vary from state to state. For example, Michigan developed the Children's Special Health Care Services (CSHCS) program. CSHCS is a program for children and some adults with special health care needs. The state of Maryland has the Maryland Children's Health Program (MCHP), which provides access to health insurance coverage for higher-income uninsured children up to age 19, and Georgia has PeachCare for Kids, which is a comprehensive health program for uninsured children living in Georgia. Benefits of the program include primary, preventive, specialist, dental, and vision care. It also covers hospitalization, emergency room services, prescription medications, and mental health care.

CHIP benefits are different in each state, but all provide comprehensive coverage which includes:

- Routine check-ups
- Immunizations
- Doctor visits
- Prescriptions
- Dental and vision care
- Inpatient and outpatient hospital care
- Laboratory and x-ray services
- Emergency services

An internet link to the CHIP website has been provided at the end of this chapter under *Internet Resources.*

Medicare Savings Programs

Medicare Savings Programs (MSPs) help low-income individuals with out-of-pocket costs for Medicare, including Medicare Part A and Part B premiums, deductibles, copayments, and coinsurance. There are four types of MSPs:

- Qualified Medicare Beneficiary program
- Specified Low-Income Medicare Beneficiary program
- Qualifying Individual program
- Qualified Disabled and Working Individuals program

All four types of MSP are run by state Medicaid programs. Each program addresses a different financial category, and the monthly income figures are adjusted each year. Eligibility for the programs may differ from state to state.

Medicaid Qualified Medicare Beneficiary Program

The Medicaid Qualified Medicare Beneficiary program was introduced in the Medicare Catastrophic Coverage Act of 1988 as an amendment to the Social Security Act. In 1990, the Omnibus Reconciliation Act (**OBRA**) of 1989 allowed for assistance to qualified Medicare beneficiaries (**QMBs**, pronounced "kwimbees") who are aged and disabled, are receiving Medicare, and have annual incomes less than the FPL. Eligibility also depends on what other financial resources an individual might have.

Under this Act, states must provide limited Medicaid coverage for QMBs. The QMB program helps pay Medicare Part A premiums, Medicare Part B premiums, deductible, coinsurance, and copayments. Coinsurance is the portion of the Medicare allowed amount that the patient pays. Medicaid will not pay for the service if Medicare does not cover the service to the patient.

States are also required to pay Medicare Part A premiums but no other expenses for qualified disabled and working individuals. It is optional for states to provide full Medicaid benefits to QMBs who meet a state-established income standard.

Specified Low-Income Medicare Beneficiary Program

The Specified Low-Income Medicare Beneficiary (**SLMB**, pronounced "slim-bee") program was established in 1993 for elderly individuals whose income is 20% more than the FPL. It pays the entire Medicare Part B premium. The patient must pay the deductible and copay and must pay for noncovered items.

Qualifying Individual Program

The Qualifying Individual (**QI**) **program** was created in 1997 for qualifying individuals whose income is at least 120% but less than 135% of the FPL. This program pays for the Medicare Part B premium and automatically qualifies them for prescription drug coverage assistance. Patients who qualify for Medicaid cannot receive QI benefits.

Qualified Disabled and Working Individuals Program

The Qualified Disabled and Working Individuals (QDWI) program is different from the other three Medicare Savings Programs in that it only pays for Medicare Part A premiums. Individuals may qualify for a QDWI Program if any the following apply:

- They returned to work and lost their premium-free Medicare Part A coverage.
- They are younger than 65, disabled, and currently working.
- They are not getting state medical assistance.
- They meet the income and resource requirements of their state.

 7.2   QUICK REVIEW
Question: What category of individuals was the Children's Health Insurance Program established to assist in paying medical expenses?

MEDICAID ELIGIBILITY

As discussed earlier in this chapter, Medicaid is available to certain needy and low-income people, and eligibility is based on income and resources.

In addition to financial qualifications, an individual must also meet certain non-financial eligibility criteria. Medicaid is available only to US citizens and certain "qualified immigrants." Passports and birth certificates must be submitted for proof of citizenship. Nonimmigrants and unauthorized aliens are not eligible for most federal benefits; however, states have the option to cover nonimmigrant and unauthorized aliens who are pregnant or who are children and can meet the definition of "lawfully residing" in the United States. If a person may be eligible for Medicaid, he or she goes to the local public service welfare office, human service, or family independence agency and applies for benefits.

All Medicaid eligible individuals are assigned to one of two broad classifications—categorically needy or medically needy.

Categorically Needy

The first classification, the categorically needy group, includes all cash recipients of Temporary Assistance for Needy Families. The Temporary Assistance for Needy Families (TANF) program is a federal assistance program that began on July 1, 1997. The program provides limited cash assistance to extremely low-income parents and their children. TANF assists families with children when the parents or other responsible relatives cannot provide for the family's basic needs. The federal government provides grants to states to run the TANF program. States may have different names for this program, and it can be called welfare, public assistance, temporary assistance, general assistance, or cash assistance.

Other individuals who may be considered categorically needy are most cash recipients of the Supplemental Security Income (SSI) program; other SSI-related groups; QMBs; and patients in institutional, long-term care, and intermediate care facilities (see Box 7.1). A recipient is an individual certified by the local welfare department to receive benefits of Medicaid under one of the specific aid categories.

Medically Needy

In states with medically needy (MN) Medicaid programs, individuals with significant health needs may qualify for Medicaid coverage. Although their income is too high to qualify for Medicaid, they have incurred medical expenses that significantly reduce their income, therefore making them eligible. Assistance can be provided if patients' income minus their medical expenses fall below a certain limit. Most states have MN programs, allowing those with high medical expenses to still qualify for Medicaid.

States that choose to have MN programs may decide not to offer the MN option to all categories of Medicaid-eligible people. For example, a state may choose to offer the MN programs to elderly but not disabled people. However, states that offer any MN programs must offer them to most children and pregnant women.

A Medicaid recipient in this category may or may not pay a copayment or a deductible, which must be met within the eligibility month or other specified time frame before he or she can receive state benefits (also known as share of cost or *spend down*). Emergency care and pregnancy services are exempt by law from copayment requirements. This may be a component of a state's general assistance program for low-income people.

Spousal Impoverishment Protection Law

In 1988, Congress enacted provisions to prevent spousal impoverishment, which refers to leaving the spouse who is still living at home in the community with little or no income or resources. The Spousal Impoverishment Protection Law is federal legislation that affects special financial provisions in Medicaid for the elderly, blind, or disabled. Formerly, if one partner (institutionalized spouse) needed to be in a nursing facility, a couple's income and assets would become so depleted to qualify that the other

---

> ### BOX 7.1   Groups Eligible for Medicaid Benefits
>
> **Mandatory Eligibility Groups**
> - Low-income families
> - TANF–related groups
> - Non-TANF pregnant women and children
> - Infants born to Medicaid-eligible pregnant women
> - Recipients of adoption assistance or foster care assistance under Title IV-E of the Social Security Act
> - Aged, blind, and disabled
> - SSI–related groups
> - Qualified Medicare Beneficiaries
> - Persons who receive institutional or other long-term care in nursing facilities and intermediate care facilities
> - Medicare–Medicaid beneficiaries
>
> **Optional Eligibility Groups**
> - Low-income persons who are losing employer health insurance coverage (Medicaid purchase if person has Consolidated Omnibus Budget Reconciliation Act coverage)
> - Infants up to age 1 and pregnant women not covered under the mandatory rules whose family income is not more than 185% of the federal poverty level (note that the percentage may be modified by each state)
> - Children younger than age 21 who meet TANF income and resource requirements but who are otherwise not eligible for TANF
> - Persons who would be eligible if institutionalized but receive care under home- and community-based service waivers
> - Persons infected with tuberculosis who would be financially eligible for Medicaid at the SSI income level if they were within a Medicaid-covered category (limited coverage)
> - Low-income children with the State Children's Health Insurance Program
> - Low-income, uninsured women who are diagnosed through the Centers for Disease Control and Prevention's National Breast and Cervical Cancer Early Detection Program and who need treatment for breast or cervical cancer
>
> **Medically Needy Eligibility Group**
> - Medically indigent low-income individuals and families who have too much income to qualify under mandatory or optional eligibility Medicaid groups

SSI, Supplemental Security Income; *TANF*, Temporary Assistance for Needy Families.

---

spouse (community spouse) did not have a sufficient amount to live on. This protection counts assets such as cash, checking and savings accounts, life insurance policies, and certificates of deposits. It does not count the couples' home, car, household furnishings, burial assets (insurance, trust funds, or plots), clothing, or other personal items. This prevents the community spouse from being impoverished by his or her spouse's institutionalization.

Verifying Eligibility

After acceptance into the program, the patient brings a form or card to the health care provider's office that verifies acceptance into the program (Fig. 7.1), but this does not indicate proof of eligibility. It is the provider's responsibility to verify at each visit that the person present to receive care is eligible on the date on which the service is rendered and is the individual to whom the card was issued.

A patient can be on Medicaid 1 month and then off it the following month, or the patient could be on the program for

Fig. 7.1 Medicaid patient checking in with the receptionist.

several months or years; each case is different. When obtaining personal information from the patient at the time of the first visit or a follow-up visit, always check and update the patient's name and address by asking for photo identification, such as a driver's license.

Identification Card

A plastic or paper Medicaid identification card (or coupons in some states) is usually issued monthly. Each state's Medicaid identification card may look differently; however, the card typically includes the name of the individual who will use the card, their photo, sex, date of birth, signature of the individual, and an identification number. Under certain classifications of eligibility, identification cards are issued in some states on the 1st and 15th of each month, every 2 months, every 3 months, or every 6 months. Sometimes an unborn child can be issued an identification card that is used for services promoting the life and health of the fetus. Obtain a photocopy or scan of the front and back of the card; carefully check the expiration date of the card each time the patient visits the health care office to see whether eligibility is indicated for the month of service; note whether the patient has other insurance, copayment requirements, or restrictions, such as being eligible for only certain types of medical services. Remember that the presentation of an insurance ID card does not guarantee coverage. The items that must be abstracted from the card for claim submission are (1) the patient's name exactly as shown, (2) Medicaid identification number, (3) gender, and (4) date of birth.

Medicaid Eligibility Verification Systems

When professional services are rendered, eligibility for that month must be verified. Verification is done if several ways, depending on how the state has developed their process. For example, some states outsource their Medicaid eligibility verification process. The Nashville-based company Medifax provides internet Medicaid eligibility verification using real-time, online access to patient eligibility and benefit information for health care providers.

Other states provide their own Medicaid Eligibility Verification System (MEVS), which may consist of one or all of the following:
- Verification by telephone with an automated voice response system.
- A software program that allows the provider to verify eligibility.
- A point-of-service (**POS**) **machine** (Fig. 7.2), which allows the insurance billing specialist to swipe the Medicaid patient's identification card which then displays eligibility information.

Printout

Read out

Swipe card

Enter data

A

Fig. 7.2 (A) Insurance billing specialist using a point-of-service (POS) machine to check a patient's Medicaid eligibility.

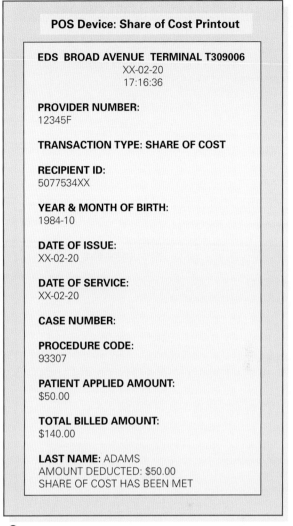

B   C

Fig. 7.2   *(Cont.)* (B) Printout from a POS machine for Medi-Service. (C) Printout from a POS machine for share of cost.

Retroactive Eligibility

Retroactive eligibility may be granted to a patient in some cases. In a situation where the patient has been referred to apply for Medicaid, the patient must ask for retroactive status; otherwise the approval effective date is the date of the application. When patients are seeking medical care, hoping to qualify for Medicaid but not accepted by the time of service, the account must be set up as a cash account until retroactive eligibility has been established. Retroactive status must be decided within 90 days of filing of the application for Medicaid. If the patient has documentation or a retroactive card confirming this and has paid for any services during the retroactive period, a refund must be made, and Medicaid billed.

 7.3   QUICK REVIEW

Question: Why is it important to verify Medicaid eligibility at every health care encounter?

MEDICAID BENEFITS

States establish and administer their own Medicaid programs and determine the type, amount, duration, and scope of services within the federal guidelines. Under federal guidelines, states are re-quired to provide mandatory Medicaid benefits. These guidelines equally allow states the choice of covering other optional benefits.

Covered Services

Covered services are reimbursable services under the state's Medicaid program. They consist of a combination of the mandatory basic benefits and optional services that the state may offer (Box 7.2).

Early and Periodic Screening, Diagnosis, and Treatment

One of the basic benefits of the Medicaid program is the Early and Periodic Screening, Diagnosis, and Treatment (EPSDT) service. This is a program of prevention, early detection, and treatment of children who are under the age of 21 and enrolled in Medicaid (Table 7.2).

In California (Medi-Cal), the EPSDT program is known as the *Child Health and Disability Prevention (CHDP) program,* and in Ohio as *Healthchek.* Because many states are changing the name of EPSDT and the services offered under the program, check with the state Medicaid vendor.

The EPSDT program covers regular screening services for infants, children, and adolescents. The purpose of the screenings

BOX 7.2   Medicaid Basic Benefits

Inpatient hospital care
Outpatient hospital care
Early and Periodic Screening, Diagnostic and Treatment services
Nursing facility services
Home health services
Physicians' care
Rural health clinic services
Federally qualified health center services
Laboratory and x-ray services
Family planning services
Nurse midwife services
Certified pediatric and nurse practitioner services
Freestanding birth center services (when recognized by the state)
Transportation to and from medical care
Tobacco cessation counseling for pregnant women
In some states, additional services might include the following:

- Allergy care
- Ambulance services
- Certain medical cosmetic procedures
- Chiropractic care
- Clinic care
- Dental care
- Dermatologic care
- Diagnostic, screening, preventive, and rehabilitative services (e.g., physical therapy)
- Emergency department care
- Eyeglasses and eye refractions
- Hospice care
- Intermediate care
- Occupational therapy
- Optometric services
- Physical therapy
- Podiatric care
- Prescription drugs
- Private duty nursing
- Prosthetic devices
- Psychiatric care
- Respiratory care
- Speech, hearing, and language disorder services

(This list may not be a comprehensive listing and is subject to variances by state.) Information taken from Medicaid.gov. (https:// www.medicaid.gov/medicaid/benefits/mandatory-optional-medicaid-benefits/index.html.)

TABLE 7.2   Explanation of Early and Periodic Screening, Diagnosis, and Treatment Benefits

Early	Identifying problems early, starting at birth
Periodic	Checking children's health at periodic, age-appropriate intervals
Screening	Doing physical, mental, developmental, dental, hearing, vision, and other screening tests to detect potential problems
Diagnosis	Performing diagnostic tests to follow up when a risk is identified
Treatment	Treating the problems found

is to identify health and developmental issues as early as possible. Covered screening services include:

- Comprehensive health and developmental history that assesses for both physical and mental health, as well as for substance use disorders.

- Comprehensive, unclothed physical exam.
- Appropriate immunizations in accordance with the schedule for pediatric vaccines established by the Advisory Committee on Immunization Practices.
- Laboratory testing (including blood lead screening appropriate for age and risk factors).
- Health education and anticipatory guidance for both the child and caregiver.
- Vision screening.
- Dental screening.
- Hearing screening.

Furthermore, states are required to provide necessary health care, diagnostic services, treatment, and other services to correct any physical or mental defects found. An internet link has been provided for the EPSDT coverage guide prepared by CMS at the end of this chapter under *Internet Resources*.

Non-Covered Services

The items or services that are non-covered by Medicaid will vary from state to state. However, it can be expected that any services that are not medically necessary, such as cosmetic services, will not be covered. Services that are considered to be experimental or investigational by the Department of Health and Human Services are also not covered.

In many states, if a service is not covered by Medicaid and it results in a denied claim, the health care organization is within their legal rights to bill the patient. It is recommended that the insurance billing specialist consult state regulations to confirm this before deciding to bill. Furthermore, some states require that the patient sign a waiver of liability agreement if the service to be provided may be a denied service from known past claim submission experiences. Write or telephone the state agency to obtain up-to-date information and details on billing patients for non-covered services.

7.4   QUICK REVIEW

Question: What does the Early and Periodic Screening, Diagnosis, and Treatment (EPSDT) program covers?

MEDICAID MANAGED CARE

Managed care began in the private insurance sector of health care, but eventually spread to federally and state-funded health care programs. In the late 1990s, a few states began applying the principles of managed health care to their Medicaid programs. Mainly this was done to control escalating health care costs by curbing unnecessary emergency department encounters and emphasizing preventive care.

Medicaid managed care plans allow the patient to choose a gatekeeper (clinic or primary care physician [PCP]), or they will be assigned one. The gatekeeper must approve all specialty care and inpatient or outpatient hospital treatment. Patients must use health care providers, clinics, and hospitals that participate in their assigned plan (Fig. 7.3).

Patients can be cared for side by side with private-paying patients. Some states have adopted capitation (a flat fee per

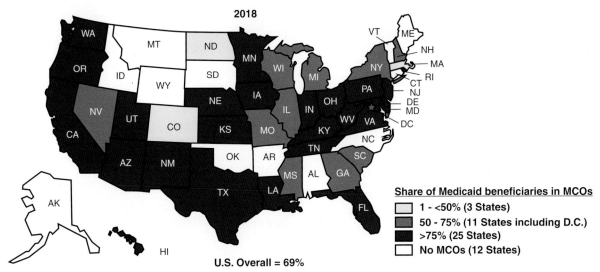

In most states with comprehensive MCOs, at least 75% of beneficiaries are enrolled in one.

2018

Share of Medicaid beneficiaries in MCOs
- 1 - <50% (3 States)
- 50 - 75% (11 States including D.C.)
- >75% (25 States)
- No MCOs (12 States)

U.S. Overall = 69%

Fig. 7.3 At least 75% of Medicaid beneficiaries are enrolled in a Medicaid Managed Care plan. (Source: Medicaid Managed Care Enrollment Report. CMS, DHSS, 2019.)

patient) rather than fee-for-service reimbursement. There may be a small copayment for services. It has been found that there is better access to primary health care, and money is saved when delivering care, if the Medicaid programs are well managed.

 7.5   QUICK REVIEW
Question: What is the role of the Medicaid managed care plan's gatekeeper?

ACCEPTING MEDICAID PATIENTS

Program Participation

A health care organization or provider must enroll for participation in the Medicaid program. The enrolling service provider must sign a written agreement with the fiscal agent as part of the application process. In the Medicaid program, a fiscal agent is an organization under contract with the state to process claims for a state Medicaid program.

Health care organizations and service providers have their own office procedures for handling Medicaid patients. The organization or provider may accept or refuse to treat Medicaid patients but must make the decision based on the entire Medicaid program, not an individual patient's personality, medical situation, or any other discriminating factor. The patient must receive quality care and be treated like the paying patient. If the health care organization decides to take Medicaid patients, they must accept the Medicaid allowance as payment in full. The Medicaid allowance is the maximum dollar amount to be considered for payment for a service or procedure by the program.

 7.6   QUICK REVIEW
Question: Are all health care providers required to accept Medicaid patients?

CLAIMS PROCEDURES

Medicaid policies and claim procedures about identification cards, prior approval regulations, claim forms, and time limits vary from state to state. General guidelines for submitting claims are stated here.

For specific state guidelines, consult the current *Medicaid Handbook* online at the state fiscal agent's website.

Copayment

There are two types of copayment requirements that may apply to a state. Some states require a small fixed copayment paid to the provider at the time services are rendered. This policy was instituted to help pay some of the administrative costs of providers participating in the Medicaid program.

Another requirement is the share of cost or *spend down* copayment. Some Medicaid recipients must meet this copayment requirement each month before Medicaid benefits can be claimed. For example, if an individual's income is too high to qualify, some states allow deduction of certain medical expenses from their income so that the income may fall within Medicaid guidelines. These spend down programs are available in some states for the elderly, the blind, or those who have a disability. Spend down eligibility is a monthly process and patients must submit proof of medical expenses that meet the spend down amount. Expenses covered by other insurances are not eligible to be used toward the spend down amount. For example, if the income is $150 more than the limit, the excess income is equal to the spend down amount, and the patient must submit $150 of acceptable medical bills or pay in the spend down amount to receive Medicaid coverage for the remainder of the month. Because the amount may change from month to month, be sure to verify the copayment each time it is collected. Obtain this copayment amount when the patient comes in for medical care and report on the claim form that it has been collected.

Prior Approval

Many times, prior approval is necessary for various goods and services, except in a bona fide emergency. **Prior approval** is the evaluation of a provider's request for a specific good or service to determine the medical necessity and appropriateness of the care requested for the patient. In some states this may be referred to as *prior authorization*. Some of the goods and services that may require prior approval are the following:

- Durable medical equipment
- Hearing aids
- Hemodialysis
- Home health care
- Inpatient hospital care
- Long-term care facility services
- Medical supplies
- Medications
- Prosthetic or orthotic appliances
- Some vision care
- Surgical procedures
- Transportation

Usually prior authorization forms are completed to obtain permission for a specific service or hospitalization (Fig. 7.4) and mailed or faxed to the Department of Health or a certain office in a region for approval. In some cases, time does not allow for a written request to be sent for prior approval, so an immediate authorization can be obtained via a telephone call to the proper department in any locale. Note the date and time that the authorization was given, the name of the person who gave the authorization, and any verbal number given by the field office. Usually a treatment authorization form indicating that the service was already authorized must be sent in as follow-up to the telephone call.

Hospital-Acquired Condition

On July 1, 2012, under the Affordable Care Act, Medicaid implemented the provision to either make a payment adjustment or prohibit payment for any hospital-acquired condition (HAC), such as foreign object retained after surgery; air embolism; blood incompatibility; stages III and IV pressure ulcers; vascular catheter-associated infection; mediastinitis after coronary artery bypass graft; falls and trauma resulting in fractures, dislocations, intracranial injury, crushing injury, burn, and other unspecified effects of external causes; manifestations of poor glycemic control; surgical site infection after spine, neck, shoulder, or elbow orthopedic procedures; surgical site infection after bariatric surgery for obesity; deep vein thrombosis and pulmonary embolism after a total knee or hip replacement, except for pediatric (individuals younger than age 21) and obstetric populations; wrong surgical procedure; correct procedure performed on the wrong patient; or correct procedure performed on the wrong body part.

Time Limit

Each state has its own time limit for the submission of a claim. The time limit can vary from 2 months to 12 or 18 months from the date that the service was rendered. A bill can be rejected if it is submitted after the time limit unless the state recognizes some valid justification. Some states have separate procedures for billing over-one-year (OOY) claims. A percentage of the claim may be reduced according to the date of a delinquent submission.

Reciprocity

Most states have reciprocity for Medicaid payments if a patient requires medical care while out of state. Contact the Medicaid fiscal intermediary in the patient's home state and ask for the appropriate forms. If the case was an emergency, state this on the form. File the papers with Medicaid in the patient's home state. Reimbursement will be at that state's rate.

Claim Form

As of October 1, 1986, federal law has mandated that the CMS-1500 Insurance Claim Form be adopted for the processing of Medicaid claims in all states.

The health care provider of service must submit a claim form to the fiscal agent for the Medicaid program. Depending on state guidelines, prescription drugs and dental services may be billed to a different fiscal agent than those that are performed by a physician or other health care provider. There may also be special cases, in which the provider of services may be directed to send a bill directly to the local public service welfare office, human service, or family independence agency. These agencies have different names in each state.

Further guidance for completion of a CMS 1500 claim form for a Medicaid patient will be explained in Chapter 14 of this textbook; however, Fig 7.5 shows an example of a completed Medicaid claim form. Note the following information included on the claim form:

- The name of the insurance carrier the claim is being prepared for is identified at the top right-hand corner of the form.
- In box #1, Medicaid has been checked to identify this patient has Medicaid coverage.
- In box #1a, the patient's Medicaid identification number has been entered.
- In box #27, the accept assignment box has been checked "yes" to indicate that the provider accepts assignment.

Because guidelines for completing the form may vary from state to state, refer to the state's fiscal agent for directions. To stay up to date, always read the current bulletins or program memos on the state's Medicaid website. Read and implement the rule changes and updates to avoid rejected claims.

Medicaid Managed Care Claims

When filing a claim for a Medicaid managed care patient, send the bill or claim form to the managed care organization (MCO) and not to the Medicaid fiscal agent. The MCO receives payment for services rendered to eligible members either via the capitation or other managed care methods.

Children's Health Insurance Program Claims

Each state's jurisdiction operates its own CHIP with its own unique administrative characteristics. Thus, each has its own system and forms for billing and related procedures. The official plans and documents are retained in the individual state offices and are not available on either a regional or a national office basis. For specific information about a state's policies, contact the state's local Department of Health.

Medicaid and Other Plans

It is possible that a person can be eligible for Medicaid and also have group health insurance coverage through an employer.

Fig. 7.4 Treatment authorization request form used in California for the Medi-Cal program (DHCS Form 50-1).

MEDICAID
NO SECONDARY COVERAGE

DRAFT - NOT FOR OFFICIAL USE

HEALTH INSURANCE CLAIM FORM

APPROVED BY NATIONAL UNIFOR MCLAIM COMMITTEE (NUCC) 02/12

		PICA							PICA		

1. MEDICARE MEDICAID TRICARE CHAMPVA GROUP HEALTH PLAN FECA BLK LUNG OTHER	1a. INSURED'S I.D. NUMBER (For Program in Item 1)
☐ (Medicare#) ☒ (Medicaid#) ☐ (ID#DoD#) ☐ (Member ID#) ☐ (ID#) ☐ (ID#) ☐ (ID#)	376435099

2. PATIENT'S NAME (Last Name, First Name, Middle Initial)	3. PATIENT'S BIRTH DATE SEX	4. INSURED'S NAME (Last Name, First Name, Middle Initial)
Bishop, George	MM 02	DD 12	YY 1985 M ☒ F ☐	Bishop, George

5. PATIENT'S ADDRESS (No., Street)	6. PATIENT RELATIONSHIP TO INSURED	7. INSURED'S ADDRESS (No., Street)
312 Eighth Street	Self ☒ Spouse ☐ Child ☐ Other ☐	

CITY	STATE	8. RESERVED FOR NUCC USE	CITY	STATE
Woodland Hills	XY		Woodland Hills	NY

ZIP CODE	TELEPHONE (Include Area Code)		ZIP CODE	TELEPHONE (Include Area Code)
12345	( )		12345	( )

9. OTHER INSURED'S NAME (Last Name, First Name, Middle Initial)	10. IS PATIENT'S CONDITION RELATED TO:	11. INSURED'S POLICY GROUP OR FECA NUMBER
a. OTHER INSURED'S POLICY OR GROUP NUMBER	a. EMPLOYMENT? (Current or Previous) ☐ YES ☒ NO	a. INSURED'S DATE OF BIRTH MM DD YY SEX M ☐ F ☐
b. RESERVED FOR NUCC USE	b. AUTO ACCIDENT? PLACE (State) ☐ YES ☒ NO	b. OTHER CLAIM ID (Designated by NUCC)
c. RESERVED FOR NUCC USE	c. OTHER ACCIDENT? ☐ YES ☒ NO	c. INSURANCE PLAN NAME OR PROGRAM NAME Medicaid
d. INSURANCE PLAN NAME OR PROGRAM NAME	10d. CLAIM CODES (Designated by NUCC)	d. IS THERE ANOTHER HEALTH BENEFIT PLAN? ☐ YES ☒ NO If yes, complete items 9, 9a, and 9d.

READ BACK OF FORM BEFORE COMPLETING & SIGNING THIS FORM.	13. INSURED'S OR AUTHORIZED PERSON'S SIGNATURE I authorize payment of medical benefits to the undersigned physician or supplier for services described below.
12. PATIENT'S OR AUTHORIZED PERSON'S SIGNATURE I authorize the release of any medical or other information necessary to process this claim. I also request payment of government benefits either to myself or to the party who accepts assignment below. SIGNED George Bishop DATE 7/14/XX	SIGNED George Bishop

14. DATE OF CURRENT: ILLNESS, INJURY, or PREGNANCY(LMP) MM DD YY QUAL.	15. OTHER DATE QUAL. MM DD YY	16. DATES PATIENT UNABLE TO WORK IN CURRENT OCCUPATION FROM MM DD YY TO MM DD YY
17. NAME OF REFERRING PROVIDER OR OTHER SOURCE	17a. 17b. NPI	18. HOSPITALIZATION DATES RELATED TO CURRENT SERVICES FROM MM DD YY TO MM DD YY
19. ADDITIONAL CLAIM INFORMATION (Designated by NUCC)		20. OUTSIDE LAB? ☐ YES ☒ NO $ CHARGES

21. DIAGNOSIS OR NATURE OF ILLNESS OR INJURY Relate A-L to service line below (24E) ICD Ind. 0	22. RESUBMISSION CODE ORIGINAL REF. NO.
A. N390 B. C. D. E. F. G. H. I. J. K. L.	23. PRIOR AUTHORIZATION NUMBER

24. A. DATE(S) OF SERVICE From To MM DD YY MM DD YY	B. PLACE OF SERVICE	C. EMG	D. PROCEDURES, SERVICES, OR SUPPLIES (Explain Unusual Circumstances) CPT/HCPCS MODIFIER	E. DIAGNOSIS POINTER	F. $ CHARGES	G. DAYS OR UNITS	H. EPSDT Family Plan	I. ID. QUAL.	J. RENDERING PROVIDER ID. #
1 07 12 XX	11	Y	99213 25	A	90 00	1		NPI	37640017XX
2								NPI	
3								NPI	
4								NPI	
5								NPI	
6								NPI	

25. FEDERAL TAX I.D. NUMBER SSN EIN	26. PATIENT'S ACCOUNT NO.	27. ACCEPT ASSIGNMENT? (For govt. claims, see back)	28. TOTAL CHARGE	29. AMOUNT PAID	30. Rsvd for NUCC Use
XX12210XX ☒ ☐	046	☒ YES ☐ NO	$ 90.00	$	$

31. SIGNATURE OF PHYSICIAN OR SUPPLIER INCLUDING DEGREES OR CREDENTIALS (I certify that the statements on the reverse apply to this bill and are made a part thereof.) Pedro Atrics MD 071420XX SIGNED Pedro Atrics MD DATE	32. SERVICE FACILITY LOCATION INFORMATION a. X950731067 b.	33. BILLING PROVIDER INFO & PH # (555) 4869002 College Clinic 4567 Broad Avenue Woodland Hills XY 123450001 a. 3664021CC b.

NUCC Instruction Manual available at: www.nucc.org   PLEASE PRINT OR TYPE   OMB APPROVAL PENDING

Fig. 7.5 Completed Medicaid CMS-1500 Claim Form.

When Medicaid and a third-party payer cover the patient, Medicaid is always considered the payer of last resort. The third-party payer (other insurance) is billed first.

After a remittance advice (**RA**) or check voucher is received from the primary carrier, Medicaid (the secondary carrier) is billed. A copy of the RA or check voucher from the primary insurance must be included with the Medicaid claim.

Government Programs and Medicaid

When a Medicaid patient has Medicare (sometimes referred to as a *crossover case* or *dual eligible case*), TRICARE, or Veterans Health Administration (CHAMPVA) coverage, always send the insurance claim first to the federal program fiscal agent servicing the region. Usually the Medicare fiscal agent automatically forwards the claim to the secondary payer, Medicaid. If this does not occurs, bill Medicaid second and attach to the claim form the RA or check voucher that has been received from the federal program. Send in a claim only if the other coverage denies payment or pays less than the Medicaid fee schedule or if Medicaid covers services not covered by the other policy.

In the past, state Medicaid programs paid the Medicare deductibles and coinsurance for dual eligible cases at the full Medicare rate. However, the Balanced Budget Act of 1997 permits states to limit payment to the amount that the Medicaid program would otherwise pay for the service. Because of the health care reform legislation passed in 2010, many states have lowered their cost-sharing obligations for these cases to no more than the Medicaid payment amount for the same service. If the Medicare payment amount equals or exceeds the Medicaid payment rate, the state Medicaid program does not pay the Medicare deductible or coinsurance. The result is that the reimbursement becomes that of a Medicare-only patient even though it is crossed over to the Medicaid program.

 7.7 QUICK REVIEW
Question: What is the time limit for submitting Medicaid claims?

AFTER CLAIMS SUBMISSION

Remittance Advice

Remittance Advices (RA) are sent with the Medicaid payment check. If providers prefer, they can receive an electronic RA, but must first complete an electronic RA request form and submit it to their fiscal agent. Claim adjudication can be detailed on an RA as approved, paid, adjustment, denial, pend, suspend or void transactions although this terminology may vary from one fiscal agent to another (Fig. 7.6). *Adjudication* or *claim settlement* is the processing of an insurance claim through a series of edits for final determination of coverage (benefits) for possible payment.

Adjustments occur from overpayments or underpayments by the fiscal agent. Approval is when an original claim or a previously denied claim is approved for payment. Denied claims are listed with a reason code on the RA. Claims that are pended or in suspense for a certain period may be listed on the RA. Accounts receivable (A/R) transactions are miscellaneous transactions as a result of cost settlements, state audits, voids, or refund checks received.

Appeals

The time limit to appeal a claim varies from state to state but is usually 30 to 60 days from the date listed on the RA. Most Medicaid offices consider an appeal filed when they receive it, not when it is sent. Usually appeals are sent on a special form or with a cover letter along with photocopies of documents applicable to the appeal (for example, claim form, RA, and preauthorization forms). Appeals go first to either the regional fiscal agent or Medicaid bureau, next, to the Department of Social Welfare or Human Services, and then to an appellate court that evaluates decisions by local and government agencies. At each level, an examiner looks at the case and makes a decision. If not satisfied, the service provider may ask for further review at the next level.

! COMPLIANCE ALERT

Medicaid Fraud Control
Each state has a Medicaid Fraud Control Unit (MFCU), which is a federally funded state law enforcement entity usually located in the state attorney general's office. The MFCU employs teams of investigators, attorneys, and auditors who investigate and prosecute cases of fraud and other violations, including complaints of mistreatment in long-term care facilities. The Office of Inspector General (OIG) oversees and assesses the MFCU for performance and compliance with federal requirements. An internet link for access to the Medicaid Integrity Program has been provided at the end of this chapter under *Internet Resources*.

 7.8 QUICK REVIEW
Question: What is the time limit for appealing a denied Medicaid claim?

 DISCUSSION POINT
Discuss the importance of preventive health services such as those provided under the CHIP and EPSDT programs to individuals with low incomes.

PROCEDURE 7.1 Determining Covered Preventive Services Under Medicaid

Objectives
Preventing disease before it starts is critical to helping people live longer, healthier lives and Medicaid promotes prevention by helping patients gain access to preventive health care services. The objective of this procedure is to determine preventive health care services that are covered under the Medicaid program.

Directions
1. Go to the Medicaid.gov link (https://www.medicaid.gov/medicaid/benefits/prevention/index.html) to access a list of preventive services offered through the Medicaid program and answer the following questions.
   a. What program is ran jointly by CMS and the Centers for Disease Control Prevention (CDC) to provide immunizations to children, adolescents, and adults?
   b. What has Medicaid done to address the prevalence of obesity over the past 20 years?
   c. Are states required to provide dental benefits to children? Are states required to provide dental benefits to adults?
   d. What measures has the Medicaid program taken to address tobacco abuse and dependence?
   e. What other preventive health measures does Medicaid offers?

PAPER REMITTANCE ADVICE SECTIONS

Exhibit 3.5.10-2

PAGE 03
DATE   08/06/07
CYCLE 1563

MAHADEHENT
INFORMATION SYSTEM
MEDICAL ASSISTANCE (TITLE IX) PROGRAM
REMITTANCE STATEMENT

ETIN:
PRACTITIONER
PROW ID: ################
REMITTANCE NO: ##########

TO: WXYZ PRACTITIONER
     12345 ELM STREET
     ANYWHERE, NEW JERSEY 88888

LN. NO	OFFICE ACCOUNT NUMBER	CLIENT NAME	CLIENT ID NUMBER	TCN	DATE OF PROC. SERVICE CODE	UNITS	CHARGED	PAID	STATUS	ERRORS
01	CPXXXXXX	LASTNAME	LL#####L	####-#########-##	MM/DD/YY 91105	1.000	14.30	14.30	PAID	
02	CPXXXXXX	LASTNAME	LL#####L	####-#########-##	MM/DD/YY 90846	1.000	14.30	14.30	PAID	
01	CPXXXXXX	LASTNAME	LL#####L	####-#########-##	MM/DD/YY 99221	1.000	14.30	52.80	PAID	
01	CPXXXXXX	LASTNAME	LL#####L	####-#########-##	MM/DD/YY 99111	1.000	66.00	66.00	PAID	
01					99285	1.000	14.30		ADJT	ORIGNAL
	CPXXXXXX	LASTNAME	LL#####L	####-#########-##	MM/DD/YY			17.60-		CLAIM PAID MM/DD/YY
01	CPXXXXXX	LASTNAME	LL#####L	####-#########-##	MM/DD/YY 99281	1.000	14.30	14.00	ADJT	

*=PREVIOUSLY PENDED CLAIM
*=NEW PEND

TOTAL AMOUNT ORIGNAL CLAIMS	PAID	147.40	NUMBER OF CLAIMS	4
NET AMOUNT ADJUSTMENTS	PAID	3.60 -	NUMBER OF CLAIMS	1
NET AMOUNT VOIDS	PAID	0.00 -	NUMBER OF CLAIMS	0
NET AMOUNT VOIDS-ADJUSTS		3.60 -	NUMBER OF CLAIMS	1

REMITTANCE ADVICE

Version 2013 - 01   7/31/2013

Fig. 7.6 New York State Medicaid remittance advice form.

KEY POINTS

This is a brief chapter review, or summary, of the key issues presented.

1. Medicaid was established by Title XIX of the Social Security Act, a federally aided, state-operated, and state-administered program that provides medical assistance for certain low-income persons in need of health and medical care.
2. Medicaid is administered by each state's government with partial federal funding.
3. The Patient Protection and Affordable Care Act (PPACA) and the Health Care and Education Reconciliation Act (HCERA) passed in 2010 affect the Medicaid program by expanding access for childless adults, nonelderly, and nonpregnant individuals, and includes preventive services and long-term care benefits.
4. Coverage and benefits vary widely from state to state.
5. Each state operates a children's health insurance program for children in families who earn too much money to qualify for Medicaid.
6. Some federal acts allow assistance to qualified Medicare beneficiaries (QMBs) and specified low-income Medicare beneficiaries (SLMBs) who are aged and/or disabled and receiving Medicare but have annual incomes below the federal poverty level (FPL).
7. A medically needy (MN) Medicaid classification may or may not pay a deductible, copayment, or share of cost (spend down) within a specific time frame before receiving state benefits.
8. Medicaid benefits identification cards are issued monthly to recipients.
9. Medicaid eligibility must be verified before providing medical services to patients. Some patients may have retroactive eligibility.
10. Sometimes prior approval is required for medical services and procedures.
11. Health care organizations and providers must enroll for participation in the Medicaid program with the fiscal agent.
12. Each state may have a different time limit for submitting a claim for reimbursement.
13. The CMS-1500 insurance claim form has been adopted for processing Medicaid claims in all states to a regional fiscal agent.
14. A remittance advice (RA) or check voucher accompanies all Medicaid payment checks sent by the fiscal agent to the provider of services.
15. Each state has a Medicaid Fraud Control Unit (MFCU) that investigates and prosecutes cases of fraud and other violations, including complaints of mistreatment in long-term care facilities.

INTERNET RESOURCES

Medicaid Program Names by State:
- https://aspe.hhs.gov/dataset/medicaid-program-names

Children's Health Insurance Program:
- https://www.medicaid.gov/chip/index.html

EPSDT Coverage Guide
- https://www.medicaid.gov/sites/default/files/2019-12/epsdt_coverage_guide.pdf

Medicaid Integrity Program
- www.cms.gov/MedicaidIntegrityProgram

STUDENT ASSIGNMENT

- Study Chapter 7.
- Complete all exercises in the *Workbook* to reinforce the theory learned in this chapter.
- Turn to the Glossary at the end of this text for a further understanding of the key terms and key abbreviations used in this chapter.

8

TRICARE and Veterans' Health Care

Linda M. Smith

OBJECTIVES

After reading this chapter, you should be able to:

1. Discuss the history of TRICARE.
2. State who is eligible for TRICARE.
3. Explain the Defense Enrollment Eligibility Reporting System.
4. Differentiate between authorized and nonauthorized providers.
5. Identify the four different types of military treatment facilities.
6. Explain the benefits of the TRICARE Select government program.
7. State the managed care features of TRICARE Prime and discuss enrollment, Primary Care Managers, preauthorization, and payments.
8. Define individuals who may enroll in the TRICARE Prime Remote program and discuss enrollment, preauthorization, and payments.
9. Discuss the TRICARE Reserve Select, TRICARE Retired Reserve, and TRICARE Young Adult programs.
10. Explain TRICARE for Life benefits and identify those who are eligible.
11. Identify out-of-pocket costs for individuals with TRICARE for Life.
12. Name individuals eligible for TRICARE Plus and discuss enrollment, preauthorization, and payments.
13. Discuss the Supplemental Health Care Program, including enrollment and payments.
14. Discuss the TRICARE Hospice Program.
15. Identify individuals who are eligible for the Veterans Health Administration program (CHAMPVA) and discuss enrollments and preauthorization.
16. Describe how to process a claim for an individual who is covered by CHAMPVA or the various types of TRICARE programs.
17. State the components of a TRICARE explanation of benefits
18. List the components of a Veterans Health Administration (CHAMPVA) Explanation of Benefits document.

KEY TERMS

Active duty service member
allowable charge
authorized provider
beneficiary
catastrophic cap
catchment area
Civilian Health and Medical Program of the Department of Veterans Affairs
Civilian Health and Medical Program of the Uniformed Services
cooperative care
coordination of benefits
cost share
Defense Enrollment Eligibility Reporting System
Department of Veterans Affairs
emergency
explanation of benefits

fiscal intermediary
health benefits advisor
health care finder
medically (or psychologically) necessary
Military Health System
Military Treatment Facility
network provider
nonparticipating provider
other health insurance
participating provider
partnership program
point-of-service option
preauthorization
Prime Service Area
primary care manager
regional contractor
service benefit program

service-connected injury
service retiree (military retiree)
sponsor
Supplemental Health Care Program
total, permanent service-connected disability
Transitional Assistance Management Program (TAMP)
TRICARE
TRICARE for Life
TRICARE Prime
TRICARE service center
TRICARE Select
urgent care
veteran
Veterans Choice Act
Veterans Health Administration
Veterans Health Care

KEY ABBREVIATIONS

ADSM	FI	OHI	TAMP
CHAMPUS	HBA	par	TFL
CHAMPVA	HCF	PCM	TMA
COB	MHS	POS	TPR
DEERS	MTF	PSA	TSC
EOB	nonpar	SHCP	VA

INSIGHTS FROM THE FIELD

Paula C.: Insurance Billing Specialist

I have worked in the health care field for over 20 years, starting on the insurance side as a TRICARE customer service representative. The most critical issue in billing TRICARE and CHAMPVA claims is getting the correct information from the patient. This is especially true when obtaining information for dependents. Without the correct information, there is a domino effect, resulting in an unpaid claim. It is important for insurance billing specialists to learn the art of asking simple and straightforward questions effectively and considerately—to get the correct information needed.

TRICARE and Veteran's Health Care (CHAMPVA) are both government medical insurance plans. The two plans are often confused but are completely separate and distinct programs. If an individual is eligible for TRICARE, they are not eligible for the Veteran's Health Care (CHAMPVA).

- **TRICARE** is a Department of Defense (DOD) benefit for active duty military, their dependents, and retired military.
- The Veteran's Health Care (CHAMPVA) is a Department of Veterans Affairs benefit for dependents of veterans who are permanently and totally disabled due to a service-connected injury or died of a service-connected disability or injury.

TRICARE

The Military Health System (MHS) is one of America's largest and most complex health care institutions. It is a federated system of uniformed, civilian and contract personnel, and additional civilian partners at all levels of the Department of Defense and beyond. The mission of the MHS is to ensure that active duty service members (ADSMs) of the United States military (Army, Navy, Air Force, Marines, Coast Guard) are healthy and able to complete their missions, are trained to provide medical care to operational forces around the world, and to provide them, their families, and retirees with medical benefits.

TRICARE is a major component of the MHS. TRICARE is the health care program provided by the Department of Defense for active duty service members (ADSMs) of the United States military and their families. Retired military service members and their families and survivors of ADSMs are also eligible for TRICARE. TRICARE is a federally funded program that provides comprehensive health coverage to all its members, including health plans, special programs, prescriptions, and dental plans.

8.1 QUICK REVIEW

Question: What category of individuals was TRICARE established for to provide health care benefits?

HISTORY OF TRICARE

The US Congress created Civilian Health and Medical Program of the Uniformed Services (CHAMPUS) in 1966 under Public Law 89-614. The purpose of the law was to assist individuals in the military who were finding it increasingly difficult to pay for the medical care required by their families. In January 1994, TRICARE became the new title for CHAMPUS. The TRICARE program is managed and administered by the TRICARE Management Activity (**TMA**) office.

TRICARE is available worldwide and managed by regional offices in three separate regions (Fig.8.1). Those regions are:

- TRICARE East
- TRICARE West
- TRICARE Overseas (anywhere outside the United States)

Each area has their own regional contractor. A regional contractor is an insurance company under agreement with the federal government to administer benefits, provide resources and assistance to beneficiaries, and handle claim processing within a particular state or country (Table 8.1).

8.2 QUICK REVIEW

Question: The TRICARE Regional Offices manage and oversee an integrated health care delivery system in the three U.S. TRICARE regions. What are those three regions?

TRICARE Eligibility

An individual who qualifies for TRICARE is known as a beneficiary; the ADSM is called the sponsor. A person who is retired from a career in the armed forces is known as a service retiree (military retiree) and remains in the TRICARE program until age 65, at which time the individual becomes eligible for the Medicare program. If an individual served as an active duty military person for 4 to 6 years and gives up their military career and leaves, no further family benefits are provided.

The following individuals are entitled to medical benefits under TRICARE:

- Active duty service members and their families
- National Guard/Reserve members and their families

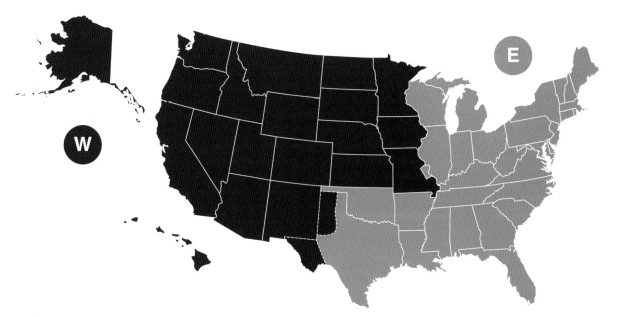

Fig. 8.1 Map of the two U.S. TRICARE regions: TRICARE East (E) and TRICARE West (W). The third region (not displayed) is TRICARE overseas for any location outside of the U.S. (From US Department of Defense, TRICARE Management Activity.)

TABLE 8.1 **Regional Contractors Effective January 1, 2018**	
Region	**Regional Contractor**
TRICARE West	Health Net Federal Services
TRICARE East	Humana Military

- Retired service members and their families
- Surviving eligible family members of deceased, active, or retired service members
- Former spouses of active or retired service members who meet certain length-of-marriage rules and other requirements.
- Medal of Honor recipients and their families
- Others registered in the Defense Enrollment Eligibility Reporting System

Defense Enrollment Eligibility Reporting System

All TRICARE-eligible persons must be enrolled in the Defense Enrollment Eligibility Reporting System (DEERS). DEERS is a computerized data base of military sponsors, families, and others worldwide who are entitled to TRICARE benefits. Sponsors are automatically registered in DEERS; however, sponsors must register eligible family members. Only sponsors can add or remove family members.

TRICARE claims processors check DEERS before processing claims to verify beneficiary eligibility. A TRICARE beneficiary may check their status by contacting the nearest personnel office of any branch of the service or by calling the toll-free number of the DEERS center.

TRICARE Identification Card

Once the sponsor has been registered into DEERS, they will be issued a TRICARE identification card. Children under the age

of 10 can usually use a parent's or guardian's ID card. At the age of 10, the sponsor will be required to get an ID card for the child. Children lose eligibility at the age of 21. An exception to this is if the child is enrolled in college, they will not lose eligibility until the age of 23.

Active duty uniformed service personnel are issued a common access card (CAC) to be used as standard identification. Military family members and retirees are issued a Uniformed Services Identification card to access health care benefits (Fig. 8.2).

Essential information must be abstracted from the front and back of the card; therefore, medical office staff should photocopy both sides of the card to retain in the patient's medical record.

> **8.3   QUICK REVIEW**
>
> Question: Under TRICARE, what is the difference between the beneficiary and the sponsor?

TRICARE Authorized Providers

TRICARE defines a provider as a person, business, or institution that provides health care. There are different types of providers the beneficiary can see; however, the type of provider will determine how much the beneficiary will pay out-of-pocket.

An authorized provider is a physician or other provider of care, a hospital, or supplier approved by TRICARE to provide medical care and supplies. Providers must pass a credentialing process to be authorized by TRICARE.

Patients should verify that the health care organization or service provider they are seeking services from are authorized to treat TRICARE beneficiaries before receiving medical services. Regional TRICARE contractors will verify a provider's authorized status before they can pay for services. If the provider is not authorized, TRICARE cannot help with paying

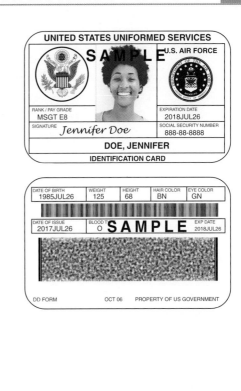

Fig. 8.2 Sample Common Access Card (CAC) and Uniformed Services ID card. From US Department of Defense and TRICARE and Humana Military Healthcare Services.

the bill. Beneficiaries who use nonauthorized providers may be responsible for their entire bill, and there are no legal limits on the amounts these providers can bill beneficiaries.

Network Providers

A network provider is any TRICARE-authorized provider that has signed a contract with a regional TRICARE contractor. Network providers will file claims on behalf of the patient and will agree to accept the TRICARE-allowable charge as payment in full. The allowable charge is the maximum amount that TRICARE can pay a provider for a procedure or service. Patients are responsible for any deductibles or cost shares. By using a network provider, patients will pay less out-of-pocket, and the provider will collect the rest of the amount directly from TRICARE.

Non-network providers are TRICARE-authorized civilian providers who have not established a contract with their regional TRICARE contractor. Non-network providers can

determine whether they are participating or nonparticipating on a claim-by-claim basis.

- Participating providers (par) have signed a contractual agreement with TRICARE to give medical care to TRICARE beneficiaries. The provider agrees to accept assignment, agrees to accept the TRICARE-determined allowable charge as payment in full, and transmits claims to the regional contractor. The provider may bill the patient for their cost share, which is the portion of the allowable charges (20% to 25%) after the deductible has been met. Beneficiaries pay only a certain amount each year for the cost share and annual deductible. This amount is known as a catastrophic cap. After the cap is reached, TRICARE pays 100% of the allowable charges for the rest of the year. The cap does not apply to noncovered TRICARE services (Table 8.2).
- Nonparticipating providers (nonpar) do not agree to accept the TRICARE-allowable charge as payment in full.

TABLE 8.2 Catastrophic Cap		
2020 Catastrophic Cap Amount for:	**Group A**	**Group B**
Active Duty Family Members (TRICARE Prime and Select)	$1000 per family, per calendar year	$1044 per family, per calendar year
Retirees and Their Family Members (TRICARE Prime and Select)	$3000 per family, per calendar year	$3655 per family, per calendar year
TRICARE Reserve Select (TRS)	$1044 per family, per calendar year	
TRICARE Retired Reserve (TRR)	$3655 per family, per calendar year	
TRICARE Young Adult (TYA)	Active Duty Family Members: $1044 per individual, per calendar year	
	Retiree Family Members: $3655 per individual, per calendar year.	

Catastrophic cap is the maximum amount paid by the patient each year. Cap amount is determined by the sponsor's initial enlistment or appointment date:
- Group A: Sponsor's enlistment or appointment date is before Jan. 1, 2018.
- Group B: Sponsor's enlistment or appointment date is on or after Jan. 1, 2018.

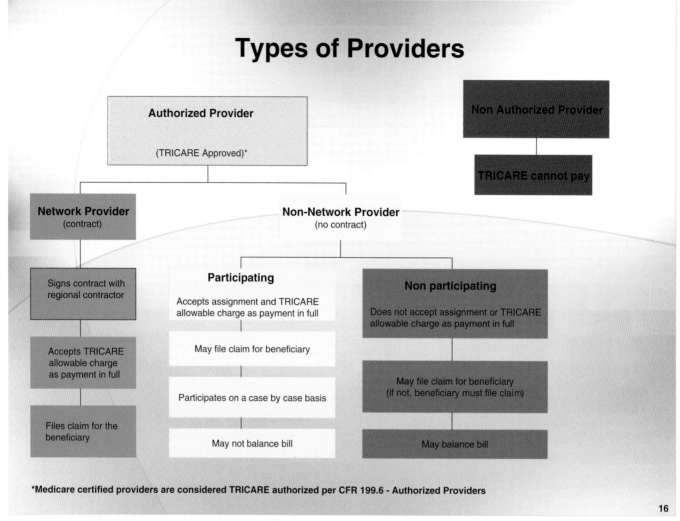

Types of Providers

Authorized Provider

(TRICARE Approved)*

Non Authorized Provider

TRICARE cannot pay

Network Provider
(contract)

Non-Network Provider
(no contract)

Signs contract with regional contractor

Participating

Accepts assignment and TRICARE allowable charge as payment in full

Non participating

Does not accept assignment or TRICARE allowable charge as payment in full

Accepts TRICARE allowable charge as payment in full

May file claim for beneficiary

Files claim for the beneficiary

Participates on a case by case basis

May file claim for beneficiary (if not, beneficiary must file claim)

May not balance bill

May balance bill

*Medicare certified providers are considered TRICARE authorized per CFR 199.6 - Authorized Providers

Fig. 8.3 Types of providers.

Nonparticipating providers may not bill the patient more than 115% of the allowable charge, which is referred to as the *limiting charge*. For example, if the TRICARE allowable charge for a procedure is $100, providers who decide not to participate in TRICARE may charge TRICARE patients no more than $115 for that procedure. The patient pays the deductible (20% or 25% of the charges determined to be allowable) and any amount more than the allowable charge up to 115% when the physician or health care organization does not accept assignment (Fig. 8.3).

Military Hospitals and Clinics

A Military Treatment Facility (MTF) is a uniformed services facility that provides inpatient, outpatient, and emergency care to eligible TRICARE beneficiaries. These military hospitals and clinics are run by the Department of Defense and operate on military bases and posts around the world. MTFs do not charge a fee for most services. There are four different types of military facilities that each provide different levels of service (Table 8.3).

TABLE 8.3	Types of Military Treatment Facilities
Multi-Service Markets	Integrated networks of military hospitals and clinics which may be composed of any combination of medical centers, hospitals, or clinics. There are 15 around the world (11 in the U.S. and 4 overseas). An internet link has been provided to identify the 15 multi-service markets at the end of this chapter under *Internet Resources*.
Medical Centers	Largest type of military facility, offering hospitalization and outpatient services. Have multiple specialties and sub-specialties. Serve as trauma centers in the community for military and civilian patients.
Hospitals	Smaller than medical centers. Offer hospitalization and outpatient services. Have multiple specialties but not sub-specialties.
Clinics	These are the smallest military facilities which offer only outpatient services. There are a limited number of specialties. Some clinics only provide primary care. Some clinics may also limit services to active service members.

Source: https://www.tricare.mil/FindDoctor/AllProviderDirectories/Military.

Catchment Area

TRICARE beneficiaries are assigned to a catchment area. The catchment area is a specific geographic region defined by zip codes and is based on an area of approximately 40 miles in radius surrounding each MTF in the United States.

 8.4   QUICK REVIEW

Question: What is the advantage of going to a provider in the TRICARE network?

TRICARE HEALTH PLANS

TRICARE offers several different health plans. Availability of the plans depends on the beneficiary's category and where they live. There are two primary TRICARE programs:

- TRICARE Select
- TRICARE Prime
  Additional TRICARE programs include the following:
- TRICARE Select Overseas
- TRICARE Prime Remote
- TRICARE Prime Overseas
- TRICARE Prime Remote Overseas
- TRICARE for Life
- TRICARE Reserve Select
- TRICARE Retired Reserve
- TRICARE Young Adult
- US Family Health Plan

TRICARE Select

The TRICARE Select program became effective January 1, 2018. It replaced the TRICARE Standard, TRICARE Extra, and TRICARE Standard Oversees programs. TRICARE Select is a fee-for-service, self-managed, preferred provider network plan. Beneficiaries enrolled in TRICARE Select can choose any TRICARE authorized provider for services.

TRICARE Select is offered to the following:
- Active duty family members
- Retired service members and their families
- Family members of activated Guard/Reserve members
- Nonactivated Guard/Reserve members and their families who qualify for care under the Transitional Assistance Management Program (TAMP). TAMP is a premium-free transitional health care benefits program lasting for 180 days after regular TRICARE benefits end
- Retired Guard/Reserve members at age 60 and their families
- Survivors
- Medal of Honor recipients and their families
- Qualified former spouses

Enrollment

Those entitled to medical benefits under TRICARE are automatically enrolled in the TRICARE Select program.

Benefits

In the TRICARE Select program, beneficiaries may receive a wide range of civilian health care services with a significant portion of the cost paid by the federal government. Patients are not limited to using network providers, and benefits include medical or psychological services or supplies that are considered appropriate care. Such services are generally accepted by qualified professionals to be reasonable and adequate for the diagnosis and treatment of illness, injury, pregnancy, and mental disorders or to be reasonable and adequate for well-baby care. These services are referred to as medically (or psychologically) necessary.

Beneficiaries also may receive urgent care and emergency care services. Urgent care is medically necessary treatment needed for an immediate illness or injury that would not result in further disability or death if not treated immediately. Treatment should not be delayed but should occur within 24 hours to avoid development of further complications. An emergency is a sudden and unexpected medical condition, or the worsening of a condition, that poses a threat to life, loss of limb, or loss of sight and requires immediate treatment to alleviate suffering (for example, shortness of breath, chest pain, or drug overdose). Emergency care is usually obtained at a hospital emergency department.

TRICARE Select patients usually seek care from a military treatment facility in their catchment area. The military health care provider may refer the patient to a civilian source if the service hospital that is managing the patient cannot provide a particular service or medical supplies. Cooperative care consists of services or supplies that may be cost-shared by TRICARE Select under certain conditions.

A partnership program is another option that allows TRICARE Select–eligible persons to receive inpatient or outpatient treatment from civilian providers of care in a military treatment facility or from uniformed services providers of care in civilian facilities. Whether a partnership program is instituted at a particular military treatment facility is up to the facility's commander, who makes the decision on an economic basis.

In addition, there are times when a specific health care service may not be available in the catchment area and a TRICARE Select beneficiary may seek care through a private health care provider or organization.

Referrals and Preauthorization

Referrals are not required in the TRICARE Select program. However, some care may require preauthorization. Preauthorization is a requirement to obtain permission for a service or procedure before it is done to determine if the regional contractor considers it to be medically necessary.

When specialty care or hospitalization is necessary, the MTF must be used if services are available. If services are not available, the health care finder (HCF) can assist with the referral or preauthorization process. A TRICARE referral/authorization form is shown in Fig. 8.4. An HCF is a health care professional, usually a registered nurse, who helps the patient to work with their primary care physician (PCP) to locate a specialist or obtain preauthorization for care. HCFs are found at a TRICARE service center (TSC), which is an office staffed by HCFs and beneficiary service representatives. All admissions, ambulatory surgical procedures, and other selected procedures require preauthorization. Certain types of health care services

Patient referral authorization form

Patient name: _____

Phone: _____   TRICARE ID: _____   DOB (mm-dd-yyyy): _____

Sponsor address: _____

Other Health Insurance: ☐ Yes ☐ No   Carrier: _____

Policy #: _____

Provider or setting: ☐ Physician's office ☐ Allied health professional's office ☐ Outpatient facility ☐ Inpatient facility

Date of service (if known; mm-dd-yyyy): _____ ☐ Evaluate only ☐ Evaluate and treat

Point of contact: _____   Phone: _____   Fax: _____

Ordering provider: _____   Phone: _____   Fax: _____

Type of service: ☐ Office visit   List specialty: _____   Specialist Tax ID/NPI: _____
☐ Surgical/Diagnostic procedure   ☐ Speech therapy ☐ Hospice ☐ Home health ☐ DME ☐ Observation ☐ PT/OT
☐ OP behavioral health   ☐ Other   ☐ Inpatient admission: ☐ Acute care   ☐ Rehab   ☐ SNF

If inpatient, please provide a diagnosis code: _____

Procedure or HCPC code: _____

Facility: _____   Tax ID/NPI #: _____

Address: _____

Rendering provider: _____   Tax ID/NPI #: _____

Address: _____

Presenting symptoms or reason for referral: _____

_____

Pertinent history, findings and specials situations include known discharge needs if inpatient admission: _____

_____

_____

Fig. 8.4 TRICARE Patient Referral Authorization Form. *ID*, Identification.

requiring prior approval from the TRICARE health contractor follow:

- Arthroscopy
- Breast mass or tumor removal
- Cardiac catheterization
- Cataract removal
- Cystoscopy
- Dental care
- Dilatation and curettage
- Durable medical equipment (DME) purchases
- Gastrointestinal endoscopy
- Gynecologic laparoscopy

- Hernia repairs
- Laparoscopic cholecystectomy
- Ligation or transection of fallopian tubes
- Magnetic resonance imaging (MRI)
- Mental health care
- Myringotomy or tympanostomy
- Neuroplasty
- Nose repair (rhinoplasty and septoplasty)
- Strabismus repair
- Tonsillectomy or adenoidectomy

TRICARE will only reimburse care received from authorized providers. For reduced cost, beneficiaries must use network providers.

Payment: Deductible and Copayment

TRICARE will pay authorized providers for covered services based on the allowable charge. TRICARE Select beneficiaries are subject to paying deductibles and copayments.

TRICARE Prime

TRICARE Prime is a managed care option available in Prime Service Areas that offers lower costs. Prime Service Areas (PSAs) are geographic areas that were created to ensure medical readiness of the active duty force by augmenting the capability and capacity of MTFs.

TRICARE Prime is offered to the following:
- Active duty family members and their families
- Retired service members and their families
- Activated Guard/Reserve members and their families
- Nonactivated Guard/Reserve members and their families who qualify for care under the Transitional Assistance Management Program (TAMP).
- Retired Guard/Reserve members at age 60 and their families
- Survivors
- Medal of Honor recipients and their families
- Qualified former spouses

Individuals on active duty can choose to enroll in TRICARE Prime or TRICARE Select. If they choose TRICARE Prime, they must enroll in the plan; enrollment is not automatic. TRICARE Prime offers fewer out-of-pocket costs than TRICARE Select, but there is less freedom of choice in providers. If the beneficiary elects to enroll in TRICARE Prime, the patient may no longer use the TRICARE Select program.

Primary Care Manager

Upon enrollment into the plan, the beneficiary has the option of choosing or being assigned a primary care manager (PCM). The PCM may be a civilian or military provider who provides the majority of patient care. The PCM is responsible for coordinating and managing the beneficiary's entire health care (except emergencies). The PCM may refer the beneficiary for additional services, when necessary, but specific referral and preauthorization requirements must be carried out. Referral patterns are evaluated to determine excessive or inappropriate referrals to specialists. A pattern of such referrals could result in termination of participation in TRICARE Prime. Enrolled beneficiaries may not use a non-network provider, except in emergencies or for pharmaceuticals, without a specific referral from an HCF.

Enrollment

An individual must complete an application and enroll for a minimum of 12 months to become a TRICARE Prime member. An annual enrollment fee is charged per person or family, except for active duty families, who may enroll for free. These members can use the local military and civilian provider network with necessary authorization.

Benefits

Covered services are the same as those for TRICARE Select patients, plus there are additional preventive and primary care services. For example, periodic physical examinations are covered at no charge under TRICARE Prime but are not covered under TRICARE Select. Prime also covers certain immunizations and annual eye examinations for dependent children of retirees that are not a benefit under the Select plan. A dental plan is available for an additional monthly premium

Preauthorization

All admissions, ambulatory surgical procedures, and other selected procedures require preauthorization. Outpatient or ambulatory surgery must be on the approved procedure list before it is performed. The list is in the *TRICARE Handbook* available at www.tricare.mil.

The health benefits advisor (HBA) at the nearest military medical facility should be called to determine whether preauthorization is required for the procedure before the surgery is scheduled in the approved facility. An HBA is a person at a military hospital or clinic who is there to help beneficiaries obtain medical care needed through the military and TRICARE. A point-of-service (POS) option is available if no authorization is obtained. This means that the individual can choose to get TRICARE-covered nonemergency services outside the Prime network of providers without a referral from the PCM and without authorization from the HCF.

Payments

Active duty service members pay nothing out-of-pocket for any type of care. Active duty family members only pay for care when they use a TRICARE Prime plan and they get care without a referral. Furthermore, there is no cost for services received at an MTF except for a small copayment amount when using inpatient care, which varies for active duty family members and retirees and their family members and survivors.

TRICARE Prime Remote

An additional TRICARE Prime option that is available is TRICARE Prime Remote (TPR). TPR is a managed care plan that is available in remote areas in the United States. TPR can only be used if both the sponsor's home and work addresses are more than 50 miles or 1 hour's drive time from a military treatment facility.

TABLE 8.4   Summary of Unique Aspects of TRICARE Prime Remote Program and Supplemental Health Care Program

	TPR	SHCP
Plan description	TPR is a program for ADSMs who live and work more than 50 miles or 1 h from an MTF. ADSMs must enroll.	SHCP is a program for • ADSMs • Inpatients at military treatment facilities who are not TRICARE eligible (e.g., eligible parents, parents-in-law) referred by an MTF to a civilian provider for care (usually for a specific test, procedure, or consultation) • Non–MTF-referred ADSMs (e.g., ROTC students, cadets/midshipmen, eligible foreign military)
Provider type	Any civilian provider	Any civilian provider
Beneficiary access to care	TPR ADSMs receive care from any civilian provider or from an MTF when available. Under TPR, ADSMs will have the same priority to care as other ADSMs at the MTF.	The beneficiary may receive services from any civilian provider in accordance with referral and preauthorization requirements (see later).
Beneficiary responsibility	TPR ADSMs have no annual deductible, cost shares, or copayments. The TPR ADSM must present his or her military ID card at the time care is received.	ADSMs and others eligible for SHCP referred to civilian providers have no copayment, deductible, or cost share. Beneficiary must present his or her military ID card at the time care is received.
POS	POS does not apply. If the ADSM receives care without a referral or preauthorization, the claim will be processed if it meets all other TRICARE requirements on a case-by-case basis.	The POS option does not apply.
Program benefits	Offers benefits similar to TRICARE Prime. Some benefits (including all behavioral health care) require preauthorization.	Offers benefits similar to TRICARE Prime. Some benefits (including all behavioral health care) require preauthorization.
Referrals and preauthorizations	*Primary care:* ADSMs can receive primary care from a provider without a referral or preauthorization. ADSMs with an assigned PCM will receive primary care from their PCM. ADSMs with no PCM can use any TRICARE-certified provider, or he or she can contact an HCF for assistance in locating a provider. *Specialty and inpatient care:* The SPOC will review requests for specialty and inpatient care.	*Specialty and inpatient care:* The MTF will review all requests for specialty and inpatient care for ADSMs. The MTF Commander or designee signature on a DD Form 2161 is required for designated patients referred for civilian care. Preauthorization for non–referred ADSMs for specialty, inpatient, and behavioral health care must be obtained from the SPOC or the HCF.

ADSMs, Active duty service members; *HCF,* health care finder; *ID,* identification; *MTF,* Military Treatment Facility; *PCM,* primary care manager; *POS,* point-of-service; *ROTC,* Reserve Officers' Training Corps; *SHCP,* Supplemental Health Care Program; *SPOC,* service point of contact; *TPR,* TRICARE Prime Remote.

TRICARE Prime Remote is available to the following:
• ADSMs
• Activated National Guard and Reserve members called or ordered to active duty service for more than 30 days in a row
• Active duty family members who live with a TPR-enrolled sponsor
• Active National Guard/Reserve family members if they live in a designated remote location when the sponsor is activated

Beneficiaries are assigned a PCM who will provide most of the patient's care. Active duty and their family members pay no copay or cost share when seen by their PCM or referred specialist.

Identification Card

ADSMs must present their military identification card to receive care from providers. Photocopy the front and reverse sides of the card so that information is available for reference when completing the insurance claim form.

Benefits

TPR program benefits are similar to TRICARE Prime. Services may be received from an MTF when available or from any

civilian provider. Primary routine care does not require prior authorization (i.e., office visits, preventive health care). The HCF must be contacted to receive authorization for referrals, inpatient admissions, maternity, physical therapy, orthotics, hearing appliances, family planning (tubal ligation or vasectomy), outpatient and inpatient behavioral health services, and transplants. Table 8.4 provides a summary of the unique aspects of TPR.

Referral and Preauthorization

Routine primary care (i.e., office visits, preventive health care) does not require prior authorization. The PCM must initiate all specialty referrals and coordinate requests through the HBA for certain outpatient services, all inpatient surgical or medical services, maternity services, physical therapy, orthotics, hearing appliances, family planning, transplants, and inpatient or outpatient behavioral health services.

Payments

Those persons covered and receiving benefits under TPR are not responsible for any out-of-pocket costs. ADSM claims for services provided by a TRICARE network provider are paid at the same contracted rate as other TRICARE beneficiary claims.

TRICARE Prime Overseas

TRICARE Prime Overseas is a managed care plan available in overseas areas near military treatment facilities.

TRICARE Prime Overseas is only available to ADSMs (including activated Guard/Reserve members) and command sponsored family members. Retirees and their families cannot enroll in TRICARE Overseas Prime.

Beneficiaries are assigned a PCM who will provide most of the patient's care. Beneficiaries will be referred to specialists as needed. Active duty and their family members pay no copay or cost share when seen by the PCM or referred specialist.

TRICARE Prime Remote Overseas

TRICARE Prime Remote Overseas is a managed care plan available in designated remote overseas locations of Eurasia-Africa, Latin American, Canada, and the Pacific.

The program is only available to ADSMs, active Guard/Reserve members, and command sponsored family members. Retirees and their families cannot enroll in TRICARE Overseas Prime.

Beneficiaries are assigned a PCM who will provide most of the patient's care. Beneficiaries will be referred to specialists as needed. ADSMs and their family members pay no copay or cost share when seen by the PCM or referred specialist.

US Family Health Plan

The US Family Health Plan is an additional TRICARE Prime option available through networks of community-based, not-for-profit health care systems in six areas of the United States. To enroll, beneficiaries must live in one of the designated US Family Health Plan service areas (Table 8.5). Care is provided through regional civilian health care networks of primary care physicians, hospitals, and affiliated specialties. The beneficiary selects their primary care provider, who will coordinate care and referrals to specialists and hospitals. Beneficiaries do not get care from military treatment facilities or from TRICARE network providers.

This plan is available to the following beneficiaries who live in a designated US Family Health Plan area:

- Active duty family members
- Retired service members and their families
- Family members of Activated National Guard/Reserve members
- Nonactivated National Guard/Reserve members and their families who qualify for care under the Transitional Assistance Management Program
- Retired National Guard/Reserve members at age 60 and their families
- Survivors
- Medal of Honor recipients and their families
- Qualified former spouses

TRICARE Reserve Select

TRICARE Reserve Select (TRS) is a premium-based health plan available worldwide for purchase by qualified members of the Selected Reserve and their families. TRS health care benefits are similar to TRICARE Select.

Members of the Selected Reserve and their families can participate in the program. Members can include the Army National Guard, Army Reserve, Navy Reserve, Marine Corps Reserve, Air National Guard, Air Force Reserve, and Coast Guard Reserve. Members must meet the following qualifications:

- Not on active duty orders
- Not covered under TAMP
- Not eligible for or enrolled in the Federal Employee Health Benefits (FEHB) program

Individuals enrolled in TRICARE Reserve Select are allowed to see a provider of their choice. If they see a network provider, they will pay less out-of-pocket expenses whereas seeing a non-network provider will result in paying a higher cost share.

TRICARE Retired Reserve

TRICARE Retired Reserve (TRR) is a premium-based health plan that qualified retired Reserve members and survivors may purchase. TRR offers coverage similar to TRICARE Select. Retired National Guard and Reserve personnel may qualify to purchase TRR coverage if they are members of the retired Reserve of a Reserve component of the armed forces, younger than age 60, and not eligible for or enrolled in the FEHB program. At age 60, TRR coverage is automatically terminated, and the retiree becomes eligible for TRICARE Prime/Select and may enroll in one of those programs.

Individuals enrolled in TRICARE Retired Reserve are allowed to see a provider of their choice. If they see a network provider, they will pay less out-of-pocket expenses whereas seeing a non-network provider will result in paying a higher cost share.

TABLE 8.5 Designated US Family Health Plan Service Areas and Designated Providers

US Family Health Plan Service Area	Designated Provider
• Maryland • Washington, DC • Delaware • Parts of Pennsylvania, Virginia, and West Virginia	• Johns Hopkins Medicine
• Maine • New Hampshire • Vermont • Upstate and Western New York	• Martin's Point Health Care
• Massachusetts, including Cape Cod • Rhode Island • Northern Connecticut	• US Family Health Plan of Southern New England
• New York City • Long Island • Western Connecticut • New Jersey • Philadelphia and area suburbs	• St. Vincent Catholic Medical Centers
• Southeast Texas • Southwest Louisiana	• CHRISTUS Health
• Puget Sound area of Washington State	• Pacific Medical Centers (Pacmed Clinics)

TRICARE Young Adult

The TRICARE Young Adult (TYA) program is a premium-based health care plan available for purchase by qualified dependents. TYA offers TRICARE Select or TRICARE Prime coverage based on the sponsor's status. It has medical and pharmacy benefits but no dental coverage. To join this program, the enrollee must be a dependent of an eligible uniformed service sponsor, unmarried, at least age 21, and not eligible to enroll in an employer-sponsored health plan. He or she can also enroll if under the age of 26 and enrolled in a full-time course of study at an approved institution of higher learning and if the sponsor provides at least 50% of his or her financial support.

TRICARE for Life

TRICARE for Life is a medical benefit program rather than an insurance program. The benefit is offered to individuals serving in the military and they pay no premiums for the coverage. TRICARE for Life (TFL) is a Medicare-wraparound coverage for TRICARE-eligible beneficiaries who have Medicare Parts A and B. The program is available worldwide and offers additional TRICARE benefits as a supplementary payer to Medicare for uniformed service retirees, their spouses, and survivors age 65 or older. In overseas areas, TRICARE is the first payer.

When beneficiaries become entitled to receive Medicare Part A and Medicare Part B at age 65, they experience no break in TRICARE coverage. The only change is that TRICARE will pay secondary to Medicare beginning on the first day of the month in which they turn 65.

Enrollment

Enrollment is not required. Coverage is automatic if the beneficiary has Medicare Part A and B. The beneficiary must pay Medicare Part B premiums.

The DEERS notifies a beneficiary within 90 days before his or her 65th birthday that the medical benefits are about to change. It asks the beneficiary to contact the nearest Social Security Administration office about enrollment in Medicare. The beneficiary must elect to enroll in Medicare Part B to be eligible for TFL benefits.

Identification Card

Beneficiaries who qualify for TFL do not need a TRICARE enrollment card. Beneficiaries will use their Medicare card and their military identification as proof of coverage.

Benefits

TRICARE for Life and Medicare cover medically necessary services. Both TFL and Medicare have special rules and limitations on certain types of care. Some types of services are not covered at all. Examples of services that are not typically covered by TFL or Medicare include (but are not limited to): acupuncture, experimental or investigational services, eye exams, and hearing aids.

In addition to medical benefits, individuals enrolled in TFL have the option to enroll in dental, vision, and pharmacy plans.

Referral and Preauthorization

There are no preauthorization requirements for the TFL program. All services and supplies must be benefits of the Medicare or TRICARE programs to be covered.

Payment

The out-of-pocket costs an individual will be responsible for are determined by the service they receive and whether or not the service is covered by Medicare and TFL (Table 8.6).

TRICARE Plus

TRICARE Plus is a primary care program offered at some military treatment facilities. The program allows patients to get primary care at their military treatment facility and pay nothing out-of-pocket. There is no enrollment fee, but beneficiaries must enroll to participate. Beneficiaries are limited to using only the treatment facility where they are enrolled. TRICARE Plus does not cover specialty care.

Enrollment

Beneficiaries are allowed to enroll in the program if they are TRICARE eligible and not enrolled in a TRICARE Prime Plan, the US Family Health Plan, or a civilian or Medicare managed care plan. Dependent parents or parent-in-laws are also eligible for enrollment; however, TRICARE will not pay for care by civilian providers, even if the military hospital or clinic refers the patient.

Identification Card

Persons enrolled in TRICARE Plus are issued an identification card and registered in the DEERS.

Benefits

The TRICARE Plus program is designed to function in the following ways:

- Enrollees use the MTF as their source of primary care; it is not a comprehensive health plan.
- Enrollees may seek care from a civilian provider but are discouraged from obtaining nonemergency primary care from sources outside the MTF.

TABLE 8.6 **TRICARE for Life Out-of-Pocket Costs**			
Type of Service	**Medicare Pays**	**TRICARE Pays**	**Patient Pays**
Covered by TRICARE and Medicare	Medicare-authorized amount	Remaining balances	Nothing
Covered by Medicare only.	Medicare-authorized amount	Nothing	Medicare deductible and coinsurance.
Covered by TRICARE only	Nothing	TRICARE-allowed amount	TRICARE deductible and cost-share.
Not covered by TRICARE or Medicare	Nothing	Nothing	Billed charges

DRAFT - NOT FOR OFFICIAL USE

CHAMPVA
NO SECONDARY COVERAGE

HEALTH INSURANCE CLAIM FORM

APPROVED BY NATIONAL UNIFOR MCLAIM COMMITTEE (NUCC) 02/12

| | PICA | | | | PICA | |

1. MEDICARE (Medicare#) □ MEDICAID (Medicaid#) □ TRICARE (ID#DoD#) □ CHAMPVA (Member ID#) X GROUP HEALTH PLAN (ID#) □ FECA BLK LUNG (ID#) □ OTHER (ID#) □

1a. INSURED'S I.D. NUMBER (For Program in Item 1) 507 XX 8111

2. PATIENT'S NAME (Last Name, First Name, Middle Initial) Walls, James, S

3. PATIENT'S BIRTH DATE MM 08 DD 10 YY 1935 SEX M X F □

4. INSURED'S NAME (Last Name, First Name, Middle Initial) Walls, James, S

5. PATIENT'S ADDRESS (No., Street) 72 Henry Drive

6. PATIENT RELATIONSHIP TO INSURED Self X Spouse □ Child □ Other □

7. INSURED'S ADDRESS (No., Street)

CITY Woodland Hills STATE XY

8. RESERVED FOR NUCC USE

CITY STATE

ZIP CODE 123450000 TELEPHONE ( )

ZIP CODE TELEPHONE ( )

9. OTHER INSURED'S NAME 10. IS PATIENT'S CONDITION RELATED TO: 11. INSURED'S POLICY GROUP OR FECA NUMBER 023

a. OTHER INSURED'S POLICY OR GROUP NUMBER a. EMPLOYMENT? X YES □ NO a. INSURED'S DATE OF BIRTH SEX M □ F □

b. RESERVED FOR NUCC USE b. AUTO ACCIDENT? □ YES X NO PLACE (State) b. OTHER CLAIM ID

c. RESERVED FOR NUCC USE c. OTHER ACCIDENT? □ YES X NO c. INSURANCE PLAN NAME OR PROGRAM NAME

d. INSURANCE PLAN NAME OR PROGRAM NAME 10d. CLAIM CODES d. IS THERE ANOTHER HEALTH BENEFIT PLAN? □ YES X NO

12. PATIENT'S OR AUTHORIZED PERSON'S SIGNATURE SIGNED Signature on file DATE

13. INSURED'S OR AUTHORIZED PERSON'S SIGNATURE SIGNED Signature on file

14. DATE OF CURRENT ILLNESS QUAL. 15. OTHER DATE QUAL. 16. DATES PATIENT UNABLE TO WORK FROM TO

17. NAME OF REFERRING PROVIDER DN Gerald Practon MD 17a. 17b. NPI 46278897XX 18. HOSPITALIZATION DATES FROM 07 29 20XX TO 07 31 20XX

19. ADDITIONAL CLAIM INFORMATION 20. OUTSIDE LAB? □ YES X NO $ CHARGES

21. DIAGNOSIS ICD Ind. 0 A. K4031 22. RESUBMISSION CODE ORIGINAL REF. NO. 23. PRIOR AUTHORIZATION NUMBER

24. A. DATE(S) OF SERVICE From / To	B. PLACE	C. EMG	D. CPT/HCPCS MODIFIER	E. DIAG PTR	F. $ CHARGES	G. UNITS	H.	I. QUAL	J. RENDERING PROVIDER ID #
04 20 XX	22		49505	A	570 00	1		NPI	25678831XX
								NPI	
								NPI	
								NPI	
								NPI	
								NPI	

25. FEDERAL TAX I.D. NUMBER XX12210XX SSN EIN X 26. PATIENT'S ACCOUNT NO. 8681 27. ACCEPT ASSIGNMENT? X YES □ NO 28. TOTAL CHARGE $ 570 00 29. AMOUNT PAID $ 30.

31. SIGNATURE OF PHYSICIAN Gene Ulibarri MD 073020XX SIGNED Gene Ulibarri MD DATE 32. SERVICE FACILITY College Hospital 4500 Broad Avenue Woodland Hills XY 123450001 a. X950731067 33. BILLING PROVIDER (555) 4869002 College Clinic 4567 Broad Avenue Woodland Hills XY 123450001 a. 3664021CC

NUCC Instruction Manual available at: www.nucc.org PLEASE PRINT OR TYPE OMB APPROVAL PENDING

Fig. 8.7 Completed CHAMPVA CMS 1500 Claim Form.

electronically transmit claims to TRICARE subcontractors for services given to beneficiaries. Referral and preauthorization numbers are required when applicable.

TRICARE Prime Remote and Supplemental Health Care Program

Outpatient professional services are electronically transmitted, or paper claims may be submitted using a CMS-1500 claim form. Primary care service claims are processed and paid without a referral or preauthorization from a network or non-network provider. A referral number provided by the HCF must be included for specialty medical or surgical care and for behavioral health counseling and therapy sessions.

TRICARE for Life

If the beneficiary receives care from a civilian provider, the provider electronically transmits claims to Medicare. Medicare pays its portion and then electronically forwards the claim to TRICARE for the remaining amount. TRICARE sends its payment directly to the provider. The beneficiary receives a TRICARE explanation of benefits that indicates the amount paid to the provider.

TRICARE/Veterans Health Administration and Other Insurance

By law, TRICARE/Veterans Health Administration (CHAMPVA) is usually the second payer when a beneficiary is enrolled in other health insurance (OHI). OHI may be coverage through an employer, an association, a private insurer, or any other non-military organization. However, two exceptions are as follows:

- Bill TRICARE or Veterans Health Administration (CHAMPVA) claims first when the beneficiary is a recipient of the Medicaid program.
- Bill TRICARE or Veterans Health Administration (CHAMPVA) claims first when coverage is specifically designed to supplement TRICARE benefits (i.e., Medigap [MG] health plan). When the patient has OHI that is primary, electronically transmit or send a paper claim using the CMS-1500 insurance claim form. Attach the explanation of benefits (EOB) from the primary carrier. If the patient is submitting their own claim to the other insurance, take these steps:
- Bill the other insurance carrier with the form it has supplied.
- Bill TRICARE or Veterans Health Administration (CHAMPVA) by completing the top section of the CMS-1500 after receiving payment and an EOB from the other third-party payer. Submit the health care provider's itemized statement, which must contain the following:
  a. Provider's name
  b. Date on which the services or supplies were provided
  c. Description of each service or supply
  d. Place of treatment
  e. Number or frequency of each service
  f. Fee for each item of service or supply
  g. Procedure code number(s)
  h. Diagnostic code number(s) or description of condition(s) for which treatment is being received
  i. Billing statements showing only total charges, canceled checks, or cash register receipts (or similar-type receipts) are not acceptable as itemized statements.

1. Attach a photocopy of the EOB from the other third-party payer.
2. Electronically transmit the TRICARE or Veterans Health Administration (CHAMPVA) claim to the local contractor (claims processor/regional contractor).

Medicare and TRICARE

TRICARE is considered secondary to Medicare for persons younger than age 65 who have Medicare Part A as a result of a disability and who have enrolled in Medicare Part B. Those eligible for Medicare Part A are not covered by TRICARE unless disabled. Claims should be electronically transmitted to Medicare, then to TRICARE with a copy of the Medicare remittance advice. Services covered by TRICARE but not covered by Medicare (i.e., prescriptions) are paid by TRICARE.

Medicare and Veterans Health Administration (CHAMPVA)

The Veterans Health Administration (CHAMPVA) program is considered secondary to Medicare for persons younger than age 65 who are enrolled in Medicare Parts A and B. Claims first must be transmitted electronically to Medicare because the Veterans Health Administration (CHAMPVA) is a secondary payer.

Dual or Double Coverage

A claim must be filed if a patient has an additional private insurance policy that provides double coverage. Refusal by the beneficiary to claim benefits from OHI coverage results in a denial of TRICARE benefits. In double coverage situations, TRICARE pays the lower of the following:

- The amount of TRICARE-allowable charges remaining after the double coverage plan has paid its benefits
- The amount TRICARE would have paid as primary payer
  When patients have double coverage and there are two insurance carriers providing benefits, there must be coordination of benefits (COB). The insurance carriers must work together and coordinate the payment of their benefits so there is no duplication of payments between the primary and secondary insurance carrier.

Third-Party Liability

If the patient is in an automobile accident or receives an injury that may have third-party involvement, the following two options are available for reimbursement:

1. **Option 1:** TRICARE Form DD 2527 (Statement of Personal Injury, Possible Third-Party Liability) must be sent with the regular claim form for cost sharing of the civilian medical care. All five sections of the form should be completed by the patient. This form allows TRICARE to evaluate the circumstances of the accident and the possibility that the government may recover money for medical care from the person who injured the patient. If a CMS-1500 claim form is submitted without TRICARE Form DD 2527, a request is made to complete it. This form must be returned within 35 days of the request or the claims processor will deny the original and all related claims. Then the regional contractor submits a claim to the third party for reimbursement or files a lien for reimbursement with the liability insurance carrier, the liable party, or the attorneys or court involved.

2. **Option 2:** The provider can submit claims exclusively to the third-party liability carrier for reimbursement. Claims submitted with *International Classification of Diseases, Tenth Revision, Clinical Modification* (ICD-10-CM) diagnostic codes between S00 and T88 (Injuries, Poisonings, and External Causes) trigger the fact that there might be third-party litigation and the claims processor may request the completion of DD Form 2527.

Workers' Compensation

If a TRICARE or Veterans Health Administration (CHAMPVA) beneficiary is injured on the job or becomes ill because of his or her work, a workers' compensation claim must be filed with the compensation insurance carrier. TRICARE or the Veterans Health Administration (CHAMPVA) can be billed when all workers' compensation benefits have been exhausted.

In some situations, it must be decided whether a case that involves an accident or illness is work related and the claim might be transmitted electronically to the TRICARE or Veterans Health Administration (CHAMPVA) claims regional contractor. In those instances, the claims processor files a lien with the workers' compensation carrier for recovery when the case is settled.

TRICARE and CHAMPVA Claim Offices

When submitting TRICARE claims and billing for medical care received in the U.S. or U.S. Territories, claims are sent to the claims address for the region where the patient resides. For medical care received in all other overseas areas, claims are sent to the address where the care is received. An internet link has been provided for finding TRICARE claims addresses at the end of this chapter under *Internet Resources*.

Health care providers should submit CHAMPVA claims to the central claims processing center at: The Veterans Health Administration (CHAMPVA); Department of Veteran's Affairs, PO Box 469063, Denver, CO 80246-9063.

TRICARE and CHAMPVA Time Limits for Claim Filing

Both TRICARE and CHAMPVA claims must be filed within 1 year from the date a service is provided or (for inpatient care) within 1 year from the patient's date of discharge from the inpatient facility. If a claim covers several different medical services or supplies that were provided at different times, the 1-year deadline applies to each item on the claim.

When a claim is electronically transmitted on time, but the contractor returns it for more information, the claim should be retransmitted with the requested information so that it is received by the contractor no later than 1 year after the medical services or supplies were provided or 90 days from the date the claim was returned to the provider, whichever is later.

A contractor may grant exemptions from the filing deadlines for several reasons. A request that includes a complete explanation of the circumstances of the late filing, all available documentation supporting the request, and the claim denied for late filing should be transmitted electronically to the contractor.

8.7 QUICK REVIEW
Question: What is the time limit for filing both TRICARE and CHAMPVA claims?

AFTER CLAIM SUBMISSION

Explanation of Benefits

An **Explanation of Benefits (EOB)** is a primary method of communication between health insurance carriers, health care providers, and the individuals that they provide benefits to.

For each TRICARE and CHAMPVA claim submitted, the claims processor issues an explanation of benefits (EOB) that is an itemized statement of the action they have taken (Fig. 8.8). The EOB details the payment of the claim (that is, service or supplies received, allowable charges, amount billed, amount paid, how much deductible has been paid, and patient's cost share amount). When the health care provider participates (accepts assignment), the EOB is sent to the health care organization with the check. Patients also have access to the EOB statement, which are either made available online by their regional contractor or they are mailed a copy of it.

Claims Inquiries and Appeals

For both TRICARE and CHAMPVA, providers may issue claim inquiries to the regional contractor. They may also request reconsideration of denied claims through the appeals process. See Chapter 16 for inquiring about the status of a claim and to learn the procedures for how to file reviews and appeals.

8.8 QUICK REVIEW
Question: What is the definition of an explanation of benefits?

DISCUSSION POINT

TRICARE and CHAMPVA are both government medical insurance plans. The two plans are often confused but are completely separate and distinct programs. Why is it important to understand the separate and distinct programs, and what special skills are required to manage the plans?

PROCEDURE 8.1 Determining TRICARE Eligibility Based on Beneficiary's Category

Objectives
TRICARE offers many different health plans. Availability of the plans depend on the beneficiary's category and where they live. To help you and the other insurance billing specialists in your health care organization, you have been asked to create a table outlining what plans are available to the specific categories of individuals.

Directions
1. Using the information provided in the textbook, create a table. Make one column the "TRICARE beneficiary categories" and add a second column for "Program Options" those individuals have.
   a) Beneficiary categories should include: Active duty service members, active duty family members, retired service members and eligible family members, activated national guard and reserve members and family members, deactivated national guard and reserve members and family members.
   b) Program options should include: TRICARE Select, TRICARE Reserve Select, TRICARE Select Overseas, TRICARE Prime, TRICARE Prime Remote, TRICARE Prime Overseas, TRICARE Prime Remove Overseas, TRICARE for Life, US Family Health Plan, TRICARE Young Adult
   c) Complete the table by matching which programs are available to each beneficiary category.

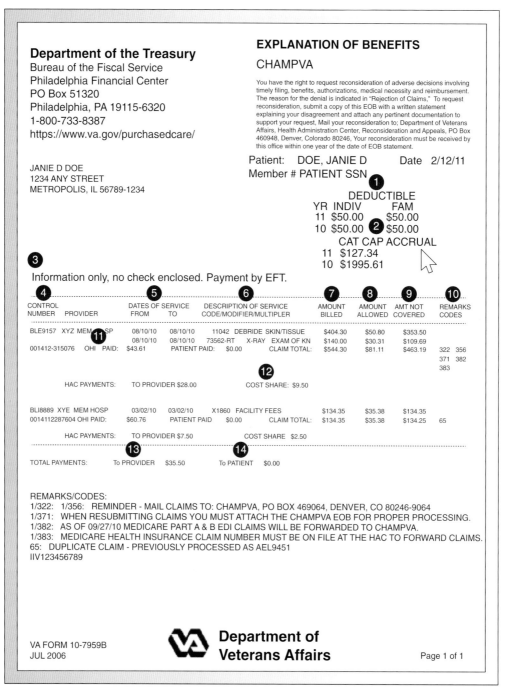

Department of the Treasury
Bureau of the Fiscal Service
Philadelphia Financial Center
PO Box 51320
Philadelphia, PA 19115-6320
1-800-733-8387
https://www.va.gov/purchasedcare/

JANIE D DOE
1234 ANY STREET
METROPOLIS, IL 56789-1234

EXPLANATION OF BENEFITS

CHAMPVA

You have the right to request reconsideration of adverse decisions involving timely filing, benefits, authorizations, medical necessity and reimbursement. The reason for the denial is indicated in "Rejection of Claims." To request reconsideration, submit a copy of this EOB with a written statement explaining your disagreement and attach any pertinent documentation to support your request. Mail your reconsideration to: Department of Veterans Affairs, Health Administration Center, Reconsideration and Appeals, PO Box 460948, Denver, Colorado 80246. Your reconsideration must be received by this office within one year of the date of EOB statement.

Patient: DOE, JANIE D   Date   2/12/11
Member # PATIENT SSN ❶

DEDUCTIBLE
YR INDIV   FAM
11 $50.00 $50.00
10 $50.00 ❷ $50.00
CAT CAP ACCRUAL
11 $127.34
10 $1995.61

❸
Information only, no check enclosed. Payment by EFT.

❹ CONTROL NUMBER PROVIDER	❺ DATES OF SERVICE FROM TO	❻ DESCRIPTION OF SERVICE CODE/MODIFIER/MULTIPLER	❼ AMOUNT BILLED	❽ AMOUNT ALLOWED	❾ AMT NOT COVERED	❿ REMARKS CODES
BLE9157 XYZ MEM ❶ SP	08/10/10 08/10/10	11042 DEBRIDE SKIN/TISSUE	$404.30	$50.80	$353.50	
	08/10/10 08/10/10	73562-RT X-RAY EXAM OF KN	$140.00	$30.31	$109.69	
001412-315076 OHI PAID: $43.61	PATIENT PAID: $0.00	CLAIM TOTAL:	$544.30	$81.11	$463.19	322 356 371 382 383

HAC PAYMENTS: TO PROVIDER $28.00   ❷ COST SHARE: $9.50

| BLI8889 XYE MEM HOSP | 03/02/10 03/02/10 | X1860 FACILITY FEES | $134.35 | $35.38 | $134.35 | |
| 0014112287604 OHI PAID: $60.76 | PATIENT PAID $0.00 | CLAIM TOTAL: | $134.35 | $35.38 | $134.25 | 65 |

HAC PAYMENTS: TO PROVIDER $7.50   COST SHARE $2.50

TOTAL PAYMENTS: ❸ To PROVIDER $35.50   ❹ To PATIENT $0.00

REMARKS/CODES:
1/322: 1/356: REMINDER - MAIL CLAIMS TO: CHAMPVA, PO BOX 469064, DENVER, CO 80246-9064
1/371: WHEN RESUBMITTING CLAIMS YOU MUST ATTACH THE CHAMPVA EOB FOR PROPER PROCESSING.
1/382: AS OF 09/27/10 MEDICARE PART A & B EDI CLAIMS WILL BE FORWARDED TO CHAMPVA.
1/383: MEDICARE HEALTH INSURANCE CLAIM NUMBER MUST BE ON FILE AT THE HAC TO FORWARD CLAIMS.
65: DUPLICATE CLAIM - PREVIOUSLY PROCESSED AS AEL9451
IIV123456789

VA FORM 10-7959B
JUL 2006

Department of Veterans Affairs

Page 1 of 1

Fig. 8.8 (1) **Deductible:** The amounts you have paid toward your annual deductible. (2) **CAT Cap Accrual:** The amounts you have paid toward your annual catastrophic cap, up to $3,000 per calendar year. (3) **Payment Information:** Indicates who the payment was sent to, if any, and the method of payment for reference. (4) **Control Number:** The CHAMPVA claim specific identifier. This number is needed to look up the specific claim in our system. (5) **Dates of Service (DOS):** The day or range of days the physician or hospital provided the service. (6) **Description of Service:** A description of the type of service rendered; e.g., office visit, immunization, etc., or the drug or durable medical equipment purchased. (7) **Amount Billed:** The amount your physician or the hospital charged the health insurance plan for providing services to you or your covered dependents. (8) **Amount Allowed:** This is the maximum dollar amount that CHAMPVA will reimburse a provider for a procedure, drug, or service. (You may owe a portion of this amount). (9) **Amount Not Covered:** The portion of the physician or hospital charge that is NOT covered or eligible for payment by your health insurance plan. (10) **Remarks/Codes:** Codes associated with the description of service. A code in this column relates to the narrative description at the bottom of the EOB. (11) **OHI:** The amount paid by other health insurance toward the amount billed, including adjustments applied as a result of agreements between the provider and the OHI. (12) **Cost Share:** The amount you are required to pay to the provider unless there is an OHI. (13) **Totally Payments: To Provider:** The amount CHAMPVA has paid to the provider or hospital on your behalf. (14) **Total Payments: To Patient:** The amount of money CHAMPVA has paid you, the beneficiary. (From Veterans Health Administration (Civilian Health and Medical Program of the Department of Veterans Affairs [CHAMPVA]) explanation of benefits document).

KEY ABBREVIATIONS

AME	LHWCA	PD	SIF
C and R	ND	POR	TD
ERISA	OSHA	QME	WP
FECA	OWCP	ROM	
IME	P and S	SCIF	

INSIGHTS FROM THE FIELD

Tina G.: Billing Manager for Orthopedic Practice
Credentials: CPC, CPMA, COC, COSC, CMBS

The most challenging part of billing Workers' Compensation claims is that there are so many parties to deal with. Accurate information must be obtained from the patient and the employer. Many times, there are third-party vendors who do authorizations for diagnostic testing, surgeries, medications, and other ancillary services on behalf of the insurance carrier. Then all of the information must go to the insurance carrier, the workers' compensation board, and sometimes there are even attorneys involved. It is not a simple process because the Workers' Compensation does not follow industry standards; they have their own rules, their own forms, and their own fee schedules. The insurance billing specialist must be able to understand the process, must be highly organized, and, most importantly, must be diligent in completing all parts of the process.

WORKERS' COMPENSATION DEFINED

Workers' compensation insurance is the most important coverage written to insure work-related injuries and illnesses. Previously this form of insurance was known as "workmens' compensation." The term *workmen* was changed to *workers* for a more generic title and to avoid sexual bias in language.

Workers' compensation was developed to protect both employers and employees. Workers' compensation insurance provides payment of medical expenses, lost wages, and rehabilitation costs to employees who are injured or become ill in the course and scope of their job. It also pays death benefits to families of employees who are killed while executing their job. Furthermore, workers compensation laws protect employers from lawsuits by injured employees. Under state and federal workers' compensation laws, business owners are required to purchase workers' compensation for their employees. Businesses that fail to provide workers' compensation coverage can face severe and costly repercussions including payment of claims out of pocket, fines, and possible imprisonment, as well as possibly losing the right to conduct business in that state.

HISTORY

Before the establishment of a workers' compensation program in the United States, the employer was responsible for an employee's work-related medical bills or the employee paid for their own medical expenses. Employees are individuals working for another, generally for wages, in exchange for labor or services. Originally the worker had to prove legally that injury was caused by negligence on the part of the employer. By the end of the nineteenth century, the number of accidents had increased, and legal processes were uncertain; therefore, federal and state legal provisions were required. In the early 1900s, employers' liability laws were adopted by many states, but there was still a great need for improvement. In 1911, the first workers' compensation laws that allowed injured employees to receive medical care without first taking employers to court were enacted. All states currently have workers' compensation laws.

Workers' Compensation Statutes

There are two kinds of statutes under workers' compensation: federal compensation laws and state compensation laws. Federal laws apply to miners, maritime workers, and those who work for the government; they do not apply to state and private business employees. State compensation laws apply to employers and employees within each state. State laws vary from state to state.

The workers' compensation statutes relieve the employer of liability for injury received or illness contracted by an employee in a work situation, except in gross negligence cases. They also enable the employee to get compensated for loss of wages and medical expenses easily and quickly. Most workers recover from their job injuries, but some continue to have problems. If the treatment provider determines that the patient will never recover completely or will always be limited in the work they can do, this is considered a permanent disability (PD). The workers' compensation laws assist the patient who is permanently disabled to receive disability income benefits without an extended delay.

Workers' Compensation Reform

By 1994, dysfunctional workers' compensation systems were costing companies more than $65 billion annually in many US cities. Some employers began moving their businesses to states requiring lower premiums. Other companies closed their doors because of the high cost of workers' compensation coverage. Widespread legal and medical corruption had evolved throughout the system in the form of record-high medical treatment and legal expenses. Reforms of the compensation of health care workers became necessary because of these problems. Reform laws have been introduced in a number of states that deal with the following issues:

- Antifraud legislation and increased penalties for workers' compensation fraud
  - Anti-referral provisions (for example, restrictions of physicians referring patients for diagnostic studies to sites where the physician has a financial interest)

- Proof of the medical necessity for treatment (or tests) as well as appropriate documentation. If guidelines are not adhered to, the carrier may refuse to pay the entire fee.
- Preauthorization for major operations and expensive tests
- Caps on vocational rehabilitation
- Use of a disabled worker in another division of the company where he or she was employed so that the worker may be gainfully employed while not using the injured part of the body
- Increase in occupational safety measures
- Employers offering a variety of managed care plans from which employees can choose, with some of these restricting their choice of provider
- Development of fee schedules specifically for workers' compensation claims
- Medical bill review to identify duplicate claims and billing errors
- Use of mediators instead of lawyers to reach agreement between employers and the injured employee
- Prosecution of health care organizations, physicians, lawyers, and employees who abuse the system

Although the system is far from perfect or complete, much progress has been made toward reducing high costs by trimming reimbursement for medical services and minimizing abuses of the system.

Purposes of Workers' Compensation Laws

Workers' compensation laws have been developed for a variety of reasons and accomplished much, including the following:

1. Provide the best available medical care necessary to ensure a prompt return to work of any injured or ill employee as well as achieving maximum recovery.
2. Provide income to the injured or ill worker or to their dependents, regardless of fault.
3. Provide a single remedy and reduce court delays, costs, and workloads arising out of personal injury litigation.
4. Relieve public and private charities of financial drains resulting from uncompensated work-related injuries and illnesses.
5. Eliminate payment of fees to attorneys and witnesses as well as time-consuming trials and appeals.
6. Encourage maximum employer interest in safety and rehabilitation through an appropriate experience-rating mechanism.
7. Promote the study of causes of accidents and reduce preventable accidents and human suffering rather than concealing fault.

9.1   QUICK REVIEW
Question: Explain who is protected by workers' compensation laws?

WORKERS' COMPENSATION INSURANCE PROGRAMS

Although workers' compensation systems vary from state to state, all workers' compensation benefits are paid for by the employer in some manner. Each state has its own rules about where an employer may buy workers' compensation insurance. There are typically three ways that workers' compensation premiums may be purchased by an employer:

- through a state-run program or State Compensation Insurance Fund.
- from a private insurance company plan.
- through a self-insurance plan.

State Compensation Insurance Fund

The largest provider of workers' compensation in most states is through their own state-run programs, referred to as a State Compensation Insurance Fund (SCIF). These state government insurance carriers are self-sufficient, funding their own operations with insurance policy premiums and investments rather than taxpayer money. Small and medium-sized businesses often rely on state-run programs. The mission of a SCIF is to ensure that all businesses have workers' compensation programs available to them at a fair price. SCIFs compete with private insurance carriers and are required to provide the lowest possible premiums to maintain their solvency. The state's department of labor or industrial relations typically administer the program. It should be noted that not all states have a SCIF, and in some states the SCIF is only offered as an insurer of last resort for a business that cannot find coverage from a private insurer. A link to the listing of the state compensation insurance funds has been provided under *Internet Resources* at the end of this chapter.

Private Insurance Workers Compensation Carriers

There are many private insurance carriers who offer workers' compensation coverage to businesses of all sizes. Insurers must meet state mandates for workers' compensation coverage. Some insurers are specialty companies that focus on specific businesses such as agricultural businesses, education-related businesses, or sports-related businesses. Examples of large private insurance carriers include the Travelers Group, Hartford Group, Zurich Insurance Group, and Liberty Mutual Group.

Encouraged by the success of managed care in the medical insurance market, increasing numbers of employers are seeking managed care contracts with preferred provider organizations (PPOs) and health maintenance organizations (HMOs) to insure their workers against work-related accidents and illnesses. Some states have adopted laws authorizing managed care programs. Managed care contracts are not uniform and may limit the choice of providers, use fee schedule–based payments, require precertification for certain procedures, implement hospital and medical bill review, and incorporate utilization review of medical services.

Self-Insurance

A large employer with sufficient capital can save money by self-insuring employees for work-related injuries and illnesses. The self-insuring employer does not pay insurance premiums; instead the employer sets aside a state-mandated percentage of funding to cover medical expenses, wage compensation, death benefits, and other benefits related to work injuries or illnesses. Employers who self-insure may also purchase a large deductible insurance policy for catastrophic problems. Benefits are variable from plan to plan, and precertification for certain services may be required. Self-insured employers are governed by the Employee Retirement Income Security Act (ERISA). This federal law sets minimum requirements for group health plans and ensures that injured employees are taken care of in a fair manner. ERISA provides a safety net for injured workers by making sure their needs are met. Sometimes a self-insured plan may have stop-loss or reinsurance that becomes active on large claims or a set dollar limit per policy year or employee, depending on how it is structured. Such provisions give the insurer an excuse to delay claims until the reinsurer decides to fund the claim. In such cases it may be necessary to become aggressive and ask for the name, address, and telephone number of the reinsurer to learn the claim status. Prompt processing and payment should be demanded because delaying claims is a violation of federal laws and ERISA regulations.

A form of self-insurance designed to serve smaller or medium-size companies is known as *captive insurance.* Captive insurance is owned by its policyholders. This is best for companies that have good safety records and those willing to implement worker safety programs to keep claims to a minimum. Members of captive self-insurance programs may hire an outside firm to process claims and purchase extra insurance for major claims. They share overhead expenses and investment income if any remains after paying expenses and claims.

Second-Injury Fund (Subsequent-Injury Fund)

The second-injury fund, also known as the subsequent-injury fund (SIF), was established to meet problems arising when an employee has a preexisting injury or condition and is subsequently injured at work. The preexisting injury combines with the second injury to produce disability that is greater than that caused by the latter alone.

Two functions of the fund are:
1. to encourage hiring of the physically disabled and
2. to allocate more equitably the costs of providing benefits to such employees.

Second-injury employers pay compensations related primarily to the disability caused by the second injury, even though the employee receives benefits relating to the combined disability. The difference is made up from the SIF.

SCENARIO: SECOND-INJURY FUND

Bob Evans lost his left thumb while operating machinery. Then, 2 years later, Bob lost his left index finger in a second work-related accident. A question could arise of whether the second injury added to a preexisting condition or was related to the prior injury. This case illustrates that the existence of the former injury or disability substantially increased (added to) the disability caused by the latter injury. The employer would pay compensation related to the second injury and funds would come from a second-injury fund to pay for the difference between the first and second injuries.

 9.2   QUICK REVIEW
Question: What are the three ways that private employer's typically purchase workers' compensation programs for their workers?

ELIGIBILITY

Individuals are entitled to workers' compensation insurance coverage if they meet several basic requirements:

- The patient's employer must have workers' compensation insurance. Most states require any employer with at least one employee to have coverage, but some states set a minimum of two to five employees. A few states have different requirements for agricultural or construction businesses, and some allow charities to opt out of the workers' compensation system.
- The patient must be an employee of the company holding the workers' compensation insurance. Not all workers are employees when it comes to workers' compensation eligibility. For example, independent contractors, freelancers, and consultants are generally not entitled to workers' compensation benefits.
- The patient must have been injured at work or became ill as a result of job-related duties. Generally speaking, if they were doing something for the benefit of their employer and were injured or became ill as a result, then it is work-related.

It is not always clear whether an injury that seems related to the job is actually covered under workers' compensation eligibility rules. For an injury to be considered work related, the individual must be injured while working within the scope of their job description, or there must be a clear connection between the illness and the individual's employment. For example:

- An individual who amputates a finger while operating a drill press at work is considered a work-related injury.
- The posttraumatic stress disorder that a firefighter develops as a result of on-the-job experiences is considered work related.
- An employee who breaks his leg during an official company retreat at a ski resort would have an injury considered to be work related.
- An injury that occurs during the morning commute to work is *not* considered work related.
- An independent contractor, who is not actually an employee, is *not* covered by the company he or she is contracted with.
- An employee that receives an injury during a fight at work that he started with another employee would *not* be considered work related.
- An injury sustained by an employee at work due to being intoxicated would *not* be covered as work related.

Work-Related Accident

An accident is an unplanned and unexpected happening traceable to a definite time and place and causing injury (damage or loss).

Workers' compensation accidents do not necessarily occur at the customary work site. For example, an individual may be asked to obtain cash for the petty cash reserve during the lunch hour. He or she may misstep off the curb while walking to the bank and suffer a fractured ankle. This person is considered to be working, although not at the customary work site, and the injury is covered under workers' compensation insurance.

Occupational Illness

Occupational illness or disease is any abnormal condition or disorder caused by exposure to environmental factors associated with employment, including acute and chronic illnesses or diseases that may be caused by inhalation, absorption, ingestion, or direct contact. Occupational diseases usually become apparent soon after exposure. However, some diseases may be latent for a considerable amount of time. Therefore, some states have extended periods during which claims may be filed for certain slowly developing occupational diseases. These diseases include silicosis, asbestosis, pneumoconiosis, berylliosis, anthracosilicosis, radiation disability, deafness, cumulative trauma, and repetitive motion illnesses (for example, carpal tunnel syndrome).

Volunteer Workers

Volunteers are not paid employees; therefore, they are not typically covered under workers' compensation in most states. Instead the volunteer is more likely to be covered under the company's general liability insurance. Each state handles workers' compensation for volunteers differently. Therefore, each state's law should be reviewed to determine whether a volunteer qualifies for workers compensation benefits. Several states have laws to compensate civil defense and other volunteer workers, such as firefighters who are injured in the line of duty.

Agricultural Workers

In some states there are workers' compensation exemptions for employers of agricultural or farm workers. This exemption is based on the historical concern that a small farming operation may not have the financial means to maintain the necessary records, insurance, and accounting to properly comply with the workers' compensation system. State exemptions vary widely and may be affected by the number of employees on the payroll, the average payroll wages, seasonal labor, or employment of family members. Each state's law should be reviewed to determine if agricultural workers qualify for workers compensation benefits.

 9.3 QUICK REVIEW

Question: What are the requirements an individual must meet to be entitled to the workers' compensation insurance coverage?

FEDERAL AND STATE LAWS

As stated earlier in this chapter, there are two kinds of statutes under workers' compensation: federal compensation laws and state compensation laws.

Federal Laws

Employees who work for federal agencies are covered by a number of federal workers' compensation laws. These programs are provided through an exclusive funding system and are administered through the Office of Workers' Compensation Programs (OWCP). The mission of the OWCP is to protect the interest of workers who are injured or become ill on the job, their families, and their employees by making timely, appropriate, and accurate decisions on claims, providing prompt payment of benefits, and helping injured workers return to gainful work as early as it is feasible.

- *Federal Coal Mine Health and Safety Act of 1969.* This Act, also referred to as the *Black Lung Benefits Act,* provides compensation to coal miners who are totally disabled by pneumoconiosis arising out of coal mine employment and to survivors of coal miners whose deaths are attributable to the disease. The Act also provides eligible miners with medical coverage for the treatment of lung diseases related to pneumoconiosis. The Division of Coal Mine Workers' Compensation (DWMWC) administers claims filed under the Black Lung Benefits Act.
- *Federal Employees' Compensation Act.* The Federal Employees' Compensation Act (FECA) was instituted on May 30, 1908. The Act provides benefits for on-the-job injuries and occupational illnesses to any federal employee throughout the world. Federal employees include executive, legislative, and judicial branch employees; civilian defense workers; medical workers in veterans' hospitals; and employees of the US Postal Service.
- *Longshore and Harbor Workers' Compensation Act (LHWCA).* This Act became effective on March 4, 1927 and provides benefits for private or public employees engaged in maritime work nationwide. This includes occupations such as longshore workers, ship repairers, shipbuilders or ship breakers, and harbor construction workers. The injury must occur on the navigable waters of the United States or in the adjoin areas, including piers, docks, terminals, wharves, and areas used in loading and unloading vessels.
- *Energy Employees Occupational Illness Compensation Program Act (EEOICPA).* The EEOICPA became effective on July 31, 2001. This program provides compensation to current or former employees, or their survivors, of the Department of Energy (DOE), its predecessor agencies, and contractors and subcontractors who were diagnosed with diseases resulting from an exposure to radiation, beryllium, or silica while employed at covered facilities.
- An additional provision of the EEOICPA, enacted October 28, 2004, compensates DOE contractor and subcontractor employees, eligible survivors of such employees, and uranium miners, millers, and ore transporters, as defined by the Radiation Exposure Compensation Act (RECA), for any occupational illnesses that are causally linked to toxic exposures in the DOE or mining work environment. The OWCP oversees administration of claims for this program.

State Laws

State compensation laws cover those workers not protected by the previously mentioned federal statutes. Federal law mandates that states set up laws to meet minimum requirements. If an employer does not purchase workers' compensation insurance from a private insurance company, the employer must self-insure and have enough cash in reserve to cover the cost of medical care for all workers who suffer work-related injuries.

An employer may be reluctant to file a workers' compensation report with the state in some instances, preferring to pay medical expenses out of pocket rather than have premium rates increase. It is illegal for an employer to fail to report a work-related accident when reporting is required by state law, and some states consider it a misdemeanor. Different penalties can be imposed, depending on state law, such as imprisonment or assessment of fines of $500 to $100,000 or more.

Statutes require that employers have employers' liability insurance in addition to workers' compensation protection. The difference between workers' compensation insurance and employers' liability insurance is that the latter is coverage that protects against claims arising out of bodily injury to others (nonemployees) or damage to their property when someone is on business premises. It is not considered insurance coverage for someone who is working at a business site.

Workers' compensation requirements vary by state, by industry, by size, by structure of businesses, and by payrolls (Table 9.1). State compensation laws are compulsory or elective, which may be defined as follows:

1. **Compulsory Law.** Each employer is required to accept its provisions and provide for specified benefits. Failure to carry compulsory workers' compensation insurance can face severe fines, a heavy lawsuit, or even criminal charges.
2. **Elective Law.** The employer may accept or reject the law. If the statute of the law is rejected, the employer loses the three common-law defenses, which are the following:
   a. Assumption of risk
   b. Negligence of fellow employees
   c. Contributory negligence

Each state has a **Worker's Compensation Board** that is responsible for administering the law. Specific services include:

- Conduct hearings to ensure injured workers are provided benefits they are entitled to
- Provide an appeal process to resolve disputes
- Monitor businesses to ensure they have acceptable coverage
- Monitor insurance carrier's performance
- Investigate complaints and health care provider issues
- Establish medical treatment guidelines in certain areas to support health care providers in their efforts to treat patients

- Provide educational outreach to employers and workers who may need assistance navigating the workers' compensation system.

A link has been provided at the end of this chapter, under *Internet Resources*, which lists all states' Workers' Compensation Boards.

Minors

Every state requires children who are injured on the job to be entitled to the same workers' compensation benefits as other injured workers. However, most states provide additional workers' compensation protection over and above the standard workers' compensation benefits paid to adults. For example, in some states, if a minor is injured on the job and is determined to be permanently disabled, the wage loss benefits may be calculated at a level higher than an adult worker to produce the maximum compensation rate.

Interstate Laws

Questions may arise as to which state's law determines payment of compensation benefits if a worker's occupation takes him or her into another state (for example, truck drivers). Most compensation laws are extraterritorial, which means they are effective outside the state, by either specific provisions or court decisions. When billing, follow the rules and fee schedule of the state in which the workers' compensation claim was originally filed. This may or may not be the same as the patient's current state of residence. The only exception is workers' compensation for federal employees, which has nationwide rules. For railroad workers, most states abide by nationwide rules, but some states have theirs.

Waiting Periods

There are no waiting periods for workers' compensation to pay for medical bills resulting from a workplace injury or illness. However, each state has a defined waiting period (WP) required for the injured employee to receive wage benefits. The WP is defined as the number of days an employee must be unable to work (as a result of a workplace injury or illness) before income benefits are payable. In most states the WP begins on the first day wages are lost. WPs were instituted to reduce paperwork for the claim administrator and ensure that wage benefits are not granted for a minor injury that typically should not keep an employee out of the workplace. If an injury results in disability that goes on for some time, the injured worker is retroactively paid wages that were lost during the waiting period.

TABLE 9.1	Example of State Compensation Laws (Compulsory vs. Elective)	
Alabama	Compulsory for employers of 5 or more	Elective for partners, corporate affairs, and sole proprietors
Connecticut	Compulsory	Elective to officers and partners
Massachusetts	Compulsory	No exceptions
New York	Compulsory	Elective to partners, officers, self-employed
South Dakota	Compulsory	Elective to farm labor, employer
Texas	Not Compulsory	Elective
Vermont	Compulsory	Elective for officers, partners, sole proprietors

Source: https://www.nfib.com/content/legal-compliance/legal/workers-compensation-laws-state-by-state-comparison-57181/.

 9.4 QUICK REVIEW
Question: Give examples of categories of employees who would be covered under federal workers' compensation laws?

TYPES OF STATE COMPENSATION BENEFITS

Workers' compensation pays for medical treatment and care for those who suffer a work-related illness or injury. It also provides additional benefits if the individual is disabled or the injury/illness results in death.

Five principal types of state compensation benefits that may apply in ordinary cases are the following:

1. *Medical treatment.* This includes compensation for hospital, medical, surgical services, medications, and prosthetic devices. Treatment may be rendered by a medical doctor, osteopath, dentist, or chiropractor.
2. *Temporary disability indemnity.* This compensation is in the form of weekly cash payments for lost wages made directly to the injured or ill person.
3. *Permanent disability indemnity.* This compensation may consist of either weekly or monthly cash payments for lost wages based on a rating system that determines the percentage of PD or a lump sum award. The payment amount depends on how much the individual earned before the injury/illness and is typically capped at two-thirds of their wages.
4. *Death benefits for survivors.* This compensation consists of cash payments to dependents of employees who are fatally injured. A burial allowance is also given in some states.
5. *Rehabilitation benefits.* Compensation for rehabilitation services for individual who may be temporarily or permanently disabled. Although an ill or injured individual may not be able to return to their previous position, the purpose of rehabilitation (medical or vocational) is to retrain employees so they can return to the workforce with some capacity.

Fig. 9.1 Health care provider interacting with an injured worker in the examination room.

TYPES OF STATE WORKERS' COMPENSATION CLAIMS

There are three types of state workers' compensation claims: nondisability claims, temporary disability (**TD**) claims, and PD claims. Each type is discussed in details to provide a clear definition and understanding of the determination process.

Nondisability Claim

The simplest type of claim is a nondisability (ND) claim. In these cases, an individual has a work-related injury or illness, but is treated and goes back to work. The individual does not lose time from their job and continues working (Fig. 9.1).

Temporary Disability Claim

Temporary disability occurs when a worker has a work-related injury or illness and is unable to perform the duties of their occupation for a specific time or range of time. The time period of TD can extend from the date of injury until the worker returns to full duty without residual ratable disability. TD may also occur when the patient returns to modified work or has ratable residual disability that the physician states is permanent and stationary (P and S). A condition is considered P and S when the patient reaches a point where their medical condition is not improving and not getting worse. This is referred to as the point in time when the patient has reached maximal medical improvement (MMI).

An insurance adjuster is a person at the workers' compensation insurance carrier who oversees the work-related injury or illness case. The insurance adjuster is responsible for keeping in contact with the health care organization about the patient's ongoing progress. The insurance adjuster must evaluate the injury or illness, predict in advance the amount of money reserves needed to cover medical expenses, and calculate as accurate a reserve as possible for weekly TD payments to the injured. This is often a challenging task because a seemingly minor injury or illness can become very complex. For example, a simple back strain ultimately may require fusion, or a small cut may become gangrenous and lead to an amputation. The insurance carrier wants to provide the best possible medical care for the patient. Usually workers' compensation weekly TD income payments are based on a percentage of the employee's earnings at the time of the injury. Compensation benefits are not subject to income tax.

Sometimes a patient is released from disability to light duty or a modified work program before returning to full duty, especially when heavy work is involved. Other times an employee is returned to the company and placed in a different department or division so that he or she is gainfully employed while not using the injured body part. This topic is further detailed in the next section.

Vocational Rehabilitation

Many states provide vocational rehabilitation in the form of retraining, education, job guidance, and placement to assist an injured individual in finding work before TD compensation benefits expire. In any successful rehabilitation program, the insurance carrier, health care organization, physician, physical therapist, employer supervisor, and personnel department must act as a team with the common goal of getting an injured employee back to light duty or regular work as soon as possible. It is believed that the longer a person remains out of work, the less chance there is that he or she will return to the workplace. The employer and insurance adjuster must remain in communication with the rehabilitation center therapists to determine when the injured person will be able to resume some form of work. The physician may suggest a rehabilitation center that provides good care, or the employer may have an in-house program.

Work Hardening

Sports medicine therapy and physical medicine rehabilitation are often used to strengthen the injured worker. Another type of therapy, called work hardening, is an individualized program using simulated or real work tasks to build up strength and improve the worker's endurance toward a full day's work.

Ergonomics

Ergonomics is the applied science of designing and arranging things people use so they can interact more efficiently and safely. In some cases, an ergonomic evaluation of the work site is performed and modifications may be instituted to the job or work site to lessen the possibility of future injury and to get the employee back to gainful employment. Injured individuals may also be retrained into another career field if their disability prevents them from returning to their former occupation.

Permanent Disability Claim

In a PD claim the patient or injured party is usually on TD benefits for a time and then concludes that they are unable to return to their former occupation. The physician states in the report that the patient has residual disability that will hamper their opportunity to compete in the open job market. Examples of residual disability include loss of a hand, an eye, or a leg, and neurologic problems. Each patient who has PD is rated according to the severity of the injury, the age of the injured person, and the patient's occupation at the time of the injury. The older the person, the greater the PD benefit. One might think that a younger person deserves higher compensation because they will be disabled for a longer period of their working career. However, the workers' compensation laws assume that a young person has a better chance of being rehabilitated into another occupation.

In a PD claim the physician's final report must include the words "permanent and stationary." The case is rated for PD, and a settlement called a compromise and release (C and R), is made. This is an agreement between the injured party and the insurance company on a total sum. The case can then be closed.

Reasons that may delay closing a workers' compensation case include the following:

1. Unanswered questions or incomplete answers to data required on workers' compensation forms by the employee, employer, or physician.
2. Vague terminology used by the physician or service provider in medical reports.
3. Omitted signatures on forms or written reports by the employee, employer, or health care provider.
4. Incorrect billing by the health care organization's office
5. Inadequate progress reports (for example, the physician or service provider fails to send in a medical report routine ly to update the insurance carrier when the injured employee is seen in subsequent visits)

Rating

Final determination of the issues involving settlement of a work-related accident is known as adjudication, or the rating of a case. A health care provider does not rate disability but renders a professional opinion on whether the injured individual has TD or PD that prevents him or her from gainful employment. The rating proper is carried out by the state's industrial accident commission or workers' compensation board. Wage loss, earning capacity, and physical impairment are three categories that may be taken into consideration to rate temporary partial, permanent partial, or total disabilities.

In addition, permanent partial disabilities may be rated by using a scheduled or nonscheduled injury award system. This system is based on a set number of weeks of compensation for a specific loss, such as 288 weeks for the loss of a leg. Scheduled injuries may be loss of a body part, disfigurement, permanent hearing loss, and so on. Nonscheduled injuries are more general, such as disability caused by injury to the back or neck.

If an injured person is dissatisfied with the rating after the case has been declared P and S, he or she may appeal the case by submitting a formal request in writing. The request is referred to as a petition and is sent to the Workers' Compensation Board or the Industrial Accident Commission.

Surveillance

Sub rosa is a Latin term meaning "under the rose," which is a symbol of secrecy. In Workers' Compensation, the term *sub rosa* refers to the secret act of surveillance of a person. Sub rosa films are provided occasionally when rating a case to document the extent of a patient's PD. Videotapes are made over a period of 2 to 3 days without the patient's knowledge. This surveillance is expensive and is used as a last resort, especially in a case in which a person receiving workers' compensation benefits is suspected of making exaggerated complaints. It is also used in cases when a worker has been off work for a long time and supposedly is unable to perform any work activity, even light duty.

Investigators have been known to carry a camera in a gym bag and videotape a supposedly disabled claimant bench pressing at the gym. Patients also have been videotaped going into the health care provider's office for an appointment wearing a neck brace and removing the brace after returning to their car.

9.5 QUICK REVIEW
Question: What are the three types of state workers' compensation claims?

FRAUD AND ABUSE

Workers' compensation fraud occurs when an individual or organization makes a false statement or conceals information to receive workers' compensation benefits. It is also considered fraud to prevent someone from receiving benefits to which they are entitled to. Workers' compensation fraud can be committed by an employee, an employer, a health care provider, or a lawyer.

Increases in the number of fraudulent workers' compensation claims were noted throughout many large metropolitan cities in the 1990s. An increasing number of states have enacted some kind of antifraud legislation and stiffened penalties for workers' compensation fraud, making it a felony.

Physicians are responsible for determining the legitimacy of work injuries and reporting findings accurately. If a report is prepared with the intention of using it to support a fraudulent claim or if a fraudulent claim is knowingly submitted for payment under an insurance contract, the physician may be subject to fines or imprisonment and revocation or suspension of their medical license. Some physicians sign and send a disclosure statement with the medical report certifying that they personally performed an evaluation. The physician may list the total time spent in reviewing records, face-to-face time with the patient, preparing a report, and other relevant activities.

It is the responsibility of all individuals who deal with workers' compensation cases to notify the insurance carrier of any suspicious situation. By doing so, action can be taken to have the case investigated further by personnel from the fraud divisions or referred to the district attorney's office. Perpetrators and signs of workers' compensation fraud and abuse are listed in Box 9.1.

> ### 9.6 QUICK REVIEW
> Question: Who is responsible for determining the legitimacy of work injuries and reporting findings accurately?

LEGAL SITUATIONS

Medical Evaluator

Physicians who conduct medical–legal (ML) evaluations of injured workers must pass a complex medical examination. They are then certified by the Industrial Medical Council (IMC) and may be referred to as one of the following titles:

- Agreed medical evaluator (**AME**)
- Independent medical evaluator (**IME**)
- Qualified medical evaluator (**QME**)

The medical evaluator is hired by the insurance company or appointed by the referee or appeals board to examine an individual, independent from the attending physician, and render an unbiased opinion about the degree of disability of an injured worker. When the physician performs an evaluation on an injured worker, the workers' compensation fee schedule may have specific procedure codes to bill for the examination.

BOX 9.1   Perpetrators and Signs of Workers' Compensation Fraud and Abuse

Employee
- Symptoms are all subjective.
- Misses the first health care provider's visit or cancels or repeatedly reschedules appointments.
- Cannot describe the pain or is overly dramatic, such as an employee who comes to the health care provider's office limping on the left leg, suddenly starts limping on the right leg, and then goes back to limping on the left leg.
- Delays in reporting the injury.
- Does not report Friday's injury until Monday morning.
- First reports an injury to a legal or regulatory agency.
- Reports an injury after missing several days of work.
- Changes health care providers frequently.
- Is a short-term worker.
- Has a curious claim history.
- Fabricates an injury.
- Exaggerates a work-related injury to obtain larger benefits, such as an injured employee who has a back pain and claims inability to bend over or lift. Surveillance cameras capture the individual at work on weekends repairing cars in the driveway at home—a task he is supposedly unable to perform.
- Blames an injury that occurred off the job on the employer.
- Adds symptoms in response to efforts to return the person to work.

Employer
- Misrepresents the annual payroll to get lower premium rates.
- Misrepresents the number of workers employed.
- Gives a false address with the least expensive premium rates.
- Falsely classifies the job duties of workers (as not hazardous), such as stating the job title as a clerical worker when in fact the employee is using a lathe every day.
- Conspires with the employee to defraud.
- Insurer.
- Refuses to pay valid medical claims.
- Forces the injured worker to settle by using unethical tactics. For example, an insurance agent tells an employee that he has a back sprain. Relying on that

information, the worker settles the case. Later, a myelogram reveals a herniated intervertebral disk. The patient is left with a permanent partial disability.

Medical Provider
- Makes immediate referral for psychiatric care despite the worker's report of a trauma injury.
- Orders or performs unnecessary tests.
- Treatment dates fall on weekends and holidays.
- Renders unnecessary treatment.
- Lists a diagnosis that is not consistent with the course of treatment.
- Charges the insurance carrier for services never rendered.
- Prolongs treatment for what appears to be a minor injury.
- Participates in a provider mill scheme (see explanation under "Lawyer").
- Makes multiple referrals from a health care organization regardless of type of injury.
- Sends medical reports that look photocopied with the same information typed in (for example, employer's address, description of injury) or that read almost identical to other reports.
- Sends in many claims in which injuries are of a subjective nature, such as stress, emotional distress, headaches, and inability to sleep.
- Sends in claims from one employer showing several employees with similar injuries, using the same health providers and/or attorneys.
- Bills both the workers' compensation carrier and the health insurer for the same service.

Lawyer
- Overbills clients.
- Participates in a medical provider mill scheme. For example, an individual is solicited while in the unemployment line by a recruiter known as a "capper." The capper tells the worker it is possible to obtain more money on disability than through unemployment. The worker is referred to an attorney and a "provider mill" clinic, which help the individual to fabricate a claim by claiming stress or an on-the-job injury. In some states, such acts may be considered a public offense and are punishable as a misdemeanor or felony.

Depositions

When a case involves a medical evaluation, a deposition may be taken of the medical evaluator's testimony. A deposition is a proceeding in which an attorney asks a witness questions about a case and the witness answers under an oath but not in open court. It may take place in the attorney's office or often in the health care provider's office. In PD workers' compensation cases, depositions are usually taken from the health care provider and the injured party by the attorney representing the workers' compensation insurance company. The injured party's attorney is also present if the witness is the defendant. Direct questioning and cross-examination may be done by both attorneys.

Exhibits may be entered into evidence. The witness is allowed to read the transcript and make corrections or changes. The witness may be asked to sign the transcript but can waive a signature if their attorney recommends against signing it. The deposition is used when the case comes to trial.

Depositions may be taken to find out additional information, the health care provider's version of the facts, the patient's version of the facts, the kind of witnesses the health care provider and patient will be, and so on. Another use for a deposition is to challenge the credibility of a witness on cross-examination. If the witness takes the stand and the testimony is inconsistent with the deposition, the attorney will make this known to the jury.

Medical Testimony

In a workers' compensation situation, a third-party liability claim is not made against a worker's employer, but against some separate person or company who may be responsible for the worker's injury. Third-party claims often arise when a worker is injured by a defective product or by someone other than the worker's boss or co-workers, such as a customer, a worker from another company, or a member of the public. In the instance of an accident case with third-party liability, the health care provider may have to testify as an expert witness, take time to give a deposition, or attend a pretrial conference. There should be a clear understanding of the terms of testimony and payment to eliminate future misunderstandings. A written agreement from the patient's lawyer should be obtained stating exactly what compensation the health care provider will receive for research (preparation), time spent waiting to testify (if appointments must be canceled), and actual testimony time (Fig. 9.2). In some cases, the health care provider may want to ask for partial payment in advance. If the health care provider is subpoenaed, he or she must appear in court regardless of whether an agreement exists.

Fig. 9.2 Example of a medical testimony agreement between a health care provider and an attorney. This is signed by the provider and sent to the attorney for signature. A copy is retained by the attorney and the original is kept by the health care provider.

SCENARIO: FILING A LIEN

Problem 1: Suppose Attorney Blake advises client Roger Reed not to pay the health care provider until after the trial. Or what happens if payment is not made for Dr. Practon's courtroom testimony and the case is lost? Suppose that medical reports are ordered and Attorney Blake neglects to pay for them. What happens if Roger Reed forgets about the physician's bill?

Solution: If a lien had been signed, then once the case has been settled the money would be paid to the physician; otherwise, the settlement would belong to the patient, Roger Reed, and he could take any action with the money that he wanted.

Problem 2: Suppose that Dr. Practon had an oral agreement covering his fee. The patient, Katie Crest, was unable to pay for medical treatment except on legal monetary recovery. When Katie Crest settled her case, the proceeds went almost entirely to welfare agencies because she received retroactive Medicaid. Dr. Practon sued the patient's attorney and lost.

Solution: If Dr. Practon had gotten a written assignment of the proceeds, the lawyer could have been held liable for the fee.

This agreement should be signed by the health care provider and sent to the attorney. The attorney should return the original to the health care provider, retaining a copy for their files.

Liens

In some cases, a health care provider may render services to a patient but may not receive reimbursement due to pending litigation related to the work-related injury or illness. In those cases, it may be advantageous to file a lien. The word lien derives from the same origin as the word *liable*, and the right of lien expresses legal claim on the property of another for the payment of a debt. To file a lien, the health care organization must obtain permission from the patient (Fig. 9.3). Liens sometimes are called *encumbrances* and may be filed for several reasons.

The advantages of filing a lien are as follows:
- It is a written agreement and is recognized in court.
- It is a source of protection in the event of litigation.

Fig. 9.3 Patient's authorization to release information to an attorney and grant lien to the health care provider against proceeds of settlement in connection with a work-related injury/illness or third-party litigation cases.

- It ensures that payment for previously rendered medical services are received when the attorney and patient have reached a settlement with the insurance company in an accident case.
- It is an inexpensive method of collecting the fee. The health care organization can file suit and try to get a judgment against the patient, but this is relatively expensive compared with filing a lien.
- The health care organization will collect the full fee. If the delinquent account is turned over to a collection agency, the health care organization may lose as much as 50% of the fee when it is collected.
- If the health care organization wishes to bill more than what is allowed for a given service or services, a lien can be filed, and the judge will determine whether it is reasonable.
- It avoids harassment in trying to collect the bill.

The chief disadvantage of not filing a lien is that there is no legal documentation if the case goes to court as far as collecting monies owed to the health care organization. A case could be settled, the attorney would get their fee, and the health care organization's fee may be placed last on the list for payment or remain unpaid.

A time limit should be specified when a lien form is completed; reaching a settlement may involve several years of litigation. Some patients may be persuaded to pay before a legal settlement is made or at least make payments until a settlement is reached. The lien becomes null and void at the end of the time limit.

The health care organization's fee should be protected by having the attorney sign the lien, thereby indicating that he or she will pay the service provider directly from any money received in a settlement. This makes the attorney responsible for the fee. The patient's file must be placed in a Hold for Settlement category until the case comes up in court. In some states the health care organization's fee owed by the patient constitutes a first lien against any such money settlement, and the attorney must first satisfy that lien before the patient or attorney receives any money from the settlement. State laws should be checked. The office of the patient's attorney should be called at least quarterly for an update.

If there is a third-party litigation involved in a workers' compensation case or a decision has not been reached as to whether an accident is work related, both a regular lien and a workers' compensation lien should be filed. In most states a special lien form for workers' compensation filing is available and should be used. A copy of the lien should be completed and sent to all concerned parties, including the following:
- Appeals board
- Employer of the patient
- Employee (the patient)
- Insurance carrier
- Health care organization or provider's files (lien claimant or one who is filing for the lien)

The patient/employee consents to the lien by their signature. Do not accept a lien form unless it is also signed by the patient's attorney. Check with the local Division of Industrial Accidents for forms pertinent to filing a lien and instructions on the formalities, number of copies required, and where they are to be sent.

Third-Party Subrogation

Subrogation is a workers' compensation insurance company's right to legally pursue a third party that caused an insurance loss to the employer. This is done in order to recover the amount of the claim paid by the workers' compensation insurance carrier to the injured worker. Third-party subrogation means "to substitute" one party for another. When applied to workers' compensation cases, it means a transfer of the claims and rights from the original creditor (workers' compensation insurance carrier) to the third-party liability carrier. Generally, there are three types of workers' compensation claims potentially caused by a third party:
- The direct action or inaction of a third party (i.e. auto accident).
- Defective or malfunctioning machinery, equipment or products owned or maintained by a third party
- A claim involving a workplace injury on property owned by a third party

In any of these instances, subrogation may be used to help the workers' compensation insurance provider recoup the costs of an injured employee's claims.

SCENARIO: THIRD-PARTY SUBROGATION

Scenario: As Monica Valdez, a secretary, went to the bank to deposit some money for her employer, her car was rear-ended by another automobile and she was injured.

Subrogation Solution: In such a case there is no question of fault and no question of cause. Monica was hurt during the performance of her work and the workers' compensation insurance carrier is liable. The carrier must adjust the claim, provide all medical treatment, and pay all temporary disability and permanent disability benefits.

However, the insurance carrier does have legal recourse. It may send a representative to visit with Monica, explain to her that she has a good subrogation case, encourage her to seek the advice of an attorney and sue the third party (other automobile driver) in civil court. This is sometimes referred to as *litigation,* which is the process of carrying on a lawsuit. If Monica agrees to sue, the insurance carrier files a demand with the court for repayment of all money it has paid out. This is called a *lien,* which is discussed earlier in this chapter. When the case is settled, if an award is made to Monica, the insurance carrier is reimbursed for all that it has paid, and Monica receives the balance. In some states, such as California, the patient is legally prevented from collecting twice.

 9.7 QUICK REVIEW
Question: What is the role of the workers' compensation medical evaluator?

MEDICAL RECORD MANAGEMENT

Health Information Record Keeping

If a private patient comes to the office with a work-related injury or illness, a separate medical record (chart) and financial record (ledger) should be set up for the work-related injury. A private medical record should never be combined with a workers' compensation case record because separate disclosure laws apply to each and the workers' compensation case may go to court.

It is preferable that a patient should not be scheduled to see a health care provider of services for a workers' compensation follow-up examination and an unrelated complaint during the same appointment. Separate appointments (back to back, if necessary) should be arranged. This allows for separate dictation without intermixing the required documentation for each chart.

⚠ COMPLIANCE ALERT
Workers' Compensation and HIPAA Compliance

It is important to note that workers' compensation programs are not included under the definition of a "health plan" as identified in the Health Insurance Portability and Accountability Act (HIPAA). Therefore, workers' compensation programs are not required to comply with HIPAA standards; however, it is beneficial to workers' compensation insurance payers and health care providers to use the adopted HIPAA Transaction and Code Set (TCS) to work harmoniously within the claims processing activities used throughout the industry.

⚠ COMPLIANCE ALERT
Privacy and Confidentiality

The Health Insurance Portability and Accountability Act (HIPAA) Privacy Rule allows for the disclosure of protected health information (PHI) to workers' compensation insurers, state administrators, and employers to an extent necessary to comply with laws relating to workers' compensation. The HIPAA Privacy Rule recognizes the legitimate need of insurers and other entities involved in the workers' compensation systems to have access to individuals' health information as authorized by state or other law. Because of the significant variability among such laws, the HIPAA Privacy Rule permits disclosures of health information for workers' compensation purposes in several different ways.

1. *Disclosures without Individual Authorization.* The HIPAA Privacy Rule permits covered entities to disclose PHI to workers' compensation insurers, state administrators, employers, and other persons or entities involved in workers' compensation systems without the individual's authorization. This relates to workers' compensation injuries or illnesses and federal programs, such as; Black Lung Benefits Act, Federal Employees' Compensation Act (FECA), the Longshore and Harbor Workers' Compensation Act (LHWCA), and Energy Employees Occupational Illness Compensation Program Act. The disclosure must comply with and be limited to what the state law requires. Disclosure is allowed for purposes of obtaining payment for any health care provided to the injured or ill worker.

2. *Disclosures with Individual Authorization.* Covered entities may disclose PHI to workers' compensation insurers and others involved in workers' compensation systems to which the individual has provided their authorization for the release of the information to the entity. For example, if a patient's attorney calls the health care provider's office for information, it is only ethical and legal to get a signed authorization from the patient and to ask permission from the insurance carrier before giving out any medical information. The contract exists between the health care provider and insurance carrier, not the health care provider and patient.

3. *Minimum Necessary.* Covered entities are required to limit the amount of PHI disclosed to the minimum necessary to accomplish the workers' compensation purpose. Under this requirement, PHI may be shared for such purposes to the full extent authorized by state or other law.

Documentation

In workers' compensation cases, it is important for the service provider to document how the injury occurred and where the injury occurred. Diagnosis codes will be assigned to relay this information on the claim form. For example, if a machinist receives a large cut on his hand because of operating a machine, this should be clearly documented; even the type of machine (saw, lathe, drill) should be specified. Where the injury occurred should also be documented in detail.

BOX 9.2 Terms that Describe Intensity of Pain and Frequency of Occurrence of Symptoms

Definitions that describe intensity of pain and frequency of symptoms were developed to assist the health care provider when documenting subjective complaints.

- A *severe* pain would preclude the activity causing the pain.
- A *moderate* pain could be tolerated but would cause marked handicap in the performance of the activity precipitating the pain.
- A *slight* pain could be tolerated but would cause some handicap in the performance of the activity precipitating the pain.
- A *minimal (mild)* pain would constitute an annoyance but would cause no handicap in the performance of the particular activity. It would be considered a non-ratable permanent disability (PD).
- *Occasional* means approximately 25% of the time.
- *Intermittent* means approximately 50% of the time.
- *Frequent* means approximately 75% of the time.
- *Constant* means 90% to 100% of the time.

Terminology

Most workers' compensation cases involve accidents causing body injuries. Therefore, one should become familiar with anatomic terms, directional and range-of-motion words, types of fractures, body activity terms, and words that describe pain and symptoms (Box 9.2). This terminology appears in progress chart notes and workers' compensation injury reports. The more knowledgeable one becomes about the meaning of the documentation, the more proficient one will be in knowing whether the procedure and diagnostic codes assigned are substantiated or if code selection is deficient and should be enhanced for better payment. The insurance billing specialist should learn how to spell the words and find the definitions of the words in the dictionary.

Directional terms are commonly used when a case is being rated for PD. A range-of-motion (ROM) test determines whether the body part can move to the full extent possible. Often, after an injury to an extremity or joint, there is restriction of motion and loss of strength (for example, grip). ROM can be improved with activity and therapy. It is measured with special measurement devices and documented each time a patient is examined. Fractures can occur from falling, blows, impact hits, a disease process, or direct violence, such as in an automobile accident. Healing may take months and depends on the location and severity of the injured part, associated injury, and complications or infections.

9.8 QUICK REVIEW
Question: How should medical records for work-related injuries or illnesses be organized in the patient's file?

REPORTING REQUIREMENTS

Each state has its own reporting requirements for workers' compensation claims. It is important for the insurance billing specialist to understand the forms that are used in their state and the process for filing them.

Employer's Report of Injury

The laws clearly state that the injured person must promptly report the work-related injury or illness to their employer or immediate supervisor, which may be a safety officer in some businesses. Most states require, by law, that the employer must send an Employer's Report of Occupational Injury or Illness form (Fig. 9.4) to the insurance company. The time limit for

State of California **EMPLOYER'S REPORT OF OCCUPATIONAL INJURY OR ILLNESS**	Please complete in triplicate (type if possible) Mail two copies to: XYZ Insurance Company P.O. Box 5 Woodland Hills XY 12345	OSHA CASE NO. # 18
		FATALITY ☐

Any person who makes or causes to be made any knowingly false or fraudulent material statement or material representation for the purpose of obtaining or denying workers compensation benefits or payments is guilty of a felony.

California law requires employers to report within **five days** of knowledge every occupational injury or illness which results in lost time beyond the date of the incident **OR** requires medical treatment beyond first aid. If an employee subsequently dies as a result of a previously reported injury or illness, the employer must file within **five days** of knowledge an amended report indicating death. In addition, every serious injury, illness, or death must be **reported immediately** by telephone or telegraph to the nearest office of the California Division of Occupational Safety and Health.

EMPLOYER

	Please do not use this column
1. FIRM NAME The Conk Out Company	Ia. Policy Number B12345
2. MAILING ADDRESS: (Number, Street, City, Zip) 45 South Gorman St. Woodland Hills, XY 12345	2a. Phone Number (555) 430-3488	CASE NUMBER
3. LOCATION if different from Mailing Address (Number, Street, City and Zip)	3a. Location Code	OWNERSHIP
4. NATURE OF BUSINESS; e.g.. Painting contractor, wholesale grocer, sawmill, hotel, etc. Plumbing Repair	5. State unemployment insurance acct.no	
6. TYPE OF EMPLOYER: ✓ Private ☐ State ☐ County ☐ City ☐ School District ☐ Other Gov't, Specify: _____		INDUSTRY
7. DATE OF INJURY / ONSET OF ILLNESS (mm/dd/yy) 04/03/20	8. TIME INJURY/ILLNESS OCCURRED __ AM 2:00 PM	9. TIME EMPLOYEE BEGAN WORK 8:00 AM __ PM	10. IF EMPLOYEE DIED, DATE OF DEATH (mm/dd/yy)	OCCUPATION
11. UNABLE TO WORK FOR AT LEAST ONE FULL DAY AFTER DATE OF INJURY? ✓ Yes ☐ No	12. DATE LAST WORKED (mm/dd/yy) 04/03/20	13. DATE RETURNED TO WORK (mm/dd/yy)	14. IF STILL OFF WORK, CHECK THIS BOX: ✓	
15. PAID FULL DAYS WAGES FOR DATE OF INJURY OR LAST DAY WORKED? ✓ Yes ☐ No	16. SALARY BEING CONTINUED? ☐ Yes ✓ No	17. DATE OF EMPLOYER'S KNOWLEDGE /NOTICE OF INJURY/ILLNESS (mm/dd/yy) 04/03/20	18. DATE EMPLOYEE WAS PROVIDED CLAIM FORM FORM (mm/dd/yy) 04/03/20	SEX

INJURY OR ILLNESS

19. SPECIFIC INJURY/ILLNESS AND PART OF BODY AFFECTED, MEDICAL DIAGNOSIS if available, e.g.. Second degree burns on right arm, tendonitis on left elbow, lead poisoning Ankle Injury. Swelling, possible fracture.	AGE
20. LOCATION WHERE EVENT OR EXPOSURE OCCURRED (Number, Street, City, Zip) 45 Gorman St. Woodland Hills, XY 12345	20a. COUNTY	21. ON EMPLOYER'S PREMISES? ✓ Yes ☐ No	DAILY HOURS
22. DEPARTMENT WHERE EVENT OR EXPOSURE OCCURRED, e.g., Shipping department, machine shop. Stock Room	23. Other Workers injured or ill in this event? ☐ Yes ✓ No	DAYS PER WEEK
24. EQUIPMENT, MATERIALS AND CHEMICALS THE EMPLOYEE WAS USING WHEN EVENT OR EXPOSURE OCCURRED, e.g.. Acetylene, welding torch, farm tractor, scaffold 6 Foot Ladder	WEEKLY HOURS
25. SPECIFIC ACTIVITY THE EMPLOYEE WAS PERFORMING WHEN EVENT OR EXPOSURE OCCURRED, e.g.. Welding seams of metal forms, loading boxes onto truck. Climbed ladder to remove a ream of paper from top shelf; Fell	WEEKLY WAGE
26. HOW INJURY/ILLNESS OCCURRED. DESCRIBE SEQUENCE OF EVENTS. SPECIFY OBJECT OR EXPOSURE WHICH DIRECTLY PRODUCED THE INJURY/ILLNESS, e.g.. Worker stepped back to inspect work and slipped on scrap material. As he fell, he brushed against fresh weld, and burned right hand. USE SEPARATE SHEET IF NECESSARY Worker climbed ladder to remove a ream of paper from the top shelf in stock room. She was descending and mis-stepped falling to the floor. She tried to land upright and her leg took the brunt of the fall.	COUNTY
27. Name and address of physician (number, street, city, zip) Raymond Skeleton, MD 4567 Broad Ave., Woodland Hills, XY 12345	27a. Phone Number	NATURE OF INJURY
28. Hospitalized as an inpatient overnight? ☐ No ☐ Yes If yes then, name and address of hospital (number, street, city, zip)	28a. Phone Number	PART OF BODY
	29. Employee treated in emergency room? ✓ Yes ☐ No	

ATTENTION This form contains information relating to employee health and must be used in a manner that protects the confidentiality of employees to the extent possible while the information is being used for occupational safety and health purposes. See CCR Title 8 14300.29 (b)(6)-(10) & 14300.35(b)(2)(E)2.

Note: Shaded boxes indicate confidential employee information as listed in CCR Title 8 14300.35(b)(2)(E)2*.

EMPLOYEE

30. EMPLOYEE NAME Ima B. Hurt	31. SOCIAL SECURITY NUMBER	32. DATE OF BIRTH (mm/dd/yy)
		EVENT
33. HOME ADDRESS (Number, Street, City, Zip)	33a. PHONE NUMBER	SECONDARY SOURCE
34. SEX ☐ Male ☒ Female	35. OCCUPATION (Regular job title, NO initials, abbreviations or numbers)	36. DATE OF HIRE (mm/dd/yy)
37. EMPLOYEE USUALLY WORKS ____ hours per day, ____ days per week, ____ total weekly hours	37a. EMPLOYMENT STATUS ☐ regular, full-time ☐ part-time ☐ temporary ☐ seasonal	37b. UNDER WHAT CLASS CODE OF YOUR POLICY WHERE WAGES ASSIGNED	EXTENT OF INJURY
38. GROSS WAGES/SALARY $ ____ per ____	39. OTHER PAYMENTS NOT REPORTED AS WAGES/SALARY (e.g. tips, meals, overtime, bonuses, etc.)? ☐ Yes ☐ No	
Completed By (type or print)	Signature & Title	Date (mm/dd/yy)

• Confidential information may be disclosed only to the employee, former employee, or their personal representative (CCR Title 8 14300.35), to others for the purpose of processing a workers' compensation or other insurance claim; and under certain circumstances to a public health or law enforcement agency or to a consultant hired by the employer (CCR Title 8 14300.30). CCR Title 8 14300.40 requires provision upon request to certain state and federal workplace safety agencies.

FORM 5020 (Rev7) June 2002   FILING OF THIS FORM IS NOT AN ADMISSION OF LIABILITY

Fig. 9.4 Employer's Report of Occupational Injury or Illness. This form complies with Occupational Safety and Health Administration (OSHA) requirements and California State Workers' Compensation laws.

submission of this form varies from immediately to as long as 30 days in different states. The insurance billing specialist should contact their state's Workers' Compensation Board to determine the time limit applicable to their health care organization. Many states have adopted the Employer's Report of Occupational Injury or Illness form shown in see Fig. 9.4 to meet the requirements of the federal Occupational Safety Health Administration (OSHA) Act of 1970 and for state statistical purposes. OSHA was established to protect employees against on-the-job health and safety hazards. Work standards were designed to minimize exposure to on the job hazards, such as faulty machinery, noise, dust, and toxic chemical fumes. Employers are required by law to meet these health and safety standards. Failure to do so can result in fines against the employer.

Medical Service Order

In addition to the employer's report, the employer may complete and sign a medical service order, giving this to the injured employee to take to the health care organization or health care provider's office (Fig. 9.5). This authorizes the health care organization to treat the injured employee. The form should be photocopied, and the copy retained by the health care organization. The original should be attached to the Doctor's First Report of Occupational Injury or Illness (preliminary report). An employer may prefer to write the service order on their business letterhead, on billhead, or simply on a piece of scratch paper.

Authorizations may also be obtained over the telephone. However, if a patient arrives for an appointment without written authorization, the employer can be telephoned and asked to have the authorization e-mailed or faxed to give permission for treatment. Subsequently, if payment is not received or the claim is disputed, it may be easier to collect if a copy of the written authorization is included when sending collection follow-up correspondence.

A copayment is not collected for a workers' compensation patient who submits a completed Employer's Report of Occupational Injury or Illness form. If a patient was injured on the job but does not have this form, standard protocol is to bill the patient's primary health insurance and collect the appropriate copayment. The patient may decide to bring in the Employer's Report of Occupational Injury or Illness at a later time. The health care provider has the right to reevaluate the patient under the workers' compensation policy and submit a medical service order (Fig. 9.6).

If outside testing or treatment is necessary, authorization should be obtained from the employer or the adjuster for the insurance company. When this is done by telephone, the name of the procedure or test and the medical necessity for it should be stated. The name and title of the person giving authorization should be obtained and written in the patient's chart and on the order form along with the date. No authorization numbers are issued in workers' compensation cases.

WORKERS' COMPENSATION
MEDICAL SERVICE ORDER

To: Dr./Clinic _____ Martin Feelgood, MD _____

Address _____ 4567 Broad Avenue, Woodland Hills, XY 12345 _____

We are sending _____ Mrs. Ima Hurt _____

Address _____ 300 East Central Ave., Woodland Hills, XY 12345 _____

Social Security No. __120-XX-6542__ Date of birth _3-4-1966_
  to you for treatment in accordance with the terms of the Workers'
  Compensation Laws. Please submit your report to the
  _____ XYZ Insurance Company _____
  at once. Compensation cannot be paid without complete medical
  information.
Insurance carrier __ XYZ Insurance Company __

Address P.O. Box 5, Woodland Hills, XY 12345 Telephone 555-271-0562

Employer _____ The Conk Out Company _____

Address 45 S. Gorman St. Woodland Hills, XY 12345 Telephone 555-430-3488

Signature ____ *J.D.HAWKINS, MD* ____ Date ____ 4-3-20XX ____
  If patient is able to return to work today or tomorrow, please
  show date and time below — sign and give to patient to return to
  employer. If there are any work restrictions indicate on the back
  of this form. Please submit your usual first report in any case.

Date/Time _____ By _____

Fig. 9.5 Medical service order.

Fig. 9.6 Receptionist receiving a medical service order via telephone for the worker to receive medical services.

The insurance adjuster handling the case should be contacted if a translator is necessary for a workers' compensation patient. He or she should make arrangements for an official translator to be present for all appointments. A member of the patient's family or the patient's friend should not be allowed to serve as a translator because there may be no legal recourse for the health care organization if miscommunicated information leads to a bad outcome.

SCENARIO: MULTIPLE INJURIES AND DATES OF INJURY

Problem: A patient has a workers' compensation claim for the left wrist and the right big toe. The patient needed to address pain in the left wrist on 10/4/20YY for carpel tunnel syndrome and was injured on 6/8/20YY when a steel bar crushed the patient's big toe.

Solution: Be sure to keep accurate records and file the medical claims for both injuries separately. If by chance the big toe injury was billed with the date of injury for the wrist, the claim will automatically be rejected. The insurance billing specialist should be accurate in posting the correct reimbursed amounts for the correct corresponding injury.

Health Care Provider's First Report of Injury

A physician of record (POR) is commonly used to identify the health care provider directing care in an injured or ill worker's claim. After the POR sees the injured person for the first time, he or she completes the Doctor's First Report of Occupational Injury or Illness form.

The Doctor's First Report of Occupational Injury or Illness form should be sent with a completed CMS-1500 claim form for the service provided. Each state will have their own First Report of Injury form which can typically be found on the state's Worker's Compensation website. Unlike other insurance types, individuals covered by workers' compensation are not typically issued an identification card. It is extremely important that the health care office staff collect all information needed to complete the first report of injury form. In addition to patient information, providers will need to answer questions on the report such as:

- Date of injury or onset of illness
- Patient's job description
- Patient's usual job activities
- Employer's name, address, and phone number
- Employer's workers' compensation insurance carrier's name, address, and phone number

If the POR prefers to submit a narrative letter, the medical report should include the components, if relevant, shown in Table 9.2. Once the first report of injury has been received by the insurance carrier, they will assign a claim number to the case.

Time limits for filing the health care provider's first report vary from state to state. Failure to file the report can be a misdemeanor. Copies of the report form go to the insurance carrier and the state. Because the report is a legal document, each copy *must be signed in ink* by the health care provider. The insurance company waits for the health care provider's report and bill, then issues payment to the provider. The case can be closed if there is no further treatment or disability.

TABLE 9.2	Narrative Medical Report Issues, if Relevant
History	• Outline all specific details of accident, injury, or illness. • Health care provider should state whether there is a causal connection between the accident and conditions that may appear subsequently but are not obvious sequelae (diseased conditions following and usually resulting from a previous disease). If facts were obtained by reviewing prior records or x-ray films, the source should be mentioned. When a history is obtained through an interpreter, include that person's name.
Present complaints	Usually given as subjective complaints. *Subjective* refers to statements made by the patient about symptoms and how he or she feels. Subjective disability is evaluated by the following: • A description of the activity that produces the disability • The duration of the disability • The activities that are precluded by and those that can be performed with the disability • The means necessary for relief
Past history	Description of any previous, current, or subsequent medical information relevant to this injury or illness and whether there is a preexisting defect that might entitle the injured person to benefits from the subsequent injury fund or represent the actual cause of the present condition.
Examination findings	Usually given as objective findings. State all significant physical or psychiatric examination, testing, laboratory, or imaging findings.
Diagnostic impression	State all diagnostic findings and opinion as to relationship, if any, between the injury or disease and the condition diagnosed. Use diagnostic terminology that corresponds to the diagnostic code book.
Disability and prognosis	• Period during which the patient has been unable to work because of the injury or illness. • Opinion as to probable further temporary disability and a statement as to when the patient will be able to return to work or has returned to work. • Statement indicating whether the condition is currently permanent and stationary as well as the probability of future permanent disability. • Statement indicating that "All objective tests for organic pathology are negative. There is obviously a strong functional or emotional overlay," when a patient has multiple complaints but no clinical objective findings.
Work limitations	Description of any limitations to all activities.
Causation	Description of how the permanent disability is related to the patient's occupation and the specific injury or cumulative events causing the illness.

Health Care Provider's Progress or Supplemental Report

In a TD case, a supplemental report is sent to the insurance carrier after 2 to 4 weeks of treatment to give information on the status of the patient. If there is a significant change in the prognosis, a detailed progress report, referred to as a reexamination report, is sent to the insurance carrier. Subsequent progress or supplemental reports should be sent to the insurance carrier after each hospitalization and health care encounter to update the progress of a case (Fig. 9.7). Every evaluation and

---

ATTENDING PHYSICIAN'S REPORT

Employee: __Mrs. Ima B. Hurt__   Claim number: __120 XX 6542__

Employer: __The Conk Out Company__   Date of injury(ies): __4-3-20XX__   Date of next exam: __4-24-20XX__

Date of this exam: __4-10-XX__   Patient Social Security No: __120 XX 6542__

Current diagnosis: __S82.852A closed fracture; L. trimalleolar ankle__
(include ICD•10 code)

PATIENT STATUS

Since the last exam, this patient's condition has:

[X] improved as expected.   [ ] improved, but slower than expected.   [ ] not improved significantly.

[ ] worsened.   [ ] plateaued, no further improvement is expected.   [ ] has been determined to be non-work related.

Briefly, describe any change in objective or subjective complaint: _____

TREATMENT

Treatment plan: (only list changes from prior status)   [ ] No change   [ ] Patient is/was discharged from care on _____

Est. discharge date: __5-18-20XX__   Medications: __Tylenol for pain__

Therapy: Type _____   Times per week _____   Estimated date of completion _____

Diagnostic studies: __X-ray, L. ankle 3 views__

Hospitalization/surgery: _____

Consult/other service: _____

WORK STATUS

The patient has been instructed to:

[ ] return to full duty with no limitations or restrictions.

[ ] remain off the rest of the day and return to work tomorrow:

_____ with no limits or restrictions. _____ with limits listed below.

[ ] return to work on _____
   work limitations: _____

[X] remain off work until __5-17-20XX — discharge exam scheduled__

Estimated date patient can return full duty: __5-18-20XX__

DISABILITY STATUS

[ ] Patient discharged as cured.

Please supply a brief narrative report if any of the below apply:

[ ] Patient will be permanently precluded from engaging in his/her usual and customary occupation.

[ ] Patient's condition is permanent and stationary.

[ ] Patient will have permanent residuals.

[ ] Patient will require future medical care.

Physician name: __Martin Feelgood, MD__   Address: __4567 Broad Avenue, Woodland Hills, XY 12345__

Date: __April 10, 20XX__   Telephone: __(555)__ __482-9002__

Signature: __Martin Feelgood, MD__

reference initials

Fig. 9.7 Health care provider's supplemental report form.

report submitted must be mailed promptly to the insurance company along with a CMS-1500 form. If the disability is ongoing over time, monthly progress reports should be submitted. A follow-up report must contain the following information:

- Patient name and workers' compensation case number
- Date of most recent examination
- Present condition and progress since last report
- Measurements of function
- X-ray or laboratory report since last examination
- Treatment (give type and duration)
- Work status (patient working or estimated date of return to work if patient is still temporarily disabled)
- PD to be anticipated

Final Report

TD ends when the health care provider tells the insurance carrier that the patient is able to return to work or if the disability is longer than 24 months. When the TD case is closing, the health care provider will submit a final evaluation report that provides an overview of the care provided and the patient's progress with the disability. When the patient resumes work, the insurance carrier closes the case and the TD benefits cease.

A health care provider's final report indicating any impairment or PD should be submitted with a CMS-1500 claim form. Detailed guidance for completion of a Workers' Compensation CMS 1500 claim forms will be explained in chapter 14 of this textbook. Examples of completed claim forms are provided in Fig. 9.8. Note the following information included on the claim form:

- In box #1, "Other" has been checked to identify the type of coverage.
- In box #1a., the patient's employee identification number has been entered.
- In box #4, the name of the patient's employer has been entered.
- In box #6, "Other" has been checked.
- In box #7, the address of the employer has been entered.
- In box #10.a, the employment box has been checked as "yes".
- In box #27, the accept assignment box has been checked "yes" to indicate that the provider accepts assignment.

 9.9 QUICK REVIEW
Question: Explain how an insurance billing specialist would determine the time limit for submission of workers' compensation reports and claims?

CLAIM SUBMISSION

When the patient first seeks treatment for a work-related illness or injury, the claim for services will be submitted on a CMS-1500 form along with the first report of injury. Once the case has been established, a claim number will be assigned. The date of injury and the claim number should be included on all future CMS 1500-claim forms for services related to the work-related illness or injury.

In addition, to understanding the claim submission guidelines and processes, the medical billing specialist must also be

knowledgeable of fee schedules pertinent to their state. They should also understand the steps to take in the event that claim processing is delayed, the claim is denied, or only partial payment is made.

Financial Responsibility

When an individual is being treated as a workers' compensation case, the financial responsibility is between the health care organization and the workers' compensation insurance company. As long as treatment is authorized by the insurance carrier, the insurance company is responsible for payment. A health care organization that agrees to treat a workers' compensation case must agree to accept payment in full according to the workers' compensation fee schedule. For workers' compensation cases, patients are not financially responsible so deductibles, copayments or coinsurances cannot be collected.

An injured worker is under obligation to be evaluated by the employer's health care provider. However, the patient has the right to choose a different provider to seek care; in this case, the request needs to be approved by the employer.

Some states have a medical program wherein employers can reduce their workers' compensation rates by paying the first $1000 in medical bills. This is similar to a deductible for the employer's policy. The health care provider will first file the insurance claim with the workers' compensation insurance plan. The explanation of benefits will then direct the health care provider to bill the employer for the deductible amount. The statement should be sent to the employer for payment in this situation; it should not be sent to the patient.

Health insurance information should always be obtained in case services provided are determined to be unrelated to work injury or illness. To assist in informing patients of financial responsibility for nonrelated illness, the worker should sign an agreement for nonrelated medical expenses, as shown in Fig. 9.9. If the workers' compensation carrier declares that the case is not work related, bill the patient's health insurance, attaching a copy of the refusal by the workers' compensation carrier.

When examining the injured or ill worker, the health care provider may discover a problem unrelated to the workers' compensation injury or illness. For example, the provider may discover that the patient has high blood pressure that is unrelated to the work injury or illness for which the patient is being examined. In that case, the health care provider may bill the workers' compensation carrier for the examination but should code the claim carefully with regards to treatment of the injury. If treatment is initiated for the patient's high blood pressure, that portion of the examination becomes the financial obligation of the patient (or their private insurance plan) and not of the workers' compensation carrier.

Fee Schedules

Each state has its own workers' compensation fee schedule. Some states have developed a workers' compensation fee schedule using a relative value scale, which is then adjusted with a conversion factor. The relative value scale considers the time, skills, and extent of the service provided by the health care

WORKERS' COMPENSATION

DRAFT - NOT FOR OFFICIAL USE

HEALTH INSURANCE CLAIM FORM
APPROVED BY NATIONAL UNIFOR MCLAIM COMMITTEE (NUCC) 02/12

| | | PICA | | | | | | | | PICA | | |

1. MEDICARE MEDICAID TRICARE CHAMPVA GROUP HEALTH PLAN FECA BLK LUNG OTHER	1a. INSURED'S I.D. NUMBER (For Program in Item 1)
(Medicare#) (Medicaid#) (ID#DoD#) (Member ID#) (ID#) (ID#) [X] (ID#)	120-xx-6542

2. PATIENT'S NAME (Last Name, First Name, Middle Initial)	3. PATIENT'S BIRTH DATE SEX	4. INSURED'S NAME (Last Name, First Name, Middle Initial)
Hurt, Ima, B	MM 03	DD 04	YY 1966 M [ ] F [X]	The Conk Out Company

5. PATIENT'S ADDRESS (No., Street)	6. PATIENT RELATIONSHIP TO INSURED	7. INSURED'S ADDRESS (No., Street)
300 East Central Avenue	Self [ ] Spouse [ ] Child [ ] Other [X]	1212 Hardrock Place

CITY	STATE	8. RESERVED FOR NUCC USE	CITY	STATE
Woodland Hills	XY		Woodland Hills	XY

ZIP CODE	TELEPHONE (Include Area Code)		ZIP CODE	TELEPHONE (Include Area Code)
123450000	(555) 476-9989		123450000	(555) 4277777

9. OTHER INSURED'S NAME (Last Name, First Name, Middle Initial)	10. IS PATIENT'S CONDITION RELATED TO:	11. INSURED'S POLICY GROUP OR FECA NUMBER
		12345

a. OTHER INSURED'S POLICY OR GROUP NUMBER	a. EMPLOYMENT? (Current or Previous)	a. INSURED'S DATE OF BIRTH SEX
	[X] YES [ ] NO	MM	DD	YY M [ ] F [ ]

b. RESERVED FOR NUCC USE	b. AUTO ACCIDENT? PLACE (State)	b. OTHER CLAIM ID (Designated by NUCC)
	[ ] YES [X] NO	

c. RESERVED FOR NUCC USE	c. OTHER ACCIDENT?	c. INSURANCE PLAN NAME OR PROGRAM NAME
	[ ] YES [X] NO	XYZ Insurance Company

d. INSURANCE PLAN NAME OR PROGRAM NAME	10d. CLAIM CODES (Designated by NUCC)	d. IS THERE ANOTHER HEALTH BENEFIT PLAN?
		[ ] YES [ ] NO If yes, complete items 9, 9a, and 9d.

READ BACK OF FORM BEFORE COMPLETING & SIGNING THIS FORM.

12. PATIENT'S OR AUTHORIZED PERSON'S SIGNATURE I authorize the release of any medical or other information necessary to process this claim. I also request payment of government benefits either to myself or to the party who accepts assignment below.	13. INSURED'S OR AUTHORIZED PERSON'S SIGNATURE I authorize payment of medical benefits to the undersigned physician or supplier for services described below.
SIGNED Signature on file DATE	SIGNED

14. DATE OF CURRENT: ILLNESS, INJURY, or PREGNANCY(LMP)	15. OTHER DATE	16. DATES PATIENT UNABLE TO WORK IN CURRENT OCCUPATION
MM 04	DD 03	YY 20XX QUAL. 431	QUAL.	MM	DD	YY	FROM MM 04	DD 03	YY 20XX TO MM	DD	YY

17. NAME OF REFERRING PROVIDER OR OTHER SOURCE	17a.	18. HOSPITALIZATION DATES RELATED TO CURRENT SERVICES
	17b. NPI	FROM MM	DD	YY TO MM	DD	YY

19. ADDITIONAL CLAIM INFORMATION (Designated by NUCC)	20. OUTSIDE LAB? $ CHARGES
	[ ] YES [ ] NO

21. DIAGNOSIS OR NATURE OF ILLNESS OR INJURY Relate A-L to service line below (24E) ICD Ind. 0	22. RESUBMISSION CODE ORIGINAL REF. NO.
A. S82852A B. C. D.	
E. F. G. H.	23. PRIOR AUTHORIZATION NUMBER
I. J. K. L.	

24. A. DATE(S) OF SERVICE		B. PLACE OF SERVICE	C. EMG	D. PROCEDURES, SERVICES, OR SUPPLIES (Explain Unusual Circumstances)		E. DIAGNOSIS POINTER	F. $ CHARGES	G. DAYS OR UNITS	H. EPSDT Family Plan	I. ID. QUAL.	J. RENDERING PROVIDER ID. #
From MM DD YY	To MM DD YY			CPT/HCPCS	MODIFIER						
1 04 03 XX		11		99204		A	180 00	1		NPI	12678547XX
2										NPI	
3										NPI	
4										NPI	
5										NPI	
6										NPI	

25. FEDERAL TAX I.D. NUMBER SSN EIN	26. PATIENT'S ACCOUNT NO.	27. ACCEPT ASSIGNMENT? (For govt. claims, see back)	28. TOTAL CHARGE	29. AMOUNT PAID	30. Rsvd for NUCC Use
XX12210XX [ ] [X]	633	[X] YES [ ] NO	$ 180 00	$	$

31. SIGNATURE OF PHYSICIAN OR SUPPLIER INCLUDING DEGREES OR CREDENTIALS (I certify that the statements on the reverse apply to this bill and are made a part thereof.)	32. SERVICE FACILITY LOCATION INFORMATION	33. BILLING PROVIDER INFO & PH # (555) 4869002
Martin Feelgood, MD		College Clinic
040320xx		4567 Broad Avenue
SIGNED Martin Feelgood, MD DATE	a. NPI b.	Woodland Hills XY 123450000
		a. 3664021CC b.

NUCC Instruction Manual available at: www.nucc.org   PLEASE PRINT OR TYPE   OMB APPROVAL PENDING

Fig. 9.8 Example of a completed CMS-1500 (02-12) Health Insurance Claim Form for a workers' compensation case. (From National Uniform Claim Committee, NUCC Instruction Manual www.nucc.org.)

PATIENT AGREEMENT

Patient's Name _____James Doland_____ Soc. Sec. # _431-XX-1942_

Address _67 Blyth Dr., Woodland Hills, XY 12345_ Tel. No. _555-372-0101_

WC Insurance Carrier _____Industrial Indemnity Company_____

Address _____30 North Dr., Woodland Hills_____ Telephone No. _555-731-7707_

Date of illness _2-13-20XX_ Date of first visit _2-13-20XX_

Emergency Yes __X__ No _____

Is this condition related to employment Yes _X_ No _____

If accident: Auto _____ Other _____

Where did injury occur? ___Construction site___

How did injury happen? ___fell 8 ft from scaffold suffering fractured right tibia___

Employee/employer who verified this information _____Scott McPherson_____

Employer's name and address _Willow Construction Company_

Employer's telephone no. ___555-526-0611___

In the event the claim for workers' compensation is declared fraudulent for this illness or condition or it is determined by the Workers' Compensation Board that the illness or injury is not a compensable workers' compensation case, I _James Doland_, hereby agree to pay the physician's fee for services rendered.

I have been informed that I am responsible to pay any services rendered by Dr. _Raymond Skeleton_ with regard to the discovery and treatment of any condition not related to the workers' compensation injury or illness. I agree to pay for all services not covered by workers' compensation and all charges for treatment and personal items unrelated to my workers' compensation illness or injury.

Signed _____James Doland_____ Date _2-13-20XX_

Fig. 9.9 Patient agreement to pay the health care provider's fees if the case is declared not work related or an illness is discovered and treated that is not work related.

provider of services. Each procedure is rated on how difficult it is, how long it takes, the training a health care provider should perform, and expenses the health care organization incurs, including the cost of malpractice insurance. A conversion factor is then applied that sets a specific dollar amount for each of the sections of the fee schedule. Conversion factors may be adjusted to reflect regional differences and in some states are recalculated annually (Box 9.3).

Other states pay medical claims based on the Medicare fee schedule plus a certain percentage or have implemented managed care.

All claims are sent to the workers' compensation insurance, and no billing statements are sent to the patient. Fee schedules assist with the following:

1. They limit the amount that health care providers will be paid.
2. They make the allowable charges and procedures more consistent.
3. They provide follow-up procedures in case of a fee dispute.

Most workers' compensation fee schedules list the maximum reimbursement for all covered health care services, and service providers are expected to accept as payment in full. Service providers may ask for exceptions to the maximum reimbursement if any of the following factors can be supported:

- Provider's medical training, qualifications, and time in practice may warrant a higher reimbursement.
- Nature of services provided was more complex than what reimbursement allows for.

BOX 9.3 2020 Conversion Factors of the Utah Labor Commission Industrial Accident Division Medical Fee Standards

$62/unit	Anesthesia
$65/unit	Surgery
$58/unit	Radiology
$56/unit	Pathology
$52/unit	Medicine
$50/unit	Restorative Services
$52/unit	Evaluation and Management

Scenario 1: If the state has assigned a relative value of 5.2 for a specific surgical procedure, it is multiplied by the conversion factor for surgery (65.00/unit), and the amount the health care provider would be reimbursed for the procedure would be: $338.00.

Scenario 2: If the state has assigned a relative value of 2.8 for a specified radiological procedure, it is multiplied by the conversion factor for radiology ($58.00/unit), and the amount the health care provider would be reimbursed for the procedure would be $162.40.

- Reimbursements for the same services in other regions are typically higher than what are allowed in the fee schedule.
- There are other relevant economic factors of the health care organization.
- Any unusual circumstances in the case.

The insurance carrier may pay the additional amount if documentation is sent validating the fee and noting any of the aforementioned considerations.

Reviews or audits may be performed by the following entities to enforce fee schedules:

- The state agency or state fund responsible for overseeing workers' compensation (bill review)
- The payer, employer, or insurance carrier (bill review)
- The payer (bill review) and state agency (compliance audit)

Helpful Billing Tips

The following are helpful hints for billing workers' compensation claims.

1. Ask whether the injury occurred within the scope of employment and verify insurance information with the benefits coordinator for the employer. This will promote filing initial claims with the correct insurance carrier.
2. Obtain the date of injury. This date will be associated with the patient's care for the duration of patient care for the specific episode.
3. Either ask the employer the name of the claims adjuster or request that the patient obtain the claim number of their case when he or she comes in for the initial health care encounter.
4. Educate the patient on the health care organization's billing policies for workers' compensation cases by having him or her complete the patient agreement form shown in see Fig. 9.9.
5. Verify whether prior authorization is necessary before a surgical procedure is performed.
6. Document in the patient's record all data for authorization of examination, diagnostic studies, or surgery (for example, date, name of individual who authorizes, response).
7. Obtain the workers' compensation fee schedule for the relevant state.
8. Use appropriate procedural codes and modifiers to ensure prompt and accurate payment for services rendered.
9. Documentation should include a description of how the injury occurred and where it occurred.
10. Complete the Doctor's First Report of Occupational Injury or Illness form for the relevant state.
11. Ask whether there is a state-specific insurance form or if the CMS-1500 form is acceptable.
12. Determine which procedural (*Current Procedural Terminology* [CPT]) and diagnosis (*International Classification of Diseases* [ICD]) coding manuals the insurance carrier uses. Some carriers use outdated coding manuals that do not reflect the deletion or addition of some procedures and diagnostic codes.
13. Clearly define any charges in excess of the fee schedule. Attach any x-ray reports, operative reports, discharge summaries, pathology reports, and any other medical reports that can clarify excess charges.
14. Itemize in detail and send invoices for drugs and dressings furnished by the health care provider.
15. Call the insurance carrier and talk with the claims examiner. The claims examiner may also be referred to as the claims adjuster or claims representative and would be familiar with the patient's case.
16. Search the internet for a website or write to the workers' compensation state plan office in each state for booklets, bulletins, forms, and legislation information.
17. Follow up and track the date on which the claim was filed. If no payment has been received or payment has been received beyond the 30- to 45-day deadline, determine whether it meets eligibility requirements for interest.

Out-of-State Claims

Guidelines for billing for out-of-state claims vary from state to state. When billing for an out-of-state claim, insurance billing specialists must follow all workers' compensation regulations from the jurisdiction (state) in which the injured person's claim was originally filed. These guidelines can be obtained from the state's Workers' Compensation Board.

Companies that have employees who travel to other states are required to obtain workers' compensation insurance in those states unless they have a policy that covers out-of-state employees. Sometimes a patient may request care from a health care organization or provider in an adjacent state because they are seeking a higher quality of care or the patient needs a specialized type of surgery, expensive diagnostic tests, or treatment. Referral requirements should be met before the patient is seen (e.g., letter of referral or preauthorization from the managing doctor with a copy to the workers' compensation carrier). When a patient crosses a state line for treatment, they may be liable for some balance billing and the patient should be informed of this fact.

When the claim is billed, the out-of-state fee schedule should be obtained to determine the proper procedure codes, modifiers, and amounts. It should be determined whether the claimant's jurisdiction accepts electronic submission of the CMS-1500 claim form or another form and whether other documents (e.g., the operative report) are required to be submitted with the bill.

Delinquent or Slow Pay Claims

If payment of a workers' compensation claim is slow or the claim becomes delinquent (no payment for more than 45 days after the date of service), the insurance billing specialist should use an organized standard follow-up procedure.

1. Contact the human resources department at the patient's employer. Note the name of the person with whom you speak; the name, address, and telephone number of the workers' compensation carrier; and the claim number. Verify the employer's address.
2. Send a copy of the claim form and the service provider's First Report of Occupational Illness or Injury form to the insurance carrier. Send a letter and include details of the

Martin Feelgood, MD
4567 Broad Avenue
Woodland Hills, XY 12345
555-486-9002

June 20, 20XX

XYZ Insurance Company
P. O. Box S
Woodland Hills, XY 12345

Dear Madam or Sir:

Re: Case No.:   120 XX 6542
     Injured: Mrs. Ima B. Hurt
     Date of Injury: April 3, 20XX
     Employer: The Conk Out Company
     Amount: $148.92

Our records indicate that our final statement for the above case
dated ___5/18/20XX___ remains unpaid.

Your cooperation in furnishing us the present status of this
statement will be appreciated. A notation on the bottom of
this letter will be sufficient.

Very truly yours,

Martin Feelgood ,MD

ref initials

_____ No Employer's Report on file
_____ No Doctor's First Report on file
_____ Did not receive itemized billing statement
_____ Payment was made. Check No. ___ Date _____
_____ Other reason(s) _____

Fig. 9.10 Letter sent to the insurance carrier when a workers'
compensation claim becomes 45 days delinquent.

Martin Feelgood, MD
4567 Broad Avenue
Woodland Hills, XY 12345
555-486-9002

June 20, 20XX

The Conk Out Company
45 South Gorman Street
Woodland Hills, XY 12345

Dear Madam or Sir:

Re: Case No.:   120 XX 6542
     Injured: Mrs. Ima B. Hurt
     Date of Injury: April 3, 20XX

I have been informed by your workers' compensation insurance
carrier that they have not as yet received the employer's report
in regard to the above injured person.

Unless you have already done so, may I ask your cooperation in
completing and sending this report so that the case may be
closed.

Should you have any questions or if I can be of assistance to
you in any way, please do not hesitate to call on me.

Very truly yours,

Martin Feelgood , MD

ref initials

Fig. 9.11 Letter sent to the employer when the insurance company notifies the health care provider's office that the employer's preliminary report of injury has not been received.

accident if necessary (Fig. 9.10). For problem claims, it may
be wise to obtain and complete a Certificate of Mailing form
from the US Postal Service.

3. Contact the insurance carrier after 45 working days and
request the expected date of payment.
4. Be reminded of the expected payment date by using a com-
puter-automated reminder or a note on the desk calendar. If
payment is not received on or before that day, call the carrier
again and ask for payment on a day determined by the facility's expectations.
5. Contact the patient's employer and explain that there is difficulty with the carrier. Ask the employer to contact the carrier and have him send payment immediately. The insurance
billing specialist might also talk to the patient and suggest
that they discuss the problem with their employer to see if
this will bring positive action.

6. Send the employer a copy of the financial account statement
showing the outstanding balance. If the carrier is not paying,
ask the employer for payment. An employer's legal obligation
to pay may vary from case to case.
7. Contact the patient only if given information by the carrier
or employer that the injury is not work related.
8. Develop office policies that address when an outstanding
account should be reviewed (perhaps after 90 or 120 days),
whether to continue collection efforts internally, and at which
point the account should be turned over to a collection agency.

It may be necessary to send subsequent letters to the
employer after receiving a response from the insurance carrier.
For example, a letter should be sent to the employer (Fig. 9.11)
if the insurance company notifies the health care organization
that the employer's preliminary report of injury has not been
received.

If 30 days have elapsed from the date on which the letter was sent requesting the Employer's Report of Work Injury and the employer has not responded, a letter should be sent to the state Workers' Compensation Board or Industrial Accidents Commission (Fig. 9.12).

9.10 QUICK REVIEW

Question: In the case of a workers' compensation claim, is the health care organization allowed to bill the patient?

DISCUSSION POINT

It is the responsibility of all individuals, including the insurance billing specialist, to notify the insurance carrier of any suspicious activity related to a workers' compensation case. Review the list of signs of workers' compensation fraud and abuse in see Box 9.1 and discuss a course of action that could be taken by the insurance billing specialist if they identify a red flag.

Martin Feelgood, MD
4567 Broad Avenue
Woodland Hills, XY 12345
555-486-9002

July 15, 20XX

Division of Industrial Accidents
State Office Building
107 South Broadway, Room 4107
Woodland Hills, XY 12345

Dear Madam or Sir:

Re: Failure of employer to follow Section No. 3760

Your office is being solicited to help secure an Employer's Report of Work Injury from the employer listed below.

Case No.:	120 XX 6542
Name of Employer:	The Conk Out Company
Address:	45 South Gorman Street
	Woodland Hills, XY 12345
Name of Injured:	Mrs. Ima B. Hurt
Address:	300 East Central Avenue
	Woodland Hills, XY 12345
Date of Injury:	April 3, 20XX
Name of Insurance Carrier:	XYZ Insurance Company
Amount of Unpaid Bill:	$148.92

Your cooperation in this matter will be greatly appreciated. If you need further information, please feel free to contact my office.

Sincerely yours,

Martin Feelgood , MD

ref initials

Fig. 9.12 Letter sent to the Workers' Compensation Board or Industrial Accident Commission if the employer does not respond to a request for the Employer's Report of Work Injury after 30 days have elapsed from the date of the letter.

PROCEDURE 9.1   Completing the Doctor's First Report of Occupational Injury or Illness

Objective: Accurately complete a Doctor's First Report of Occupational Injury or Illness form for the State of California.

Step 1: Download a blank Doctor's First Report of Occupational Injury or Illness form for the State of California [Form 5021 (Rev.5) 10/2015]. It can be accessed at: https://www.dir.ca.gov/OPRL/dlsrform5021.pdf

Step 2: Create a workers' compensation scenario with a classmate as the injured employee. Ask the classmate to provide information needed to complete fields 1 thru 26 for form 5021 as identified below.

Step 3: When completing the form, a completed form from the chapter (see Fig. 9.7) can be accessed for reference.

1. Enter the workers' compensation insurance carrier's complete name, street address, city, state, and zip code.
2. Enter the employer's full name and policy number if known. Some insurance carriers file by employer and then by policy number. Sometimes the employer's telephone number is necessary on this line.
3. Enter the employer's street address, city, state, and zip code.
4. Enter the type of business (for example, repairing shoes, building construction, retailing men's clothes).

5. Enter the patient's complete first name, middle initial, and last name.
6. Enter a check mark in the appropriate box to indicate the patient's gender.
7. Enter the patient's birth date and list the year as four digits.
8. Enter the patient's street address, city, state, and zip code.
9. Enter the patient's home telephone number.
10. Enter the patient's specific job title. Be accurate in listing the occupation with the job title so that the insurance carrier may be certain the patient was doing the job for which he or she was insured.
11. Enter the patient's Social Security number. Some insurance carriers use the Social Security number as the workers' compensation case number.
12. Enter the exact location where the patient was injured. Many times, the injury may occur off the premises of the company or factory, depending on the type of job on which the employee was working. List the county where the patient was injured.
13. Enter the date the patient was injured and time of the injury. List the year as four digits.
14. Enter the date the patient last worked. This date should coincide with the date the patient reported to work and worked any portion of their shift

PROCEDURE 9.1 *cont'd*

(workday). This may be the same date of injury. This item is important because it informs the insurance carrier of the working status of the patient or whether the patient has been disabled and cannot return to work. List the year as four digits.

15. Enter the date and hour of the health care provider's first examination. The insurance carrier should know the time that elapsed after the accident before the patient sought medical attention. List the year as four digits.

16. Enter a check mark in the appropriate box indicating whether the health care provider or an associate, treated the patient previously.

17. Have the patient completed this section? if possible, in their own words, stating how the illness or injury occurred. The health care provider also may dictate this information after obtaining it from the patient.

18. Enter the answers to these questions about the patient's complaints and medical findings, which may be found in the patient's medical record. List all the patient's subjective complaints.

19. 19.a. Enter all objective findings from physical examination.
    19.b. Enter all x-ray and laboratory results. If none, state "none" or "pending."

20. Enter a check mark in "yes" or "no" to indicate if chemical or toxic compounds are involved. Enter the diagnosis and diagnostic code number. Specify etiologic agent and duration of exposure if occupational illness.

21. Enter a check mark in "yes" or "no" to indicate if the findings and diagnosis are consistent with the history of injury or onset of illness. Insert an explanation if "yes."

22. Enter a check mark in "yes" or "no" to indicate if there is any other current condition that will impede or delay the patient's recovery. Insert an explanation if "yes."

23. Enter a full description of what treatment was rendered.

24. Enter an explanation if further treatment is necessary and, if so, specify the treatment plan. Indicate if physical therapy is necessary, specify its frequency and duration.

25. Enter the name and location of the hospital, admission date, and estimated stay if the patient is to be hospitalized.

26. Enter a check mark in "yes" or "no" to indicate whether the patient is able to work as usual. If the answer is "no," give the date when it is estimated that the patient will be able to return to regular or modified work. List the year as four digits. Specify any work restrictions. It is important for the insurance company to anticipate how long the patient will be off work so that money may be set aside for TD benefits, medical benefits, and, if necessary, PD benefits. If the estimated date of return to work should change after the form is submitted, a supplemental report or progress note should be sent to the insurance carrier to change the date of the disability.

Bottom of Form: If not preprinted, enter the health care provider's name and degree (for example, MD, DC), complete address, state license number, federal tax identification number, and telephone number. Indicate the date when the report is submitted. The insurance billing specialist should type reference initials in the lower left-hand corner of the form. This form must be signed in ink by the health care provider. Any carbon copies or photocopies must be signed in ink, too. A stamped signature will not be accepted because sometimes these cases go into litigation or are presented for a PD rating. Only those documents that are considered original medical records will be accepted; this means that a handwritten signature by the attending health care provider is necessary.

KEY POINTS

This is a brief chapter review, or summary, of the key issues presented.

1. Federal and state regulations require that employers have workers' compensation insurance coverage against on-the-job injury or illness and pay the premium for each of their employees.

2. There are two kinds of statutes under workers' compensation: federal compensation laws and state compensation laws.

3. State workers' compensation laws vary from state to state.

4. Employees who work for federal agencies are covered by a number of federal workers' compensation laws.

5. The second-injury fund, also known as the *subsequent-injury fund,* was established to meet problems arising when an employee has a preexisting injury or condition and is subsequently injured at work.

6. Individuals are entitled to workers' compensation insurance coverage if they have been injured at work or become ill as a result of job-related duties,

7. Each state's legislation lists a waiting period (WP) that must elapse before income benefits are paid. However, medical and hospital care for work-related injuries or illnesses is provided immediately.

8. Workers' compensation benefits consist of medical treatment, temporary disability (TD) indemnity, permanent disability (PD) indemnity, death benefits for survivors, and rehabilitation benefits.

9. A nondisability (ND) claim involves a minor injury in which the patient is seen by the health care provider but is able to continue to work.

10. A TD claim occurs when a worker has a work-related injury or illness and is unable to perform the duties of their occupation for a period time.

11. A PD consists of an illness or injury (impairment of the normal use of a body part) that is expected to continue for the lifetime of the injured worker and prevents the person from performing the functions of their occupation, therefore impairing their earning capacity.

12. In a PD case the health care provider's final report must contain the words "permanent and stationary" so that the case can be adjudicated or rated, settlement can be reached (called a *compromise and release [C and R]*), and the case can be closed.

13. It is the responsibility of all individuals who handle workers' compensation cases to notify the insurance carrier of any fraudulent or suspicious situation.

14. The Occupational Safety and Health Administration (OSHA) is the federal agency that regulates and investigates safety and health standards at work sites for the protection of employees.

15. Depositions from the health care provider and the injured individual by the attorney representing the workers' compensation insurance company are usually taken in PD cases.
16. The health care organization should consider filing a lien in a workers' compensation case that has gone into third-party litigation or if there is a question whether the case is compensable.
17. A private medical record should never be combined with a work-related injury/illness case record because separate disclosure laws apply to each and the workers' compensation case may go to court.
18. The first report of a work-related injury/illness must be completed by the employer and the health care provider and is required by law in most states.
19. A medical service order given to the employee by the employer authorizes the health care organization or provider to treat the injured worker.
20. In workers' compensation cases, all medical reports and forms are legal documents and must be signed in ink by the treatment provider.
21. When an individual is being treated as a workers' compensation case, the financial responsibility is between the health care organization and the workers' compensation insurance company.

INTERNET RESOURCES

US Department of Labor WC Boards:
- https://www.dol.gov/owcp/dfec/regs/compliance/wc.htm

State Compensation Insurance Fund Listing:
- https://classcodes.com/list-workers-compensation-state-funds-state/

STUDENT ASSIGNMENT

- Study Chapter 9.
- Complete all exercises in the *Workbook* to reinforce the theory learned in this chapter.
- Turn to the Glossary at the end of this text for a further understanding of the key terms and key abbreviations used in this chapter.

Disability Income Insurance and Disability Benefit Programs

Linda M. Smith

OBJECTIVES

After reading this chapter, you should be able to:

1. Define key terms associated with disability income insurance.
2. Discuss the history of disability income insurance.
3. List the ways an individual can purchase disability income insurance.
4. Describe benefits and exclusions contained in individual and group disability income insurance.
5. Name and describe federal disability benefit programs.
6. Differentiate between Social Security Disability Insurance (SSDI) and Supplemental Security Income (SSI).
7. State eligibility requirements, benefits, and limitations of SSDI and SSI.
8. Explain disability benefit programs for disabled active military personnel, veterans, and their dependents.
9. Name states that have state disability insurance plans and paid family and medical leave insurance programs.
10. State eligibility requirements, benefits, and limitations of state disability plans.
11. Explain voluntary disability insurance plans.
12. Describe data necessary to complete the attending physician's report for proof of disability.
13. List guidelines for federal disability claims.
14. Explain procedures for state disability claims.
15. Recognize forms used for processing state disability plans.

KEY TERMS

accidental death and dismemberment
benefit period
Civil Service Retirement System
consultative examiner
cost-of-living adjustment
Department of Defense Disability
disability
Disability Determination Services
disability income insurance
double indemnity
exclusions
Family and Medical Leave Act
Federal Employees Retirement System

future purchase option
guaranteed renewable
hearing
indemnity benefits
long-term disability insurance
non-cancelable clause
Paid family and medical leave insurance
partial disability
reconsideration
residual benefits
residual disability
short-term disability insurance
Social Security Administration

Social Security Disability Insurance program
State Disability Insurance
supplemental benefits
Supplemental Security Income
temporary disability
temporary disability insurance
total disability
Unemployment Compensation Disability
Veterans Affairs disability program
voluntary disability insurance
waiting period
waiver of premium

KEY ABBREVIATIONS

CE	FERS	SSDI	VA
COLA	FMLA	SSI	WP
CSRS	PFML	TD	
DDS	SDI	TDI	
DoD	SSA	UCD	

INSIGHTS FROM THE FIELD

Cathy C.: Medical Office Assistant for Orthopedic Practice

In a busy health care office, completion of disability income insurance forms may not seem like a priority with everything else that is going on. What may seem inconvenient to the physician or the staff is of great importance to the patient. A patient who has become disabled and whose livelihood is on the line should be the first consideration. The best approach is to complete the forms while the patient is in the office. The information will be accurate and complete, as the patient was just seen by the physician, and the patient will be able to move forward in the process of obtaining disability benefits.

DISABILITY INCOME INSURANCE DEFINED

Disability income insurance does not pay for medical services. The insurance billing specialist will not file a CMS-1500 claim form for disability income insurance. However, it is essential for the insurance billing specialist to understand what disability income insurance is, how it affects the patients in their health care organization, how they can assist them, and what is expected from the health care provider.

The broad definition of a disability is "a limitation in a range of major life activities which includes activities such as seeing, hearing, walking, and tasks such as thinking and working due to physical or mental illness, disease or injury." According to the World Health Organization, about 15% of the world's population has some form of disability with rates of disability increasing due to an aging population and increases in chronic health conditions.

Disability income insurance is a form of insurance that provides reimbursement for lost income when the insured is unable to work because of illness, disease, or injury—not as a result of a work-related accident or condition. For example, a patient may have been diagnosed with pancreatic cancer and is unable to work because of the illness. This patient may be able to apply for disability income benefits.

Health care providers receive requests for medical records to support disability claims. Frequently, the insurance billing specialist will be assigned the task of abstracting information from the patient's medical record to assist the provider in completion of the disability claim form. Disability insurance plays an important role in the financial planning and safeguarding of an individual's future. Accurate and prompt completion of the attending physician's portion of the disability insurance form or any associated medical record request assists the patient in obtaining disability income when he or she is unable to work because of a non–work-related illness or injury

Types of Disability

A disability may be partial, temporary, or total. There is no standard definition for total disability, and the definition stated in each disability income policy varies. For example, a liberal definition might read as follows: "The insured must be unable to perform the major duties of their specific occupation."

The terms residual disability and partial disability are defined as occurring "when an illness or injury prevents an insured person from performing one or more of the functions of their regular job"—in other words, when a person cannot perform all of their usual job duties.

Temporary disability (TD) exists when a person cannot perform all of the functions of their regular job for a limited period.

Waiting Period

The period from the beginning of disability to receiving the first payment of benefits is called an *elimination period* or *waiting period (WP)*. During this initial period, a disabled individual is not eligible to receive benefits even though he or she is unable to work. This period varies by policy, but it is usually 30 to 45 days before the first benefit payment processes.

Benefit Period

A benefit period is the maximum amount of time that benefits will be paid to the injured or ill person for the disability (for example, 2 years, 5 years, to age 65, or lifetime).

 10.1   QUICK REVIEW
Question: Explain what disability income insurance is.

HISTORY

Before the late 1800s, disability income insurance provided only accident protection. Some life insurance contracts had disability income riders attached to them that offered limited benefits. In the early 1880s, insurance companies began selling disability income policies that offered coverage for accident and illness. The Paul Revere Life Insurance Company introduced the first "noncancelable" disability income policy in the early 1900s. The noncancelable clause guaranteed that the contract would be in force for a certain period and the premium would not be increased. By 1956, the Congress had enacted legislation under the Social Security program that provided disability income protection to disabled individuals older than 50 years of age. This program was expanded in 1965 to cover all workers, regardless of age, if certain eligibility standards were met. Today, disability income insurance is available from private insurance companies (individual policies) and employer-sponsored plans (group policies). Government-funded and state benefit programs are also available for disabled persons. These plans and programs are discussed in this chapter, along with the role of the insurance billing specialist in dealing with this type of insurance.

DISABILITY INCOME INSURANCE POLICIES

There are several ways to purchase disability income insurance. In some cases, individuals will fall under a state or federal government sponsored disability income insurance plan. Other individuals may have a disability income insurance policy through an employer's group plan. Although employers are not required to offer disability income insurance, some offer it as fringe benefit to their employees. For those who are not covered by a state or federal government plan or an employer group plan, they can purchase individual disability income insurance coverage on their own.

Individual Policies

Individual disability income insurance is coverage that provides a specific monthly or weekly income when a person becomes unable to work, temporarily or totally, because of an illness or injury. The disability cannot be work related. As explained in the previous chapter, an illness or accident that is work related is covered by "workers' compensation insurance."

For individuals who are self-employed, this insurance is particularly important because a business could not meet its financial obligations if the owner became injured or too ill to work. For example, if an individual is self-employed with a home-based business and faced with a repetitive stress injury (RSI), the condition would not allow that individual to use the computer for several months. He or she would have no income. The main purpose of these policies is to provide some benefits while the person is unable to work. To collect benefits, the individual must meet the policy's criteria of what constitutes partial, temporary, or total disability. These policies end or are valid until the individual retires or reaches a certain age, usually 65 years.

Benefits

Compensation paid to the insured disabled person is called indemnity benefits and can be received daily, weekly, monthly, or semiannually, depending on the policy. Premiums and benefits depend on several risk factors, such as age, gender, health history and physical state, income, and occupational duties. Some policies include residual or partial disability income benefits. Benefits are not taxable if premiums are paid by the individual.

Residual benefits pay is a partial benefit when the insured is not totally disabled. If one becomes partially disabled or can work only part time or in a limited capacity, the residual benefits make up the difference between what an individual can earn at present and what he or she would have earned working full time.

Supplemental benefits may consist of insurance provisions that will increase monthly indemnity, such as a future purchase option or a cost-of-living adjustment. Cost-of-living adjustment (**COLA**) means to increase monthly benefits in disability income benefit, pension benefit, or life income benefit to make up for a change in the cost of living. This is also known as future purchase option or cost-of-living rider. Provisions also distribute a percentage of the policy premiums if an individual keeps a policy in force for 5 or 10 years or does not file any claims.

An accidental death and dismemberment benefit is written into some contracts. This offers the insured person protection when loss of sight or loss of limb occurs. In some policies (for example, life insurance), a special provision known as double indemnity applies if an unintended, unexpected, and unforeseeable accident results in death. This feature provides for twice the face amount of the policy to be paid if death results from accidental causes.

Clauses

Certain clauses may be written into disability income insurance policies. With a guaranteed renewable policy, the insurer is required to renew the policy as long as premium payments are made for a specified number of years or to a specified age, such as 60, 65, or 70 years, or for life. However, the premium may be increased when it is renewed. When the policy has a noncancelable clause, the premium cannot be increased.

If a waiver of premium is included in the insurance contract, the policy pays all premiums while the employee is disabled; the employee does not have to pay. Usually, this provision is used as a total and permanent disability benefit and may be available in certain other cases.

Exclusions

Exclusions are provisions written into the insurance contract denying coverage or limiting the scope of coverage. Examples of preexisting conditions that may be written into a contract are:

- disability because of war or riot
- disability due to self-inflicted injury or attempted suicide
- disability due to mental or nervous conditions
- disability while legally intoxicated or under the influence of narcotics (unless prescribed by a licensed health care professional); the phrase "legally intoxicated" means intoxication in an individual whose blood alcohol level, when tested, exceeds limits set by state law
- conditions arising from normal pregnancy
- conditions that are work related and patient is receiving benefits under workers' compensation or a government program.

Group Policies

Some employers elect to offer group disability income insurance as a fringe benefit. These contracts are drawn up between the insurer and the employer. Premiums may be paid by the employer with or without contributions from the employee. Employees hold certificates of insurance and are covered under the employer's policy. When the employee leaves the company, the insurance is no more valid unless the employee is disabled. A few group policies allow conversion to a limited benefit individual policy.

Benefits

Group policy benefits vary from one plan to another but are usually for short-term disability insurance (13 weeks to 24 months) or long-term disability insurance (to age 65). To qualify for benefits, an individual must be unable to perform the major duties of their occupation during the initial period of disability (for example, the first 2 years). Benefits cease when the employee returns to work, even part time. However, some of these policies offer the worker partial disability income benefits to motivate a disabled individual to return to work on a part-time basis. Monthly benefits are usually paid directly to the employee and are taxable if the employee is not making any contribution toward the premiums.

> **10.2   QUICK REVIEW**
> Question: What are common examples of "exclusions" that may be written into a disability insurance contract?

FEDERAL DISABILITY PROGRAMS

As mentioned earlier, some individuals will fall under a federal government sponsored disability income insurance plan. Federal disability programs serve people of all ages, but most disability programs tend to be targeted either on children or on adults in their working years, typically defined from 18 through 64 years of age.

Work-Related Disability

The federal government has several programs that cover workers from loss of income because of work-related disability. These programs are mentioned in Chapter 9 because work-related disabilities fall under workers' compensation laws. When an individual is eligible under more than one program, coordination of benefits is used so that a worker cannot receive benefits that result in an amount greater than what the person receives when working. Coordination of benefits is a provision preventing double payment for expenses by making one of the programs the primary payer and ensuring that no more than 100% of the costs are covered.

Disability Benefit Programs

The government's major non–work-related disability programs are as follows:
- Social Security Disability Insurance (SSDI) program
- Supplemental Security Income (SSI)
- Civil Service Retirement System (CSRS)
- Federal Employees Retirement System (FERS)
- Department of Defense (DoD) Disability
- Veterans Affairs (VA) disability program

The Social Security Administration (SSA) is a United States federal agency that administers Social Security retirement benefits. It also manages two programs that pay monthly disability income benefits to people younger than age 65 who cannot work for at least 1 year because of a severe disability: Social Security Disability Insurance and Supplemental Security Income. Medical requirements are the same for both programs.

Social Security Disability Insurance Program

Social Security Disability Insurance (SSDI) is part of the Social Security program that also pays retirement benefits to older Americans. It is funded through payroll taxes that have been collected through workers' payroll deductions and matching employer contributions. SSDI is a long-term disability program that pays monthly income benefits to workers who are no longer able to work because of a significant illness or impairment that is expected to last at least a year or to result in death within a year.

Disability Definition. Disability under Social Security has a strict definition: "the inability to engage in any substantial gainful activity due to any medically determinable physical or mental impairment which can be expected to result in death or which has lasted or can be expected to last for a continuous period of not less than 12 months."

Eligibility. Individuals are eligible for SSDI if they have worked for a certain number of years and have made contributions to the Social Security trust fund in the form of Federal Insurance Contribution Act (FICA) and paid Social Security Taxes.

The following is a list of individuals who meet eligibility requirements for SSDI:
- Disabled workers younger than age 65 years and their families
- Individuals who become disabled before age 22 years, and/or if a parent (or in certain cases, a grandparent) who is covered under Social Security retires, becomes disabled, or dies
- Disabled widows or widowers, age 50 years or older, if the deceased spouse worked at least 10 years under Social Security
- Disabled surviving divorced spouses older than age 50 years, if the ex-spouse was married to the disabled person for at least 10 years
- Blind workers whose vision in the better eye cannot be corrected to better than 20/200 or whose visual field in the better eye, even with corrective lenses, is 20 degrees or less

Workers must be fully insured in accordance with standards set by the SSA in terms of age, number of quarters worked, and amount of wages earned per quarter. The processing of eligibility application forms may take up to 2 months.

Benefits. Monthly benefits are paid to qualified individuals. There is a 5-month waiting period (WP) for benefits, which means the individual will not receive SSA benefits for the first 5 months they become disabled. The amount of the monthly benefit will depend on the worker's past earning records. After 24 months of disability payments, the disabled individual also becomes eligible for Medicare. The benefits convert to retirement benefits when an individual reaches age 65.

Supplemental Security Income

The Supplemental Security Income (SSI) program pays monthly income benefits to people (adults and children) with limited income and resources who are disabled, blind, or age 65 or older. The SSI program is overseen and managed by the SSA and is funded by general fund taxes, not from the Social Security trust fund. The SSI program differs from the SSDI program in that it has nothing to do with work history. Eligibility for the SSI program is based strictly on financial need.

Eligibility. Eligibility for SSI benefits is based on income and assets.

No prior employment is necessary to receive SSI benefits. Many SSI recipients also qualify for Medicaid, a state assistance program. The following individuals may qualify for SSI disability payments:
- Disabled persons younger than 65 years who have limited income and resources
- Disabled children younger than age 18 years, if the disability compares in severity with one that would prevent an adult from working and has lasted or is expected to last at least 12 months or result in death

- Blind adults or children who have a visual acuity no better than 20/100 or have a visual field of 20 degrees or less in the better eye, with the use of corrective lenses

Disability Determination Process. Individuals applying for disability will initiate the process by applying in person, by telephone, or by completing an application online or to be sent through the mail. This information is usually processed through a network of local Social Security field offices. The field office is responsible for verifying eligibility requirements including factors such as income, age, employment, citizenship, and marital status. Once all information has been collected, the case is forwarded to the Disability Determination Services (DDS), who will determine if the claimant is or is not disabled under the definition of the law. A health care professional may be involved in the determination process in one of these three ways:

1. as a treating source who provides medical evidence on behalf of their patients;
2. as a consultative examiner (CE) who is paid a fee and examines or tests the applicant; or
3. as a full- or part-time medical or psychological consultant reviewing claims for a state or regional office.

Final determination of disability is made by a DDS team composed of a physician or a psychologist and a disability examiner (DE), not by the applicant's health care provider. Upon making their disability determination, DDS will return the case to the field office. The field office will take appropriate action depending on whether the claim is allowed or denied.

Appeals of the Evaluation Process. If a claimant does not agree with the determination of disability, the following four-level appeals process is available:

1. A reconsideration, which is a complete review of the claim by a medical or psychological consultant or DE team who did not take part in the original disability determination.
2. The second level of appeals for a disability claim is a hearing before an administrative law judge who had no part in the initial or reconsideration determinations of the claim. The hearing is held within 75 miles of the claimant's home. The claimant and their representative are permitted to present their case in person and present a written statement. They are also permitted to review information the judge will use to make a decision and question any witnesses.
3. A review by the Appeal Council, which considers all requests for review but may deny a request if it believes that the decision by the administrative law judge was correct. If the Appeal Council decides that the case should be reviewed, it will make a decision on the case or return it to an administrative law judge for further review.
4. A review by the federal court for which the claimant may file an action where they reside.

Disability cases are reviewed from time to time to be sure that the individuals are still disabled. The frequency depends on the nature and severity of the impairment, the likelihood of improvement, rehabilitation, ability to work, and so on.

Benefits. Social Security disability programs are designed to give long-term protection and benefits to individuals totally disabled who are unable to do any type of work in the national economy.

Work Incentives. Special rules allow disabled or blind people presently receiving Social Security or SSI to work and still receive monthly benefits as well as Medicare or Medicaid (e.g., an SSDI recipient who is given a 90-day trial of work and at the end of that time either continues to work and loses SSDI coverage or leaves the temporary employment and remains on SSDI). A limit exists as to how much the person can earn in a calendar year. These are referred to as "work incentives"; the rules are different for Social Security beneficiaries and SSI recipients. Occasionally a person may be working and receiving SSDI benefits, as illustrated by the earlier example.

Civil Service and Federal Employees Retirement Systems

There are two types of federal retirement, Civil Service Retirement System (CSRS) and Federal Employees Retirement System (FERS). CSRS began in 1920, and a second system, FERS, was introduced in 1984. People who began working for the federal government in 1984 or later are covered by FERS instead of CSRS. Some workers who had been covered by the CSRS program changed to the FERS program when it became available.

Eligibility. Federal employees who work in civil service fall under the CSRS. This system has provisions for those who become totally disabled. This program is a combination of federal disability and Social Security disability. Both portions of the program must be applied for by the worker. The disability cannot be work related, and 5 years of service is necessary before benefits are payable. Eighteen months of service is necessary under the FERS.

Benefits. Those who qualify are entitled to benefits that are payable for life. For example, an individual who works for the Internal Revenue Service (IRS) performing clerical and filing job duties is involved in an automobile accident on the weekend. The head injuries are so severe that the person is unable to return to gainful employment at any job. He or she could apply for benefits under either CSRS or FERS, depending on their eligibility status.

Department of Defense Disability

The Department of Defense *(DoD)* gives military disability benefits to all active duty service members and reservists who leave the military with service-connected medical conditions that make the service member unfit for duty.

Eligibility. Individuals covered under the DoD Disability program must be members of the armed services on active duty who suffer a disability or illness. To receive DoD disability, the service member must first go through a DoD disability process, which includes a case review by the Medical Evaluation Board and the Physical Evaluation Board. The boards will determine type and quantity of DoD disability the service member will receive.

Benefits. DoD disability compensation is calculated based on the individual's service time, rank (basic pay rate), and disability rating.

Veterans Affairs Disability

A veteran is an individual who served in the active military service and was discharged or released under honorable conditions.

Veterans Affairs (VA) Disability compensation pays a monthly tax-free payment to veterans who got sick or injured while serving in the military and to veterans whose service made an existing condition worse.

Eligibility. An individual may qualify for VA disability benefits for physical conditions and mental health conditions that developed before, during, or after service. Examples of conditions that are often covered by these benefits are:

- Chronic back pain resulting in a diagnosed back disability
- Breathing problems resulting from a current lung condition or disease
- Severe hearing loss
- Scar tissue
- Loss of range of motion
- Ulcers
- Cancers caused by contact with toxic chemicals
- Traumatic brain injury
- Posttraumatic stress disorder
- Depression and anxiety

Benefits. The basic rate of compensation varies depending on the individual's degree of disability. If the disabled veteran has dependents, an additional allowance may be added.

In addition to the basic rate of compensation, a special monthly compensation may also be payable when the severity of certain disabilities or a combination of disabilities involves:

- Loss or loss of use of specific organs, sensory function, or extremities
- Disabilities that may confine the individual to their residence
- Disabilities that render the individual permanently bedridden or in need of aid and attendance
- A combination of severe disabilities that significantly affect walking
- Existence of multiple, independent disabilities each rated at 50% or 100%
- Existence of multiple disabilities that, in total, render the individual in need of such a degree of special skilled assistance that without it they would be permanently confined to a skilled-care nursing home.

 10.3   QUICK REVIEW

Question: List the federal government's major nonwork-related disability programs.

STATE DISABILITY INSURANCE

In 1944, Rhode Island began a **State Disability Insurance (SDI)** program that proved successful. This form of insurance is part of an employment security program that provides temporary cash benefits for workers suffering a wage loss because of off-the-job illness or injury. It can be referred to as **Unemployment Compensation Disability (UCD)** or **temporary disability insurance (TDI)**. California became the second state to add nonindustrial disability coverage to the Social Security protection afforded to its citizens by appending Article 10 to the Unemployment Insurance Act. This became law on May 21, 1946; when the legislation

took effect on December 1, 1946, this article diverted the 1% tax formerly paid by workers for unemployment insurance to a disability insurance fund. New York and New Jersey soon followed with similar programs. Two decades later, in 1969, Puerto Rico and Hawaii passed nonindustrial disability insurance laws. To date, these five states (California, Hawaii, New Jersey, New York, Rhode Island) and Puerto Rico are the only jurisdictions to operate non–work-related statutory SDI Programs.

Another nine jurisdictions (California, Colorado, Connecticut, District of Columbia, Massachusetts, New Jersey, Oregon, Rhode Island, and Washington) are now operating, or will soon be operating, **paid family and medical leave (PFML) insurance** programs. PFML insurance is a state-offered benefit, which provides paid leave for medical or family reasons. Eligibility and benefits may vary from state to state. Individuals who do not reside in those states are allowed to take time off work for health, disability, or caregiving reasons under **the Family and Medical Leave Act (FMLA)**. The FMLA is a federal law that gives eligible employees the right to take time off work, *unpaid*, to recover from serious medical conditions and care for ailing family members, among other things.

Funding for SDI programs varies by state. In some states, a small percentage of wages are deducted from the employees' paychecks each month, or the employer may elect to pay all or part of the cost of the plan as a fringe benefit for employees. The money is then sent in quarterly installments to the state and put in a special fund.

Eligibility

To receive SDI benefits, an employee must meet the following criteria:

- Employed fully or part time, or actively looking for work when disability begins
- Suffering a loss of wages because of disability
- Eligible for benefits, depending on the amount withheld during a previous period before disability began
- Under the care and treatment of a physician who certifies that the employee is disabled
- Disabled at least 7 calendar days
- Filing a claim within the time limit

If the worker was employed at the time of disability, benefits are not subject to federal income tax. An employee who retires is no longer eligible for the insurance.

Types of workers not covered are employees of school districts, community college districts, and churches, state workers; federal employees, interstate railroad workers, employees of nonprofit organizations, and domestic workers.

Benefits

Weekly benefits are determined by the wages earned in a base period or based on a percentage of average weekly wages (Table 10.1). Benefits begin after the seventh consecutive day of disability.

Limited Benefits

In some states, a patient may qualify for benefits if he or she is a resident of an approved alcoholic recovery facility or an approved drug-free residential facility.

TABLE 10.1 State Disability Information Summary
Statutory Disability Matrix by State, Effective January 1, 2020

State	Maximum Benefit Period (Weeks)	Waiting Period	2020 Employee Contribution from Salary (%)	Benefits
California	52	7-day waiting period. Benefits begin on eighth day	1.0% of annual taxable wage base: $122,909	60% of average weekly earnings in highest quarter of base period (maximum weekly benefit: $1300)
Hawaii	26	7-day waiting period Benefits begin on eighth day	0.5%; maximum weekly wage base: $1119.44	Based on 58% of average weekly wage (maximum weekly benefit: $650)
New Jersey	26	7-day waiting period Benefits begin on eighth day	0.26% of annual taxable wage base. $134,900	66 2/3% of average weekly wage (maximum $667/week)
New York	26	7-day waiting period Benefits begin on eighth day	0.5% of weekly taxable wage base: $120	Based on 50% of average weekly wage (maximum $170/week)
Puerto Rico	26	7-day waiting period Benefits begin on eighth day	0.2% of annual taxable wage base: $9000	Based on 65% of weekly earnings (maximum weekly benefit: $113)
Rhode Island	30	No waiting period Must be unemployed for at least 7 days because of non–job-related illness or injury	1.3% of annual taxable wage base: $72,300	4.62% of total high base period quarter wages (maximum weekly benefit: $867)

Reduced Benefits

An individual may be entitled to partial benefits if he or she is receiving certain types of income, such as the following:

- Sick leave
- Vacation
- Wages paid by employer
- Insurance settlement for the disability
- Workers' compensation benefits
- Unemployment benefits

Time Limits

A claim for SDI should be filed within the time limit of the state laws. There is usually a grace period of 7 or 8 days after the deadline. After the claim is approved, basic benefits become payable after the seventh day of disability. A person may continue to draw disability insurance for a maximum of 26 weeks in Hawaii, New Jersey, New York, and Puerto Rico; 30 weeks in Rhode Island; and 52 weeks in California for the same illness or injury or overlapping disabilities. An employee is also entitled to disability benefits 15 days after recovery from a previous disability or illness. For example, if a patient is discharged by the health care provider to return to work and is on the job 15 calendar days and then becomes ill with the same ailment, he or she may file a new claim.

Medical Examinations

The claimant may be required to submit to an examination or examinations by an independent medical examiner to determine any mental or physical disability. The state department that handles disability insurance pays fees for such examinations. *Current Procedural Terminology* (CTP) code 99450 for billing these medical examinations may be found in the Special Evaluation and Management Services section of the CPT manual.

Restrictions

Disability insurance has many restrictions. A few of the major situations in which a claim could be denied are listed here.

1. Conditions covered by workers' compensation unless the rate is less than the disability insurance rate. In this case, the state pays the difference between the two rates.
2. Applicants receiving unemployment insurance benefits that are more than a certain specified amount. *Exception:* If the applicant is on unemployment insurance and then becomes ill or injured, he or she is put on TDI until able to go on a job interview.
3. Disabilities beginning during a trade dispute. If an employee is on strike and is injured while walking a picket line, he or she is considered to still be employed. If injured while picketing, it may be considered workers' compensation. However, if the union is on strike and an individual member remains at home and then becomes ill or injured, he or she can claim disability and will receive benefits.
4. Confinement by court order or certification in a public or private institution as an alcoholic, drug addict, or sexual psychopath.
5. When the pursuit of legal custody of a child is the cause of inability to work.
6. When the employing company has a voluntary disability plan and is not paying into a state fund.
7. Religious exemption certificate on file by employee or company with no payment being made into a state fund.
8. Pregnancy-related disability, unless the pregnancy is complicated (for example, cases in which the patient has diabetes, varicose veins, ectopic pregnancy, or cesarean section). *Exceptions:* California, Hawaii, New Jersey, New York, and Rhode Island have maternity benefits that may be applied for at the time the health care provider tells the patient to stop working.

Voluntary Disability Insurance

Persons residing and working in states that do not have SDI programs may elect to contact a local private insurance carrier to arrange for coverage under a **voluntary disability insurance** plan. If these persons become ill or disabled, they receive a fixed weekly or monthly income, usually for approximately 6 months. If the disability or illness is permanent and the individual is unable to return to work, there is sometimes a small monthly income for the duration of the person's life. Some of the state laws provide that a "voluntary plan" may be adopted instead of the "state plan" if a majority of company employees consent to private coverage.

 10.4   QUICK REVIEW

Question: List the six jurisdictions that currently operate nonwork-related SDI programs.
    List the nine jurisdictions that are now operating or will soon be operating PFML insurance.

DISABILITY INCOME CLAIMS SUBMISSION GUIDELINES

For disability income claims, the insured must file a proof of loss form, and the attending physician must complete a section to confirm the disability. The report must show that the patient's disability meets the policy's definition of disability or benefits will be denied. Because the definition of disability varies among policies, the critical issues are the content and wording on the claim form.

The portion of the form that is completed by the attending physician generally requires the following data:
- Medical history
- Date on which patient became disabled
- Subjective symptoms (patient's own words about their chief complaints)
- Objective findings on physical examination (for example, rashes, lacerations, abrasions, or contusions)
- Severity of the illness or injury (range-of-motion [ROM] tests)
- Photocopies of laboratory tests, x-ray studies, or hospital discharge report
- Medication
- Treatment dates
- Diagnosis
- Prognosis (outcome of the disease or injury)
- Names of any other treating physician or health care service provider
- Date on which the patient is expected to return to work
- Description of job duties and patient's ability to perform work

Providing this information helps to verify the disability. In some cases, the health care provider may wish to dictate a medical report and attach it to the claim form instead of completing a portion of the form. The insurance billing specialist must be prepared to extract data from source documents, such as medical and financial records, to complete the claim form. In such situations, the health care provider should be asked to read the information carefully before signing the document. The patient should always be asked to sign an authorization form to release medical information. Reasons for denial of benefits often include improper choice of words or inadequate medical information.

The insurance company may request information from other places, such as employer's records, employee's wage statements or tax forms, or the patient's medical records from the attending physician, to justify payment of benefits. A company representative may interview the insured if conflicting information exists.

If disability continues, additional claim forms should be completed monthly or more frequently by the insured and attending physician. Other sources of information may be requested, for example, records from medical specialists or Social Security records.

If the validity of the case is in question, an independent medical examiner may be asked by the insurance company to examine the disabled individual. If the claimant neglects to return claim forms, refuses telephone calls, misses appointments, or engages in questionable activities, the insurance company will discreetly engage in surveillance of the insured through the services of a professional investigation firm.

Federal Disability Claims

The SSA division called *Disability Determination Services* has a tele-dictation service so that the physician or psychologist can dictate the medical report over the telephone instead of completing a medical report form. The service is available at any time, including nights and weekends. A typed transcript is sent to the physician to review, sign, and return to the SSA state agency, or a report may be typed on the health care provider's stationery. The physician may photocopy relevant portions of the patient's chart and submit that information, but it should be legible. An authorization signed by the patient to release information should be on file. Copies of consultation reports and hospital summaries are also helpful. By law, only data no more than 1 year old are allowed.

A medical report must include the following:
- Relevant medical history, social history, or family history
- Subjective complaints (patient's symptoms)
- Objective findings on physical examination (for example, results of physical or mental status examination, blood pressure)
- Laboratory and x-ray findings
- Diagnostic studies (for example, treadmill tests, pulmonary function tests, and electrocardiogram [ECG] tracings)
- Diagnosis (statement of disease or injury based on signs and symptoms)
- Treatment prescribed, with patient's response and prognosis
- Medical prognosis about disability based on medical findings

A description of the individual's ability to perform work-related activities, such as standing, sitting, lifting, carrying, walking, handling objects, hearing, speaking, and traveling, is necessary. For cases of mental impairment, the statement should present the individual's capacity for understanding and remembering, sustained concentration and persistence, social interaction, and adaptation.

State Disability Claims

Residents of a state that provides state disability benefits may call or write to the nearest office that handles SDI to obtain a claim form and insurance pamphlet. See the state disability websites for detailed information about each state's benefits, claim procedures, and claim forms.

In some states, the claim form is in three parts and must be completed by the claimant, employer, and health care provider.

In other states, the form is in two parts and is completed by the claimant and the health care provider (Fig. 10.1). In either instance, the case must be substantiated by a physician before the applicant may begin receiving benefits. All information from the SDI office should be read carefully and the directions

Fig. 10.1 Form DB-450: New York State Notice and Proof of Claim for Disability Benefits.

PART B - HEALTH CARE PROVIDER'S STATEMENT (Please Print or Type)

THE HEALTH CARE PROVIDER'S STATEMENT MUST BE FILLED IN COMPLETELY. THE ATTENDING HEALTH CARE PROVIDER SHALL COMPLETE AND RETURN TO THE CLAIMANT WITHIN SEVEN (7) DAYS OF RECEIPT OF THIS FORM. For item- 7-d, you must give estimated date. if disability is caused by or arising in connection with pregnancy, enter estimated delivery date in item 7-e. **INCOMPLETE ANSWERS MAY DELAY PAYMENT OF BENEFITS.**

1. Last Name: _____ First Name: _____ MI: ___

2. Gender: ☐ Male ☐ Female   3. Date of Birth: ___ / ___ / ____

4. Diagnosis/Analysis: _____ Diagnosis Code: _____

   a. Claimant's symptoms: _____

   b. Objective findings: _____

5. Claimant hospitalized?: ☐ Yes ☐ No   From: ___ / ___ / _____   To: ___ / ___ / _____

6. Operation indicated?:   ☐ Yes ☐ No   a. Type _____   b. Date ___ / ___ / _____

7. ENTER DATES FOR THE FOLLOWING	MONTH	DAY	YEAR
a. Date of your first treatment for this disability			
b. Date of your most recent treatment for this disability			
c. Date Claimant was unable to work because of this disability			
c. Date Claimant will again be able to perform work (Even if considerable question exists, estimate date. Avoid use of terms such as unknown or undetermined.)			
e. If pregnancy related, please check box and enter the date ☐ estimated delivery date OR ☐ actual delivery date			

8. In your opinion, is this disability the result of injury arising out of and in the course of employment or occupational disease?: ☐ Yes ☐ No   If "Yes", has Form C-4 been filed with the Board? ☐ Yes ☐ No

I certify that I am a:

_____
(Physician, Chiropractor, Dentist, Podiatrist, Psychologist, Nurse-Midwife)   Licensed or Certified in the State of _____   License Number _____

_____
Health Care Provider's Printed Name   Health Care Provider's Signature   Date

_____
Health Care Provider's Address   Phone #

IMPORTANT NOTICE TO CLAIMANT - READ THESE INSTRUCTIONS CAREFULLY

PLEASE NOTE: Do not date and file this form prior to your first date of disability. In order for your claim to be processed, Parts A and B must be completed.

1. If you are using this form because you became disabled **while employed** or you became disabled **within four (4) weeks after termination of employment**, your completed claim should be mailed **within thirty (30) days of your first date of disability to your employer or your last employer's insurance carrier**. You may find your employer's disability insurance carrier on the Workers' Compensation Board's website, www.wcb.ny.gov, using Employer Coverage Search.

2. If you are using this form because you became **disabled after having been unemployed for more than four (4) weeks**, your completed claim Must be mailed to: **Workers' Compensation Board, Disability Benefits Bureau, PO Box 9029, Endicott, NY 13761-9029.** If you answered "Yes" to question 13.B.3, please complete and attach form DB-450.1.

If you do not receive a respose within 45 days or if you have questions about your disability benefits claim, please call your employer's insurance carrier. For general information about disability benefits, please visit www.wcb.ny.gov or call the Board's Disability Benefits Bureau at (877) 632--4996.

DB-450 (1-20) Page 2 of 2

Fig. 10.1, cont'd.

followed precisely. The data requested should be provided and the health care provider and patient should sign the forms. The form should be submitted within the stated time limits.

All follow-up correspondence should include the patient's name and Social Security number. The insurance billing specialist should promptly report any change of address, telephone number, or return-to-work date to the SDI office.

 10.5 QUICK REVIEW

Question: List the information that is typically required in the attending physician's medical record when filing a federal disability income claim form.

DISCUSSION POINT

Accurate and prompt completion of the attending physician's portion of a disability claim form assists the patient in obtaining disability income when they are unable to work. What steps can the insurance billing specialist take to ensure that income assistance is not delayed?

PROCEDURE 10.1 Completing the Notice and Proof of Claim for Disability Benefits

Objective: Accurately complete a Notice and Proof of Claim for Disability Benefits form from the State of New York

Step 1: Download a blank Notice of Proof of Claim for Disability Benefits form from the State of New York. [Form DB-450] (1-20). It can be accessed at: https://www.standard.com/eforms/sny9457.pdf

Step 2: Create a disability scenario with a classmate as the claimant. Ask the classmate to provide information needed to complete the first page of the form (Claimant's Information).

Step 3: Review information that will be needed to complete page 2 of the form (Health Care Provider's Statement). Highlight all fields of the claim form that will require abstraction of information from the patient's medical record or must be obtained by the health care provider.

Step 4: Determine your strategy for ensuring that the health care provider's statement will be completed promptly, and patient's income benefits will not be delayed.

Step 5: Review the bottom portion of the claim form that refers to false statements made on the claim.

KEY POINTS

This is a brief chapter review, or summary, of the key issues presented.

1. Disability income insurance is a type of insurance that provides periodic wage replacement payments under certain conditions when the insured is unable to work because of illness, disease, or injury, not as a result of a work-related accident or condition.
2. The types of disability are temporary, residual, partial, or total.
3. While disabled, benefits begin after an elimination or waiting period (WP).
4. There are several ways to purchase disability income insurance.
5. Disability policies may be guaranteed renewable for a specific number of years to a certain age.
6. The Social Security Administration (SSA) manages two programs that pay monthly disability benefits to people younger than age 65 who cannot work for at least 1 year because of a severe disability: Social Security Disability Insurance (SSDI) program and Supplemental Security Income (SSI) program.
7. Federal employees who have put in a certain number of years of service and who become disabled not by work-related means may be eligible for Civil Service Retirement System (CSRS) and Federal Employees Retirement System (FERS) programs.
8. Individuals on active duty fall under the Department of Defense (DoD) Disability program if they become disabled while serving in the military.
9. The Veterans Affairs (VA) disability program provides benefits for veterans who have suffered a service-connected disability.
10. Five states plus Puerto Rico have a State Disability Insurance (SDI) program for those who suffer a wage loss because of off-the-job illness or injury.
11. Claims for SDI must be filed within the time limits of each state's laws.
12. For disability income claims, the insured must file a proof of loss form, and the attending physician must also complete a section to verify the disability.
13. For federal disability cases, the physician must submit details about the individual's disabled condition.
14. State disability claim forms must be completed by the attending physician to substantiate the claimant's condition to receive benefits.

STUDENT ASSIGNMENTS

- Study Chapter 10.
- Complete all exercises in the *Workbook* to reinforce the theory learned in this chapter.
- Turn to the Glossary at the end of this text for a further understanding of the key terms and key abbreviations used in this chapter.

UNIT 3

Documentation and Coding for Professional Services

Medical Documentation and the Electronic Health Record

Cheryl Fassett

OBJECTIVES

After reading this chapter, you should be able to:

1. Identify the most common documents found in the health record.
2. Understand why complete documentation is important.
3. Discuss health record systems and list the advantages and disadvantages of an electronic health record system.
4. Define the various titles of physicians as they relate to health record documentation.
5. Explain the purpose of Clinical Documentation Improvement (CDI).
6. Explain the reasons that legible documentation is required.
7. Describe signature requirements for documentation.
8. Describe common documentation errors found in health records and define medical necessity.
9. Formulate a procedure for termination of care.
10. Define common terminology related to medical, diagnostic, and surgical services and describe proper documentation for each.
11. Respond appropriately to the subpoena of a witness and records.
12. Identify principles for the retention of health records.
13. Abstract information from the health record to complete a life or health insurance application.
14. Describe the difference between prospective, concurrent, and retrospective review of records.

KEY TERMS

acute
attending physician
back up
chief complaint
chronic
clinical documentation
  improvement
cloned note
computed tomography
concurrent care
concurrent review
consultation
consulting physician
continuity of care
counseling
critical care
deep
degaussing
documentation
electronic health record
emergency care
eponym
established patient
external audit
family history

gross examination
health record
history of present illness
internal review
laboratory services
lateral
legible
magnetic resonance imaging
medial
medical decision making
medical necessity
microscopy
modality
morbidity
mortality
new patient
non-physician practitioner
occupational therapy
ordering provider
past history
pathology
physical examination
physical therapy
preoperative
prepayment (prospective) audit

postoperative
primary care provider
prone
prospective review
proximal
query
referral
referring provider
resident physician
retrospective review or audit
review of systems
social history
speech-language pathology
subacute
subpoena
subpoena duces tecum
superficial
supine
teaching physician
transfer of care
treating, or performing, provider
ultrasound
x-ray
zeroization

KEY ABBREVIATIONS

ARRA	EMR	MRI	RCU
CC	FH	PACU	RLQ
CDI	HIM	PCP	ROS
CCU	HIV	PE or PX	RUQ
CT	HPI	PFSH	SH
dx or Dx	ICU	PH	SOAP style
ED or ER	LLQ	POMR system	SOR system
EHR	LUQ	Preop	U/S
E/M	MDM	Postop	WNL

INSIGHTS FROM THE FIELD

Patricia S.: Registered Health Information Technician (RHIT), Certified Professional Coder (CPC), Certified Interventional Radiology Cardiovascular Coder (CIRCC)

I have worked in the health care field for over 30 years. Currently, I am a hospital billing supervisor and oversee the department responsible for sending out clean inpatient and outpatient claims for all areas of the hospital. The most valuable skill a new billing specialist can have is critical thinking and a desire to continue learning. There are so many variables in each type of billing scenario. Each insurance company offers a large variety of plans and requires something different on their electronic or paper claim. Payer contracts can also dictate what is required to be submitted to an insurance carrier. Knowing what to look for and who to contact to rectify payer issues is key. It's important to realize that no one can sit you down and just teach you everything you will need to know in your career. I go to work each day excited that I am going to learn something new. This field is ever changing. The level of skill required continues to increase. There are growth opportunities in the field for those willing to put the time in and the effort needed to be successful.

THE DOCUMENTATION PROCESS

Health Record

The health record is the most important tool in clinical care and communication. Documentation is the process of chronologically recording pertinent facts and observations about the patient's health. A health record is the written or graphic documentation of facts and events during the patient care encounter. It may be kept in either a paper or an electronic format. Some health care organizations use different terminology when referring to the health record, such as medical information, medical report, progress or chart note, or facility record.

Complete documentation is important, as it allows health care providers to evaluate their patient's treatment and condition over time. It acts as a communication between various providers who may be involved in a patient's care.

Contents of a health record vary from case to case, but some of the most common health care organization documents are as follows:
- Patient demographic information
- Medication record
- History and physical examination notes or report
- Progress or chart notes
- Consultation reports
- Imaging and x-ray reports
- Laboratory reports
- Immunization records
- Consent and authorization forms
- Operative reports
- Pathology reports

In a health care facility setting, there will also be provider's orders, discharge summaries, and dates of admission and discharge. Supporting documentation is the key to substantiating procedure and diagnostic code selections for claim submission and to ensuring appropriate reimbursement. Proper documentation can prevent penalties and refund requests in the event that the health care organization is reviewed or audited.

Health Record Systems

An electronic health record (EHR) is an electronic version of a patient's medical history that is immediately available to multiple providers who have authorized access. EHRs create a timely and accessible record that can assist in patient care decisions. An EHR can be organized and displayed depending on user preference. For example, data can be organized using a problem-oriented medical record (POMR) system or a source-oriented record (SOR) system.

The POMR system is designed to organize patient information by the presenting problem. This allows the provider to obtain a quick and structured overview of the patient's history when the patient presents for care. The record consists of flow sheets, charts, or graphs that allow a service provider to quickly locate information and compare evaluations. These data sheets are commonly used to record blood sugar levels, blood pressure readings, weight, immunizations, medication refills, and so on. Using this type of system assists the provider in focusing on the patient's problems, his or her evolution, and the relationship between clinical events.

In the SOR system, documents are arranged according to the type of document. For example, history and physical sections, progress notes, laboratory tests, radiology reports, or surgical operations are grouped together. Documents are typically filed in reverse chronological order.

Electronic Health Records

Though paper-based records still exist to capture a variety of data, the electronic format has grown in popularity. The ability to share patient health records among care team members has become increasingly important to providing patient care.

An EHR is a collection of medical information about the past, present, and future of a patient, which resides in a centralized electronic system. This system receives, stores, transmits, retrieves, and links data from many information systems. This enables information such as laboratory test results, radiology reports and x-ray images, pathology reports, and financial documents to be shared between various departments.

The terms *EHR* and *EMR* may be used interchangeably; however, they are not the same. The electronic medical record (EMR) is an individual provider's record for the patient, including medical history, allergies, and appointment information. In comparison, the EHR is all patient medical information from many information systems, including all components of the EMR.

In an EHR system, medical information software may allow the service provider to type or dictate (free-text) the entire record for each encounter. Software may also allow providers to use built-in templates. A template is a sample document that has some of the details already in place but requires the service provider to fill in the blanks either by hand or through an automated checklist. Templates help structure documentation through a process of answering a series of questions and entering data.

Electronic Health Records in the Billing Process

Many EHR programs allow the insurance billing specialist to perform insurance verification automatically during the preregistration process. The electronic verification then becomes part of the health record.

The selection of procedure and diagnostic codes by the provider may be computer-assisted before final review by a medical coding specialist. These codes are then used for interpretation by the insurance company when processing a claim. When billing the insurance company, the date of service (DOS), place of service (POS), diagnosis (dx or Dx), and procedures are recorded and transmitted in electronic format according to HIPAA standards. Electronic signatures are applied to documents when they are reviewed and authenticated by the creator. Insurance claims are generated and transmitted to a clearinghouse or to the insurance carrier. In this way, the revenue cycle is managed completely online.

Advantages of Electronic Health Records

An EHR system has several advantages over a paper-based system. The greatest advantage of the EHR is the accessibility of health records between providers and health care organizations. Providers have full access to a patient's complete record in an EHR system. This type of access can improve the quality of care and patient safety.

Other EHR advantages include cost savings and decreased workplace inefficiencies. The EHR system requires less physical space because the files remain in an electronic database and are available online. The health record is accessible from remote sites, and retrieval of information at almost any work site is nearly immediate. Chart chasing is eliminated. The EHR can decrease charting time and charting errors, thus increasing the productivity and effectiveness of providers.

The need for staff to select information from a patient's EHR for completion of an insurance claim is often eliminated because data may be captured automatically from various documents via dictation or templates. The EHR is expected to increase patient safety through built-in safety features by use of medical alerts and reminders that can capture things such as medication allergies. The EHR reduces the likelihood of errors since there is no illegible handwriting to decipher.

Disadvantages of Electronic Health Records

The greatest drawback to EHRs is startup costs, which can be extremely high. Usability can also be a major obstacle in the implementation of an EHR. Learning curves vary depending on the user's technical abilities and knowledge.

With increased accessibility comes greater concern with confidentiality and security issues. These issues are the primary focus of the HIPAA Privacy and Security Rules. As discussed in Chapter 2, health care organizations must maintain a higher level of integrity in these areas.

Although EHR is designed to save providers time and improve the quality and legibility of their documentation, the use of EHR has also led to a new problem with health records related to copied and templated documentation. These are referred to as cloned notes. The process may also be referred to as "copy and paste" or information that is "carried over." The Centers for Medicare and Medicaid Services (CMS) considers documentation to be cloned when each entry in the health record for a patient is worded exactly the same as or similar to the previous entries. Cloning also occurs when medical documentation is exactly the same from patient to patient.

Cloned notes increase the risk for medical errors and can result in the loss of crucial clinical details that may be omitted from a patient's assessment or treatment plan. All documentation in the health record must be specific to the patient and his or her situation at the time of the encounter. Payers are refusing to pay for services when the documentation for those services appears to be cloned. This process has come under increased scrutiny by the Office of Inspector General (OIG) and is a red flag for fraud investigations.

Incentive Programs for Adoption of Electronic Health Records

Federal legislation established by the American Recovery and Reinvestment Act of 2009 (ARRA) created programs to help the health care industry change from paper to electronic health records. Legislation affecting Medicare and Medicaid programs was established to provide more than $27 billion in payouts of incentives to eligible providers who implement electronic health records. The programs provided a reimbursement incentive for health care organizations that adopted, implemented, upgraded, and demonstrated meaningful use (MU) of certified EHR technology. It was anticipated that compliance with MU would result in the following:

- Better clinical outcomes
- Improved population health outcomes
- Increased transparency and efficiency

- Empowered patients
- More robust research data on health systems

Starting in 2015, these incentive programs began transitioning into reimbursement penalties for those who have not adopted EHR. Medicare payments were reduced by 1% for those who were not using EHR in the previous year. Penalties rose to 2% in 2016 and 3% in 2017.

During the last decade, Medicare implemented additional programs such as the Physician Quality Reporting System (PQRS) and the Merit-based Incentive Payment System (MIPS). These programs link reimbursement directly to the documentation of quality measures. Like the MU incentives, failure to adopt these documentation and reporting measures will result in reimbursement penalties.

Further legislation in the Medicare Modernization Act created the Commission on Systemic Interoperability, which was tasked with developing a strategy that would make health care information available at all times to patients and providers. To reach a goal of having electronic records for all Americans, the adoption of health information standards and increased funding for these projects have begun.

It is important for insurance billing specialists to be familiar with all incentive programs. They will be involved in the submission of qualifying data, collection of incentive payments, and analysis of incentive program outcomes as they affect the organization's accounts receivable.

 11.1   QUICK REVIEW
Question: What is the difference between an EMR and an EHR?

 11.2   QUICK REVIEW
Question: What are the advantages of an EHR over a paper records system?

 11.3   QUICK REVIEW
Question: What is cloning?

GENERAL PRINCIPLES OF HEALTH RECORD DOCUMENTATION

Documentation is the core of the revenue cycle in any health care organization. To bill for any health care services, the medical billing specialist will refer to the documentation to identify the services provided and to complete the claim form. Documentation must be accurate and complete. Supporting documentation is critical to ensure accurate and timely payment of services furnished. As with patient care, the driving criteria for proper documentation should always be medical necessity. Just like a provider should not order unnecessary lab tests, a provider should not document a more in-depth exam in an effort to get paid more.

Additionally, clear and concise documentation of health records is critical to providing patients with quality care. Documentation of health records assists health care professionals in evaluating and planning the patient's immediate treatment and monitoring the patient's health care over time.

Documenters

All individuals providing health care services may be referred to as documenters because they record pertinent facts and observations about the patient's health. Documentation (charting) may be electronic, handwritten, or dictated and transcribed. Regardless of the method used, it is the health care provider's responsibility to ensure the final documentation is accurate and complete.

Some documenters use a speech recognition system to dictate health information. These computerized voice recognition systems make it possible for a computer system to respond to spoken words. When a dictation software speech recognition system is used, many health care organizations use a medical editor or correctionist who proofreads and edits the computer-generated documents. There are two basic categories of speech recognition systems:

- Navigation or command control systems allow an individual to launch and operate software applications with spoken directions.
- Dictation software systems make it possible for a computer system to recognize spoken words and automatically convert them into text.

Some organizations use printed checklists for typical examinations. The health care provider notes his or her findings on the checklists and gives this document to an employee for input to the EMR system.

Health care service providers are not the only documenters in a health care organization. The receptionist obtains the first document completed by the patient, called the patient registration information form. The medical assistant or a front desk staff member is often the one who records entries for no-show appointments, prescription refills, and telephone calls. The insurance billing specialist uses the information in the health record for billing purposes. It is their responsibility to bring any substandard documentation to the provider or office manager's attention, depending on office policy. In the health care facility setting, a trained health information management (HIM) professional maintains the health record for completeness.

When referring to guidelines for documentation of the health record and completion of the insurance claim form, a service provider's role and title may change, depending on the circumstances of each patient encounter. This can get confusing at times. To clarify the various roles, some of these titles are defined as follows:

- **Attending physician** refers to the facility staff member who is legally responsible for the care and treatment given to a patient.
- **Consulting physician** is a provider whose opinion or advice regarding evaluation or management of a specific problem is requested by another provider.
- **Non-physician practitioner** is a nurse practitioner, clinical nurse specialist, licensed social worker, nurse midwife, physical therapist, speech therapist, audiologist, or physician assistant who furnishes a consultation or treats a patient for a specific medical problem. Non-physician practitioners are also known as *physician extenders*.
- **Ordering provider** is the individual in the health care organization directing the selection, preparation, or administration of tests, medication, or treatment.

- **Primary care provider (PCP)** oversees the care of patients in a managed health care plan and refers patients to see specialists for services as needed.
- **Referring provider** is one who sends the patient for tests or treatment.
- **Resident physician** is a physician who has finished medical school and is performing 1 or more years of training in a specialty area on the job at a health care facility. A resident performs the elements required for an evaluation and management (E/M) service or another service in the presence of or jointly with the teaching physician. The resident documents the service.
- **Teaching physician** is a doctor who has responsibilities for training and supervising medical students, interns, or residents and who takes them to the bedsides of patients in a teaching facility to review course and treatment. Teaching physicians must document that they supervised and were physically present during key portions of the service provided to the patient when performed by a resident.
- **Treating, or performing, provider** is the health care provider who renders a therapeutic or evaluation service to a patient.

Clinical Documentation Improvement

Clinical documentation improvement (CDI) is the process of ensuring the creation of accurate and effective patient health records. CDI programs were developed in response to CMS's transition to quality-based reimbursement systems. The goal of any CDI program is to improve patient outcomes, provide accurate data for quality measurement reporting, and ensure proper reimbursement.

A **query** is a tool used by coding and CDI specialists to request additional clarification from the provider. Queries should include the clinical indicators that prompted the request and should not be leading. In other words, the coding specialist or auditor should not attempt to direct the provider's response based on their interpretation of the data. The query should not introduce new information not contained in the health record. Queries and query forms often become part of the permanent health record. It is beneficial if a CDI program has a health care provider who advises and provides education to the CDI specialist and serves as a liaison between them and the medical staff. Box 11.1 for examples of compliant and noncompliant queries.

Often, service providers are unfamiliar with the documentation requirements for proper coding. On the other hand, many coding specialists lack the clinical knowledge that explains procedures and tests. A CDI specialist links the two, providing documentation education to both. For those interested in pursuing a career focusing on this area, the American Health Information Management Association (AHIMA) offers a clinical documentation improvement practitioner (CDIP) certification. The American Association of Professional Coders (AAPC) also offers a clinical documentation expert outpatient (CDEO) certification. The Association of Clinical Documentation Improvement Specialists (ACDIS) offers the clinical documentation specialist (CCDS) certification, as well as one aimed at outpatient clinical documentation (CCDS-O).

> **! COMPLIANCE ALERT**
>
> If handwritten, entries in the patient's record must be legible. Illegible entries should be returned to the health care provider for clarification or to be rewritten.

Documentation Requirements
Documentation Must Be Legible

Health record documentation details pertinent facts, findings, and observations about an individual's health history, examinations, tests, treatments, and outcomes. It enables the health care professional to evaluate and plan the patient's immediate treatment and monitor the patient's health care over time. It also helps health care providers communicate with each other regarding a patient's diagnosis and treatment. A health record also acts as a legal document for evidence if the need arises. It is a basic and important element in providing the highest level quality of care.

The documentation guidelines issued by CMS state that the health record should be complete and legible. The CMS definition of legible is that the data must be easily recognizable by someone outside the health care organization who is unfamiliar with the handwriting. It is important that providers have comprehensive and legible documentation describing what occurred during the patient's encounter for the following reasons:

- To avoid denial or delay of payments by insurance carriers
- To avoid misdiagnosing patients
- To avoid dispensing incorrect medications

BOX 11.1   Examples of Compliant and Noncompliant Queries

Noncompliant Queries	Compliant Queries
Patient has diabetes and retinopathy. Did you mean to say diabetic retinopathy?	Patient has diabetes and retinopathy. Please addend office note to document the relationship, if any, between the diabetes and the retinopathy.
There is contradictory information in the office note. History states patient has never smoked, but assessment states patient was educated about smoking cessation. Please update the history to indicate patient is a smoker.	There is contradictory information in the office note. History states patient has never smoked, but assessment states patient was educated about smoking cessation. Please addend the office note to resolve the contradiction.
Office note indicates hyperglycemia and hypoglycemia. Based on the lab results, I think you meant hyperglycemia.	Office note indicates both hyperglycemia and hypoglycemia. Please clarify.
Patient's chart indicates past history of breast cancer, but patient is being prescribed Tamoxifen. I have coded it as a current cancer diagnosis.	Patient's chart indicates past history of breast cancer, but patient is being prescribed Tamoxifen. Can you clarify if cancer is resolved or current? If resolved, please indicate reason for Tamoxifen prescription.

SIGNATURE LOG

Name	Position	Signature or Initials	
Ann M. Arch	Receptionist	*Ann M. Arch*	*AMA*
John Bortolonni	Office manager	*John Bortolonni*	*JB*
Gerald Practon, MD	Provider	*Gerald Practon, MD*	*GP*
Rachel Vasquez, CPC	Insurance billing specialist	*Rachel Vasquez, CPC*	*RV*
Mary Ann Worth	Clinical medical assistant	*Mary Ann Worth*	*MAW*

Fig. 11.1 Example of a signature log for paper-based records.

- To ensure proper treatments are given
- To ensure continuity of care when multiple providers are involved with the patient
- To comply with insurance carrier payment policies requiring documentation to support procedural and diagnostic codes submitted on claims
- For subpoena of health records by state investigators or the court for review
- For the defense of any professional liability claims
- For the execution of the health care provider's written instructions to the patient or the caregiver
- To avoid charges of negligence and malpractice

Documentation Must Be Signed

Medicare also requires that all documentation be signed by the provider who performed the service. Signatures should be dated and include the provider's credentials. A signature shows that the record entry has been reviewed and authenticated by the provider. Some private payers may not require signatures, but since all health care documentation may become legal documents, it is a best practice to ensure the provider has reviewed and signed off on the documentation as being an accurate description of services provided. Signature stamps are not secure and can easily be misused. Stamps are not allowed by CMS. See Box 11.2 for examples of compliant and noncompliant signatures.

If a signature log has been established for paper-based records, initials are acceptable because these would be defined in the log (Fig. 11.1). A signature log is a list of all staff members' names, job titles, signatures, and initials. It is used to establish signature legibility. In regard to paperless documents, if passwords are used for restricted access, electronic or digital signatures may be acceptable.

Documentation Must Support Medical Necessity

A health care provider's documentation is the basis for determining appropriate medical care. It outlines the provider's rationale in choosing tests, procedures, and other treatment options. To appropriately treat patients, providers must have access to accurate and timely health records from all providers the patient has seen. Proper documentation ensures that patient care will be consistent from provider to provider and specialty to specialty. It can also act as proof of proper care in the case of a lawsuit.

Complete documentation is required not only to support high-quality care but also to support the bills submitted to the services. Proper documentation must reflect the medical necessity of the services provided. It must be sufficient to support the accuracy of the CPT, HCPCS, and ICD-10 codes submitted to third-party and government payers.

Common Documentation Errors

Understandably, health care providers put patient care first. The documentation process is secondary and is oftentimes hurried and treated as an afterthought. Providing excellent patient care is often used as an excuse for poor documentation. It is important to help health care providers understand the link between quality care and documentation.

The following is a list of common errors found in health records:

- Medication lists are not updated with new or discontinued medications.
- Incorrect dosages of prescription medications are documented.
- Duplicate prescriptions are documented for both brand-name and generic medications.
- Over-the-counter medications the patient is taking are not documented.
- Information related to medication allergies is not documented.
- Treatment outcomes are often incorrect. For example, a condition is noted as being resolved when it is still being treated.
- Laboratory information is missing or not updated.
- Important information related to the patient's illness and symptoms, as stated by the patient, are not documented.

BOX 11.2 Compliant and Noncompliant Signatures

Noncompliant Signatures	Compliant Signatures
John Smithfield (handwritten with no credential or date)	Electronically signed by John Smithfield, MD, 05/21/XX
Dictated by John Smithfield, MD	Verified by J. Smithfield, MD 05/21/XX
JOHN SMITHFIELD, MD (signature stamp)	Authenticated by John Smithfield, MD, 05/21/XX
Signed, but not read by, John Smithfield, MD	John Smithfield, MD, 05/21/XX (handwritten)

- There are inaccuracies in diagnosis and incomplete documentation related to the plan of care for the condition.
- Information from other providers is missing.
- Evidence of cloning.
- Incorrect dates of service.
- Incomplete dictation.
- Unsigned records.

> **! COMPLIANCE ALERT**
>
> Third-party payers and federal programs have a responsibility to ensure that professional services provided to patients were medically necessary. Documentation must support the level of service and each procedure rendered.

Insurance carriers have become stricter in enforcing accurate coding substantiated by documentation. It is not uncommon for carriers to perform random prepayment and postpayment audits or to monitor the accuracy of providers' use of medical services and procedure codes. Medicare administrative contractors and other carriers have "walk-in rights" that they may invoke to conduct documentation reviews, audits, and evaluations. This means that they have access to a health care organization without an appointment or search warrant.

Termination of Care

A health care provider may wish to withdraw formally from further care of a patient because of patient noncompliance. There are many reasons for this, such as the following:

- The patient discharged the health care provider.
- The patient did not follow instructions.
- The patient did not take the recommended medication.
- The patient failed to return for an appointment.
- The patient discontinued payment on an overdue account.

Termination of patient care should always be made in writing. If the health care provider is terminating the relationship, the patient should be sent a letter of withdrawal via certified mail with a return receipt so that proof of termination is in the patient's health record (Fig. 11.2).

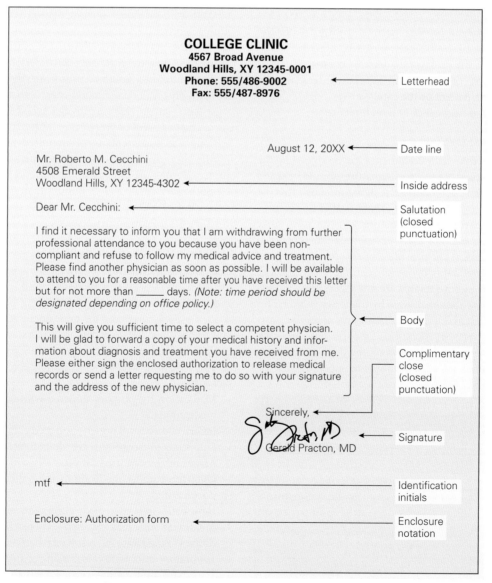

Fig. 11.2 Example of letter of withdrawal from a case.

COLLEGE CLINIC
4567 Broad Avenue
Woodland Hills, XY 12345-0001
Phone: 555/486-9002
Fax: 555/487-8976

September 3, 20XX

Mrs. Gregory Putnam
4309 North E Street
Woodland Hills, XY 12345-4398

Dear Mrs. Putnam:

This will confirm our telephone conversation today during which you discharged me from attending you as your physician in your present illness. In my opinion, your medical condition requires continued treatment by a physician. If you have not already obtained the services of another physician, I suggest you do so without further delay.

You may be assured that, upon your written authorization, I will furnish your new physician with information regarding the diagnosis and treatment you have received from me.

Very truly yours,

Gerald Procton, MD

mtf

Fig. 11.3 Letter to confirm discharge of a patient.

If the patient terminates the relationship, the health care provider should send a letter of confirmation of discharge when the patient states that they no longer desire care (Fig. 11.3). This should also be sent by certified mail with a return receipt requested.

If the patient leaves a health care facility against medical advice, the provider should send a letter confirming this. If there is a signed statement in the patient's facility records to this effect, it is not necessary to send a letter. If a letter is sent, a copy of the letter and return signature card from the post office must be filed with the patient's records.

If a noncompliant patient refuses a certified dismissal letter and it is returned unopened, file the returned letter and refusal notice in the patient's chart. Then, in a plain envelope, another copy of the letter should be sent to the patient. Document the date and time it was posted and the location of the mailbox used. Place these in the patient's chart and initial them. After 10 days, telephone the patient to confirm receipt of the correspondence. If the patient denies receiving it, read it over the telephone. In most regions, this will provide immunity against medical abandonment of a case, which is the discontinuance of medical care by a provider without proper notice. All record of notification attempts should be main-

tained in the patient's health record. This record should be retained per the health care organization's records retention policy.

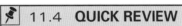

11.4 QUICK REVIEW
Question: What is the purpose of CDI?

11.5 QUICK REVIEW
Question: What is a query? How should one be performed?

11.6 QUICK REVIEW
Question: What are the three requirements for all types of documentation?

DOCUMENTATION GUIDELINES FOR DIAGNOSES

Problems can occur with documentation because of missing or misused essential words. Consider these two phrases: "heart failure due to diastolic dysfunction" or "diastolic dysfunction." The first statement gives more complete documentation of the medical condition. Always query the service provider if in doubt about the documentation to obtain the most specific, accurate terminology for the record.

Some providers document "imp" for impression or "Dx" for diagnosis, which usually serves as the diagnosis when completing the claim. If the diagnosis is not in the health record or there is doubt about the diagnosis, always ask the provider to review it. If the patient has been in a health care facility, request the electronic file of the discharge summary, which contains the admitting and discharge diagnoses.

The health care field uses many abbreviations and acronyms that can save time and aid in communication. However, they may be confusing in their interpretation. Often an abbreviation can be translated into several meanings. Official American Hospital Association (AHA) policy states that "abbreviations should be totally eliminated from the more vital sections of the health record, such as final diagnosis, operative notes, discharge summaries, and descriptions of special procedures." Many providers are not aware of this policy, and the final diagnosis may appear as an abbreviation in the patient's record.

The Joint Commission is an agency that provides accreditation status to health care organizations that comply with their standards of patient care. The Joint Commission has made it a mission to research what health care organizations provide the best health care to patients and has hundreds of performance standards with which organizations must comply. Its National Patient Safety Goal was initiated to improve communication between caregivers and has stated that health care facilities must take reasonable approaches to standardize abbreviations, acronyms, and symbols. For example, health care organizations can develop a standardized list of abbreviations or use a published reference source. When providers use multiple abbreviations, symbols, or acronyms for the same term, the organization must identify what they should use to eliminate any ambiguity.

In 2004 the Joint Commission created its "do not use" list of abbreviations (Table 11.1) for all organizations accredited through it. Use a medical dictionary to interpret an abbreviation or ask the provider when clarification is necessary—most list abbreviations alphabetically with the unabbreviated words.

If a lay term appears in a patient record, the correct medical term should be substituted to locate the correct diagnostic code. For example, use the term *contusion* when coding for bruise.

An *eponym* is a term including the name of a person, such as Graves' disease. Eponyms should not be used when a comparable anatomic term can be used in its place. A few examples of eponyms that describe medical conditions and their more appropriate documentation are included in Example 11.1.

EXAMPLE 11.1 Eponyms and Medical Terms

Eponym	Comparable Medical Term
Buerger disease	Thromboangiitis obliterans
Graves' disease	Exophthalmic goiter
Wilk's syndrome	Myasthenia gravis
Hartmann's procedure	Proctosigmoidectomy

The word *acute* refers to a condition that runs a short but relatively severe course. Acute conditions typically last 3 to 5 days. The word *chronic* means a condition persisting over a long period, often more than 3 months. *Subacute* refers to a condition that is both acute and chronic. When the terms *acute* and *chronic* are listed in the diagnostic statement, always search for these terms in the code description.

An abnormal or unexpected finding without elaboration in the health record is insufficient documentation and should be described. For example, if the provider documents that "the patient presents for review of abnormal labs," this would be insufficient. The provider should document more specifically, such as "the patient presents today for abnormally high blood sugar test results."

Commonly used phrases or abbreviations that may not support billing of services are "WNL" (within normal limits), "noncontributory," "negative/normal," "other than the above, all systems were normal," and so on. For example, phrases used to document findings, such as "all extremities are within normal limits," do not indicate how many extremities or which ones were examined. Documentation must indicate exactly which limb was examined. Providers who document that the patient's family history is "noncontributory" do not give any family background at all. Abbreviated wording will not pass an external audit. If it is determined that such phrases are copied from a template, it can mean that no assessment was actually performed. This is fraud.

TABLE 11.1 Do Not Use Abbreviations

Do Not Use	Potential Problem	Use Instead
U, u (unit)	Mistaken for "0" (zero), the number 4 (four), or "cc"	Write "unit"
IU (International Unit)	Mistaken for IV (intravenous) or the number 10 (ten)	Write "International Unit"
Q.D, QD, q.d., qd (daily) Q.O.D., QOD, q.o.d., qod (every other day)	Mistaken for each other. Period after the Q mistaken for "I" and the "O" mistaken for "I"	Write "daily" Write "every other day"
Trailing zero (X.0 mg) Lack of leading zero (.X mg)	Decimal point is missed	Write X mg Write 0.X mg
MS MSO$_4$ and MgSO$_4$	Can mean morphine sulfate or magnesium sulfate. Confused for one another	Write "morphine sulfate" Write "magnesium sulfate"

From "Facts About the Official 'Do Not Use' List of Abbreviations," Joint Commission, June 9, 2017, https://www.jointcommission.org/facts_about_do_not_use_list/.

Another word commonly used when a patient is examined, and the findings are within normal limits, is "negative." The note may contain phrases like "ears, nose, and throat negative" or "chest x-rays negative." The provider needs to document that there were no abnormalities in the system being examined. Detailed documentation justifies billed services by providing verification and provides supporting documentation when an external audit is performed.

11.7 QUICK REVIEW
Question: What is an eponym?

11.8 QUICK REVIEW
Question: What is the difference between acute, chronic, and subacute?

11.9 QUICK REVIEW
Question: What are some phrases that are not recommended in documentation?

DOCUMENTATION GUIDELINES FOR EVALUATION AND MANAGEMENT SERVICES

Terminology for Evaluation and Management Services

While learning the complexities of medical documentation and how important it is to coding and billing, a billing specialist must have a good foundation of medical terminology. A solid foundation of language, abbreviations, and symbols is important to use the diagnostic and procedure code books efficiently.

In the early 1990s, the American Medical Association (AMA) modified the term *office visits* and replaced this phrase with *office and other outpatient services*. The AMA also adopted the phrase *evaluation and management (E/M)* to describe the section of *Current Procedural Terminology* (CPT) in which those procedure codes appear. This wording better reflects the components involved when performing an office visit. However, E/M services are also performed in other settings, such as inpatient health care facilities and nursing homes.

New Versus Established Patient

In coding E/M services, two categories of patients are considered: the new patient and the established patient. A new patient is one who has not received any professional services within the last 3 years from the provider or another provider of the same specialty who belongs to the same health care organization. An established patient is one who has received professional services within the last 3 years from the provider or another provider of the same specialty who belongs to the same health care organization. Refer to the decision tree in Fig. 11.4 to help decide whether a patient is considered new or established.

A provider may determine a course of action to evaluate and manage a patient who is seeking medical care. Some of the options include the following:
- Refer to a specialist for consultation.
- See a referral from another provider.
- Give concurrent care as one of several providers.
- Render continuity of care for a provider who is out of town.
- Administer critical care.

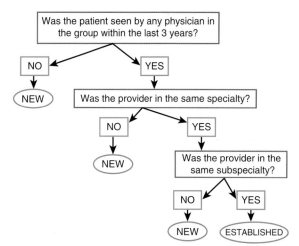

Decision Tree for New vs. Established Patients

Fig. 11.4 Decision tree for determining if a patient is a new patient versus established patient.

- Direct emergency care.
- Counsel the patient and/or the patient's family regarding diagnosis and treatment options.

Consultation

A consultation occurs when a provider is asked to provide an opinion or advice in the evaluation or treatment of a patient's illness or a suspected problem. The requesting provider must document the request in the patient's health record and the consulting provider should state: "Patient is seen at the request of Dr. John Doe for a … reason." Consultations may occur in a home, office, hospital, extended care facility, or other location. A consulting provider recommends diagnostic or therapeutic services and may initiate these services if requested by the referring provider. The opinion must be in writing, documented in a consultation report, and communicated to the referring physician. The consulting provider may order a diagnostic or therapeutic service to formulate the opinion at an initial or subsequent encounter.

Remember the four Rs: There must be a *requesting* physician, and the consultant must *render* an opinion and send a *report*. The requesting physician must document the reason for a consult in the patient's health *record*. A possible fifth R of consultations is *return*. The consulting physician must return the patient to the requesting physician for treatment of the problem so that no transfer of care is shown. Transfer of care is defined in the CPT manual as the process whereby a provider who is providing management for some, or all, of a patient's problems relinquishes this responsibility to another provider who agrees to accept this responsibility and is not merely providing a consultation.

Concurrent Care

Concurrent care occurs when one or more service providers deliver similar services to the same patient on the same day. For example, two internists, a general internist and a cardiologist, see the same patient in the hospital on the same day. The general internist admits the patient for diabetes and requests that the cardiologist also follows the patient's periodic chest pain and arrhythmia. If the second provider is not identified in carrier records as a different type of specialist, the claim may be denied. This is because the services appear to be duplicated by providers of the same specialty.

When billing insurance companies, providers giving concurrent care may be cross-referenced on the claim form. Medicare has a list that includes 99 specialties and subspecialties to help carriers more accurately judge whether concurrent care is necessary. Periodically, the provider should check with the carrier's provider service representative to determine whether the provider has updated its subspecialty status so that claims for concurrent care are not denied.

Continuity of Care

If a case involves continuity of care, there are two service providers who are both treating the patient's condition. For example, if a PCP refers a patient to a cardiologist, both providers should give the other a copy of the patient's records of care. In this way, the two providers will be aware of the treatments and medications being prescribed by the other. If the patient received treatment in a health care facility, the facility's health records department should provide copies of reports after treatment or after the patient's discharge to the patient's primary care provider.

Critical Care

Critical care refers to the intensive care provided for a variety of acute, life-threatening conditions requiring constant full attention by a provider. Critical care may sometimes, but not always, be rendered in a critical care area, such as a coronary care unit (CCU), intensive care unit (ICU), respiratory care unit (RCU), or emergency department (ED), also called an emergency room (ER). A critical illness or injury acutely impairs one or more vital organ systems. There is a high probability of imminent and life-threatening deterioration in the patient's condition. Examples of vital organ system failure include, but are not limited to, the following:

- Central nervous system failure
- Circulatory failure
- Shock
- Renal, hepatic, metabolic, or respiratory failure

For critical care services, time spent providing critical care must be documented.

Referral

A referral is the transfer of the total or specific care of a patient from one provider to another for known problems. It is not a consultation. For example, a patient is referred by a PCP to an orthopedist for the care of a fracture.

However, when dealing with managed care plans, the term *referral* is also used when requesting an authorization for the patient to receive services elsewhere (for example, referral for laboratory tests, radiology procedures, or specialty care). In most cases, the PCP must obtain authorization for the referral to ensure that the managed care plan will pay for the specialist's services. Appropriate documentation of the referral and authorization are needed to substantiate approval of the referral.

Emergency Care

Emergency care is care provided to acutely ill patients that may or may not involve organ system failure but does require immediate medical attention. An emergency may take place in any medical setting, not just an ED. In physician-directed emergency care advanced life support, the physician is located in a hospital emergency or critical care department and is in two-way voice communication with ambulance or rescue personnel outside the hospital. The physician directs the performance of necessary medical procedures.

According to CMS, an emergency medical condition is one that manifests itself by acute symptoms of sufficient severity. It is one that without immediate medical attention could lead to impairment of body functions, dysfunction of any body organ or part, or death. Examples of a medical emergency are as follows:

- Severe pain
- High fever
- Difficulty breathing
- Uncontrolled bleeding
- Chest pain
- Poisoning
- Broken bones
- Sudden facial drooping, slurred speech, or weakness in limbs
- Severe trauma (gunshot wound or crush injury from a car accident)
- Loss of consciousness

Counseling

Counseling is a discussion with a patient, family, or both. Counseling may concern diagnostic results, impressions, or recommended diagnostic studies. A health care provider may also counsel a patient or family about the prognosis, risks and benefits of treatment options, instructions for treatment or follow-up, or the importance of compliance with chosen treatment options. Counseling may also provide education, particularly in discussing lifestyle risk factors. For example, a provider may counsel a patient regarding weight loss or smoking cessation.

Documentation Guidelines for Evaluation and Management Services

The Center for Medicare and Medicaid Services (CMS) developed documentation guidelines for E/M services. The various E/M categories of services, such as Office and Outpatient Visits, Observation Care, Inpatient Hospital Care, Consultations, Emergency Department Services, and others, are coded based on what is referred to as the 1995 or 1997 documentation guidelines. To determine the appropriate level of service, a coding specialist relies on the health care provider's complete and accurate documentation to support the required elements for that category of services. Examples of required elements can include:

- Number of problems addressed at the encounter
- Severity and complexity of the presenting problem(s)
- Status of patient
- Level of history
- Level of examination
- Level of medical decision making
- Time spent on the date of the encounter and/or time spent counseling and coordinating care

The AMA released, and CMS approved, a modification of these guidelines that became effective January 1, 2021. The modification applies only to code selection for office and other outpatient visits. It did not change the requirements for proper documentation; however, it modified the required elements used to determine the appropriate levels of service.

Chief Complaint

The health record should be accurate, complete, and legible. The documentation of each patient encounter should include the chief complaint or reason for the encounter. The chief complaint (CC) is a concise statement, usually in the patient's own words, describing the symptom, problem, condition, diagnosis, provider-recommended return, or other factors that are the reason for the encounter. The chief complaint or presenting problem(s) are identified by five types which are: minimal, self-limited or minor, low severity, moderate severity, or high severity.

History

The record of the encounter must also include a medically appropriate history. It is dependent upon clinical judgment and on the nature of the presenting problem(s). There are four types of history: a problem-focused history, an expanded problem-focused history, a detailed history, or a comprehensive history.

History of present illness. The history should include a relevant history of present illness (HPI). This is a chronologic description of the development of the patient's present illness from the first sign or symptom or from the previous encounter to the present. If the health care provider is unable to obtain a sufficient diagnosis for the patient's condition, the health record documentation must reflect this. The history may include one or more of the following eight descriptive elements:

1. Location—Area of the body where the symptom is occurring.
2. Quality—Character of the symptom or pain. Examples of this may be burning, gnawing, stabbing, fullness.
3. Severity—Degree of symptom or pain on a scale from 1 to 10. Severity also can be described with terms such as *severe*, *slight*, and *persistent*.
4. Duration—How long the symptom or pain has been present and how long it lasts each time the patient experiences it.
5. Timing—When the pain or symptom occurs. For example, symptoms may occur in the morning/evening or after/before meals.
6. Context—The situation associated with the pain or symptom. For example, a patient may have pain after he ingests dairy products or big meals or at times of increased activity.
7. Modifying factors—Things done to make the symptom or pain worse or better. For example, a patient may state, "If I eat spicy foods, I get heartburn, but if I drink milk afterward, the pain is not as bad."
8. Associated signs and symptoms—The symptom or pain and other things that happen when the symptom or pain occurs. For example, a patient may note that her chest pain leads to shortness of breath.

See Fig. 11.5 for an example of history documentation.

Review of systems. The history should also include an appropriate review of systems (ROS). An ROS is an inventory of body systems obtained through a series of questions used to identify signs or symptoms that the patient might be experiencing or has experienced. It is important to note that an ROS is not an examination. The provider does not physically examine the patient in this section but merely asks questions. For example, if a patient has lost his or her balance and fallen and now presents for a laceration of the head as a result of the fall, the provider may question the patient as to whether they have had any dizziness or headaches. This would be considered a neurologic review of symptoms. The provider is asking the questions to determine the reason for the fall and identify any associated or underlying conditions. Checklists are permitted, but if a body system is not considered, it should be crossed out. For an ROS, constitutional symptoms (e.g., fever, weight loss) and the following systems are recognized: eyes, ears, nose, mouth, throat, cardiovascular, respiratory, gastrointestinal, genitourinary, musculoskeletal, integumentary (skin or breast), neurologic, psychiatric, endocrine, hematologic, lymphatic, allergic, and immunologic.

Past, family, social history. Another important part of a patient's history includes the past, family, and social histories (PFSH). This consists of a review of three areas:

1. Past history (PH)—The patient's past experiences with illnesses, operations, injuries, and treatments. E/M documents should also include active problem lists as well as a history of significant past diagnoses such as cancer. Medications prescribed and taken should be listed, specifying frequency and dosage.
2. Family history (FH)—A review of medical events in the patient's family, including diseases that may be hereditary or place the patient at risk.
3. Social history (SH)—An age-appropriate review of past and current activities, including smoking, drug use, and consumption of alcohol.

Physical Examination.

The record of the encounter must also include a medically appropriate physical examination (PE or PX) of the patient. The extent of the examination performed is dependent upon clinical judgment and the nature of the presenting problem(s). There are four types of examination which include a problem-focused exam, an expanded problem-focused exam, a detailed exam, or a comprehensive exam.

For purposes of examination, the following body areas and organ systems are recognized.

- Constitutional (vital signs, general appearance)
- Eyes
- Ears, nose, mouth, and throat
- Neck
- Respiratory
- Cardiovascular
- Chest, including breasts and axillae
- Gastrointestinal (abdomen)
- Genitourinary (male)
- Genitourinary (female)
- Lymphatic
- Musculoskeletal
- Skin

Hospital number: 00-83-06

Scott, Aimee

Rex Rumsey, MD

HISTORY

CHIEF COMPLAINT: Pain and bleeding after each bowel movement for the past 3 to 4 months.

PRESENT ILLNESS: This 68-year-old white female says she usually has three bowel movements a day in small amounts, and there has been a change in the last 3 to 4 months in frequency, size, and type of bowel movement. She has slight burning pain and irritation in the rectal area after bowel movements. The pain lasts for several minutes, then decreases in intensity. She has had no previous anorectal surgery or rectal infection. She denies any blood in the stool itself or associated symptoms. Bright red blood occurs after stools have passed.

PAST HISTORY:
ILLNESSES: The patient had polio at age 8 from which she has made a remarkable recovery. Apparently, she was paralyzed in both lower extremities and now has adequate use of these. She has no other serious illnesses.

ALLERGIES: ALLERGIC TO PENICILLIN. She denies any other drug or food allergies.
MEDICATIONS: None.
OPERATIONS: Right inguinal herniorrhaphy 25 years ago.

SOCIAL HISTORY: She does not smoke or drink. She lives with her husband who is an invalid and for whom she cares. She is a retired former municipal court judge.

FAMILY HISTORY: One brother died of cancer of the throat (age 59), and another has cancer of the kidney (age 63).

REVIEW OF SYSTEMS:
SKIN: No rashes or jaundice.
HEENT: Head normocephalic. Normal TMs. Normal hearing. Pupils equal, round, reactive to light. Deviated septum. Oropharynx clear.
CR: No history of chest pain, shortness of breath, or pedal edema. She has had some mild hypertension in the past but is not under any medical supervision nor is she taking any medication for this.
GI: Weight is stable. See present illness.
OB-GYN: Gravida II Para II. Climacteric at age 46, no sequelae.
EXTREMITIES: No edema.
NEUROLOGIC: Unremarkable.

mtf
D: 5-17-20XX
T: 5-20-20XX

_____
Rex Rumsey, MD

Fig. 11.5 Example of a medical report showing documentation of history.

- Neurologic
- Psychiatric

See Fig. 11.6 for an example of how exam documentation compares to ROS documentation in an office note.

Medical Decision Making

Medical decision making (MDM) is a health care management process done after performing a history and PE on a patient that results in a plan of treatment. MDM is documented as the provider's assessment, clinical impression, or diagnosis, as well as the plan for care. MDM refers to the complexity of managing the conditions presented. It is measured by:

- The number of possible diagnoses and/or the number of management or treatment options that are considered.
- The amount or complexity of medical records, diagnostic tests, or other information obtained, reviewed, or analyzed, and the risk of complications or associated morbidity or mortality.

Morbidity is a diseased condition or state, whereas *mortality* refers to death. It is also based on any comorbidities the patient may have which affect management options.

There are four types of MDM recognized which are: straightforward MDM, low complexity, moderate complexity, and high complexity MDM.

Example of ROS

CONSTITUTIONAL: The patient denies fever, fatigue, weakness, weight gain or weight loss.

HEAD, EYES, EARS, NOSE AND THROAT: The patient denies ringing in the ears, post nasal drip, sore throat, hoarseness.

CARDIOVASCULAR: The patient denies chest pain, shortness of breath.

RESPIRATORY: The patient denies cough, wheezing.

GASTROINTESTINAL: The patient denies decreased appetite, nausea, vomiting.

MUSCULOSKELETAL: The patient denies joint or muscle pain.

NEUROLOGIC: The patient denies headache.

Example of
Exam

CONSTITUTIONAL: The vital signs showed that the patient was afebrile; blood pressure and heart rate were within normal limits. The patient appeared alert.

EYES: The conjunctiva was clear. The pupil was equal and reactive. There was no ptosis. The irides appeared normal.

EARS, NOSE AND THROAT: The ears and the nose appeared normal in appearance. Hearing was grossly intact. The oropharynx showed that the mucosa was moist. There was no lesion that I could see in the palate, tongue. tonsil or posterior pharynx.

NECK: The neck was supple. The thyroid gland was not enlarged by palpation.

RESPIRATORY: The patient's respiratory effort was normal. Auscultation of the lung showed it to be clear with good air movement.

CARDIOVASCULAR: Auscultation of the heart revealed S1 and S2 with regular rate with no murmur noted. The extremities showed no edema.

BREASTS: Breast inspection showed them to be symmetrical with no nipple discharge. Palpation of the breasts and axilla revealed no obvious mass that I could appreciate.

GASTROINTESTINAL: The abdomen was soft, nontender with no rebound, no guarding, no enlarged liver or spleen. Bowel sounds were present.

GU: The external genitalia appeared to be normal. The pelvic exam revealed no adnexal masses. The uterus appeared to be normal in size and there was no cervical motion tenderness.

LY1\1PHATIC: There was no appreciated node that I could feel in the groin or neck area.

MUSCULOSKELETAL: The head and neck by inspection showed no obvious deformity. Again, the extremities showed no obvious deformity. Range of motion appeared to be normal for the upper and lower extremities.

SKIN: Inspection of the skin and subcutaneous tissues appeared to be normal. The skin was pink, warm and dry to touch.

NEUROLOGIC: Deep tendon reflexes were symmetrical at the patellar area. Sensation was grossly intact by touch.

PSYCHIATRIC: The patient was oriented to time, place and person. The patient's judgment and insight appeared to be normal.

Fig. 11.6 Review of systems (ROS) compared to physical exam documentation.

Supporting documentation for MDM includes documentation of any findings and prior diagnostic test results. Patient and family education and specific instructions for follow-up should also be noted. Providers should outline the patient's progress, response to and changes in treatment, planned follow-up care, and instructions. Any patient refusal to follow medical advice should be documented and a letter sent to the patient about this noncompliance.

All laboratory and medical tests ordered should be documented in the health record. When the report is received, the provider should initial the report, indicating that it has been read.

Requests for consultations from the attending or treating physician and the reason for consultation must be documented. The consultant's opinion and any services ordered or performed must be documented and communicated to the requesting physician.

Treatment must be consistent with the working diagnosis. Procedure and diagnostic codes reported on the health insurance claim form or billing statement should be supported by the documentation in the health record and be at a level sufficient for a clinical peer to determine whether services have been coded accurately. See Fig. 11.7 for an example of a complete E/M document for an office visit.

Patient: **Ryan Egbert**   **Date of service: 8/6/20XX**
DOB: **4/2/20XX**

CHIEF COMPLAINT: A 5-month-old boy with cough.

HISTORY OF PRESENT ILLNESS: A 5-month-old boy brought by his parents because of 2 days of cough. Mother took him when cough started 2 days go to Clinic where they told the mother he has viral infection and gave him Tylenol, but yesterday at night cough got worse and he also started having fever. Mother did not measure it.

REVIEW OF SYSTEMS: No vomiting. No diarrhea. He had runny nose started with the cough two days ago. No skin rash. No cyanosis. Pulling on his right ear. Feeding, he is bottle-fed 2 ounces every 2 hours. Mother states he urinates like 5 to 6 times a day, stools 1 time a day. He is still feeding good to mom.

IMMUNIZATIONS: He received first set of shot and due for the second set on 01117/2008.

BIRTH HISTORY: He was premature at 33 weeks born at Hospital kept in NICU for 2 weeks for feeding problem as the mother said. Mother had good prenatal care at 4 weeks for more than 12 visits. No complications during pregnancy. Rupture of membranes happened two days before the labor. Mother received the antibiotics, but she is not sure, if she received steroids also or not.

FAMILY HISTORY: No history of asthma or lung disease.

SOCIAL HISTORY: Lives with parents and with two siblings, one 18-year-old and the other is 14-year-old in house, in Corrales. They have animals, but outside the house and father smokes outside house. No sick contacts as the mother said.

PAST MEDICAL HISTORY: No hospitalizations. History of 2 previous ear infection, last one was in last November treated with ear drops, because there was pus coming from the right ear as the mother said.

ALLERGIES: NO KNOWN DRUG ALLERGIES.

MEDICATIONS: No medications.

PHYSICAL EXAMINATION:

VITAL SIGNS: Temperature 100.1, heart rate 184, respiratory rate 48. Weight 7 kg.

GENERAL: In no acute distress.

HEAD: Normocephalic and atraumatic. Open, soft, and flat anterior fontanelle.

NECK: Supple.

NOSE: Dry secretions.

EAR: Right ear full of yellowish material most probably pus and necrotic tissue. Tympanic membrane bilaterally visualized.

MOUTH: No pharyngitis. No ulcers. Moist mucous membranes.

CHEST: Bilateral audible breath sound. No wheezes. No palpitation.

HEART: Regular rate and rhythm with no murmur.

ABDOMEN: Soft, nontender, and nondistended.

GENITOURINARY: Tanner I male with descended testes.

EXTREMITIES: Capillary refill less than 2 seconds.

LABS: White blood cell 8.1, hemoglobin 10.5, hematocrit 30.9, and platelets 380,000. CRP 6, segments 41, and bands 41. RSV positive. Chest x-ray evidenced bronchiolitis with hyperinflation and bronchial wall thickening in the central hilar region. Subsegmental atelectasis in the right upper lobe and left lung base.

ASSESSMENT: A 5-month-old male with 2 days of cough and 1 day of fever. Chest x-ray shows bronchiolitis with atelectasis, and RSV antigen is positive.

DIAGNOSES: Respiratory syncytial virus bronchiolitis with right otitis extema.

PLAN: Plan was to admit to bronchiolitis pathway, and ciprofloxacin for right otitis extema eardrops twice daily.

Electronically signed by: Olivia Jones, MD; 8/6/20XX

Fig. 11.7 Example of a complete evaluation and management (E/M) office note.

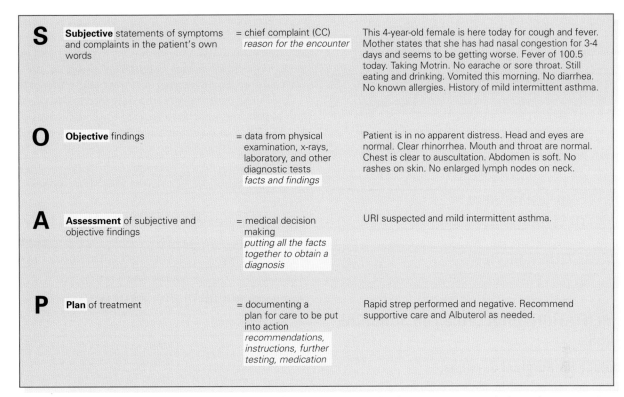

S	**Subjective** statements of symptoms and complaints in the patient's own words	= chief complaint (CC) *reason for the encounter*	This 4-year-old female is here today for cough and fever. Mother states that she has had nasal congestion for 3-4 days and seems to be getting worse. Fever of 100.5 today. Taking Motrin. No earache or sore throat. Still eating and drinking. Vomited this morning. No diarrhea. No known allergies. History of mild intermittent asthma.
O	**Objective** findings	= data from physical examination, x-rays, laboratory, and other diagnostic tests *facts and findings*	Patient is in no apparent distress. Head and eyes are normal. Clear rhinorrhea. Mouth and throat are normal. Chest is clear to auscultation. Abdomen is soft. No rashes on skin. No enlarged lymph nodes on neck.
A	**Assessment** of subjective and objective findings	= medical decision making *putting all the facts together to obtain a diagnosis*	URI suspected and mild intermittent asthma.
P	**Plan** of treatment	= documenting a plan for care to be put into action *recommendations, instructions, further testing, medication*	Rapid strep performed and negative. Recommend supportive care and Albuterol as needed.

Fig. 11.8 Explanation of the acronym SOAP (*s*ubjective, *o*bjective, *a*ssessment, *p*lan) used as a format for progress notes defining subjective and objective information, the assessment, and the treatment plan.

E/M Charting Procedures

Charting procedures for progress notes should be standardized. For office visits, the majority of health care providers in a paper-based system use a method called the SOAP (*s*ubjective, *o*bjective, *a*ssessment, *p*lan) style of documentation (Fig. 11.8). Some providers prefer to document using a narrative or more detailed descriptive style when creating a medical report such as history and physical report, operative report, radiologic report, or pathology report. Whatever method is used, the provider must ensure that it is detailed enough to support current documentation requirements.

When the insurance billing or coding specialist questions any procedure or diagnostic codes marked on the encounter form, the health care provider should approve a different code before a claim is transmitted to the insurance carrier (Fig. 11.9). Retain all billing records until they are no longer necessary by conforming to federal and state laws as well as to the health care organization's wishes.

> **! COMPLIANCE ALERT**
>
> Ensure that all health record entries are signed or electronically verified by the health care provider with his or her title or position. This offers clear evidence that the provider reviewed the note and ensures that they are aware of all test results, both normal and abnormal. Documented provider review of test results can be factored in when determining appropriate coding levels for service.

Record a patient's failure to return for needed treatment by noting it in the health record, in the appointment book, and on the financial record or ledger card. Follow up with a telephone call or send a letter to the patient advising him or her that further treatment is indicated.

For electronic health records, the software program should make an electronic record entry permanent when originally completed and authenticated. To make a correction, note that a section is in error with the date and time and enter the correct information with a notation of when and why the health care provider changed the entry. Authenticate the correction via electronic signature and date. Never delete or key over incorrect data in a computerized file. Another method for correcting a health record is to flag it as amended or obsolete and create an addendum either typed as a separate document or with a chart note inserted below in the next space available.

For paper-based records, use a permanent, not water-soluble, ink pen to cross out an incorrect entry on a patient's record. Mark

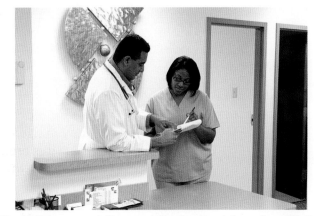

Fig. 11.9 Insurance billing specialist checking information with the health care provider before recording it on the insurance claim.

it with a single line and write the correct information, then date and initial the entry. Never erase, white out, or use self-adhesive paper over any information recorded on a patient record.

 11.10 QUICK REVIEW
Question: What is the difference between a new and established patient?

 11.11 QUICK REVIEW
Question: What is the difference between a consultation and a referral?

 11.12 QUICK REVIEW
Question: What are the criteria for determining medical decision making?

 11.13 QUICK REVIEW
Question: How should a provider make a correction to a medical record?

DOCUMENTATION GUIDELINES FOR SURGICAL SERVICES

Terminology for Surgical Services

There are many terms used in surgical documentation that a coding specialist will need to learn. For example, lateral is a positional term that means toward the sides, whereas medial means toward the center. Proximal means nearer the point of attachment, and distal means farther from the point of attachment. Superficial means external or closer to the surface, whereas deep means internal or closer to the center of the body.

The following terms are commonly used to describe the location of pain and injuries to areas of the abdomen, as shown in Fig. 11.10A (four quadrants) and Fig. 11.10B (nine regions):

Right upper quadrant (RUQ) or right hypochondriac	Liver (right lobe), gallbladder, part of the pancreas, parts of the small and large intestines
Epigastric	Upper middle region above the stomach
Left upper quadrant (LUQ) or left hypochondriac	Liver (left lobe), stomach, spleen, part of the pancreas, parts of the small and large intestines
Right and left lumbar	Middle, right, and left regions of the waist
Umbilical	Central region near the navel
Right lower quadrant (RLQ) or right inguinal	Parts of the small and large intestines, right ovary, right uterine (fallopian) tube, appendix, and right ureter
Hypogastric	Middle region below the umbilical region contains urinary bladder and female uterus
Left lower quadrant (LLQ) or left inguinal	Parts of the small and large intestines, left ovary, left uterine tube, and left ureter

A   B

Fig. 11.10 Regions of the abdomen. (A) Four quadrants. (B) Nine regions. (From Herlihy, B., & Maebius, N. K. [2011]. *The human body in health and illness* [4th ed.]. St. Louis: Elsevier.)

Two commonly used terms are *preoperative* and *postoperative*. Preoperative (preop) pertains to the period before a surgical procedure. Commonly the preoperative period begins with the first preparation of the patient for surgery and ends with the introduction of anesthesia in the operating suite. Postoperative (postop) pertains to the period after surgery. It begins with the patient's emergence from anesthesia and continues through the time required for the acute effects of the anesthetic and surgical procedures to decrease.

A billing specialist may type reports to be submitted with insurance claims to help justify the claims. Being familiar with the terms for various operational incisions is helpful (Fig. 11.11).

Terms such as *undermining* (cut in a horizontal fashion), *take down* (to take apart), or *lysis of adhesions* (destruction of scar tissue) appear in many operations. Note the position of the patient during the operation. For example, supine means the patient is placed face up, and prone means the patient is face down. The surgical approach should also be noted. Examples of surgical approaches would be *vaginal* or *abdominal*—these help to determine the proper code selection. Major errors can occur when an insurance billing specialist is not familiar with the medical terms being used. Ask the provider to clarify the case if there is a ques-

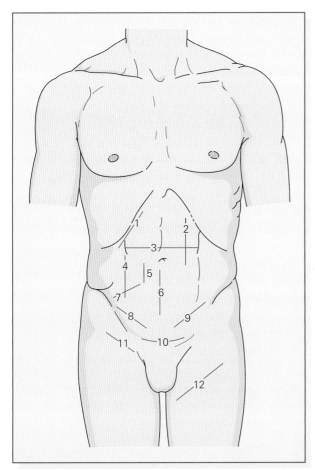

Fig. 11.11 Operational incisions. Anterior (front) view: *1,* Subcostal incision; *2,* paramedian incision; *3,* transverse incision; *4,* upper right rectus incision; *5,* midrectus incision; *6,* midline incision; *7,* lower right rectus incision; *8,* McBurney or right iliac incision; *9,* left iliac incision; *10,* suprapubic incision, *11,* hernia incision; *12,* femoral incision.

tion because medical terminology is technical and can puzzle even the most knowledgeable insurance billing specialist.

Documentation of Surgical Services

Prior to performing a surgery or medical procedure, the health care provider must obtain an informed consent for the procedure. Consent is required and should include written documentation that is kept in the medical record indicating that the diagnosis and procedure were discussed with the patient. A provider should also review potential risks of the procedure as well as any alternative procedures the patient may consider.

An operative report (Fig. 11.12) is dictated by a health care provider to describe the surgery or procedure performed. The report should be timely and dictated or written immediately after the procedure. There are usually four main sections in the report.

The header contains patient identifiers such as name, date of birth, account number and/or medical record number. It also contains the date of service, preoperative and post-operative diagnoses, the procedure performed, and the name of the provider. If the procedure is surgical, it will also list anesthesia and the anesthesia provider.

Next is a section that outlines the indication or reason for the surgery or procedure. This will outline the patient history and medical necessity for the service.

In the body of the report, the provider describes the procedure performed. This includes preparation for the procedure, approach, step-by-step details of the procedure, removal of any body parts or specimens, and any complications they encountered.

The final section of the operative report describes the findings, including estimated blood loss and how the patient did during and after the procedure.

If unusual circumstances cause surgery to take longer than usual and additional reimbursement is requested, time must be documented. If state-of-the-art instruments or equipment are used, document the equipment as well as the time spent using it.

Therapeutic or cosmetic surgical procedures should be broken down into two categories—state how much of the procedure was functional and how much was cosmetic or therapeutic. Generally, the insurance carrier pays for the functional portion of the procedure even if there is no coverage for cosmetic or therapeutic procedures. For example, if a surgeon performs an abdominoplasty (cosmetic) and an inguinal hernia, he will need to indicate how much of the time was dedicated to each procedure. Most insurance companies will not pay for cosmetic procedures, and the physician will need to collect his reimbursement for the abdominoplasty from the patient.

11.14 QUICK REVIEW
Question: What do preoperative and postoperative mean?

11.15 QUICK REVIEW
Question: What is an informed consent?

11.16 QUICK REVIEW
Question: What is documented in the header of an operative report?

XYZ Hospital

PATIENT: Rachel Smith
DATE OF BIRTH: 12/2 1/20XX
DATE OF SERVICE: 03/14/20XX
PREOPERATIVE DIAGNOSIS: Adenoid and tonsillar hypertrophy and recurrent pharyngitis.
POSTOPERATIVE DIAGNOSIS: Adenoid and tonsillar hypertrophy and recurrent pharyngitis.
PROCEDURE PERFORMED: Tonsillectomy and Adenoidectomy.
SURGEON: Martin Hall, .tv1D
ANESTHESIA: General endotracheal.
ANESTHESIA TEAM: Samuel Hawley, .tv1D and Melissa Reynolds, CRNA
SURGICAL FINDINGS: A 4+/4+ cryptic and hypertrophic tonsils with 2+/3+ hypertrophic adenoid pads.
INDICATIONS:

We were requested to evaluate the patient for complaints of enlarged tonsils, which cause difficulty swallowing, recurrent pharyngitis, and sleep-induced respiratory disturbance. She was evaluated and scheduled for an elective procedure.

DESCRIPTION OF PROCEDURE:

The patient was brought to the operative suite and placed supine on the operating room table. General anesthetic was administered. Once appropriate anesthetic findings were achieved, the patient was intubated and prepped and draped in the usual sterile manner for a tonsillectomy. He was placed in semi-Rose position and a Crowe Davis-type mouth gag was introduced into the oropharynx. Under an operating headlight, the oropharynx was clearly visualized. The right tonsil was grasped with the fossa triangularis and using electrocautery enucleation technique, was removed from its fossa. This followed placing the patient in a suspension position using a Mclvor-type mouth gag and a red rubber Robinson catheter via the right naris. Once the right tonsil was removed, the left tonsil was removed in a similar manner, once again using a needle point Bovie dissection at 20 watts. With the tonsils removed, it was possible to visualize the adenoid pads. The oropharynx was irrigated and the adenoid pad evaluated with an indirect mirror technique. The adenoid pad was greater than 2+/4 and hypertrophic. Itwas removed with successive passes of electrocautery suction. The tonsillar fossa was then once again hemostased with suction cautery, injected with 0.5% ropivacaine with 1:100,000 adrenal solution and then closed with 2-0 Monocryl on an SH needle. The redundant soft tissue of the uvula was removed posteriorly and cauterized with electrocautery to prevent swelling of the uvula in the postoperative period. The patient's oropharynx and nasopharynx were irrigated with copious amounts of normal saline contained with small amount of iodine, and she was recovered from her general endotracheal anesthetic. She was extubated and left the operating room in good condition to the postoperative recovery room area.

FINDINGS:

Estimated blood loss was minimal. There were no complications. Specimens produced were right and left tonsils. The adenoid pads were ablated with electrocautery. The patient tolerated the procedure well and left the operating room in good condition.

Electronically Signed: Martin Hall, .tvm; 03/l 4/20XX

Fig. 11.12 Example of an operative report.

DOCUMENTATION GUIDELINES FOR ANESTHESIA SERVICES

Terminology in Anesthesia Services

There are various types of anesthesia that coding and billing specialist should understand.

Local or topical anesthesia involves numbing a specific part of the body to prevent any feeling of pain during surgical procedures. This type of anesthesia is often applied in an office setting or by the surgeon and does not require anesthesia providers. This is a common choice for in-office dermatology procedures or lesion removal.

Moderate or conscious sedation is a drug-induced depression of consciousness during which patients can respond purposefully to verbal commands, either alone or accompanied by light tactile stimulation. Patients may remember little to none of the procedure. This type of anesthesia is often provided by surgeons or surgical staff, but sometimes an anesthesia provider.

Regional anesthesia is medication injected near a cluster of nerves to numb only the area of the body that requires surgery. The patient may remain awake or may be given a sedative. Spinal anesthetics is administered into the cerebral spinal fluid. This is a common choice for procedures occurring below the waist, such as total knee replacements, and is also used in c-sections. Epidurals are placed in the epidural space of the spine that corresponds with the area being treated. Probably the most common example would be the epidural catheter placed for labor and delivery.

General anesthesia is a medically induced state of unconsciousness and loss of protective reflexes. This is used for cases requiring deep sedation, such as complicated abdominal surgery or mastectomies. The anesthesia provider usually inserts a breathing tube to help protect the patient's airway. The patient is not able to communicate or follow commands. Several types of medication are used during a general anesthetic plan, such as analgesics for pain, sedation, amnesiacs to lessen awareness, and paralytics to prevent movement and reflexive actions.

Anesthesia providers may also use invasive monitoring devices to help them keep an eye on their patients, particularly during complex surgeries or those performed on high-risk patients. These include A-lines, central lines, and Swan Ganz.

An *arterial line (A-line)* is a catheter that allows measurement of your blood pressure on a continuous basis directly from an artery. A-lines are placed either percutaneously through a needle puncture in the skin or cutdown through an incised opening over a vein.

A *central line* is a long catheter placed in your neck veins, either the internal jugular or subclavian veins, reaching down to where the superior vena cava enters the heart. It is like a large IV line that is always placed under sterile conditions. It is used to administer medications or large amounts of fluid and to replace blood.

A *Swan-Ganz* is a flow-directed pulmonary artery catheter. It is introduced through a large neck vein, similar to a central line. It is primarily a diagnostic device, allowing doctors to measure the pressure inside the heart chambers and lung vessels, as well as the amount of blood being pumped out of the heart. It also helps monitor the effects of heart and blood pressure medications during surgery. A temperature sensor at the tip of the catheter measures blood temperature.

Anesthesia services may also include procedures like *nerve blocks* for postoperative or chronic pain management. When an anesthesia provider performs a nerve block, they inject an anesthetic close to a nerve that supplies the body part that is in pain. This produces a loss of sensation and provides pain relief.

Documentation of Anesthesia Services

Anesthesia documentation is different than most other specialties as it is not usually presented in narrative form. Some anesthesia services, such as line placement and postoperative nerve blocks of pain management, should be explained in a detailed paragraph like an operative report. However, when documenting anesthesia services for surgeries, documentation is often in a grid format where the provider uses hash marks to notate various vital signs, such as temperature, heart rate, and oxygen levels, that are monitored throughout the procedure. See Fig. 11.13 for an example of a blank anesthesia record. Anesthesia providers must meet pre-anesthesia, anesthesia, and post-anesthesia documentation requirements.

Like most other types of documentation, anesthesia records must include the patient's name and other appropriate identifiers, date of service, and the signature of the anesthesia provider. It must also contain the name of the surgeon, surgical procedure, type of anesthesia, anesthesia start and stop times, postoperative diagnosis, any underlying conditions that make the patient higher risk, and any medications given with dosages and times. Complete documentation for anesthesia providers must include the following:

- Pre-anesthesia
  - The reason for the procedure or service (diagnosis)
  - Any additional conditions warranting the use of anesthesia such as age, mental status, etc.
  - A preanesthetic examination and evaluation
  - A written anesthesia plan
- Anesthesia
  - Indication that anesthesia provider was present throughout the procedure
  - Intraoperative evaluation of the patient
  - Check of equipment, drugs, and so on
  - Intraoperative monitoring of the patient
  - Patient vital signs including temperature, oxygenation, ventilation, and circulation
  - Amounts of all drugs and agents used, including times given
  - Unusual events occurring during the anesthesia monitoring period
  - Total time, specifying anesthesia start, time in the operating room, time leaving operating room, and anesthesia end
- Post-Anesthesia
  - Evaluation on admission to the postanesthesia care unit (PACU)
  - Time-based record of vital signs and level of consciousness in PACU
  - Drugs provided to the patient in PACU, including the dosage and time

Date: _____ OR#: _____   Inpatient   Oupatient   **XYZ Hospital**

Anesthesia type: _____

Procedure: ☐Rt ☐Lt ☐Bilateral

_____   **Anesthesia Record**

_____

Surgeon(s): _____

Patient Label

ASA Level: 1 2 3 4 5 E ☐add on case

Hx: _____   Post-op Dx: _____

Emergency   Transfer care to: ☐PACU ☐ASU

Dx: _____   B/P: _____ P: _____ RR: _____ SaO₂: _____

IV Abx ☐None ordered ☐Med & Time: _____   Total IV fluids: _____ Urine Output: _____

Anes. start: _____ Time in OR: _____ Anes. End: _____   Blood Products: _____ EBL: _____

Position: ☐ Prone ☐ Lateral ☐ Beach Chr. ☐ Arms abducted less than 90° ☐ Controlled Hypotension

TIME																		Total Meds
O2 L/min																		
N2O Air L/min																		
Midazolam mg																		
Fentanyl ml																		
Propofol mg																		
Reglan mg																		
Succinylcholine mg																		
Rocuronium mg																		
Ondansetron mg																		
Lidocaine mg																		
Sa O2																		
ETCO2																		
EKG																		
Temp																		
BP, P																		
200																		
180																		
160																		
140																		
120																		
100																		
90																		
60																		
40																		
20																		
0																		

☐A-line site: _____
☐Indwelling
  ☐placed in OR
  ☐U/S
☐Distal pulse intact

☐CVP site: _____
☐Indwelling
  ☐placed in OR
  ☐U/S

IV Arm/hand/foot
☐Rt ☐Lt size: _____
☐Indwelling
  ☐placed in OR
☐Other:

☐Anes. Machine checked
☐ECG ☐PNS
☐BP cuff ☐Rt ☐Lt
☐Pulse Oximetry
☐Capnometer
☐Oxygen Analyzer
☐Humidifier/Humivent
☐Blood/Fluid Warmer
☐Thermal warming unit

☐Oro/NG tube
☐Natural Airway
☐O₂ Nasal Cannula
☐Oral/Nasal Airway
☐Mask
☐LMA # _____
☐Intubation
  ☐Oral _____
  ☐Nasal _____
  ☐Cuff _____
☐ETT _____ cm lips
☐Xylocaine jelly
☐LTA
☐RSI w/cricoid
☐Bil. Br. Sounds
☐+ ETCO₂
☐Smooth ☐Atraumatic
☐Difficult: _____

☐OLV
☐Eye care oint/tape

Remarks:

MD/DO directed anesthetic and was present for all key portions

Sign in / Sign out	Signature

Fig. 11.13 Example of a blank anesthesia record.

- Any unusual post-anesthesia events or complications
- Post-anesthesia visits and follow-up
- Initiation of any pain management services
- Patient's outcome/response/tolerance

 11.17 QUICK REVIEW

Question: What is the difference between regional and general anesthesia?

 11.18 QUICK REVIEW

Question: What makes anesthesia documentation different than documentation for other types of services?

DOCUMENTATION GUIDELINES FOR RADIOLOGY SERVICES

Terminology for Radiology Services

Radiology involves using medical imaging to diagnose and/or treat disease. There are various methods used to visualize areas of the body, including the following:

- **Ultrasound** uses sound waves to visualize internal structures such as organs, muscles, and tendons.
- **X-ray** uses x-rays to visualize solid, dense internal structures like bone.
- **Computed Tomography (CT)** uses a series of X-rays to visualize a cross-section of the body.
- **Magnetic Resonance Imaging (MRI)** uses a magnetic field and protons in the body to produce a cross-section image of ligaments, the brain, spinal cord, heart, and other internal organs.

Other types of services in the radiology specialty include radiation oncology, guidance, and nuclear medicine.

Radiology services use a number of terms to describe the position of the patient and the direction of the image. The following is a list of common terms.

Anteroposterior (AP)	Front to back
Oblique (OBL)	Angled
Posteroanterior (PA)	Back to front
Stereo	Two views taken at different angles
Anatomical position	Standing upright, feet flat, and directed forward
Coronal (Frontal) plane	Divides the body into front and back sections
Sagittal plane	Divides the body into left and right sides
Transverse plane	Divides the body into top and bottom portions

Fig. 11.14 shows the various planes.

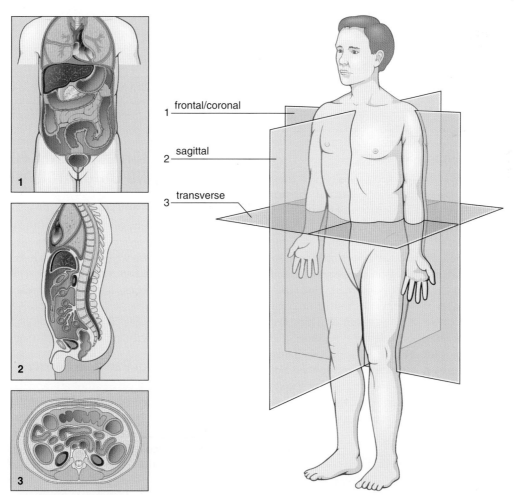

Fig. 11.14 Planes of the body. The figure is in the anatomic position. 1, Frontal (Coronal) plane; 2, Sagittal plane; 3, Transverse plane. Note the views of the body represented by each plane. (Modified from Chabner, E. [2021]. *The language of medicine* [12th ed.]. St. Louis: Elsevier.)

Southview Radiology Group

Patient: Jane Goodson

Date of Birth: 01/05/19XX

Date of Service: 08/22/20XX

Ordering Provider: X. A. Zanderhoven, MD

EXAM: Chest X-Ray, PA & Lateral.

REASON FOR EXAM: Shortness of breath, evaluate for pneumothorax versus left-sided effusion.

INTERPRETATION: There has been interval development of a moderate left-sided pneumothorax with near complete collapse of the left upper lobe. The lower lobe appears aerated. There is stable, diffuse, bilateral interstitial thickening with no definite acute air space consolidation. The heart and pulmonary vascularity are within normal limits. Left-sided port is seen with Groshong tip at the SVC/RA junction. No evidence for acute fracture, malalignment, or dislocation.

IMPRESSION:

1. Interval development of moderate left-sided pneumothorax with corresponding left lung atelectasis.

2. Rest of visualized exam nonacute/stable.

3. Left central line appropriately situated and stable.

4. Preliminary report was issued at time of dictation. Dr. X. A. Zanderhoven was called with results.

Authenticated and Electronically Signed: Jeffrey Rockefeller, MD; 8/22/20XX; 18:32

Fig. 11.15 Example of a radiology report.

Documentation of Radiology Services

All radiology services require a written order. This request must include the patient's name, the service being requested, the reason for the request, and the name and signature of the ordering provider.

A radiology report (Fig. 11.15) must be dictated after the service is performed. To be complete, the report must include the date and time of the service, the reason for the service, and a detailed statement about the service performed. This statement should include whether the exam was limited or complete and the number and type of views taken. If a contrast material is used, the report must include the type, dose, and method of administration. If there are prior studies available, any comparison should be noted. The radiologist's conclusions and findings must also be included. The radiologist should also note any discussions with the ordering provider, as well as any follow-up studies they recommend. Lastly, the report must be signed.

> **11.19   QUICK REVIEW**
> Question: What are the coronal, sagittal, and transverse planes?

> **11.20   QUICK REVIEW**
> Question: What must be documented if contrast is used?

DOCUMENTATION GUIDELINES FOR PATHOLOGY AND LABORATORY SERVICES

Terminology in Path/Lab Services

Pathology is the study of tissue and cells to determine the disease process. These services include biopsies on tissue removed from living patients as well as those who have died to determine the cause of death. Laboratory services, in contrast, refer to medical tests performed for diagnosis, treatment, and prevention of disease. A gross examination looks at the entire specimen with the bare eye. Microscopy slices the specimen into slides and examines them under a microscope.

Documentation of Path/Lab Services

Like radiology services, pathology and laboratory services cannot be performed without a written order. When an ordering provider uses lab results to determine a patient's diagnosis, the results must be documented in the E/M record. The provider should document the type of test ordered, the normal range of the test, and whether the result is normal or abnormal.

In order for a pathology or laboratory report to be complete, it must contain the patient's name and other appropriate identifiers, the name of the laboratory and the ordering provider, the date and time of collection, and the date and time the laboratory

Southside Pathology Associates

Patient: Joshua Martin
Date of Birth: 07/15/ 19XX
Date of Service: 11/01/20XX

SPECIMENS:
1. Pelvis-right pelvic obturator node.
2. Pelvis-left pelvic obturator node.
3. Prostate.

POST-OPERATIVE DIAGNOSIS: Adenocarcinoma of prostate, erectile dysfunction.

DIAGNOSTIC OPINION:
1. Adenocarcinoma, Gleason score 9, with tumor extension to periprostatic tissue, margin involvement, and tumor invasion to seminal vesicle, prostate.
2. No evidence of metastatic carcinoma, right pelvic obturator lymph node.
3. Metastatic adenocarcinoma, left obturator lymph node; see description.

CLINICAL HISTORY: None listed.

GROSS DESCRIPTION:

Specimen #1 labeled "right pelvic obturator lymph nodes" consists of two portions of adipose tissue measuring
2.5 x 1x 0.8 cm and 2.5 x 1x 0.5 cm. There are two lymph nodes measuring 1 x 0.7 cm and 0.5 x 0.5 cm. The entire specimen is cut into several portions and totally embedded.

Specimen #2 labeled "left pelvic obturation lymph nodes" consists of an adipose tissue measuring 4 x 2 x 1 cm. There are two lymph nodes measuring 1.3 x 0.8 cm and 1 x 0.6 cm. The entire specimen is cut into 1 cm. The entire specimen is cut into several portions and totally embedded.

Specimen #3 labeled "prostate" consists of a prostate. It measures 5 x 4.5 x 4 cm. The external surface shows very small portion of seminal vesicles attached in both sides with tumor induration. External surface also shows tumor induration especially in right side. External surface is stained with green ink. The cut surface shows diffuse tumor induration especially in right side. The tumor appears to extend to excision margin. Multiple representative sections are made.

MICROSCOPIC DESCRIPTION:

Section #1 reveals lymph node. There is no evidence of metastatic carcinoma.

Section #2 reveals lymph node with tumor metastasis in section of large lymph node as well as section of small lymph node.

Section #3 reveals adenocarcinoma of prostate. Gleason's score 9 (5+4). The tumor shows extension to periprostatic tissue as well as margin involvement. Seminal vesicle attached to prostate tissue shows tumor invasion. Dr. XXX reviewed the above case. His opinion agrees with the above diagnosis.

SUMMARY:

A. Adenocarcinoma of prostate, Gleason's score 9, with both lobe involvement and seminal vesicle involvement (T3b).

B. There is lymph node metastasis (N1).

C. Distant metastasis cannot be assessed (MX).

D. Excision margin is positive and there is tumor extension to periprostatic tissue.

Electronically Signed: Colette Baker, MD; 11 101/20XX; 17:25

Fig. 11.16 Example of a pathology report.

received the specimen. Once tests are run, a detailed description of the test performed and the result must also be included. There should be a signature and the date and time of the report. See Fig. 11.16.

11.21 QUICK REVIEW

Question: What is the difference between pathology and laboratory services?

DOCUMENTATION GUIDELINES FOR MEDICAL SERVICES

The medicine section of the CPT has a variety of tests and procedures for all specialties. Examples of types of services covered in this section range from injections and immunizations to infusions and dialysis to psychiatric services. Coding and billing specialists who are working with each type of service should search the CMS website for specific documentation guidelines to ensure compliance. Each area has its own documentation requirements. Outpatient therapy services will be outlined as an example.

Outpatient Therapy Services

Outpatient therapy services include occupational therapy, physical therapy, and speech-language pathology therapy. Patients may be referred for these services for a variety of reasons ranging from acute injury to arthritis, side effects from myocardial or cerebrovascular infarction (heart attack or stroke), or dementia. The goal of these types of services is to restore function, reduce pain, and improve daily life activities for the patient following an injury, surgery, or illness.

Physical therapy services focus on improving strength, mobility, range of motion, and flexibility. These include a variety of modalities, some requiring constant attendance from the therapist, others that the patient can do independently without one-on-one supervision. A modality is defined in the CPT as any physical agent applied to produce therapeutic changes to biological tissue. Examples of modalities used in therapy services include heat, ice, traction, infrared light, ultraviolet light, electrical stimulation, and massage. Therapists also use various exercises, both assisted and independent, to help strengthen and stretch muscles, tendons, and ligaments.

Occupational therapy evaluates performance deficits a patient may have in day-to-day life activities. These may be from physical, cognitive, or psychological impairments. An occupational therapist will assist a patient in learning to adapt to these impairments and perform daily tasks. For example, if a patient has a physical limitation due to a stroke, the therapist may help them learn a new way to hold a fork or button their shirt, or they may help an elderly patient learn how to prevent falls in their home.

Speech-language pathology services involve assisting patients with communication deficits. Some of these patients may have a developmental impairment that they were born with, while others may have acquired their impairment following an injury or due to age-related dementia. A communication deficit may mean a patient cannot produce sound, has a learning disability, or may not be able to think of the correct word. Perhaps the patient has a stammer or has social interaction disabilities. The therapist may also assist patients with eating, drinking, and swallowing. Therapeutic exercises may involve problem-solving, memory and organization skills, communication techniques, and breathing exercises.

In addition to patient identification, date of service, name of referring provider, and signature of therapist, documentation requirements for therapy services include the following:

- history
- physical examination
- medical decision making
- plan of treatment including measurable objectives
- assessment of performance
- modalities and exercises used in treatment including time
- any changes in patient's clinical status since the last visit
- patient tolerance to treatment and improvement
- patient education
- expected outcome of treatment
  See Fig. 11.17 for an example of a physical therapy note.

 11.22 QUICK REVIEW
Question: What is the difference between physical, occupational, and speech-language pathology therapy services?

RELEASE AND RETENTION OF RECORDS

In an electronic system, health records are stored in the computer. Paper-based records are either stored in color-coded file folders containing a collection of paper documents or are scanned into multiple electronic databases and displayed in a variety of formats via computer access. Many health care organizations have a combination of both paper records and electronic records to consider when they are creating a records retention policy. Regardless of the system used, general guidelines must be followed to record information correctly, use it according to law, and retain it. A sample retention policy is shown in Table 11.2.

Subpoena

Subpoena literally means "under penalty." In legal language, it is a writ requiring the appearance of a witness at a trial or other proceeding. Strictly defined, a *subpoena duces tecum* requires the witness to appear and bring or send certain records in his or her possession. For a *subpoena duces tecum* for health information to be valid under the HIPAA Privacy Rule, it must be accompanied by a court order. If there is no court order, the covered entity must receive satisfactory assurance from the party seeking the information that reasonable efforts have been made to ensure that the patient or legal guardian was given notice of the request. If no notice was given, the party must show that reasonable efforts were made to secure a qualified protective order that meets the requirements of the HIPAA Privacy Rule. A subpoena is a legal document signed by a judge or an attorney in the name of a judge. If an attorney signs it, they must attest it is in the name of a judge, the court clerk, or another proper officer. In some states in which a pretrial of evidence or deposition is set up, the subpoena may be issued by a notary public, in which event it is called a *notary subpoena*.

It is possible for a state investigator to subpoena patient records and then file administrative charges against the provider or health care organization, not because of the practice of shoddy medicine, but rather because the case was inadequately documented for the treatment provided. Health records also may be subpoenaed as proof in a medical malpractice case. Complete documentation and well-organized patient records help to establish a strong defense in a medical professional liability claim.

ABC Physical Therapy Associates

Patient: Elizabeth Bennett Date of **Birth: 09/01/19XX**

Date of Service: 02/01/20XX
Referring Provider: Michael Walker, MD

DIAGNOSIS: Status post brain tumor removal.

HISTORY: The patient is a 64-year-old female referred to physical therapy following complications related to brain tumor removal. The patient reports that on 10/24/08 she had a brain tumor removed and had left-sided weakness. The patient was being seen in physical therapy from 11/05/20XX to 11/14/20XX then she began having complications. The patient reports that she was admitted to Hospital on 12/05/20XX. At that time, they found massive swelling on the brain and a second surgery was performed. The patient then remained in acute rehab until she was discharged to home on 01/05/20XX. The patient's husband, Al, is also present and he reports that during rehabilitation the patient did have a DVT in the left calf that has since been resolved.

PAST MEDICAL HISTORY: Umemarkable.

MEDICATIONS: Coumadin, Keppra, Decadron, and Glucophage.

SUBJECTIVE: The patient reports that the pain is not an issue at this time. The patient states that her primary concern is her left-sided weakness as related to her balance and her walking and her left arm weakness.

PATIENT GOAL: To increase strength in her left leg for better balance and walking.

OBJECTIVE:

RANGE OF MOTION: Bilateral lower extremities are within normal limits.

STRENGTH: Bilateral lower extremities are grossly 5/5 with one repetition, except left hip reflexion 4+/5.

BALANCE: The patient's balance was assessed with a Berg balance test. The patient has got 46/56 points, which places her at moderate risk for falls.

GAIT: The patient ambulates with contact guard assist. The patient ambulates with a reciprocal gait pattern with good bilateral foot clearance. However, the patient has been reports that with increased fatigue, left footdrop tends to occur. A 6-minute walk test will be performed at the next visit due to time constraints.

ASSESSMENT: The patient is a 64-year-old female referred to Physical Therapy status post brain surgery. Examination indicates deficits in strength, balance, and ambulation. The patient will benefit from skilled physical therapy to address these impairments.

TREATMENT PLAN: The patient will be seen three times per week for 4 weeks and then reduce it to two times per week for 4 additional weeks. Interventions include:

1. Therapeutic exercise.
2. Balance training.
3. Gait training.
4. Functional mobility training.

SHORT TERM GOAL TO BE COMPLETED IN 4 WEEKS:

1. The patient is to tolerate 30 repetitions of all lower extremity exercises.
2. The patient is to improve balance with a score of 50/56 points.
3. The patient is to ambulate 1000 feet in a 6-minute walk test with standby assist.

LONG TERM GOAL TO BE ACHIEVED IN 8 WEEKS:

1. The patient is to ambulate independently within her home and standby to general supervision within the community.
2. Berg balance test to be 52/56.
3. The patient is to ambulate a 6-minute walk test for 1500 feet independently including safe negotiation of comers and busy areas.
4. The patient is to demonstrate safely stepping over and around objects without loss of balance.

Prognosis for the above-stated goals is good. The above treatment plan has been discussed with the patient and her husband. They are in agreement.

Electronically Signed: Alexander Smith, PT; 02/01/20XX; 1215pm

Fig. 11.17 Example of a physical therapy note.

TABLE 11.2 Sample Records Retention Schedule

Record	Retention Period	Reference
Accounts receivable (patient ledger)	7 years	IRS
Appointment sheets	3 years	False Claims Amendment Act
Bank deposit slip (duplicate)	1 years	IRS
Bank statements and canceled checks	7 years	IRS
Cash receipt records	6 years	IRS
Contracts (expired)	7 years	IRS
Correspondence, general	6 years	IRS
Correspondence, legal	retain indefinitely	IRS
Daysheets (balance sheets and journals)	5 years	False Claims Amendment Act
Health records (active patients)	retain indefinitely	False Claims Amendment Act
Health records (inactive patients)	retain indefinitely	False Claims Amendment Act
Health records (expired patients)	5 years	HIPAA
Income tax returns and documents	retain indefinitely	IRS
Insurance policies and records	retain indefinitely	IRS
Inventory records	3 years	IRS
Invoices	6 years	IRS
Medicare financial records	7 years	CMS
Remittance advice documents	10 years	False Claims Amendment Act
Payroll records	7 years	IRS
X-ray films	retain indefinitely	False Claims Amendment Act

CMS, Centers for Medicare and Medicaid Services; *HIPAA,* Health Insurance Portability and Accountability Act; *IRS,* Internal Revenue Service.

Subpoena Process

A subpoena must be personally served or handed to the prospective witness or keeper of the health records. The acceptance of a document by someone authorized to accept it is the equivalent of personal service. The subpoena cannot be left on a counter or desk. Never accept a subpoena or give records to anyone without the provider's prior authorization. The medical office should designate one person as keeper of the health records. If the subpoena is only for health records or financial data, the representative for the specific doctor can usually accept it, and the provider will not be called to court.

If a service provider is on vacation and there is no designated keeper of the records, tell the deputy that the provider is not in and cannot be served. Suggest that the deputy contact the provider's attorney and relay this information.

The health care organization is given a prescribed time in which to produce the records. It is not necessary to show them at the time the subpoena is served unless the court order so states. The attorney usually employs a person or copy service to copy records that are under subpoena. At the time the subpoena is served, a date is usually agreed upon when the representative will return and copy the portion of the record that is named in the subpoena. Often only the portion of the health record requested is removed from the original chart and put in a copy folder. Items such as the patient registration information sheet, encounter form, and explanation of benefits should not be included. The

attorney who sent the subpoena can be called to see whether the records can be mailed. If so, mail them by certified mail with a return receipt requested. Retain a copy of the records released. A billing specialist will have to appear in court if specified in the subpoena. Verify with the court that the case is actually on the calendar. Failing to appear places the employee in contempt of court and subject to a penalty, possibly several days in jail.

Financial Documents

According to income tax regulations on record retention, accounting records should be kept for a minimum of 4 to 7 years after the due date for filing the tax return or the date the tax is paid, whichever is later. Always contact an accountant before discarding records that may determine tax liability.

A federal regulation mandates that assigned claims for Medicaid and Medicare be kept for 7 years; the health care organization is subject to auditing during that period. The federal False Claims Amendments Act of 1986 allows a claim of fraud to be made up to 10 years from the date a violation was committed. Documentation must be available for inspection and copying by the investigator of the false claim (31 US Code §3729–3733). Retention policies for billing records should reflect this.

Health Records

Preservation of health records is governed by federal and state laws. Under federal legislation, the HIPAA Administrative

Simplification Rules require a covered entity to retain documentation for 6 years from the date of its creation or the date when it last was in effect, whichever is later. However, individual states have their own laws for health record retention. Whichever law is more stringent (federal or state) is the law that should be adhered to.

CMS maintains that the health record needs to be in its original form or in a legally reproduced form, which may be electronic, so that health records may be reviewed and audited by authorized entities. Providers must have a record system that ensures that the record may be accessed and retrieved promptly. Guidance concerning record retention after these time periods should be obtained through legal advice based on laws applicable to the state in which the health care organization resides.

Effective December 1, 2006, changes to the Federal Rules of Civil Procedure make requests for electronic data a standard part of the discovery process during federal lawsuits. This includes health records, accounting documents, cellphone records, instant messaging, and electronic mail that might be needed for future litigation.

Under the federal False Claims Act, a claim may be filed 7 to 10 years after the date of service. Cases that involve radiologic injury claims (for example, leukemia from radiation) may begin running the statute of limitations after discovery of the injury, which may occur 20 or 30 years after radiation exposure.

A patient's health record may be of value not only to the patient in later years but also to the patient's children. In some states, a minor may file suit after they have attained legal age for any act performed during childhood that the person believes to be wrong or harmful. Sometimes a suit may be permitted even 2 to 3 years after the child has reached legal age. Thus, it is important to keep pediatric records until patients are 3 to 4 years beyond the age of majority.

Many factors must be considered when developing a retention policy for health records. Different types of health care facilities may have different retention requirements. For example, research facilities are required to maintain patient records permanently. All record retention policies should be reviewed and approved by a health care attorney who would be most knowledgeable of the laws in their state.

Data Storage

A paperless office requires an organized and efficient system for keeping files that have been saved to the hard drive. The data storage needs to be protected from accidental destruction. Keep financial records on computer disks or tapes and store them in an area that does not have temperature extremes or magnetic fields.

When data is entered into a computer system, it is wise to back up (save data) frequently, preferably daily. Automated backup is possible, and the computer can be set to regularly initiates the process. Most financial software programs display a screen prompt instructing the operator to back up before quitting the program. If there is no automated backup, always back up files at the end of the day or several times a week so that information is not lost during a power outage or computer breakdown.

About once a week, a verification process should be done that compares the original records with the copies. This can take 20% to 30% longer than ordinary backup, but if a comparison is not made, there is no way to ensure that the data has been backed up. Store backup copies away from the office in case of fire, flood, or theft.

Maintain a log of the documents stored on computer disks or CDs with an index located at the front of the logbook. The log enables the health care organization to keep track of files and should list when the files were backed up last so they can be located quickly. Note the code for accessing these documents and date revisions when updating old documents. Do not put anything related to protected health information (PHI) in this log.

Data Disposal

In a paper-based system, it is recommended that documents that are no longer needed be shredded in a secure manner. Electronic storage media, such as CD-ROMs, floppy disks, or flash drives, containing confidential or sensitive information may be disposed of only by approved destruction methods. These methods should be outlined in the health care organization's HIPAA Security Plan and may include burning, shredding, pulverizing, or some other approach that renders the media unusable. Two methods of destroying electronic storage media are degaussing, which uses electromagnetic fields to erase data, or zeroization, which is a process of writing repeated sequences of ones and zeros over the information. CD-ROMs and other media storage devices must be physically destroyed.

Some health care organizations prefer to use health record storage companies. When records are disposed of by a professional company, be sure to obtain a certificate of destruction verifying the method of disposal. This document should be indefinitely retained in the office. Permanently retain a log of destroyed records showing the patient's name, Social Security number, date of the last encounter, and treatment.

HIPAA's security rule requires the establishment of policies and procedures for final disposal of electronic PHI (ePHI) and the hardware or electronic media on which it is stored. It is easy to recover ePHI from hard drives, CD-ROMs, and other media storage devices if it is not properly erased or destroyed. Simply deleting files or formatting drives is not sufficient to keep ePHI from being accessed. Covered entities must implement reasonable safeguards when disposing of information.

 11.23 QUICK REVIEW
Question: How long should health records be retained?

 11.24 QUICK REVIEW
Question: What are three ways to destroy electronic media?

ABSTRACTING FROM HEALTH RECORDS

The insurance billing specialist may be required to abstract information from health records. Procedure 11.1 at the end of the chapter details how to accurately pull data from a health record. Abstraction of technical information from patient records may be requested for three situations:

1. To complete insurance claim forms
2. When sending a letter to justify a health insurance claim form after professional services are rendered
3. When a patient applies for life, mortgage, or health insurance

Any information abstracted from a health record for one of these reasons should be confirmed and signed off by the provider of the services.

Life or Health Insurance Applications

When a patient applies for insurance, the insurance company may request information from the patient's provider, require a physical examination, or both. Before completing the forms, the patient must sign a release of information form. Insurance companies will typically include a check when requesting medical information. The amount of the check may vary, depending on how much information is requested. If no payment is included, the health care organization should request fee payment before sending in the completed report form. Be sure the service provider checks the documentation thoroughly before signing it to ensure that the information is accurate and properly stated.

Be extremely accurate when abstracting medical information from the patient's record. Abbreviations on the chart must be understood, and only the requested information should be provided. If the form has questions about high blood pressure, kidney infection, or heart problems, the patient could be prohibited from obtaining life, health, or mortgage insurance if the answers are derogatory.

When abstracting information related to HIV, minors, and other specific situations, it is recommended that approval be obtained from the medical records director as there are often state regulations regarding the release of this information.

In some situations, it is preferable to submit a narrative report dictated by the provider instead of completing the form, which has numerous check-off columns and no space for comments. It may be necessary to attach a copy of an operative, pathology, laboratory, or radiology report and an electrocardiogram (ECG) tracing.

A life insurance company may ask a copy service to visit the health care organization's office to photocopy the patient's record. Usually, this is done at the convenience of the office staff and an appointment should be made. The insurance company should be reminded that an authorization form signed by the patient is necessary to release medical information. An appropriate fee for this service is charged and quoted at the time of the telephone request. The provider should review the records in advance to ensure that they are in proper order.

 11.25　QUICK REVIEW
Question: When does a coding specialist abstract information from a health record?

REVIEW AND AUDIT OF HEALTH RECORDS

An audit assists the health care organization in determining whether the reported services were actually rendered and the level of service was warranted. Health record review and audits target ICD-10, CPT, and HCPCS code selection based on the documentation. These are done to identify compliance issues in documentation, coding, billing, and reimbursement and thus, identify potential areas of fraud and abuse risk to the health care provider and organization.

Internal Reviews

An internal review of medical records is a tool for health care organizations to identify areas that require education. It can identify documentation deficiencies and errors, as well as coding errors. Internal audits should be performed each year, more frequently if there are errors. Specific items in the documentation that should be audited include:

- Is the documentation legible?
- Is the documentation signed and dated?
- Is the patient properly identified on each page of the record?
- Is the documentation appropriate for the diagnosis?
- Is the treatment medically necessary?
- Are there errors or inconsistencies in the record?
- Are the services and diagnosis coded properly?
- Is the reimbursement correct?

Prospective Review

The first type of internal review is a prospective review, also termed *prebilling audit* or *review,* which is done before billing is submitted. This may be done by some health care organizations daily, weekly, or monthly.

Stage 1 of a prospective review is done to verify that completed encounter forms match patients seen according to the appointment schedule and have been posted on the daysheet. A prospective review is begun by obtaining the encounter forms and locating the dates in question for the review in the appointment schedule, printing the schedule as verification. The appointment schedule is then compared with the encounter forms to match patients for the date in question. Next, check to see if all procedures or services have been posted and the charges on the daysheet are complete.

Stage 2 of a prospective review is done to verify that all procedures or services and diagnoses listed on the encounter form match data on the insurance claim form. To perform this stage, use the completed claim form or print an insurance billing worksheet. Match the information on the claim or worksheet with the date of service, procedure or service, and diagnosis on the encounter form. It is possible that one or more diagnoses may not match. A common reason is that an active diagnosis has not been entered in the computer system, the computer defaults to the last diagnosis given for an established patient. Another problem occurs when the diagnosis is not linked to the procedure. Such problems must be found before billing and corrected before claims are printed.

Retrospective Review

The second type of internal review is called a retrospective review, which is done after billing insurance carriers. A coding or insurance billing specialist may be asked to perform a retrospective review to determine whether there is appropriate documentation or any errors in coding and/or reimbursement. To accomplish this, pull 15 to 20 health records per provider from the past 2 to 4 months at random. The following are recommended internal audit tools:

- Internal record review worksheets
- Current codebooks: CPT, HCPCS, ICD-10-CM, and/or ICD-10-PCS
- Medical dictionary
- Abbreviation reference book
- Drug reference book (e.g., *Physicians' Desk Reference*)
- Laboratory reference book
- Provider's manual for insurance program or plan
- Insurance carrier's newsletters
- Provider or health care organization's contract with insurance carrier

Standard forms may be used as tools to gather information from the patient's record, laboratory reports, pathology reports, radiology reports, operative reports, and other diagnostic tests. If the health care provider's documentation is inadequate, errors or deficiencies will appear as the review is being conducted. Doing an internal review of this type is not an exact science, and critical thinking skills are needed. Because documentation guidelines and code policies are updated and refined periodically, it is extremely important to read and keep bulletins from all insurance carriers, especially those from the local Medicare Administrative Contractor. An audit should only be performed using the most up-to-date policies. Advise the service provider of any new requirements. This resource may be the only notification of changes unless health care employees routinely attend local or national workshops.

Concurrent Review

The third type of internal review is concurrent review. These are frequently conducted by hospital facilities for inpatient stays. The reviewer validates each condition documented as being actively treated. They also query the providers if there are conditions that are clinically supported but not documented, or those that are documented but not clinically supported. They may also evaluate if the tests and procedures performed on the patient are medically necessary for the stated conditions. Often a concurrent review will be used to determine if the patient is getting the right treatment in a timely and cost-effective way.

External Reviews

An external review is an audit of health and financial records by an outside contractor or by an external reviewer. The external audit may be performed by an insurance carrier, a Medicare Administrative Contractor, or other Centers for Medicare and Medicaid Services (CMS) representative to investigate suspected fraud or abusive billing practices.

Health care organizations and facilities may initiate their own external review and request an outside contractor to perform an audit as part of its compliance program. This is a way to pinpoint areas needed for education and training. External reviews will also provide a third-party opinion for claims processing and may help an organization appeal trends in denials. External reviewers may provide objectivity, whereas internal reviewers may feel pressure to downplay errors made by their employer.

An external review may also be requested by a health care organization to evaluate the policies and procedures related to a particular service and ensure proper guidelines and regulations are being adhered to. This will point out areas for improvement and prepare the organization for an external audit by Medicare or another insurance company.

External audits can also be performed as prepayment (prospective) audits or as retrospective audits. When a health care provider is placed on a prepayment audit review by an insurance company, each time the provider submits a claim, the claim is pended by the insurance carrier. The health care provider must submit a copy of his or her patient's health record to support the claim. On receipt of the health record, the insurance carrier will review the record and determine whether the claim should be paid or not. This process can be very time-consuming and can have a significant impact on the health care organization's cash flow.

Retrospective audits are performed by insurance carriers after a claim has been paid. If it is determined that incorrect payment was made, a request will be made for monies to be refunded. Most insurance companies perform routine audits on unusual billing patterns, such as the same diagnosis code for every encounter or billing the same procedure code repeatedly. Additional red flags to auditors include the following:

- Lack of documentation for health care facility admissions
- Canned template documentation
- Illegible documentation
- Blank documentation
- Tests documented but not performed

Insurance companies have computer software programs capable of editing and screening insurance claims to identify billing excesses or potential abuses before payment is rendered. Insurance carriers may hire undercover agents who visit health care providers' offices if overuse and abuse of procedure codes are suspected. Health care organizations that charge fees that are higher than others in their geographic area are routinely audited by most carriers. Insurance carriers spot-check claims by sending questionnaires to patients and asking them if they received medical care from a provider and, if so, to verify the services rendered. The answers are then compared with what the service provider billed.

Many insurance companies have installed antifraud telephone hotlines for patients. Investigations can result from such calls, depending on the circumstances. Tips also come from peer review organizations, state licensing boards, whistle-blowing providers, former staff members, and patients. If there is any suspicion of fraud, the insurance company will notify the health care organization, specify a date and time at which they will come to the office, and indicate which records they wish to audit.

Investigators question the patient, look at the documentation in the health record, and interview the staff and all health care providers who have participated in the care of the patient. Auditors also look at appointment books and add up the hours the health care provider sees patients on any given day when a health care organization uses time-based procedure codes when submitting insurance claims.

Software Edit Checks

An edit check is a good audit prevention measure to have in place. Many software programs have edits in their software programs that automatically screen insurance claims for errors and conflicting code entries prior to submission. For example, if the diagnosis does not match the service provided, the claim will be thrown out by the edit, and it can be corrected before being billed.

 11.26 QUICK REVIEW

Question: What is the difference between an internal and external review?

 DISCUSSION POINT

What is the purpose of complete documentation? How can a coding or billing specialist assist their providers in meeting the requirements for documentation?

PROCEDURE 11.1   How to Abstract Data From a Health Record

Follow these steps, including rationales to learn this skill, and practice it by completing the *Workbook* assignment.

1. Confirm the patient's identification using name and date of birth.
2. What is the location of the services? For example, inpatient, emergency department, outpatient, ICU, etc. This will impact billing.
3. Confirm provider's name. Is the document signed, dated, and authenticated by the provider? Were any other providers involved in the care of the patient, such as an anesthesiologist, assistant surgeon, and so on?
4. What is the patient's diagnosis? This gives the reason for the encounter.
5. What professional services were provided?
6. Did the patient undergo surgery? What surgical procedure was performed?
7. Read and review the patient's health record thoroughly to learn all parts of the case.
8. What medication was prescribed, if any?
9. Does the patient have any past history (PH) indicating anything of importance?
10. Does the patient have any food or drug allergies? If so, what are they?
11. What is the etiology (cause) of the present disease, injury, or illness?
12. What is the prognosis (prediction) for this patient's medical condition?
13. What laboratory tests were ordered or performed?
14. What x-rays were ordered or obtained?
15. Define every abbreviation listed in the patient's chart notes or history and physical examination.
16. What documents assisted you in locating the answers to these questions?

KEY POINTS

This is a brief chapter review of the key issues presented. To further enhance your knowledge of the technical subject matter, review the key terms and key abbreviations for this chapter by locating the meaning for each in the Glossary at the end of this text, which appears in a section before the Index.

1. The key to substantiating procedure and diagnostic code selection for appropriate reimbursement is supporting documentation in the health record.
2. The electronic health record (EHR) is becoming the norm as the ability to share patient health records among other professionals who constitute the patient's health care team has become increasingly important.
3. Federal legislation has established programs to help the health care industry change to electronic health records (EHR) and has offered incentives to those who participate in the programs. These incentive programs will transition to reimbursement penalties for organizations that have not adopted EHRs.
4. Every patient seen by a service provider must have comprehensive legible documentation about what occurred during the encounter for the following reasons: (1) avoidance of denied or delayed payments by insurance carriers investigating the medical necessity of services; (2) enforcement of health record-keeping rules by insurance carriers requiring accurate documentation that supports procedure and diagnostic codes; (3) subpoena of health records by state investigators or the court for review; (4) defense of a professional liability claim.

5. Consultation and referral are not the same. A consultation service is rendered at the request of opinion or advice by another provider, whereas a referral is the transfer of the total or specific care of a patient for a known problem.
6. Health record abbreviations should be eliminated from the more vital sections, such as final diagnosis, operative notes, discharge summaries, and descriptions of special procedures.
7. An eponym should not be used when a comparable anatomic term can be used in its place.
8. When a patient does not comply with a health care organization's office policy, the service provider may wish to withdraw formally from further care of the patient. The service provider must send a formal letter of termination or withdrawal by certified mail with a return receipt to the patient.
9. Different types of health care services require specific elements in their documentation.
10. Abstraction of technical information from patient records may be requested to complete insurance claim forms; when sending letters to justify a health insurance claim form; or when a patient applies for life, mortgage, or health insurance.
11. When health records are subpoenaed, produce only the records requested and nothing more. Retain a copy of the records released.
12. The Health Insurance Portability and Accountability Act (HIPAA) requires documents to be retained for 6 years

from the date of creation or the date when it was last in effect, whichever is later. However, if the state requires a longer retention period, the law that is most stringent should be adhered to.

13. The two types of internal and external review of records are (1) prospective (prepayment) review and (2) retrospective (after payment) review.

14. External and internal audit of health records shows where deficiencies occur in health record documentation and substantiates proper use of diagnostic and procedural codes.

15. An edit check is a good audit prevention measure because the software program automatically screens transmitted insurance claims and electronically examines them for errors and conflicting code entries.

INTERNET RESOURCES

CMS Specialty Codes

- https://www.cms.gov/Medicare/Provider-Enrollment-and-Certification/MedicareProviderSupEnroll/Downloads/TaxonomyCrosswalk.pdf

AMA MDM Guidelines for Office Visits and Other Outpatient E/M Services

- https://www.ama-assn.org/system/files/2019-06/cpt-revised-mdm-grid.pdf

CMS General E/M Guidelines for all other E/M Services

- https://www.cms.gov/outreach-and-education/medicare-learning-network-mln/mlnproducts/downloads/eval-mgmt-serv-guide-icn006764.pdf

CMS Guidelines for Surgery Documentation

- https://www.cms.gov/Medicare-Medicaid-Coordination/Fraud-Prevention/Medicaid-Integrity-Education/Downloads/docmatters-casestudy-guide.pdf

Guidelines for Documenting Anesthesia Services

- https://www.aana.com/docs/default-source/practice-aana-com-web-documents-(all)/documenting-anesthesia-care.pdf?sfvrsn=ac0049b1_4

Radiology Documentation Guidelines

- https://med.noridianmedicare.com/web/jea/topics/documentation-requirements/radiology

Pathology/Laboratory Documentation Guidelines

- https://www.cms.gov/Outreach-and-Education/Medicare-Learning-Network-MLN/MLNProducts/Downloads/ProviderComplianceLabServices-Fact-Sheet-ICN909221.pdf

Therapy Services Documentation Guidelines

- https://www.cms.gov/Outreach-and-Education/Medicare-Learning-Network-MLN/MLNProducts/Downloads/OutptRehabTherapy-Booklet-MLN905365.pdf

STUDENT ASSIGNMENT

- Study Chapter 11.
- Complete all exercises in the *Workbook* to reinforce the theory learned in this chapter.

- Turn to the Glossary at the end of this text for a further understanding of the key terms and key abbreviations used in this chapter.

12

Diagnostic Coding

Cheryl Fassett

OBJECTIVES

After reading this chapter, you should be able to:

1. Explain the reasons for and importance of coding diagnoses.
2. Discuss the history of diagnostic coding.
3. Discuss the benefits of the ICD-10 coding system and differentiate between ICD-10-CM and ICD-10-PCS.
4. Identify and describe the Alphabetic and Tabular Index of the ICD-10-CM coding manual.
5. Describe the importance of matching the correct diagnostic code to the appropriate procedural code.
6. Differentiate between primary (first listed), principal, and secondary diagnoses and discuss admitting diagnoses.
7. Describe how medical necessity is supported by the diagnosis code.
8. Define and demonstrate an understanding of diagnostic code conventions, symbols, and terminology.
9. Apply general coding guidelines to translate written descriptions of conditions into diagnostic codes.
10. Apply chapter-specific coding guidelines to reporting of specific illnesses and conditions.
11. Relate additional coding guidelines specific to reporting of outpatient services.
12. Describe methods of becoming more familiar with codes commonly encountered in a specific health care organization and discuss computer-assisted coding.
13. Anticipate future changes to the diagnosis coding system, known as ICD-11.

KEY TERMS

adverse effect
benign tumor
carcinoma in situ
chief complaint
combination code
complication
computer-assisted coding
conventions
eponym
essential modifiers
etiology
exacerbation
Excludes 1
Excludes 2
external causes of morbidity
International Classification of Diseases, Tenth Revision, Clinical Modification

International Classification of Diseases, Tenth Revision, Procedure Coding System
intoxication
late effect
laterality
malignant tumor
manifestation
medical necessity
metastasis
morbidity
mortality
neoplasm
nonessential modifiers
not elsewhere classifiable
not otherwise specified
Official Guidelines for Coding and Reporting

ordinality of encounter
placeholder
poisoning
primary diagnosis
principal diagnosis
prophylaxis
residual subcategories
rule out
secondary diagnosis
sequela
sequencing
status asthmaticus
syndrome
uncertain behavior
Z codes

KEY ABBREVIATIONS

AHA	CPT	ICD-10-PCS	NEC
AHIMA	DM	ICD-11	NOS
CAC	HIV	MRI	SNOMED CT
CC	ICD-10-CM	NCHS	WHO

INSIGHTS FROM THE FIELD

Tammy F.: Certified Professional Coder (CPC)

I have been in the health care field for 27 years. I am currently an accounts receivable auditor for a Durable Medical Equipment supplier. I oversee this for 25 regional offices in New York and New Jersey. My job involves reviewing denials, adjustments, and electronic claims errors. I find common claim errors and educate the clinics and collection department. A billing specialist needs to have knowledge in coding and understand what is medically necessary and what is and is not billable. One of the greatest challenges is keeping up with the revolving changes and requirements of ALL the payers. Getting a clean claim out the door the first time is key.

DIAGNOSIS CODING OVERVIEW

This chapter deals with diagnostic coding for outpatient professional services. The rules for coding inpatient cases can differ and are covered more thoroughly in Chapter 19 of this text. Health care providers and outpatient facilities use diagnosis codes on insurance claims to explain the reason the patient sought health care services. Using a code eliminates the need to write out the diagnostic description on the claim form and creates a common language for all health care providers and payers.

Diagnosis codes must be used on all claims and must be accurately assigned. Appropriate diagnosis coding can mean the financial success or failure of a health care organization. To assign diagnosis codes accurately, the billing and coding specialist must have knowledge of the current approved coding guidelines and a working knowledge of medical terminology. This includes having knowledge of anatomy and physiology, clinical disease processes, and medical terminology. There are many consequences of inaccurate assignment of diagnosis codes. For example, claims can be denied, fines or penalties can be levied, sanctions can be imposed, and the health care provider's level of reimbursement for claims may be affected.

Further guidance for completion of a Centers for Medicare and Medicaid Services (CMS) 1500 claim form will be explained in Chapter 14 of this textbook; however, Fig. 12.1 is an example of a completed claim form. Note the following information included on the claim form:

- Box 21 has space for up to 12 diagnosis codes per claim.
- Box 24E for the diagnosis pointer. This reflects the procedure code back to the appropriate primary diagnosis code. This is how medical necessity is established on the CMS 1500 claim form.

12.1   QUICK REVIEW

Question: What is the benefit of health care providers, organizations, and payers using a common coding system?

INTERNATIONAL CLASSIFICATION OF DISEASES

Diagnosis coding is performed using the World Health Organization's (WHO's) *International Classification of Diseases* (ICD). The coding system classifies morbidity and mortality information for (1) statistical purposes, (2) indexing of hospital records by disease and operations, and (3) data storage and retrieval. Morbidity refers to disease, and mortality refers to death. These are important to track in terms of how they affect a population.

History

From the earliest days of medical treatment, people have tried to name and classify diseases. The ICD had its beginning in England during the seventeenth century.

In 1948, the WHO developed the official version of the ICD in Geneva, Switzerland. The system was designed to compile and present statistical data on morbidity and mortality rates and frequency. WHO assumed responsibility for preparing and publishing revisions to the coding system every 10 years. The United States began using the ICD to report causes of death and prepare mortality statistics in the latter half of the twentieth century. Hospitals began using the ICD in 1950 to classify and index diseases.

The eighth revision of the ICD was constructed in 1966 and was adapted for use in the United States in 1968 by the United States Public Health Service. This became known as ICDA-8 and served as the basis for coding diagnostic data for both official morbidity and mortality statistics in the United States.

In 1979, the ninth revision of the *International Classification of Diseases* (ICD-9) was published by the WHO. Passage of the Medicare Catastrophic Coverage Act in 1988 then placed requirements on providers and health care organizations to submit appropriate diagnosis codes on all claims when billing for services provided to Medicare beneficiaries on or after April 1, 1989. The CMS designated *International Classification of Diseases, Ninth Revision, Clinical Modification (ICD-9-CM)* as the coding system health care providers were required to use.

In 1992, the WHO published the tenth revision of the *International Classification of Diseases* (ICD-10). The NCHS further developed a clinical modification to the WHO's system, which is referred to as International Classification of Diseases, Tenth Revision, Clinical Modification (ICD-10-CM). On January 16,

MEDICARE/MEDICAID
(primary)   (secondary)
CROSSOVER CLAIM

DRAFT - NOT FOR OFFICIAL USE

HEALTH INSURANCE CLAIM FORM
APPROVED BY NATIONAL UNIFOR MCLAIM COMMITTEE (NUCC) 02/12

| | PICA | | | | | | | | PICA | |

1. MEDICARE ☐ (Medicare#) MEDICAID ☐ (Medicaid#) TRICARE ☐ (ID#DoD#) CHAMPVA ☐ (Member ID#) GROUP HEALTH PLAN ☒ (ID#) FECA BLK LUNG ☐ (ID#) OTHER ☐ (ID#)

1a. INSURED'S I.D. NUMBER (For Program in Item 1)
65428A12

2. PATIENT'S NAME (Last Name, First Name, Middle Initial)
Smith, Joseph

3. PATIENT'S BIRTH DATE 01 15 1984 SEX M ☒ F ☐

4. INSURED'S NAME (Last Name, First Name, Middle Initial)
Smith, Joseph

5. PATIENT'S ADDRESS (No., Street)
14 Magnolia Lane

6. PATIENT RELATIONSHIP TO INSURED
Self ☒ Spouse ☐ Child ☐ Other ☐

7. INSURED'S ADDRESS (No., Street)
14 Magnolia Lane

CITY Woodland Hills STATE XY

8. RESERVED FOR NUCC USE

CITY Woodland Hills STATE XY

ZIP CODE 123450000 TELEPHONE (555) 6825555

ZIP CODE 123450000 TELEPHONE (555) 6825555

9. OTHER INSURED'S NAME (Last Name, First Name, Middle Initial)

10. IS PATIENT'S CONDITION RELATED TO:

11. INSURED'S POLICY GROUP OR FECA NUMBER

a. OTHER INSURED'S POLICY OR GROUP NUMBER

a. EMPLOYMENT? (Current or Previous) YES ☐ NO ☒

a. INSURED'S DATE OF BIRTH 01 15 1984 SEX M ☒ F ☐

b. RESERVED FOR NUCC USE

b. AUTO ACCIDENT? YES ☐ NO ☒ PLACE (State)

b. OTHER CLAIM ID (Designated by NUCC)

c. RESERVED FOR NUCC USE

c. OTHER ACCIDENT? YES ☐ NO ☒

c. INSURANCE PLAN NAME OR PROGRAM NAME
Aetna

d. INSURANCE PLAN NAME OR PROGRAM NAME

10d. CLAIM CODES (Designated by NUCC)

d. IS THERE ANOTHER HEALTH BENEFIT PLAN? YES ☐ NO ☒ If yes, complete items 9, 9a, and 9d.

READ BACK OF FORM BEFORE COMPLETING & SIGNING THIS FORM.
12. PATIENT'S OR AUTHORIZED PERSON'S SIGNATURE I authorize the release of any medical or other information necessary to process this claim. I also request payment of government benefits either to myself or to the party who accepts assignment below.
SIGNED Joseph Smith DATE 10/1/XX

13. INSURED'S OR AUTHORIZED PERSON'S SIGNATURE I authorize payment of medical benefits to the undersigned physician or supplier for services described below.
SIGNED Joseph Smith

14. DATE OF CURRENT: ILLNESS, INJURY, or PREGNANCY(LMP) QUAL.

15. OTHER DATE QUAL. MM DD YY

16. DATES PATIENT UNABLE TO WORK IN CURRENT OCCUPATION FROM TO

17. NAME OF REFERRING PROVIDER OR OTHER SOURCE
DN Brady Coccidioides MD

17a.
17b. NPI 64211067XX

18. HOSPITALIZATION DATES RELATED TO CURRENT SERVICES FROM TO

19. ADDITIONAL CLAIM INFORMATION (Designated by NUCC)

20. OUTSIDE LAB? YES ☐ NO ☒ $ CHARGES

21. DIAGNOSIS OR NATURE OF ILLNESS OR INJURY Relate A-L to service line below (24E) ICD Ind. 0
A. L918 B. C. D.
E. F. G. H.
I. J. K. L.

22. RESUBMISSION CODE ORIGINAL REF. NO.

23. PRIOR AUTHORIZATION NUMBER

24. A. DATE(S) OF SERVICE From / To	B. PLACE OF SERVICE	C. EMG	D. PROCEDURES, SERVICES, OR SUPPLIES CPT/HCPCS / MODIFIER	E. DIAGNOSIS POINTER	F. $ CHARGES	G. DAYS OR UNITS	H. EPSDT Family Plan	I. ID. QUAL.	J. RENDERING PROVIDER ID. #
1 10 01 XX	24		11200	A	100 00	1		NPI	50307117XX
2								NPI	
3								NPI	
4								NPI	
5								NPI	
6								NPI	

25. FEDERAL TAX I.D. NUMBER XX12210XX SSN ☐ EIN ☒

26. PATIENT'S ACCOUNT NO. 154

27. ACCEPT ASSIGNMENT? YES ☒ NO ☐

28. TOTAL CHARGE $ 100 00

29. AMOUNT PAID $

30. Rsvd for NUCC Use

31. SIGNATURE OF PHYSICIAN OR SUPPLIER INCLUDING DEGREES OR CREDENTIALS
Cosmo Graff MD 100320XX
SIGNED Cosmo Graff, MD DATE

32. SERVICE FACILITY LOCATION INFORMATION
Woodland Hills Ambulatory Center
1229 Center Street
Woodland Hills XY 123450001
a. X950513700 b.

33. BILLING PROVIDER INFO & PH # (555) 4869002
College Clinic
4567 Broad Avenue
Woodland Hills XY 123450001
a. 3664021CC b.

NUCC Instruction Manual available at: www.nucc.org   PLEASE PRINT OR TYPE   OMB APPROVAL PENDING

Fig. 12.1 Completed CMS 1500 claim form highlighting diagnosis box and diagnosis pointer.

2009, the DHHS published the final rule in the *Federal Register* for adoption of the ICD-10-CM code set, and required health care providers to use this updated system effective October 1, 2015.

Non-covered entities, such as workers' compensation or no-fault insurance companies, were not required to shift from ICD-9-CM to ICD-10-CM. However, it is in the noncovered entities' best interest to use the ICD-10-CM coding system because of the significant value of the increased detail of diseases. Because of this, most states have adopted ICD-10-CM for workers' compensation claims processing. Coding and billing specialists should check with their state worker's compensation board to determine if the insurance carrier is using ICD-10-CM.

ICD-10 Diagnosis and Procedure Codes

There are many benefits associated with the adoption of the ICD-10 coding system. Benefits include the following:

- Greater specificity, including laterality, which defines the side of the body is affected, or ordinality of encounter, which determines whether the care encounter is the patient's first for the condition
- Expansion of clinical information and reduced cross-referencing
- Flexibility and ease of expandability of the coding system
- Updated medical terminology and classification of diseases
- The ability to compare mortality and morbidity data
- Fewer non-specific codes than in ICD-9-CM

The ICD-10-CM coding system exceeds previous versions of the ICD in the number of concepts and codes provided. The disease classification was expanded to include health-related conditions and to provide greater specificity through reporting at a sixth-digit level with a seventh-digit extension. The sixth and seventh characters are not optional and are required for use in recording the information documented in the clinical record. ICD-10-CM allows more code choices and requires greater documentation in the health record (Fig. 12.2). Many of the conventions and guidelines are the same for both ICD-9-CM and ICD-10-CM coding systems; however, there are more extensive guidelines for ICD-10-CM. The ICD-10 coding system consists of two code sets, ICD-10-CM and ICD-10-PCS.

ICD-10-CM

The Clinical Modification (CM) provides the specifics that the United States needs for collecting data on health status. This became known as the *International Classification of Diseases, Tenth Revision, Clinical Modification* (ICD-10-CM). It is used for reporting of diagnoses treated during encounters in all health care settings. Additional information on using ICD-10-CM is included in this chapter.

ICD-10-PCS

The International Classification of Diseases, Tenth Revision, Procedure Coding System (ICD-10-PCS) was developed in mid-1992 by 3M Health Information Systems under contract with the CMS. ICD-10-PCS is used by hospitals to report inpatient procedure codes. Additional information on using ICD-10-PCS is included in Chapter 19.

Selection of a Coding Manual

Many companies publish the ICD-10-CM coding manuals. Publishers very often use different styles and formats, so it is important to study and compare the features of several books before making a decision to purchase. When choosing a book, the following questions should be asked:

- Are colors used for emphasis in locating items quickly?
- Are definitions or notes included to help one interpret and gain a better understanding of difficult medical terms and phrases?
- Are coding guidelines boxed for easy reference?
- Are icons or symbols used?
- Are fonts and type styles used that can be read easily?
- Is print large enough to allow accurate coding?
  All of these special features benefit the coding specialist.

> **12.2 QUICK REVIEW**
>
> Question: What is the purpose of the *International Classification of Disease* (ICD)?

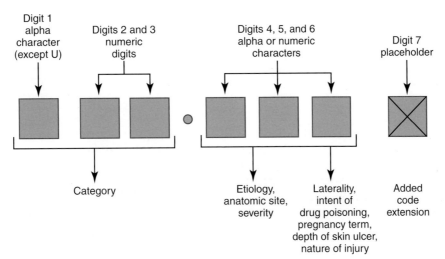

Fig. 12.2 Breakdown of a diagnosis code in the International Classification of Disease, Tenth Revision, Clinical Modification (ICD-10-CM).

ASSIGNING A DIAGNOSIS CODE

All diagnoses that are documented in the medical record for a particular health care encounter and affect management of the patient must be assigned a diagnosis code. Diagnoses that relate to a patient's previous medical problem but have no bearing on the patient's present condition are not coded. The CMS and the National Center for Health Statistics (NCHS), departments within the Department of Health and Human Services (DHHS), provide a set of Official Guidelines for Coding and Reporting. These guidelines are a set of rules that have been developed to provide instructions. Adherence to the guidelines when assigning diagnosis codes is required under the Health Insurance Portability and Accountability Act (HIPAA).

Sequencing of Diagnostic Codes

Diagnosis codes must be sequenced correctly on an insurance claim so that the reason for medical services and the severity of the disease can be understood. Sequencing codes means listing them in the appropriate order as outlined in the *International Classification of Diseases* (ICD) guidelines. The correct diagnosis code must be matched to the appropriate surgical or medical procedure code on the claim form for third-party reimbursement.

When submitting insurance claims for a health care provider or outpatient service, the primary diagnosis is the main reason for the encounter and should be listed first on the claim. In a visit with a health care professional, this is related to the chief complaint (CC), which is the patient's description of symptoms, problems, or conditions that prompted them to seek care.

Any secondary diagnoses, listed subsequently, may contribute to the condition or define the need for a higher level of care, but are not the underlying cause. The underlying cause of a disease is referred to as the etiology and, as a general rule, is sequenced in the first position.

The principal diagnosis, used in inpatient hospital coding, is defined in the ICD-10-CM Official Guidelines as the condition established after study to be chiefly responsible for occasioning the admission of the patient to the hospital for care. It is possible for the primary and principal diagnosis codes to be the same. The concept of a "principal diagnosis" is only applicable to inpatient hospital claims or cases. A principal diagnosis may be different from the admitting diagnosis, which is the diagnosis that prompted the admission. Box 12.1 outlines important differences between a primary and a principal diagnosis.

Admitting Diagnoses

Some diagnosis codes are considered problematic when used as the first diagnosis on admission of a patient to the hospital. Examples of questionable admitting diagnoses are obesity, benign hypertension, or controlled diabetes. The inpatient admission diagnosis may be expressed as one of the following:
1. One or more significant findings, symptoms, or signs representing patient distress, or abnormal findings on examination.
2. A diagnosis established on an ambulatory care basis or previous hospital admission.
3. An injury or poisoning.

BOX 12.1   Primary Versus Principal Diagnosis

	Primary Diagnosis	Principal Diagnosis
Definition	Main reason (diagnosis, condition, chief complaint) for the encounter/visit in the health record that is responsible for services provided.	Condition established after study that prompted the hospitalization.
Location	Outpatient setting only (provider office visits and hospital-based outpatient services).	Inpatient setting only.
"Probable," "suspected," "questionable," "rule out," or "working diagnosis"	May not report "probable," "suspected," "questionable," "rule out," or "working diagnosis." Codes that describe symptoms and signs, as opposed to diagnoses, are acceptable for reporting purposes when a related definitive diagnosis has not been established (confirmed) by the provider.	Code the condition as if it existed or was established at the time of discharge if it is documented on the final diagnostic statement as "probable," "suspected," "questionable," "rule out," or "working diagnosis."

---

4. A reason or condition not classifiable as an illness or injury, such as pregnancy in labor or follow-up inpatient diagnostic tests.

When a provider makes hospital visits, code the condition evaluated and managed by the provider, which might not necessarily be the reason the patient was admitted to the hospital (Example 12.1).

EXAMPLE 12.1   Coding Provider Hospital Visits

A patient is admitted to the hospital with chest pain and is being monitored in the cardiac telemetry unit. On examination, it is noted that the patient has an enlarged thyroid, and an endocrinologist is asked to see the patient in consultation.

Reason for Hospital Admission	Reason for Hospital Visit by Endocrinologist
Chest pain	Enlarged thyroid

Medical Necessity

CMS defines medical necessity as the services or supplies needed to diagnose and treat a medical condition that are consistent with the standards of good medical practice. Most health plans will not pay for health care services that they deem to be not medically necessary. The most common example is a cosmetic procedure, such as the injection of Botox to decrease facial wrinkles or tummy-tuck surgery. In those cases, a health plan may deny payment because of lack of medical necessity. In addition to certain surgical procedures, other services may have medical necessity restrictions. These include the following:

- Most imaging services (e.g., radiography, computed tomography, or magnetic resonance imaging [MRI])
- Cardiovascular services (e.g., electrocardiograms, Holter monitors, echocardiography, Doppler imaging, or stress testing)
- Neurologic services (e.g., electroencephalography, noninvasive ultrasonography)
- Many laboratory services
- Vitamin B12 injections

It is important to know exactly which diagnosis relates to the procedure being performed. Insurance carrier coverage policies will determine if the diagnosis supports medical necessity. A reference book may be helpful in this situation, and a number of manuals are available from commercial publishers. For cases dealing with CMS, consult the Medicare Administrative Carrier's (MAC) website for local coverage determinations (LCDs) and the federal government's website for national coverage determinations (NCDs), or download the manual that is updated quarterly.

 12.3   QUICK REVIEW
Question: What is medical necessity?

ORGANIZATION AND FORMAT OF ICD-10-CM

ICD-10-CM contains a Tabular List of Diseases (Volume 1), in which each disease has an assigned number and an Alphabetic Index to Diseases and Injuries (Volume 2; Figs. 12.3 and 12.4). The systematized arrangement in these books makes it possible to encode, computerize, store, and retrieve large volumes of information from the patient's health record. ICD-10-CM is used by hospitals, physicians, and other health care providers to code and report diagnostic information. This information is necessary for participation in various government programs such as Medicare, Medicaid, quality improvement organizations, and professional review organizations.

Annual updates of ICD-10-CM are published in three publications: *Coding Clinic,* published by the American Hospital Association (AHA); *American Health Information Management Association Journal,* published by American Health Information Management Association (AHIMA); and the *Federal Register,* published by the US Government Printing Office. Coding from an out-of-date manual can delay payment, result in denied claims, or cause costly mistakes that can lead to financial disaster. Annual ICD-10-CM code revisions must be in place and in use by October 1 each year.

! COMPLIANCE ALERT
ICD-10-CM Standard Code Set

A code set is any set of codes with their descriptions used to encode data elements, such as tables of terms, medical concepts, medical diagnostic codes, or medical procedure codes. Each transaction must include the use of medical and other code sets. The *International Classification of Disease, Tenth Revision, Clinical Modification* (ICD-10-CM) official guidelines for coding and reporting is the standard code set outlined under the Health Insurance Portability and Accountability Act (HIPAA) and must be used when assigning diagnostic codes.

Alphabetic Index to Diseases and Injuries

The Alphabetic Index to Diseases and Injuries (Volume 2) is placed first in most ICD-10-CM coding manuals. The Alphabetic Index

---

INDEX TO DISEASES AND INJURIES DRAFT / Anemia

Mainterm
Subterm
Subsubterm
and diagnosis
code

Anemia *(Continued)*
   deficiency *(Continued)*
      folic acid D52.9
         dietary D52.0
         drug-induced D52.1
      G SH D55.1
      G6PD D55.0
      GGS-R D55.1
      glucose-6-phosphate dehydrogenase
         D55.0
      glutathione reductase D55.1
      glyceraldehyde phosphate
         dehydrogenase D55.2
      hexokinase D55.2
      iron D50.9
         secondary to blood loss (chronic)
            D50.0
      nutritional D53.9
         with
            poor iron absorption D50.8
            specified deficiency NEC
               D53.8
      phosphofructo-aldolase D55.2
      phosphoglycerate kinase D55.2
      PK D55.2

Anemia *(Continued)*
   due to *(Continued)*
      hemorrhage (chronic) D50.0
         acute D62
      impaired absorption D50.9
      loss of blood (chronic) D50.0
         acute D62
      myxedema E03.9 *[D63.8]*
      Necator americanus B76.1 *[D63.8]*
      prematurity P61.2
      selective vitamin B12 malabsorption
         with proteinuria D51.1
      transcobalamin II deficiency D51.2
   Dyke-Young type (secondary)
      (symptomatic) D59.1
   dyserythropoietic (congenital)
      D64.4
   dyshematopoietic (congenital)
      D64.4
   Egyptian B76.9 *[D63.8]*
   elliptocytosis —*see* Elliptocytosis
   enzyme-deficiency, drug-induced
      D59.2
   epidemic (*see also* Ancylostomiasis)
      B76.9 *[D63.8]*

Anemia *(Continued)*
   hemolytic *(Continued)*
      due to *(Continued)*
         enzyme disorder D55.9
            drug-induced D59.2
            presence of shunt or other
               internal prosthetic device
               D59.4
      familial D58.9
      hereditary D58.9
         due to enzyme disorder
            D55.9
         specified type NEC D55.8
         specified type NEC D58.8
      idiopathic (chronic) D59.9
      mechanical D59.4
      microangiopathic D59.4
      nonautoimmune D59.4
         drug-induced D59.2
      nonspherocytic
         congenital or hereditary NEC
            D55.8
         glucose-6-phosphate
            dehydrogenase deficiency
            D55.0

Fig. 12.3 Excerpt from the Alphabetic Index of Diseases and Injuries of *International Classification of Diseases,* Tenth Revision, Clinical Modification (ICD-10-CM).

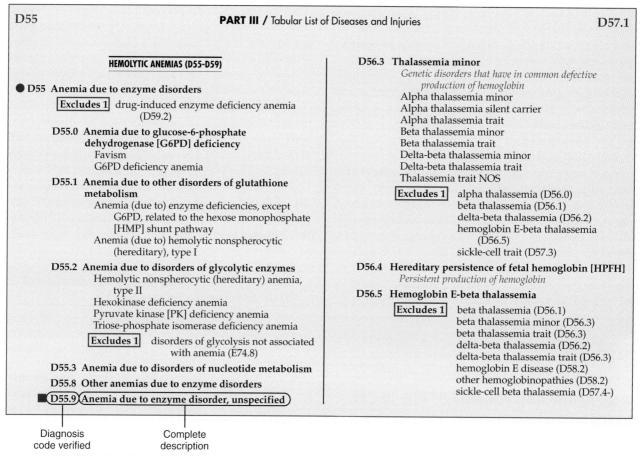

HEMOLYTIC ANEMIAS (D55-D59)

● **D55 Anemia due to enzyme disorders**

Excludes 1   drug-induced enzyme deficiency anemia
(D59.2)

D55.0 Anemia due to glucose-6-phosphate dehydrogenase [G6PD] deficiency
Favism
G6PD deficiency anemia

D55.1 Anemia due to other disorders of glutathione metabolism
Anemia (due to) enzyme deficiencies, except G6PD, related to the hexose monophosphate [HMP] shunt pathway
Anemia (due to) hemolytic nonspherocytic (hereditary), type I

D55.2 Anemia due to disorders of glycolytic enzymes
Hemolytic nonspherocytic (hereditary) anemia, type II
Hexokinase deficiency anemia
Pyruvate kinase [PK] deficiency anemia
Triose-phosphate isomerase deficiency anemia

Excludes 1   disorders of glycolysis not associated with anemia (E74.8)

D55.3 Anemia due to disorders of nucleotide metabolism

D55.8 Other anemias due to enzyme disorders

■ **D55.9 Anemia due to enzyme disorder, unspecified**

D56.3 Thalassemia minor
Genetic disorders that have in common defective production of hemoglobin
Alpha thalassemia minor
Alpha thalassemia silent carrier
Alpha thalassemia trait
Beta thalassemia minor
Beta thalassemia trait
Delta-beta thalassemia minor
Delta-beta thalassemia trait
Thalassemia trait NOS

Excludes 1   alpha thalassemia (D56.0)
beta thalassemia (D56.1)
delta-beta thalassemia (D56.2)
hemoglobin E-beta thalassemia (D56.5)
sickle-cell trait (D57.3)

D56.4 Hereditary persistence of fetal hemoglobin [HPFH]
Persistent production of hemoglobin

D56.5 Hemoglobin E-beta thalassemia

Excludes 1   beta thalassemia (D56.1)
beta thalassemia minor (D56.3)
beta thalassemia trait (D56.3)
delta-beta thalassemia (D56.2)
delta-beta thalassemia trait (D56.3)
hemoglobin E disease (D58.2)
other hemoglobinopathies (D58.2)
sickle-cell beta thalassemia (D57.4-)

Diagnosis code verified   Complete description

Fig. 12.4 Excerpt from the Tabular List of International Classification of Diseases, Tenth Revision, Clinical Modification (ICD-10-CM), Volume 1.

contains the Neoplasm Table, Tables of Drugs and Chemicals, and Index to External Cause. Main code descriptor items are in alphabetic order and indented subterms, and applicable additional qualifiers, descriptors, or modifiers are beneath the main terms.

Alphabetic Index elements are structured as follows:

• Main terms are classifications of diseases and injuries and appear as headings in bold type.

• Subterms are listings under main terms and are indented two spaces to the right under main terms. These are referred to as

essential modifiers because their presence changes the code assignment.

• Nonessential modifiers provide additional description and are enclosed in parentheses. These do not affect the code assigned and may or may not be present in the diagnosis.

• Carryover lines continue the text and are indented more than two spaces from the level of the preceding line.

• Subterms of subterms are additional listings and are indented two spaces to the right under the subterm (Fig. 12.5).

Fig. 12.5 Illustration of main terms, subterms, and nonessential modifiers. This is a diagram of the various elements for an entry in the alphabetical index.

Special Points to Remember in the Alphabetic Index

1. Notice that appropriate anatomical sites or modifiers are listed in alphabetic order under the main terms with further subterm listings as needed.
2. Examine all nonessential modifiers that appear in parentheses next to the main term. Check for nonessential modifiers that apply to any of the qualifying terms used in the statement of the diagnosis found in the patient's health record (Fig. 12.6).

Fig. 12.6 Coding with modifiers in parentheses.

3. Notice that eponyms appear as both main term entries and modifiers under main terms such as *disease* or *syndrome* and *operation*. As previously mentioned, an eponym is the name of a disease, structure, operation, or procedure, usually derived from the name of a place or a person who discovered or described it first.
4. Look for sublisted terms in parentheses that are associated with the eponym (Fig. 12.7).

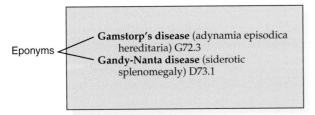

Fig. 12.7 Coding diagnoses associated with an eponym.

5. Locate closely related terms, code categories, and cross-referenced synonyms indicated by *see* and *see also* (Fig. 12.8).

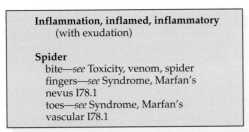

Fig.12.8 Cross-referencing synonyms, closely related terms, and code categories from the Alphabetic Index of *International Classification of Diseases*, Tenth Revision, Clinical Modification (ICD-10-CM).

Tabular List of Diseases and Injuries

The Tabular List of Diseases and Injuries (Volume 1) is placed after the Alphabetic Index (Volume 2) in most ICD-10-CM manual publications. The Tabular List contains 21 chapters and is composed of alphanumeric codes that represent diagnoses (Table 12.1). The ICD-10-CM codes can contain as few as three characters or as many as seven characters, with a decimal point after the third character. This is shown as digit 1 (alpha character), digits 2 and 3 (numeric character), and digits 4 to 7 (alpha or numeric character). The first three characters are placed to the left of the decimal point and indicate the category. The remaining digits to the right of the decimal point indicate the etiology, anatomic site, and severity. The sixth character can signify the following:

- Laterality
- Intent of a drug poisoning (intentional self-harm, assault)
- "With" or "without" a given manifestation

TABLE 12.1 Outline of Tabular List and Alphabetic Index of ICD-10-CM		
Tabular List	Chapter Headings	Codes
1	Certain Infectious and Parasitic Diseases	A00-B99
2	Neoplasms	C00-D49
3	Diseases of the Blood and Blood-Forming Organs and Certain Disorders Involving the Immune Mechanism	D50-D89
4	Endocrine, Nutritional, and Metabolic Diseases	E00-E89
5	Mental and Behavioral Disorders	F01-F99
6	Diseases of the Nervous System	G00-G99
7	Diseases of the Eye and Adnexa	H00-H59
8	Diseases of the Ear and Mastoid Process	H60-H95
9	Diseases of the Circulatory System	I00-I99
10	Diseases of the Respiratory System	J00-J99
11	Diseases of the Digestive System	K00-K95
12	Diseases of the Skin and Subcutaneous Tissue	L00-L99
13	Diseases of the Musculoskeletal System and Connective Tissue	M00-M99
14	Diseases of the Genitourinary System	N00-N99
15	Pregnancy, Childbirth, and the Puerperium	O00-O9A
16	Certain Conditions Originating in the Perinatal Period	P00-P96
17	Congenital Malformations, Deformations, and Chromosomal Abnormalities	Q00-Q99
18	Symptoms, Signs, and Abnormal Clinical and Laboratory Findings, Not Elsewhere Classifiable	R00-R99
19	Injury, Poisoning, and Certain Other Consequences of External Causes	S00-T88
20	External Causes of Morbidity	V00-Y99
21	Factors Influencing Health Status and Contact with Health Services	Z00-Z99
Alphabetic	Index	
Section 1	Index to Diseases, Alphabetic	
Section 2	Table of Drugs and Chemicals	
Section 3	Alphabetic Index to External Causes	

- Trimester of a pregnancy
- Depth of a skin ulcer
- Nature of an injury

An X is used as a placeholder to save a space for future code expansion and/or to meet the requirement of coding to the highest level of specificity (Example 12.2).

EXAMPLE 12.2 Seventh Characters and X Placeholders

S01.312A	Laceration without foreign body of left ear; initial encounter
T36.0 × 2A	Poisoning by penicillin, intentional, self-harm; initial encounter

Special Points to Remember in the Tabular List

1. Use two or more codes when necessary to describe a given diagnosis completely (Example 12.3).

EXAMPLE 12.3 Multiple Codes to Describe a Diagnosis

I25.10 + I50.9	Arteriosclerotic cardiovascular disease with congestive heart failure
I12 + N18.6 + N19	Hypertensive end stage kidney disease with renal failure

2. Follow the conventions and guidelines to determine how to code an encounter when a manifestation or a complication is present. A manifestation is an associated secondary process or disease. A complication is an evolution or consequence of a disease.
3. Use three-character category codes only if there are no subcategory codes (Example 12.4).

EXAMPLE 12.4 Category Code as Complete Code

I10	Hypertension
B20	Human Immunodeficiency Virus [HIV] disease

4. Read all instructional notes provided (Example 12.5).

EXAMPLE 12.5 Instructional Notes

G30-	Alzheimer's disease **Use additional code** to identify: delirium, if applicable (F05) dementia with behavioral disturbance (F02.81) dementia without behavioral disturbance (F02.80)
J91.0	Malignant pleural effusion **Code first** underlying neoplasm

🖋 12.4   QUICK REVIEW

Question: What is the difference between a manifestation and a complication?

OFFICIAL GUIDELINES FOR ICD-10-CM

The Official Guidelines for Coding and Reporting is a set of rules developed to accompany and complement the official conventions and instructions provided in the ICD-10-CM coding manual. The guidelines include definitions, standards, rules, general coding guidelines, and 21 chapter-specific coding guidelines. Adherence to the guidelines when assigning an ICD-10-CM diagnosis code is required under HIPAA and has been adopted for all health care settings. It is important that the health care provider and the billing/coding specialist work together to achieve complete and accurate documentation, code assignment, and reporting of diagnosis codes.

Diagnostic Code Book Conventions

To become a proficient coding specialist, it is important to develop an understanding of the conventions and terminology related to the ICD-10-CM coding system. Conventions are rules or principles for determining a diagnostic code when using diagnostic code books such as each space, typefaces, indentations, punctuation marks, symbols, instructional notes, abbreviations, cross-reference notes, and specific usage of the words *and, with,* and *due to*. These rules assist in the selection of correct codes for the diagnoses encountered. Some of the conventions for ICD-10-CM are listed in Box 12.2; however, the billing/coding specialist should read all the information included in the introduction section of the coding manual, which will provide a complete outline of all conventions used in the manual.

Placeholder Character

As mentioned, ICD-10-CM uses the placeholder character X when reporting certain codes to allow for future expansion of the code. When a placeholder is indicated, the X must be used in order for the code to be valid (Example 12.6).

EXAMPLE 12.6 Placeholder Character

T55.0 × 1A	Toxic effects of soap, unintentional; Initial encounter

Seventh Characters

Certain ICD-10-CM codes require seventh characters. If a code that requires a seventh character is not six characters, placeholder Xs must be used to fill the empty characters (Example 12.7).

EXAMPLE 12.7 Seventh Characters

S01.312A	Laceration without foreign body of left ear; Initial encounter
T36.0 × 2A	Poisoning by penicillin, intentional, self-harm; Initial encounter

Other and Unspecified Codes

The abbreviation NEC represents codes that are "not elsewhere classifiable." The Alphabetic Index will direct the coding specialist to an "other specified" code in the Tabular List. Alphabetic Index entries with NEC in the line designate "other" codes

BOX 12.2 Official ICD-10-CM Code Book Conventions

Punctuation

[]	Brackets are used in the Tabular List to enclose synonyms, alternative wording, or explanatory phrases. **Example:** J95.85- Mechanical complication of respirator [ventilator] Colons are used in the Tabular List after an incomplete term, which needs one or more of the modifiers following the colon to make it assignable to a given category. **Example:** L99 Other disorders of skin and subcutaneous tissue in diseases classified elsewhere Code first underlying disease, such as: amyloidosis (E85.-)
☑ -	Check boxes are used in the Alphabetic Index to indicate incomplete codes. These codes require additional digits. The extended codes must be found in the Tabular List for proper coding. **Example:** arteriovenous fistula, surgically created T82.9☑ Dashes are used in the ICD-10-CM the Tabular List. This symbol (-) at the end of an entry indicates an incomplete code, so additional characters are needed. Locate the referenced category or subcategory elsewhere in the Tabular List, review the options, and assign the code. **Example:** Excludes 2: cellulitis of ear (H60.1-)
()	Parentheses are used in the Tabular List to enclose supplementary words (nonessential modifiers) that may be present or absent in the statement of a disease or condition without affecting the code number to which it was assigned. **Example:** N39.3 Stress incontinence (female) (male)

Abbreviations

NEC	Not elsewhere classifiable (NEC) in the Tabular List under a code identifies it as an "other specified" code. **Example:** A85 Other viral encephalitis, not elsewhere classifiable **Includes:** specified viral encephalomyelitis **NEC**
NOS	Not otherwise specified (NOS) is equivalent to an unspecified code. **Example:** Q66.89 Other congenital deformities of feetCongenital clubfoot **NOS**

Cross-Reference Terms

and	This word represents and/or when used in a narrative statement. **Example:** B35.0 Tinea barbae **and** tinea capitis
with/without	When a condition may have two versions—with or without a specific sign, symptom, or manifestation—this is indicated by a change in one of the code characters. These words in the Alphabetic Index are sequenced after the main term, not in alphabetical order. **Example:** Epilepsy, epileptic, epilepsia intractable G40.91-**with** status epilepticus G40.911 **without** status epilepticus G40.919
see	Instruction that follows a main term in the Index indicating that another term should be referenced. Go to the main term referenced with the "see" note to find the correct code. **Example:** Postphlebitic syndrome—**see** Syndrome, postthrombotic
see also	Instruction after a main term in the Index to indicate that there is another main term that may also be referenced and may provide additional index entries that may be useful. It is not necessary to follow the "see also" note when the original main term gives the code. **Example:** Preterm delivery (**see also** Pregnancy, complicated by, preterm labor) O60.10

Instructional Notes

Code first/use additional code	Notes that certain conditions have both an underlying etiology and multiple body system manifestations due to the underlying etiology. Manifestation code titles have a phrase, "in diseases classified elsewhere." The underlying condition must be sequenced first followed by the manifestation. **Example:** E08 Diabetes mellitus due to underlying condition **Code first** the underlying condition, such as: Congenital rubella (P35.0) **Use additional code** to identify any insulin use (Z79.4), oral antidiabetic drugs or oral hypoglycemic drugs (Z79.84).
Code also	Note instructions that two codes may be needed to completely describe a condition dependent on the severity of the conditions and the reason for the encounter. **Example:** S85 Injury of blood vessels at lower leg level **Code also** any associated open wound (S81.-)
Includes	Includes appears under certain categories to add to the definition or give an example of the content of the category. **Example:** S93 Dislocation and sprain of joints and ligaments at ankle, foot, and toe level **Includes:** avulsion of joint or ligament of ankle, foot, and toe
Inclusion terms	List of terms included under some codes, such as conditions for which that code is to be used, synonyms, or various specified conditions assigned to "other specified" codes. **Example:** C46.1 Kaposi's sarcoma of soft tissue **Kaposi's sarcoma of blood vessel** **Kaposi's sarcoma of connective tissue** **Kaposi's sarcoma of fascia** **Kaposi's sarcoma of ligament**

Continued

BOX 12.2   Official ICD-10-CM Code Book Conventions—cont'd

Excludes 1	An Excludes 1 note very simply indicates "not coded here." An Excludes 1 note should never be used at the same time as the code above the Excludes 1 note. It is used when two conditions cannot occur together, such as a congenital form versus an acquired form of the same condition. **Example:** E20 **Hypoparathyroidism** **Excludes 1:** Di George's syndrome (D82.1)
Excludes 2	An Excludes 2 note very simply indicates "not included here." An Excludes 2 note indicates that the condition excluded is not part of the condition represented by the code but that a patient may have both conditions at the same time. When an Excludes 2 note appears under a code, use both the code and the excluded code together. **Example:** I10 Essential (primary) hypertension **Excludes 2:** Essential (primary) hypertension involving vessels of brain (I60-I69)

ICD-10-CM, International Classification of Diseases, Tenth Revision, Clinical Modification.

in the Tabular List. These Alphabetic Index entries represent specific disease entities for which no specific code exists, so the term is included within an "other" code (Example 12.8).

EXAMPLE 12.8   Other Specified Codes

K63.89	Other specified diseases of intestine

The abbreviation NOS represents "not otherwise specified" and means unspecified. In ICD-10-CM, a code with a fourth digit 9 or fifth digit 0 for diagnosis codes labeled "unspecified" is used when the information in the health record is insufficient to assign a more specific code. For those categories for which an unspecified code is not provided, the "other specified" code may represent both other and unspecified (Example 12.9).

EXAMPLE 12.9   Unspecified Codes

J32.9	Chronic sinusitis, unspecified Sinusitis (chronic) NOS

Punctuation and Symbols

ICD-10-CM's Alphabetic Index and Tabular List make use of certain abbreviations, punctuation, symbols, and other conventions, as shown in Box 12.2.

Brackets, [], are used in the Tabular List to enclose synonyms or alternative wording or to provide explanatory phrases (Example 12.10).

EXAMPLE 12.10   Brackets

B20	Human Immunodeficiency Virus [HIV] disease

Parentheses, (), are used in the Alphabetic Index and Tabular List to enclose supplementary words that may further define the condition but do not affect the code number assigned. These are referred to as *nonessential modifiers* (Example 12.11).

EXAMPLE 12.11   Parentheses

K55.012	Diffuse acute (reversible) ischemia of small intestine

Colons are used in the Tabular List after an incomplete term that requires additional modifiers to appropriately assign the code (Example 12.12).

EXAMPLE 12.12   Colons

D59.3	Hemolytic-uremic syndrome *Use additional code to identify associated:* E. coli infection (B96.2-) Pneumococcal pneumonia (J13)

Includes Notes

An includes note appears immediately under the three-character code title in the Tabular List and provides further definition and examples of additional content to the category (Example 12.13).

EXAMPLE 12.13   Includes Notes

I10	Essential (primary) hypertension *Includes: high blood pressure hypertension (arterial) (benign)* *(essential) (malignant) (primary) (systemic)*

Excludes Notes

There are two types of excludes notes used in the Tabular List of ICD-10-CM. An Excludes 1 note indicates certain codes that should never be used at the same time as the code selected. It is used when two conditions could not possibly occur at the same time. Excludes 2 notes indicate that the condition selected is not part of the excluded condition; however, it is possible for the patient to have both conditions at the same time. It is acceptable to report both the code and the excluded code together, when applicable (Example 12.14).

EXAMPLE 12.14   Excludes Notes

R07.0	Pain in throat *Excludes 1: chronic sore throat (J31.2)* *sore throat (acute) NOS (J02.9)* *Excludes 2: dysphagia (R13.1)* *pain in neck (M54.2)*

"And" and "With"

"And" in a code description should be interpreted as "and" or "or."

"With" or "in" should be interpreted as "associated with" or "due to" (Example 12.15).

EXAMPLE 12.15	And/With
A18.0	Tuberculosis of bones **and** joints
R11.2	Nausea **with** vomiting

"See" and "See also"

"See" indicates another term should be referenced. A "see" instruction must be followed.

"See also" suggests another term may be referenced. It is not always necessary to follow a "see also" instruction (Example 12.16).

EXAMPLE 12.16	See/See also
5.19	Cellulitis, foot—see Cellulitis, lower limb
5.20	Infarct, omentum (see also Infarct, intestine) K55.069

Default Code

A default code is shown next to a main term in the Alphabetic Index and represents the condition that is commonly associated with the main term or is the unspecified code for the condition. For example, if the electronic health record documents appendicitis but does not list acute or chronic, then the default code should be assigned (Example 12.17).

EXAMPLE 12.17	Default Code
K37	*Unspecified* appendicitis

Gender and Age Codes

Diagnostic codes must match the age and gender of the patient. If an adult male patient with breast cancer is seen, a code that matches gender must be used (Example 12.18).

EXAMPLE 12.18	Gender and Age Codes
C50.411	Malignant neoplasm of upper-outer quadrant of right *female* breast
C50.421	Malignant neoplasm of upper-outer quadrant of right *male* breast
P70.2	*Neonatal* diabetes mellitus

12.5   QUICK REVIEW
Question: What is the difference between NEC and NOS?

12.6   QUICK REVIEW
Question: What is the difference between brackets [] and parentheses () in the Tabular List?

12.7   QUICK REVIEW
Question: What is the difference between "see" and "see also?"

GENERAL CODING GUIDELINES

Locating a Code in the ICD-10-CM

To select a code that corresponds to a diagnosis or reason for a medical service, the coding specialist should first locate the term in the Alphabetic Index and then verify the code in the Tabular List. Some helpful hints to assist with finding the appropriate diagnosis code are listed in Box 12.3. Step-by-step procedures for selecting ICD-10-CM diagnostic codes are presented at the end of this chapter in Procedure 12.1.

A checked box (☑) at the end of an Alphabetic Index entry indicates that an additional character is required and can be determined by referencing the Tabular List. Even if a checked box is not present, the coding specialist must always consult the Tabular List to refer to all additional instructional notes (Example 12.19).

EXAMPLE 12.19	A Checked Box
Conjunctivitis, acute, unspecified H10.3☑	

BOX 12.3   Helpful Hints for Choosing an Appropriate Diagnosis Code

1. If the ICD-10-CM code books are not color coded, identify important references with a colored highlighter pen. Also add tabs to main sections of the Alphabetic Index, Tabular List, and Drug and Chemical Table.
2. Refer to the end of this chapter to learn how to locate and select diagnostic codes step by step. (see Procedure 2.1)
3. Many times, a cross-referenced code in the Alphabetic Index is the same when verified in the Tabular List. In some cases, indicating these codes in the Alphabetic Index with a different-colored highlighter pen will remind a billing/coding specialist that this code is correct as described in the Alphabetic Index, which saves time. However, keep in mind that the Tabular List has many instructional notes that are not indicated in the Alphabetic Index and must be followed for accurate coding.
4. Keep a list of diagnostic codes that are commonly encountered. Some insurance companies publish lists of diagnostic codes that support medical necessity and are acceptable for specific procedures. Consult payer guidelines by calling the insurance company or managed care plan to determine whether certain procedures are a covered benefit for certain diagnoses and, if not, have the patient sign a waiver. Reference books that show codes that link diagnostic and procedure codes are available. The American Medical Association (AMA) publishes a list of the most common diagnostic codes at the end of each of its mini–specialty code books.
5. In the past, some health care organizations have developed an encounter form that is an all-encompassing billing document and reference page and that acts as a shortcut to locating diagnostic codes for conditions commonly seen by a provider. Most often these types of documents are found to lack the specificity necessary to infer diagnosis details needed for accurate coding under the ICD-10-CM system. As such, it is no longer recommended that these types of billing documents be used.

A dash is used in the Tabular list to indicate an incomplete code (Example 12.20).

EXAMPLE 12.20   A Dash

| D44 | Neoplasm of uncertain behavior of endocrine glands |
| | *Excludes 1: multiple endocrine adenomatosis (E31.2-)* |

Level of Detail in Coding

ICD-10-CM codes are composed of three, four, five, six, or seven characters. Some conditions may be reported with a three-character code. However, if the code is further subdivided, it should be reported at the highest number of characters assigned. This is commonly referred to as coding to the highest level of specificity. A code is invalid if it has not been coded to the full number of characters required for that condition.

Signs and Symptoms

Codes that describe signs and symptoms are acceptable for reporting purposes when a related definitive diagnosis has not been established. This is reported using codes from Chapter 18 of the ICD-10-CM coding manual. Examples of codes found in this section are symptoms, signs, and abnormal clinical and laboratory findings, not elsewhere classified. When coding for professional or outpatient services, if the final diagnosis is qualified by any of the following terms it should not be coded as if it existed or was established:

- Apparent
- Likely
- Might
- Possible
- Probably
- Questionable
- Rule Out
- Suspected
- Suspicion Of

Instead, document the condition to the highest degree of certainty and code the chief complaint, sign or symptom, abnormal test result, or other reason for the encounter.

This is contrary to coding practices used by hospital health information management departments for coding the diagnoses of hospital inpatients. For example, if a patient is admitted and is suspected of having a heart attack, this would be coded as a confirmed case of myocardial infarction.

The following are instances in which sign and symptom codes can be used for professional or outpatient services.
- No precise diagnosis can be made (Example 12.21).

EXAMPLE 12.21   No Precise Diagnosis

The patient has an enlarged liver and further diagnostic studies may or may not be done. **Use code R16.0 for hepatomegaly.**

The patient complains of painful urination and urinalysis is negative. **Use code R30.0 for dysuria.**

- Signs or symptoms are transient or temporary and a specific diagnosis was not made (Example 12.22).

EXAMPLE 12.22   Transient Sign and Symptom Code

The patient complains of chest pain on deep inspiration. On examination, the provider finds nothing abnormal and tells the patient to return in 1 week. When the patient returns, the pain has ceased. **Use code R07.1 for painful respiration.**

- Provisional diagnosis is made for a patient who does not return for further care (Example 12.23).

EXAMPLE 12.23   Provisional Diagnosis

On examination, the provider documents abnormal percussion of the chest. The patient is sent for a chest x-ray examination and is asked to return for a recheck. The patient does not have the x-ray examination and fails to return. **Use code R09.89 for abnormal chest sounds.**

- A patient is referred for treatment before a definite diagnosis is made (Example 12.24).

EXAMPLE 12.24   Sign and Symptom Code Before Definite Diagnosis

A patient complains of nausea and vomiting and is referred to a gastroenterologist. **Use code R11.2 for nausea with vomiting.**

! COMPLIANCE ALERT

When coding for outpatient and provider services, signs and symptoms that are inherent in a disease process are not coded separately if a definitive diagnosis is documented (Example 12.25).

EXAMPLE 12.25   Conditions That Are an Integral Part of a Disease Process

The provider documents asthma with wheezing. Wheezing is a sign and symptom typically associated with asthma; therefore, the code for asthma is all that should be reported.

The provider documents nausea and vomiting due to gastroenteritis. Nausea and vomiting are signs and symptoms typically associated with gastroenteritis; therefore, only the code for gastroenteritis should be reported.

If a symptom that is not typically associated with a disease is also documented, it should be coded separately (Example 12.26).

EXAMPLE 12.26 Conditions That Are Not an Integral Part of a Disease Process

The provider documents diverticulosis with abdominal pain. Patients can have diverticulosis without having abdominal pain. By reporting abdominal pain in addition to diverticulosis, the severity of the condition is better described. Medical necessity for further study is also supported by reporting abdominal pain with diverticulosis.

The provider documents benign prostatic hypertrophy with urinary frequency. Patients can have benign prostatic hypertrophy without urinary frequency. By reporting urinary frequency in addition to benign prostatic hypertrophy, the severity of the condition is better described. Medical necessity for further study is also supported by reporting urinary frequency with benign prostatic hypertrophy.

Multiple Coding for a Single Condition

In some cases, two codes will be required to describe a single condition. "Use additional code" notes from the Tabular List will guide the coding specialist as to when it is appropriate to report a secondary code. When determining which code to sequence first, the additional code would be reported as a secondary code (Example 12.27).

EXAMPLE 12.27 Multiple Coding for a Single Condition

G30.-	Alzheimer's disease
	Use additional code to identify:
	Delirium, if applicable (F05)
	Dementia with behavioral disturbance (F02.81)
	Dementia without behavioral disturbance (F02-80)

"Code first" notes are also indicated in the Tabular List and are typically used to identify an underlying condition. The underlying condition is always reported as the primary code (Example 12.28).

EXAMPLE 12.28 "Code First" Notes

O34.-	Maternal care for abnormality of pelvic organ
	Code first any associated obstructed labor (O65.5)
131.4	Cardiac tamponade
	Code first underlying cause

Acute, Subacute, and Chronic Conditions

When the documentation mentions that a condition is both acute (subacute) and chronic and separate codes exist in the Alphabetic Index, both are coded with the acute (subacute) sequence first followed by the code for the chronic condition (Example 12.29).

EXAMPLE 12.29 Acute, Subacute, and Chronic Conditions

Appendicitis (pneumococcal) (retrocecal) K37
    Acute (catarrhal) (fulminating) (gangrenous) (obstructive) (retrocecal) (suppurative) K35.80
        Subacute (adhesive) K36
        Chronic (recurrent) K36

For documentation to support chronic conditions, the provider must discuss the chronic condition and state that the condition is pertinent to the patient's current treatment. For example, if a provider states "controlled diabetes," he or she is stating a fact. If the provider asks the patient about his blood sugar level and diet and documents the findings, then something specific has been identified about the chronic condition. This would be considered proper documentation.

Combination Code

A combination code is a situation in which a single code is used to classify two diagnoses or a diagnosis with an associated secondary process (manifestation) or a diagnosis with an associated complication. Identify a combination code by referring to subterm entries in the Alphabetic Index and by reading the inclusion and exclusion notes in the Tabular List. If the combination code does not specifically describe the manifestation or complication, use a secondary code (Example 12.30).

EXAMPLE 12.30 Combination Code

J44.0	Chronic obstructive pulmonary disease with acute lower respiratory infection
	Use additional code to identify the infection
E11.311	Type II diabetes mellitus with unspecified diabetic retinopathy with macular edema

Sequela

A sequela is a late effect or condition produced after the acute phase of an illness. There is no time limit on when a late effect code can be used. Coding of sequela generally requires two codes. The nature of the sequela is sequenced first; the sequela code is sequenced second (Example 12.31).

EXAMPLE 12.31 Sequela

R13.1-	Dysphagia
I69.991	Dysphagia following unspecified cerebrovascular disease
	Use additional code to identify the type of dysphagia, if known [R13.1-]

Impending or Threatened Condition

Codes that are described as impending or threatened should be referenced as such in the Alphabetic Index and reported accordingly. If there is no subterm under impending or threatened for the condition described, report the existing underlying condition(s) (Example 12.32).

EXAMPLE 12.32 Impending or Threatened Condition

Impending myocardial infarction I20.0
Threatened abortion O20.0

Reporting the Same Diagnosis Code More Than Once

Each unique ICD-10-CM diagnosis code may be reported only once for an encounter. This applies to bilateral conditions where there are no distinct codes to identify laterality or two different conditions are classified to the same diagnosis code.

Laterality

When reporting bilateral sites, the final character of the code in ICD-10-CM should be selected to indicate laterality. The right side is always character 1 and the left side character 2. In those situations when a bilateral code is given, the bilateral character is always 3. If the side is not identified, an unspecified code is provided, which is either 0 or 9, depending on whether it is a fifth or sixth character (Example 12.33).

EXAMPLE 12.33 Laterality

S67.0-	Crushing injury of thumb
S67.00-	Crushing injury of thumb of unspecified side
S67.01-	Crushing injury of right thumb
S67.02-	Crushing injury of left thumb

Documentation for Body Mass Index and Pressure Ulcer Stages

Information documented by clinicians, such as nurses, to indicate body mass index (BMI) or pressure ulcer stage codes can be coded and reported when documented in the medical record. The information does not need to be documented by the provider of the medical record. However, the patient's provider must document the associated diagnosis such as obesity or pressure ulcer.

Syndromes

A syndrome is another name for a symptom complex, which is a set of signs, symptoms, or other manifestations resulting from a common cause or appearing in combination, presenting a distinct clinical picture of a disease or inherited abnormality. Syndromes should be reported by following the Alphabetic Index (Example 12.34).

EXAMPLE 12.34 Syndromes

Down syndrome Q90.9
Adams-Stokes syndrome I45.9

Documentation of Complications of Care

Complications of care codes are assigned based on provider's documentation of the relationship between the condition and the care or procedure (Example 12.35).

EXAMPLE 12.35 Complications of Care

Complication of anesthesia T88.59-
Complication of colostomy K94.0

 12.8 QUICK REVIEW
Question: When should a sign or symptom be coded?

 12.9 QUICK REVIEW
Question: What is sequela?

 12.10 QUICK REVIEW
Question: What is laterality?

CHAPTER SPECIFIC CODING GUIDELINES

In addition to general diagnosis coding guidelines, there are guidelines specific to the 21 chapters of the Tabular Index. Some of the most commonly referenced chapter-specific coding guidelines are provided in this text; however, the billing/coding specialist must be familiar with the entire contents of the Official Guidelines for Coding and Reporting and refer to them when reporting all conditions. The chapter-specific guidelines are located in Section I, Subsection C of the Official Guidelines.

Human Immunodeficiency Virus

Human immunodeficiency virus (HIV) is a disease of the immune system characterized by increased susceptibility to opportunistic infections, certain cancers, and neurologic disorders. Specific guidelines for reporting HIV infections are provided in Section Ia, Chapter 1, Subsection C of the Chapter-Specific Coding Guidelines. Only confirmed cases of HIV infection or illness should be reported. The provider's documentation that the patient is HIV positive would serve as confirmation. The diagnosis code B20 is used to report HIV disease, whereas an asymptomatic HIV infection status is reported as Z21. Patients who present for testing for HIV are coded as Z11.4, encounter for screening for HIV. Once a patient is given a confirmed diagnosis of HIV, it should be coded for every subsequent admission or encounter thereafter. Sequencing is determined by the reason for the encounter.

Neoplasms

Section I, Chapter 2, Subsection C of the Chapter-Specific Coding Guidelines provides guidelines for neoplasm coding. A neoplasm is a spontaneous new growth of tissue forming an abnormal mass that is also known as a *tumor*. It may be benign or malignant. A table is provided in the Alphabetic Index to look up the condition using the main entry "Neoplasm." The table has the column headings Malignant, Benign, Uncertain Behavior, and Unspecified (Table 12.2).

First, check the index; if the term for the area in active treatment is not listed, then go to the table. Often the index entry will produce the correct code and indicate what area of the table to look in. If a coding specialist searches the table first, an incorrect code may be obtained. Code numbers for neoplasms are given by anatomic site. For each site, there are six possible code numbers, indicating whether the neoplasm in question is malignant (primary, secondary, or carcinoma in situ), benign, of uncertain behavior, or of unspecified nature. The description of the neoplasm often indicates which of the six code numbers is appropriate. For example, a melanoma of skin is malignant, a fibroadenoma of breast is benign, and a carcinoma in situ of cervix uteri is malignant by definition of the type of neoplasm (Example 12.36).

TABLE 12.2 Coding for Neoplasms

| | MALIGNANT | | | | | |
	Primary	Secondary	Carcinoma in Situ	Benign	Uncertain Behavior	Unspecified
Neoplasm, neoplastic	C80.1	C79.9	D09.9	D36.9	D48.9	D49.9
Abdomen, abdominal	C76.2	C79.8-	D09.8	D36.7	D48.7	D49.89
Cavity	C76.2	C79.8-	D09.8	D36.7	D48.7	D49.89
Organ	C76.2	C79.8-	D09.8	D36.7	D48.7	D49.89
Viscera	C76.2	C79.8-	D09.8	D36.7	D48.7	D49.89
Wall	C44.509	C79.2-	D04.5	D23.5	D48.5	D49.2
Connective tissue	C49.4	C79.8-	—	D21.4	D48.1	D49.2
Abdominopelvic	C76.8	C79.8-	—	D36.7	D48.7	D49.89
Accessory sinus—see Neoplasm, sinus						
Acoustic nerve	C72.4-	C79.49	—	D33.3	D43.3	D49.7
Adenoid (pharynx) (tissue)	C11.1	C79.89	D00.08	D10.6	D37.05	D49.0
Adipose tissue (see also Neoplasm, connective tissue)	C49.4	C79.89	—	D21.9	D48.1	D49.2
Adnexa (uterine)	C57.4	C79.89	D07.39	D28.7	D39.8	D49.5
Adrenal	C74.9-	C79.7-	D09.3	D35.0-	D44.1-	D49.7
Capsule	C74.9-	C79.7-	D09.3	D35.0-	D44.1-	D49.7
Cortex	C74.0-	C79.7-	D09.3	D35.0-	D44.1-	D49.7
Gland	C74.9-	C79.7-	D09.3	D35.0-	D44.1-	D49.7
Medulla	C74.1-	C79.7-	D09.3	D35.0-	D44.1-	D49.7
Ala nasi (external)	C44.301	C79.2-	D04.39	D23.39	D48.5	D49.2
Alimentary canal or tract NEC	C26.9	C78.80	D01.9	D13.9	D37.9	D49.0

NEC, Not elsewhere classifiable.

EXAMPLE 12.36 Adenocarcinoma of the Breast With Metastases to the Pelvic Bone

Step 1 Look up adenocarcinoma in the Alphabetic Index. Notice it states: *see also* Neoplasm, by site, malignant.

Step 2 Locate neoplasm in the table in the Alphabetic Index. At the top of the page, notice the Malignant heading with the subheadings Primary, Secondary, and Ca In Situ. *Primary* means the first site of development of the malignancy. *Secondary* means metastasis from the primary site to a second site. *Ca In Situ* means cancer confined to the epithelium of the site of origin without invasion of the basement membrane tissue of the site.

Step 3 Find the site of the adenocarcinoma (in this case the breast) and look under the Malignant and Primary headings. Note that the code given is C50.919.

Step 4 Next, find bone as a subterm in the Neoplasm Table and look for the subterm *pelvic*. Then look at the three columns under Malignant and using the Secondary column, find the correct code number C79.51. In listing these diagnoses on the insurance claim, give the following: C50.919 and C79.51.

A **benign tumor** is one that does not have the properties of invasion and **metastasis** or spread or transfer of tumor cells from one organ to another site. It is usually surrounded by a fibrous capsule. It is important to note that cysts and lesions are not neoplasms. A neoplasm is not necessarily cancer or malignant.

A **malignant tumor** has the properties of invasion and metastasis. The term *carcinoma* refers to a cancerous or malignant tumor. **Carcinoma in situ** means cancer confined to the site of origin without invasion of neighboring tissues. A *primary*

malignancy means the original malignant neoplastic site. A *secondary neoplasm* or malignancy is the site or location to which the original malignancy has spread or metastasized. If the diagnosis does not mention metastasis, code the case as a primary neoplasm (Example 12.37). Lymphomas and leukemias are not classified using the primary and secondary terminology.

EXAMPLE 12.37 Primary and Secondary Cancerous Tumors

Primary C64- Malignant neoplasm of kidney, except renal pelvis
C65- Malignant neoplasm renal pelvis

Secondary C79.0- Secondary malignant neoplasm of kidney and renal

The diagnostic statement "metastatic from" indicates primary stage carcinoma whereas "metastatic to" indicates secondary stage carcinoma. If the diagnostic statement is "malignant neoplasm spread to," code it as the primary site spread to the secondary site. The phrase "recurrent malignancy" is coded as a primary neoplasm.

The column of the neoplasm table labeled **Uncertain Behavior** is used when the lesion's behavior cannot be predicted. The pathologist has examined the specimen and found it to be benign at the present time but there is a chance it could undergo malignant transformation over time. These are well-defined neoplasms, the subsequent behavior of which cannot be predicted from the present appearance. These codes should be reported only if the pathology reports the neoplasm as "Uncertain Behavior" or an instructional note in the Alphabetic Index points toward an "Uncertain Behavior" code (Example 12.38).

If a neoplasm has been excised but no pathology report is available, it is not reported as uncertain behavior; it would be reported using the "Unspecified Behavior" column of the table. Reporting a lesion of unknown diagnosis as a lesion of uncertain behavior is a common coding error. It is always recommended that the coding specialist wait for the final pathology report after excision of a neoplasm. Although waiting for the final diagnosis may mean a delay in submission of the bill for payment, it is preferable to submit with the correct diagnosis.

Coding of Diabetes Mellitus

Diabetes mellitus (DM) is an endocrine disease; guidelines for coding DM are found in Section 1, Subsection C, Chapter 4 of the Chapter-Specific Coding Guidelines. DM is categorized as either type 1 or type 2 and should be identified in the provider's documentation for accurate reporting of the condition. Table 12.3 outlines the clinical features important in the classification of diabetes.

Type 1 DM is also known as juvenile diabetes, which commonly develops before the individual reaches puberty; however, the age of the patient is not the sole determining factor for this diagnosis. In type 1 diabetes, the patient's pancreas does not function properly and does not produce insulin. Thus, this patient's body is dependent on insulin. Do not assume that because a patient is taking insulin, he or she has an insulin-dependent diabetes; look to the service provider's documentation for clarification.

Type 2 DM used to be referred to as adult-onset diabetes. In type 2 diabetes, the patient's pancreas produces some insulin, but the insulin is ineffective in doing its job, which is to remove sugar from the bloodstream. This type of diabetes may be controlled with diet, oral medication, or insulin. If the type of diabetes is not documented in the health record, the default is E11.-, type 2 diabetes.

Patients with DM often encounter complications that affect other body systems. The diabetes codes are combination codes that include the type of diabetes, the body system affected, and the complications affecting that body system. The coding specialist should assign as many codes from categories E08-E13 as needed to identify all the associated conditions the patient has. They should be sequenced based on the reason for the particular encounter (Example 12.39).

Diabetes code categories (E08, E09, E11, and E13) have an associated instructional note in the Tabular Index that advises the coding specialist to "use additional code to identify any insulin use (Z79.4), oral antidiabetic drugs or oral hyperglycemic drugs (Z79.84)." If the patient routinely takes insulin, use diagnosis code Z79.4, long-term (current) use of insulin, but do not use this code if the patient takes insulin temporarily to control blood sugar.

If the patient receives an underdose because of pump failure, assign a code from subcategory T85.6, mechanical complication of other specified internal and external prosthetic devices, implants and grafts, followed by code T38.3 × 6-, with the appropriate code for the type of DM and any associated complications. If the pump failure causes an insulin overdose, the second diagnosis code should be T38.3 × 1-, poisoning by insulin and oral hypoglycemic drugs, accidental, with the appropriate code for the type of DM and related complications.

Diabetes is a significant complicating factor in pregnancy. When coding DM in pregnancy, assign a code from category O24, DM in pregnancy, childbirth, and the puerperium, as the primary code. The appropriate diabetes code from the category E08 to E13 should be reported as a secondary code. Gestational diabetes occurs when the diabetes was induced by the pregnancy. This can occur during the second or third trimester of pregnancy in women who were not diabetic before pregnancy. Codes from subcategory O24.4, gestational DM, are reported when this condition is documented.

Circulatory System Conditions

Diseases of the circulatory system are difficult to code because of the variety and lack of specific terminology used by service providers in stating the diagnoses. The billing/coding specialist should refer to Section 1, Subsection C, Chapter 9 of the Chapter-Specific Coding Guidelines for assistance in coding circulatory system conditions. When selecting codes, carefully read all inclusion, exclusion, and "use additional code" notations contained in the Tabular List.

Hypertension

Hypertension may be documented as benign or malignant. Malignant hypertension has nothing to do with tumor formation. Malignant hypertension is a condition of very high blood pressure with poor prognosis. It is a symptom complex of markedly elevated blood pressure and is associated with papilledema. In this disease, the term *malignant* denotes that it is life threatening. Malignant hypertension should only be coded when the provider documents

TABLE 12.3 **Features of Type 1 and Type 2 Diabetes**	
Type 1 Diabetes	**Type 2 diabetes**
Insulin-dependent diabetes mellitus	Non–insulin-dependent diabetes mellitus
Patients must be treated with insulin	Patients may be treated with insulin
Insulin levels are very low	Insulin levels may be high, "normal," or low
Ketosis prone	Non–ketosis prone
Patients usually are lean	Patients usually are obese
Usually "juvenile onset" (peak onset at early puberty)	Usually "adult onset," although occasionally seen in children
Often little family history of diabetes mellitus	Often strong family history of diabetes mellitus

it as such. *Benign hypertension* refers to high blood pressure that runs a relatively long and symptomless course. In ICD-10-CM, hypertension is reported with the code I10, regardless of whether the hypertension is documented as benign or malignant.

Hypertension can cause various forms of heart and vascular disease or it can accompany some heart conditions. There are code categories used to report these conditions as combination codes.

Code Category I11	Hypertensive heart disease
Code Category I12	Hypertensive chronic kidney disease
Code Category I13	Hypertensive heart and chronic kidney disease

When the diagnostic statement indicates a cause by stating "heart condition *due to* hypertension" or "hypertensive heart disease," assign a code from category I11. If the diagnostic statement reads "*with* hypertension" or "cardiomegaly *and* hypertension," two separate codes are needed. Whenever a patient has both HTN and chronic kidney disease, a causal relationship may be assumed.

Elevated blood pressure or high blood pressure without mention of hypertension is coded R03.0. If a patient has a single high blood pressure reading, it does not indicate there is a problem or the need for medical intervention. Sometimes, a patient simply gets nervous when seeking medical evaluation or treatment. This is referred to as *white coat syndrome*.

Secondary hypertension is due to an underlying condition and is reported from the code category I15. An additional code is required to report secondary hypertension to identify the cause of the hypertension when specified.

Myocardial Infarctions

A myocardial infarction (MI) is commonly referred to as a heart attack. During an MI, there is death to a segment of heart muscle caused by a blood clot in the coronary artery that interrupts the heart's blood supply. An MI that is equal to or less than 4 weeks old is considered acute and is reported with codes from category I21. If the patient is still receiving care related to the MI after the 4-week time frame, the appropriate aftercare code should be assigned. If the patient suffers an acute MI during the 4-week time frame, the incident should be reported with a code from category I22 to indicate a subsequent acute MI. The code I25.2 is reported for old or healed myocardial infarctions that do not require further care.

Respiratory Conditions

In the Tabular List for Chapter 10, there is a note that applies to all respiratory codes (J00-J99). It instructs coding specialists to use an additional code to identify exposure to smoke, history of tobacco use, or current tobacco use or abuse. Tobacco cessation is not only a goal for patient health but also an important quality measure that many insurance companies track.

The appropriate codes specify the following:

- exposure to environmental tobacco smoke (Z77.22)
- exposure to tobacco smoke in the perinatal period (P96.81)
- history of tobacco dependence (Z87.891)
- occupational exposure to environmental tobacco smoke (Z57.31)

- tobacco dependence (F17.-)
- tobacco use (Z72.0)

Tobacco use should not be coded if the patient is a regular smoker. If documentation states they are a smoker, or smokes a specified amount per day, coding specialists should indicate tobacco dependence. Under "smoker" in the index, a coding specialist is directed to "see Dependence, drug, nicotine." Some chronic respiratory conditions, such as asthma and chronic obstructive pulmonary disease, list exacerbations as a possible subterm. An exacerbation is an acute increase in the severity of an illness. Acute respiratory infection such as bronchitis or pneumonia would be an example of an exacerbation. Asthma also lists the subterm status asthmaticus which refers to asthma that is not responding to treatment.

Pregnancy, Delivery, or Abortion

Section 1, Subsection C, Chapter 15 of the Chapter-Specific Coding Guidelines provides guidelines for reporting pregnancy, delivery, or abortion cases. Chapter 15 codes have sequencing priority over codes from other chapters. When the provider has treated a condition unrelated to the pregnancy, but the pregnancy has been documented as incidental to the encounter, code Z33.1, pregnant state, incidental, should be used in place of a Chapter 15 code.

The following main sections are included:

O00-O08: Pregnancy with abortive outcome
O09: Supervision of high-risk pregnancy
O10-O16: Edema, proteinuria, and hypertensive disorders in pregnancy, childbirth, and the puerperium
O20-O29: Other maternal disorders predominately related to pregnancy
O30-O48: Maternal care related to the fetus and amniotic cavity and possible delivery problems
O60-O77: Complications of labor and delivery
O80-O82: Encounter for delivery
O85-O92: Complications predominantly related to the puerperium
O94-O9A: Other obstetric conditions, not elsewhere classifiable

An entire section of the Chapter-Specific Coding Guidelines is devoted to reporting obstetric cases, which are not limited to but include the following:

1. Chapter 15 codes are reported only on the maternal record, never on the newborn record.
2. Codes in Chapter 15 have a final character to indicate the trimester of pregnancy. Trimesters are counted from the first day of the last menstrual period and defined as first trimester (less than 14 weeks, 0 days), second trimester (14 weeks, 0 days to less than 28 weeks, 0 days), and third trimester (28 weeks, 0 days until delivery). Assignment of the final character should be based on the provider's documentation of the trimester. If documentation in the record is insufficient to clarify trimester, report the final character for "unspecified trimester."
3. When reporting complications in pregnancy or childbirth, a seventh character may be required in some instances to identify the fetus affected by the complications. A seventh character of "0" is reported for single gestations when the document in the record is insufficient or when it is not possible to clinically determine which fetus is affected (Example 12.40).

EXAMPLE 12.40 **Complications Related to Pregnancy**

O10.919	Preexisting hypertension complicating pregnancy, unspecified trimester
O36.5910	Pregnancy complicated by poor fetal growth, first trimester, unspecified number of gestations

4. Routine outpatient prenatal visits are reported with a code from category Z34 when no complications are present.
5. Outpatient prenatal visits for high-risk patients are reported with a code from category O09.
6. Full-term uncomplicated vaginal delivery should be reported with code O80. Code O80 is always a principal diagnosis and is not reported with any other code from Chapter 15.
7. A code from category Z37 is reported on every maternal record to report the outcome of delivery.

Injury, Poisoning, and Other Consequences of External Causes

Section 1, Subsection C of Chapter 19 of the Chapter-Specific Coding Guidelines is a large section of rules for coding of the following:

- Injuries
- Fractures
- Burns
- Poisoning
- Adult and child abuse
- Complications of care

Most categories in Chapter 19 require a seventh character extension to indicate whether the encounter is an initial encounter (identified with an A), a subsequent encounter (identified with a D), or a sequela or late effect (identified with an S).

Injuries and Late Effects/Sequela

Diagnostic codes for injuries are listed in the Alphabetic Index by the type of injury and are broken down by anatomic site. To code multiple injuries, a separate code should be assigned for each injury, unless a combination code is assigned. List the diagnosis for the conditions treated in order of importance, with the diagnosis for the most severe problem listed first. If surgery is involved, the diagnostic code for the surgical problem should be listed first unless there is a severe injury of another part of the body (Example 12.41).

EXAMPLE 12.41 **Injuries**

An intracranial injury, managed medically, and a fractured phalanx of the right hand, managed surgically

S06.9 × 0A	Intracranial injury without loss of consciousness, Initial encounter (first-listed primary diagnosis)
S62.602A	Fractured unspecified phalanx of right middle finger, Initial encounter (secondary diagnosis)

The most difficult part of assigning injury codes is to know what main terms to look for in the Alphabetic Index. Codes S00-T88 include fractures, dislocations, sprains, and other types of injury. Injuries are coded according to the general type of injury and broken down within each type by anatomic site. A list of common injury medical terms and the types of injuries included for each is shown in Table 12.4.

Use the following guidelines for coding injuries:

1. Decide whether a diagnosis represents a current injury or a late effect of an injury (Example 12.42).

EXAMPLE 12.42 **Current Injury**

S82.892A	**Current injury:** Fracture, left ankle; Initial encounter
or	
M12.572 and S82.892S	**Late effect:** Traumatic arthritis, due to old fracture, left ankle

TABLE 12.4 **Common Injury Medical Terms**

Main Term	Explanation
Contusion	Bruise and hematoma without a fracture or open wound.
Crush	Crushing injury not complicated by concussion, fractures, injury to internal organs, or intracranial injury.
Dislocation	Displacement and subluxation. Dislocation may be open or closed. Closed dislocation may be complete, partial, simple, or uncomplicated. Open dislocation may be compound, infected, or with foreign body. A dislocation not indicated as closed or open is classified as closed.
Fracture	Fractures may be open or closed. A fracture not indicated as open or closed is classified as closed. An injury described as fracture dislocation is coded as a fracture. Open fractures may be described as compound, infected, missile, puncture, or with foreign body. Closed fractures may be described as comminuted, depressed, elevated, fissured, greenstick, impacted, linear, march, simple, slipped, epiphyseal, or spiral.
Injury, blood vessel	Described as arterial hematoma, avulsion, laceration, rupture, traumatic aneurysm, or traumatic fistula.
Injury, internal	Includes all injuries to internal organs such as the heart, lung, liver, kidney, and pelvic organs. Types of injuries to internal organs include laceration, tear, traumatic rupture, penetrating wound, blunt trauma, crushing, blast injury, or open wound to internal organs with or without fracture in the same region.
Injury, intracranial	Includes concussion, cerebral laceration and contusion, or intracranial hemorrhage. These injuries may be open or closed. Intracranial injuries with skull fractures may be found under fracture.
Injury, superficial	Includes abrasion, insect bite (nonvenomous), blister, or scratch.
Sprain or strain	Injury to the joint capsule, ligament, muscle, or tendon described by the following terms: avulsion, hemarthrosis, laceration (closed), rupture, or tear. Open laceration of these structures should be coded as open wounds.
Wound, open	Includes open wounds not involving internal organs. Wounds may be to skin, muscle, or tendon, described as animal bite, avulsion, cut, laceration, puncture wound, or traumatic amputation. Open wounds may be complicated or uncomplicated. Complicated includes injuries with mention of delayed healing, delayed treatment, foreign body, or major infection.

2. Fractures are coded as "closed" if there is no indication of whether the fracture is open or closed.
3. The word *with* indicates involvement of both sites and the word *and* indicates involvement of either one or two sites when multiple injury sites are given.

As discussed, a late effect or sequela describes the residual effect or condition produced after the acute phase of an illness or injury has terminated. An injury may have a residual effect, which must be coded in a different fashion. A late effect is considered to be a sequela if the diagnosis includes any of the following terms or descriptions:

- "due to an old injury"
- "late"
- "due to"
- "following (previous illness or injury)"
- "due to" an injury or illness that occurred 1 year or more before the current admission of encounter

Residual effects can be found under the main term "sequelae." The condition or nature of the residual effect is sequenced first and the sequela is listed second (Example 12.43).

EXAMPLE 12.43 Late Effects

M17.31 + **S87.01XS**	Unilateral posttraumatic osteoarthritis, **due to crushing injury of right knee**
M81.8 + **E64.8**	Osteoporosis, **due to late effect of calcium deficiency**
O90.81 + **O94**	Anemia of the puerperium, **sequela of pregnancy, childbirth, and the puerperium**

Use the following guidelines for coding a sequela:
1. Refer to the main term "sequelae—*see also* condition" in ICD-10-CM's Alphabetic Index when coding a case with a sequela.
2. Look for the condition.
3. The Tabular Index will provide instructional notes that may indicate that two codes must be reported; code first the condition resulting from the sequela.

Burns and Corrosions

Burn codes are used for reporting thermal burns, except sunburns, that come from a heat source, such as a fire or hot appliance, or those that result from electricity or radiation. Corrosions are defined as burns caused by chemicals.

Burns are classified by depth, extent, and agent. When multiple burns are reported, a separate code for each burn site is reported. The degrees of a burn are defined as follows:
- First degree: erythema
- Second degree: blistering
- Third degree: full thickness involvement

It is important to note that burns of the eye and internal organs are coded by site, not depth. The code that reflects the highest degree of burn should be sequenced first using a code from the range T20 to T25.

An additional code from category T31 or T32 should be reported to identify the total body surface area (TBSA) for all sites. Think of the body as a whole combining it into regions. For adults, these regions break down as follows: head, 9%; arms, 9% each; trunk, 18% front and 18% back; legs, 18% each; and perineum, 1% (Fig. 12.9). Children's and infants' bodies have different regional percentages.

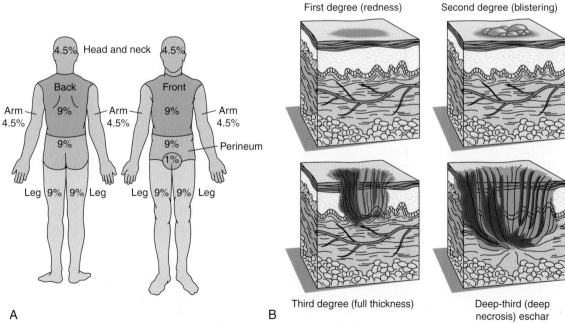

Fig. 12.9 (A) The rule-of-nines estimation of total body surface area burned. (B) The degrees of burn involving the layers of the skin: first-degree burns include the epidermis (redness), second-degree burns include the epidermis and dermis (blistering), third-degree burns include the first two layers and the subcutaneous tissues (full thickness), and deep-third burns involve all layers of the skin with resulting eschar (deep necrosis).

Adverse Effects, Poisoning, Underdosing, and Toxic Effects

Adverse effects, poisoning, underdosing, and toxic effects are reported using combination codes from the range T36 to T65. No additional external cause code is required.

The Table of Drugs and Chemicals is found after the Alphabetical Index, Section 2, and contains a classification of drugs and other chemical substances for identifying poisoning states and external causes of adverse effects.

Adverse effect is defined as an adverse or pathologic reaction to a drug that occurs when appropriate doses are given to humans for prophylaxis or prevention of disease, diagnosis, and therapy (Example 12.44). When an adverse effect occurs, such as a drug reaction, hypersensitivity, drug intolerance, or idiosyncratic reaction, a code is assigned to the diagnosis that classifies the specific reaction or symptom. For example, dermatitis, syncope, tachycardia, or urticaria can all be adverse effects. The specific reaction or symptom from use of the drug is reported as the primary code, followed by a code from the table for the correct code assignment for the adverse effect of the drug (T36–T50). The code for the drug should have a fifth or sixth character.

EXAMPLE 12.44 Coding an Adverse Effect

An inpatient had an adverse effect (ventricular fibrillation) for a medication digoxin which was prescribed by her health care provider and taken correctly.

Step 1	Refer to the Table of Drugs and Chemicals in the Alphabetic Index and look up **digoxin.**
Step 2	Because this medication was for therapeutic use, locate the correct code number under the adverse effect column.
Step 3	The correct number is **T46.0 × 5.**
Step 4	Verify the code number T46.0 × 5 in the Tabular List. Note that a seventh character is required to indicate initial encounter **T46.0 × 5A.**
Step 5	Locate the main term **fibrillation** in the Alphabetic Index to Diseases and Injuries.
Step 6	Find the subterm **ventricular.**
Step 7	The correct code number is **I49.01.**
Step 8	Verify the code number I49.01 in the Tabular List.
Sequencing	**I49.01 Ventricular fibrillation (chief complaint)** **T46.0 × 5A Therapeutic use, Digoxin**

Poisoning is defined as a condition resulting from an intentional overdose of drugs or chemical substances or from the drug or agent given or taken in error. The following situations occur and are documented in the health record to indicate poisoning:

- Taking the wrong medication
- Receiving the wrong medication
- Taking the wrong dose of the right medication
- Receiving the wrong dose of the right medication
- Ingesting a chemical substance not intended for human consumption
- Overdose of a chemical substance (drug)
- Prescription drug taken with alcohol
- Mixing prescription drugs and over-the-counter medications without the provider's advice or consent

Each of the substances listed in Table 12.5 is assigned a code according to the poisoning classification (categories T36–T50). These adverse effect codes are used when there is a state of poisoning, overdose, wrong substance given or taken, or intoxication. Intoxication is defined as an adverse effect rather than a poisoning when drugs such as digitalis and steroid agents are involved. However, whenever the term *intoxication* is used, the billing/coding specialist should clarify with the service provider the circumstances surrounding the administration of the drug or chemical before assigning the appropriate code. This must be documented in the health record. If a diagnosis is stated as possible or suspected suicide attempt, go to the column titled "Undetermined" and not to "Suicide Attempt."

Example 12.45 shows the steps for coding a case that involves poisoning.

EXAMPLE 12.45 Coding a Poisoning

Baby Kathy got into the kitchen cabinet and ingested liquid household ammonia. She was taken to the emergency room for immediate treatment.

Step 1	Refer to the Table of Drugs and Chemicals in the Alphabetic Index and look up **ammonia.**
Step 2	Find the subterm **liquid (household).**
Step 3	Because this is a case of ingesting a chemical substance not intended for human use, locate the correct code number under the **Accidental Poisoning** column.
Step 4	The correct number is **T54.3 × 1.**
Step 5	Verify the code number T54.3 × 1 in the Tabular List. Note that a seventh character is required to indicate initial encounter **T54.3 × 1A.**
Sequencing	Codes in categories T36–T65 are combination codes that include the substances related to the poisoning as well as the external cause. No additional external cause code is required for poisoning. The code from categories T36 to T65 are sequenced first, followed by any codes that specify any outcomes of the poisoning (for example, nausea and vomiting).

External Causes of Morbidity

External causes of morbidity codes are a classification of codes that describe external causes of injury rather than disease. The code description refers to the circumstances that

TABLE 12.5 Table of Drugs and Chemicals

Substance	Poisoning, Accidental	Poisoning, Intentional Self-Harm	Poisoning, Assault	Poisoning, Undetermined	Adverse Effect	Underdosing
Acetylsalicylic acid (salts)	T39.011	T39.012	T39.013	T39.014	T39.015	T39.016

INDEX TO EXTERNAL CAUSES

Fall, falling (accidental) W19
  building W20.1
    burning (uncontrolled fire) X00.3
  down
    embankment W17.81
    escalator W10.0
    hill W17.81
    ladder W11
    ramp W10.2
    stairs, steps W10.9
  due to
    bumping against
      object W18.00
        sharp glass W18.02
        specified NEC W18.09
        sports equipment W18.01
      person W03
        due to ice or snow W00.0
        on pedestrian conveyance —
          see Accident, transport,
          pedestrian, conveyance
    collision with another person W03
      due to ice or snow W00.0
      involving pedestrian conveyance —
        see Accident, transport,
        pedestrian, conveyance

Fig. 12.10 External cause coding.

caused an injury rather than the nature of the injury. The codes are also used in coding adverse reactions to medications (Fig. 12.10).

External cause codes are listed in a separate section of the Tabular List and are included in the code range V01-Y99. The external cause codes are also in a separate section, Index to External Causes of Injury and Poisoning, which follows the regular Alphabetic Index. To look up external cause codes, use Section III in the Alphabetic Index.

Use of an external cause code after the primary or other acute secondary diagnosis explains how the injury occurred. For example, if a patient falls and fractures a finger, the fracture code is primary and an external cause code after it helps explain how the accident or injury occurred (Example 12.46). This can help to speed the reimbursement process because a payer will see an acute injury code and know that a third party is responsible for payment, as in a workers' compensation injury or motor vehicle accident. External cause codes also play a role in gathering data, such as in statistical reporting, credentialing, utilization, review, and state injury prevention programs.

EXAMPLE 12.46 External Cause Codes

A patient falls off of a curb and has a closed treatment of phalangeal shaft fracture, proximal phalanx, finger; without manipulation.

S62.649A	Nondisplaced fracture of proximal phalanx of unspecified finger, Initial encounter
W10.1XXA	Fall from sidewalk curb

Although external cause codes do not generate revenue, it is recommended that they be reported in addition to the appropriate procedural and diagnostic codes. This ensures that the most specific information possible is provided regarding the patient's injury. External cause codes are billed by the initial entity seeing the patient. If the patient visits the provider's office after hospitalization for injuries sustained in a motor vehicle accident, the hospital assigns an external cause code and there is no requirement for repeating it for the office visit. An external cause code may never be sequenced as the primary diagnosis in the first position. When using external cause codes, be sure to list them last on the claim form.

External cause codes must be reported with the appropriate seventh character (initial encounter, subsequent encounter, or sequela) for each encounter for which the injury or condition is being treated. As many external cause codes as are necessary to fully explain each cause should be reported.

Codes from category Y92, place of occurrence, should be reported to identify the location of the patient at the time of injury or other condition. The place of occurrence code is reported only at the initial encounter for treatment. It should not be reported if not stated in the provider's documentation.

Factors Influencing Health Status and Contact With Health Services

Factors influencing health status and contact with health services are reported with the code range Z00-Z99 and are referred to as Z codes. All guidelines for reporting Z codes can be found in Section 1, Subsection C of Chapter 21 of the Chapter-Specific Coding Guidelines.

Z codes are included in the major section of the Alphabetic Index to Diseases and Injuries. They are used for the following four primary circumstances:

1. When a person who is not currently sick encounters health services for some specific purpose, such as to act as a donor of an organ or tissue, receive a vaccination, discuss a problem that is not in itself a disease or injury, seek consultation about family planning, request sterilization, or obtain supervision of a normal pregnancy (Example 12.47).

EXAMPLE 12.47 Supervision of First Pregnancy, Normal, First Trimester

Step 1	Find the heading **Pregnancy** in the Alphabetic Index.
Step 2	Look for the subheading **supervision.**
Step 3	Look for the second subheading **normal** and a further subheading **first,** which indicates the code Z34.0-.
Step 4	Find **Z34.0-** in the Tabular List. By Tabular List, it indicates **"Encounter for Supervision of Normal First Pregnancy."**
Step 5	Find **Z34.01** in the Tabular List, which indicates "**Encounter for Supervision of Normal First Pregnancy, First Trimester.**"

---

2. When a person with a resolving disease or injury, such as a chronic, long-term condition that needs continuous care, seeks aftercare (Example 12.48).

EXAMPLE 12.48 Aftercare

Z47.81	Encounter for orthopedic aftercare following surgical amputation *Use additional code to identify the limb amputated. (Z89.-)*

3. When a circumstance influences an individual's health status but the illness is not current (Example 12.49).

EXAMPLE 12.49 Personal History

Z85.3	Personal history of malignant neoplasm of breast

4. When it is necessary to indicate the birth status of a newborn (Example 12.50).

EXAMPLE 12.50 Newborn Birth Status

Z38.00	Single liveborn infant, delivered vaginally, born in hospital

These types of encounters are among the more common services for hospital outpatients and patients of private practitioners, health clinics, and others. Certain Z codes may appear only as a primary code and others only as secondary codes.

Some key words in patient care that indicate that a Z code might be necessary include the following:

- Exposure
- Routine annual examination
- Admission
- History of
- Encounter
- Vaccination

Z codes also are used when some circumstance or problem is present that influences the person's health status but is not in itself a current illness or injury, such as when the person is known to have an allergy to a specific drug. In this instance, the Z code cannot be used as a stand-alone code and should be used only as a supplementary code.

Additional code numbers are given for occupational health examinations and routine annual physical examinations; therefore, select specific codes depending on the circumstances (Example 12.51).

EXAMPLE 12.51 Routine Annual Adult Physical Examination, Without Abnormal Findings

Step 1	Look up **examination,** and notice **annual (adult)** as a subterm and the code **Z00.00.**
Step 2	Find **Z00.00** in the Tabular List and the wording "**Encounter for general adult medical examination without abnormal findings.**"

Encounters for Reproductive Services

Z codes are used to report family planning, contraceptive or procreative management, and counseling. Codes from the category Z30 are used only when the encounter is for contraceptive management and must be specific to the type of contraceptive managed.

Z30.011	Encounter for initial prescription of contraceptive pills
Z30.012	Encounter for prescription of emergency contraception
Z30.013	Encounter for prescription of injectable contraceptive
Z30.014	Encounter for initial prescription of intrauterine contraceptive device

Z30.015	Encounter for initial prescription of vaginal ring hormone contraceptive device
Z30.016	Encounter for initial prescription of transdermal patch contraceptive device
Z30.017	Encounter for initial prescription of implantable subdermal contraceptive device
Z30.018	Encounter for initial prescription of other contraceptives
Z30.019	Encounter for initial prescription of unspecified contraceptive
Z30.02	Counseling and instruction in natural family planning to avoid pregnancy
Z30.09	Encounter for other general counseling and advice on contraception

Codes from the category Z30.4, encounter for surveillance of contraceptives, are available for reporting encounters for continued management. The codes from category Z30.4 are also specific to the type of contraceptive being used. When sterilization is performed for the major purpose of contraception rather than being an incidental result of the treatment of a disease, code Z30.2 is reported.

 12.11   QUICK REVIEW
Question: When should a neoplasm be coded as "uncertain behavior?"

 12.12   QUICK REVIEW
Question: What is the default diabetes code if a type is not documented?

 12.13   QUICK REVIEW
Question: How is a single high blood pressure reading coding?

 12.14   QUICK REVIEW
Question: What chapter of codes have sequencing priority over the others?

 12.15   QUICK REVIEW
Question: What is the difference between an adverse effect and poisoning?

 12.16   QUICK REVIEW
Question: What are some of the key words that would indicate a Z code may be appropriate?

DIAGNOSTIC CODING AND REPORTING FOR OUTPATIENT SERVICES

Section IV of the Official Guidelines contains a set of rules specific to reporting of outpatient services with which the billing/coding specialist should be familiar. The guidelines are approved for use for reporting hospital-based outpatient services and provider-based office visits. The guidelines are used in conjunction with the general and disease-specific guidelines.

Outpatient Surgery

When patients present for outpatient surgery, the first-listed diagnosis should be the reason for the surgery. If the postoperative diagnosis is different and is confirmed, select the more specific postoperative diagnosis code.

Uncertain Diagnosis

When reporting hospital-based outpatient services and provider-based office visits, if the provider has documented a condition as "probable," "suspected," "questionable," "rule out," or "working diagnosis," do not code as if the patient has the condition. An uncertain diagnosis, or a **rule out** diagnosis, is often documented to keep an open mind about the possibility of that diagnosis. For example, a patient may have fallen and injured their wrist. The emergency room provider may request an x-ray examination to rule out a fracture. It has not been confirmed yet that the patient has a fracture; however, the provider is keeping an open mind about the possibility of that diagnosis. In cases such as this, code for the symptom, sign, or reason for the visit. In the example given, it would be best to report the diagnosis as "wrist injury" until a more definitive diagnosis has been documented. This guideline is different for health record coding specialists in the inpatient hospital setting.

Chronic Disease

Chronic diseases that are treated on an ongoing basis may be reported as long as E/M of the condition are documented.

Code All Documented Conditions That Coexist

All conditions that coexist at the time of the visit that are evaluated and managed and affect patient care should be reported. If the condition was previously treated but no longer exists, it should be reported as a history code (Z80–Z87) if the condition has an impact on the current plan of care (Example 12.52).

> **EXAMPLE 12.52 Code All Documented Conditions That Coexist**
>
> A patient is seen by her primary care provider (PCP) for management of chronic hypertension. The provider also performed a completed skin assessment, based on the patient's history of malignant melanoma in situ, which was previously excised in full.
>
> | I10 | Hypertension |
> | Z85.820 | Personal history of malignant neoplasm, skin |

Patients Receiving Diagnostic Services Only

Sequence first the diagnosis, condition, problem, or other reason for the visit for patients receiving diagnostic services. For routine laboratory or radiology testing in the absence of any signs or symptoms, assign Z01.89, encounter for other specified special examination (Example 12.53).

> **EXAMPLE 12.53 Patients Receiving Diagnostic Services Only**
>
> Patient seen in the emergency room for pain in the left leg is sent to x-ray. The x-ray is read and is negative.
>
> | M79.605 | Left leg pain |

Preoperative Evaluations

Sometimes a patient receives a consultation for a preoperative medical evaluation as an inpatient or outpatient (Example 12.54), and the majority of the results are negative for chronic or current illness. A diagnosis code indicating the patient is in good health will trigger a rejection by the third-party payer unless the insurance company allows or requires it. When reporting, sequence first a code from subcategory Z01.81-, encounter for preprocedural examination, to describe the preoperative consultation, followed by a code for the condition describing the reason for the surgery. Any additional findings related to the preoperative evaluation should also be reported.

> **EXAMPLE 12.54 Preoperative Examination**
>
> A patient to have surgery for gallstones is sent to their primary care provider and a cardiologist for a preoperative examination and clearance. The patient is actively being treated for hypertension and Type II Diabetes.
>
> | Step 1 | In the Alphabetic Index, look up **examination** and notice **preprocedural (preoperative)** and **cardiovascular** as subterms and the code **Z01.810.** Verify it in the Tabular List. |
> | Step 2 | Code the reason for the surgery—K80.20, cholelithiasis. |
> | Step 3 | Code the underlying chronic conditions that are also being evaluated—I10, hypertension and E11.9, type II diabetes mellitus, without complication. |

General Medical Examinations With Abnormal Findings

General medical examinations are reported with the category of codes Z00.0-. Subcategories provide codes for examinations with and without abnormal findings. The ICD-10-CM guidelines defines abnormal findings as a condition/diagnosis that is newly identified or a change in severity of a chronic condition (such as uncontrolled hypertension, or an acute exacerbation of chronic obstructive pulmonary disease) during a routine physical examination. A general medical examination that results in an abnormal finding should be reported with the code for general medical examination with abnormal finding assigned as the first-listed diagnosis. A secondary code for the abnormal finding should also be reported (Example 12.55).

> **EXAMPLE 12.55 General Medical Examinations**
>
> | Z00.00 | Encounter for general adult medical examination without abnormal findings |
> | Z00.01 | Encounter for general adult medical examination with abnormal findings *Use additional code to identify abnormal findings* |
> | Z00.121 | Encounter for routine child health examination with abnormal findings *Use additional code to identify abnormal findings* |
> | Z00.129 | Encounter for routine child health examination without abnormal findings |

> **12.17 QUICK REVIEW**
>
> Question: How should laboratory tests and x-rays with no confirmed diagnosis be coded?

CODING AND REPORTING GUIDELINES FOR INPATIENT HOSPITAL CARE

As discussed earlier in this chapter, choosing a diagnosis for an inpatient admission is different from choosing diagnosis codes to reflect medical necessity for an office visit, lab work, or an outpatient procedure. Section II of the ICD-10-CM Official Guidelines for Coding and Reporting states that the circumstances of inpatient admission always govern the selection of a principal diagnosis.

Signs and Symptoms

Similar to the rules for outpatient and professional services, signs and symptoms are not coded if a definitive diagnosis has been established and the symptoms are inherent to the disease.

Uncertain Diagnosis

In contrast to outpatient and provider coding, if a diagnosis is documented as uncertain at the time of discharge, it is coded as though the condition was established. Words to look for on the discharge summary include:

- probably
- suspected
- likely
- questionable
- possible
- still to be ruled out
- compatible with
- consistent with

! COMPLIANCE ALERT

When coding inpatient services, an uncertain diagnosis is coded as though it is confirmed. This is different than how uncertain diagnoses are handled in coding outpatient or provider services.

Admission After Outpatient Surgery

If a patient is admitted to inpatient care following an outpatient surgery due to a complication, the complication is the principal diagnosis. If there is no complication and no other reason stated for the admission, the reason for the outpatient surgery is the principal diagnosis. If the reason for the admission is another condition unrelated to the surgery, the unrelated condition is the principal diagnosis (Example 12.56).

EXAMPLE 12.56   Admission for Outpatient Surgery

A patient has outpatient surgery on the knee and has a myocardial infarction in the recovery room. The MI is due to a chronic heart condition, not the surgery. The patient is admitted to inpatient care.
The principal diagnosis would be myocardial infraction.

Admission for Rehabilitation

If the purpose of admission is rehabilitation, the principal diagnosis will be the condition for which the rehabilitation is being performed (Example 12.57).

EXAMPLE 12.57   Admission for Rehabilitation

A patient is admitted for rehabilitation for hemiplegia following a stroke.
The principal diagnosis would be I69.35-, with the appropriate side indicated by the 6th character, hemiplegia and hemiparesis following a cerebrovascular accident.

If the patient is admitted to rehabilitation following active treatment for a condition that is no longer present, the appropriate after care code is the principal diagnosis (Example 12.58).

EXAMPLE 12.58   Admission for Rehabilitation for a Condition No Longer Present

A patient is admitted to rehabilitation following a total hip replacement for osteoarthritis.
The principal diagnosis would be Z47.1, aftercare following joint replacement surgery.

12.18   QUICK REVIEW

Question: How are uncertain diagnoses handled in an inpatient setting vs. an outpatient setting?

COMPUTER-ASSISTED CODING

Computer-assisted coding (CAC) is a computer software that automatically generates a set of medical codes for review, validation, and use based on clinical documentation provided by health care providers. Many factors have pushed health care organizations to adopt CAC. Some of these factors are as follows:

- Shortage of coding specialists throughout the United States
- Financial need to reduce the cost of filing insurance claims
- Increased complexity of coding systems with implementation of the ICD-10-CM coding system
- Adoption of EHRs
- Advancement in natural language processing (NLP) technology
- Frequent changes in code numbers and coding rules and regulations
- Compliance liability for increased erroneous claims

CAC uses two technology options: structured input and NLP. In structured input, the health care provider inputs information on a data entry screen that has point-and-click fields, pull-down menus, or structured templates. The system prompts the health care provider for detailed information. Words and phrases selected are linked to diagnostic and procedural codes that are automatically generated when all fields are completed. Input of the detailed information results in a completed document with the appropriate level of detail. Recommended diagnostic and procedural codes are then checked and edited by a coding specialist.

The NLP system uses artificial medical intelligence. The health care provider dictates a report, handwrites a note, or inputs a picture file. The document is sent to an NLP engine that scans the health record, chooses important, relevant words, and converts them into suggested codes. A coding specialist searches and validates the diagnostic and procedural codes and makes any changes, and then the codes are transmitted to billing. NLP systems must be updated regularly to address new medical terminology and conform to changes in coding guidelines.

Automated coding software uses a statistics-based method, rules-based method, or both methods to assign codes. In a statistics-based program, also called a *data-driven method,* the software predicts the code for a word or phrase based on statistics from the past. A rules-based or knowledge-driven method applies coding rules, such as those used in logic- or rules-based encoders, and imaged coding applications, to electronic clinical documents. The codes are processed through associated established rules for refinement and code assignment.

Another feature of CAC is the use of crosswalks or *data mapping,* which gives a coding specialist the ability to input a discontinued code and find a new replacement code.

Sometimes coding specialists disagree about which codes to apply to a specific case; thus, checking and editing codes may be needed when using CAC. Usually, repetitive procedures are quick for coders to approve but complex procedures may need more time for validation. CAC technology helps coders to do their jobs faster and more efficiently and does not diminish the need for coding specialists.

 12.19 QUICK REVIEW
Question: What are some reasons for a health care organization to consider using CAC?

THE FUTURE OF DIAGNOSIS CODING

The ICD is constantly under revision to better reflect progress in health sciences and medical practices. Development of the next edition of ICD (**ICD-11**) for diagnosis coding began in April 2007 and included some very specific goals:

- To improve on the ability to function in an electronic environment
- To allow for collaborative web-based editing by interested parties while under peer review
- To incorporate international multilingual reference standards for scientific comparability

ICD-11 is alphanumeric, building on the structure of ICD-10, and will be similar in appearance. It will be a digital product that will link with terminologies (such as SNOMED CT) and support EHRs and information systems. SNOMED CT is a comprehensive health care database that incorporates terminology and clinical content with diagnostic standards in EHRs.

ICD-11 was originally scheduled for dissemination by 2012; however, the timeline was extended given the size of the task, the technical complexity of the system, and the limited funding and human resources for the project. The beta version of ICD-11 was produced in September 2013 and underwent trials and final reviews in 2018 and 2019. According to the WHO, it is expected that some countries will start reporting with ICD-11 on January 1, 2022.

 12.20 QUICK REVIEW
Question: What are the goals of ICD-11?

 DISCUSSION POINT

Discuss the differences between primary diagnosis, chief complaint, principal diagnosis, secondary diagnosis, and admitting diagnosis.

PROCEDURE 12.1 Basic Steps in Selecting Diagnostic Codes From ICD-10-CM

Objective
Accurately choose and insert diagnostic codes for electronic transmission of an insurance claim

Directions
Use a standard method and establish a routine for locating a code. Follow these steps for coding the first diagnosis. For each subsequent diagnosis in a patient's health record, repeat these steps.

1. Read the patient's health record to find the main term. To identify the main term, ask what is wrong with the patient.
2. Next, locate the main term (disease or condition), not the anatomic site, in the Alphabetic Index. The Alphabetic Index is organized by main terms and has three sections:
   - Section 1—Index to Diseases and Nature of Injury includes Neoplasm Table and Table of Drugs and Chemicals
   - Section 2—Index to External Causes of Injury
   - Section 3—Table of Drugs and Chemicals
3. Read any notes under the main term. Select and write down the code.
4. Next, go to the Tabular List, review how it is organized for the subclassification, read and be guided by any instructional terms, and then verify that the selected code gives the highest level of specificity (up to seven alphanumeric characters). Possible errors may occur when using the Tabular List and when coding diseases or conditions that begin with categories "O" and "I." These can look like the numbers "zero" and "one" (for example, I00 and O99 are correct—not 100 and 099). In these categories, special attention must be given. Always read the specific chapter guidelines and refer to the general guidelines in the code book for certain diagnoses and/or conditions in the classification before choosing a code.
5. Assign the code.

ICD-10-CM, international classification of diseases, tenth revision, clinical modification.

KEY POINTS

This is a brief chapter review of the key issues presented. To further enhance your knowledge of the technical subject matter, review the key terms and key abbreviations for this chapter by locating the meaning for each in the Glossary at the end of this text, which appears in a section before the Index.

1. Accurate diagnostic coding can mean the financial success or failure of a health care organization.
2. Payment for health care services is related to procedure codes but must be supported and justified by the diagnosis.
3. Diagnostic coding was developed for the following reasons: (a) tracking of disease processes, (b) classification of causes of mortality, (c) medical research, and (d) evaluation of hospital service use.
4. When submitting insurance claims for patients seen in a provider's office or an outpatient hospital setting, the primary diagnosis, which is the main reason for the encounter, is listed first.
5. For inpatient services, the principal diagnosis reflects the reason for admission, even if the diagnosis has not been confirmed.
6. For outpatient and provider services, signs and symptoms should only be coded if there is not a definitive diagnosis documented, or if they are not inherent in the definitive diagnosis.
7. For services provided after October 1, 2015, always use the *International Classification of Diseases, Tenth Revision, Clinical Modification* (ICD-10-CM) Alphabetic Index and then go to the Tabular (numerical) List before assigning a diagnostic code.
8. Always code to the highest degree of specificity. The more digits a code has, the more specific the description is.
9. Always code the underlying disease, the etiology, or the cause first; subsequently list the secondary diagnosis.
10. Z codes in ICD-10-CM are used when a person who is not currently sick encounters health services for some specific purpose, such as to receive a vaccination.
11. External cause codes in ICD-10-CM are used to report the causes of injury rather than the nature of the injury or disease and to code adverse reactions to medications. In ICD-10-CM, these codes begin with V, W, X, and Y.
12. Always follow coding conventions because they assist in the selection of correct codes for the diagnoses encountered. These conventions are rules or principles for determining a diagnostic code when using diagnostic code books, such as each space, typefaces, indentations, punctuation marks, symbols, instructional notes, abbreviations, cross-reference notes, and specific usage of the words *and, with,* and *due to.*

INTERNET RESOURCES

ICD-10-CM Guidelines
- https://www.cms.gov/Medicare/Coding/ICD10/2020-ICD-10-CM

WHO ICD-11 information
- https://icd.who.int/en

STUDENT ASSIGNMENTS

- Study Chapter 12.
- Complete all exercises in the *Workbook* to reinforce theory learned in this chapter.

- Turn to the Glossary at the end of this text for a further understanding of the key terms and key abbreviations used in this chapter.

13

Procedural Coding

Cheryl Fassett

OBJECTIVES

After reading this chapter, you should be able to:

1. Explain the purpose and importance of coding for professional services.
2. Define terminology used in *Current Procedural Terminology* (CPT).
3. Demonstrate an understanding of CPT code conventions.
4. Discuss the format and content of the HCPCS and CPT code books, including category I, II, and III codes.
5. Interpret the meaning of CPT code book symbols.
6. Identify and discuss the evaluation and management (E/M) services codes.
7. Explain the global surgical package.
8. Discuss the sections of the CPT book.
9. Explain correct usage of modifiers in procedure coding.
10. Explain various types of code edits.
11. Explain how to choose accurate procedure codes for descriptions of services and procedures documented in a patient's health record, including discussions on bundled codes, unbundling, downcoding, upcoding, and code monitoring.
12. Describe various methods of payment by insurance companies and state and federal programs.

KEY TERMS

bilateral
bundled codes
comorbidity
comprehensive code
conversion factor
Current Procedural Terminology
customary fee
downcoding
durable medical equipment
emergency department
fee schedule

geographic practice cost indices
global surgical package
Healthcare Common Procedure
   Coding System
modifiers
mutually exclusive code edits
National Correct Coding Initiative
never event
physical status modifiers
procedure code numbers
professional component

qualifying circumstances
reasonable fee
relative value studies
relative value unit
resource-based relative
   value scale
technical component
unbundling
upcoding
usual, customary, and
   reasonable

KEY ABBREVIATIONS

CF	E/M	HCPCS	RBRVS
CPT	EOB	NCCI	RVS
DME	FTC	PC	RVU
ECG	GAF	PS	TC
ED	GPCIs	QC	UCR

INSIGHTS FROM THE FIELD

Patricia L.: Certified Professional Coder (CPC), Certified Professional Medical Auditor (CPMA), Certified Risk Coder (CRC), Clinical Documentation Expert - Outpatient (CDEO), Certified Cardiology Coder (CCC), Certified Cardiovascular Thoracic Surgery Coder (CCVTC), Certified Evaluation and Management Coder (CEMC), Certifed Ear, Nose and Throat Coder (CENTC), Certified Family Practice Coder (CFPC), Certified Obstetrics Gynecology Coder (COBGC)

I've worked in this field for 36 years. I have been a biller and coder and currently work as a professional services auditor. I review coders' E/M levels and ICD-10 codes, giving providers feedback by using the appropriate coding guidelines. I think it is important for a new billing specialist to learn about each type of insurance policy, how their reimbursement is calculated and what needs authorization so clean claims are sent to the insurance. Understanding what CPT codes are bundled cuts down on denials too. Don't be afraid to volunteer to get your foot in the door. Some of the volunteers I work with have turned out to be the best coders!

UNDERSTANDING THE IMPORTANCE OF PROCEDURAL CODING SKILLS

The health care provider documents their care in the patient's health record. Procedure coding is the translation of these written descriptions of procedures and professional services to numeric designations or code numbers. This translation may be done by the health care provider or a billing or coding specialist. Electronic health record (EHR) systems are often implemented as a method to improve billing and coding. However, removing the human element from the coding process is not recommended. Certain features in EHR systems make it too easy for health care providers to use auto-fill and auto-prompt tools that can result in coding above the services provided (upcoding) and cloned records.

With the implementation of computer technology and stricter adherence to federal regulations, more emphasis is being placed on correct procedural coding. Coding must be correct if claims are to be paid promptly and optimally. Every procedure or service must be assigned correct and complete code numbers. Because of the complexity of procedural coding, a working knowledge of medical terminology, including anatomy and physiology, is essential.

Procedure codes are a standardized method used to precisely describe the services provided by physicians and allied health care professionals, such as chiropractors and nurse practitioners. They allow claim forms to be optically scanned by insurance companies. The general acceptance of the codes by third-party payers and government agencies assures the health care provider who uses a standardized coding system that the services and procedures they perform can be objectively identified and priced.

The Health Insurance Portability and Accountability Act of 1996 (HIPAA) requires the use of standardized code sets. The *Current Procedural Terminology* (Level I: CPT) and *Healthcare Common Procedure Coding System* (Level II: HCPCS) are the standard code sets designated for coding for professional services, equipment, and supplies.

Further guidance for completion of a CMS 1500 claim form will be explained in Chapter 14 of this textbook; however, see Fig. 13.1 for an example of a completed claim form. Note that in box #24D, there is a space for a procedure code and up to four modifiers, as needed.

A Coding Specialist's Tools

CPT and HCPCS are updated annually, with new codes, and changes going into effect on January 1. Health care organizations should always strive to use the current manuals to ensure correct codes are used. Coding and billing specialists should obtain their own manuals whenever possible so they may customize them. This can aid in code selection and make their jobs easier.

Some coding and billing specialists choose to break apart the manual into as many sections as needed on the basis of their specialty, three-hole punch it, and place it in a binder. Index tabs may be added to the frequently used section. Coding edits, Medicare updates, and notes may also be placed in the binder. Color coding any codes that typically need modifiers or that should not be chosen without reviewing criteria will also help. Customizing the CPT book annually will familiarize a coding specialist with any changes and reduce coding errors.

 13.1   QUICK REVIEW

Question: What are the two standard code sets used to report professional services, equipment, and supplies?

HEALTHCARE COMMON PROCEDURE CODING SYSTEM

The Healthcare Common Procedure Coding System (HCPCS) (pronounced "hick-picks") was developed for the Medicare program. The Medicare HCPCS consists of the following two levels of coding:

- Level I: The American Medical Association (AMA) CPT codes and modifiers. CPT is used to report professional services and procedures performed.
- Level II: The CMS-designated codes and alpha modifiers. Table 13.1 lists the Level II HCPCS code ranges with details of each alphanumeric code category. These codes are used primarily to identify products, supplies, and services not included in the Level I CPT codes, such as ambulance services, durable medical equipment.

Level I: *Current Procedural Terminology* Codes

The primary coding system used for professional services and procedures is *Current Procedural Terminology* (Level 1: CPT), published and updated annually by the AMA. Level I (CPT) uses a basic five-digit system for coding professional services and two-digit add-on modifiers to indicate circumstances in which a procedure is performed differ in some way from that described in the code. Procedure code numbers represent

MEDICARE/MEDICAID
(primary)   (secondary)
CROSSOVER CLAIM

DRAFT - NOT FOR OFFICIAL USE

HEALTH INSURANCE CLAIM FORM

APPROVED BY NATIONAL UNIFOR MCLAIM COMMITTEE (NUCC) 02/12

| | PICA | | | | | | | | | | | PICA | | |

1. MEDICARE (Medicare#) □ **MEDICAID** (Medicaid#) □ **TRICARE** (ID#DoD#) □ **CHAMPVA** (Member ID#) □ **GROUP HEALTH PLAN** (ID#) [X] **FECA BLK LUNG** (ID#) □ **OTHER** (ID#) □   **1a. INSURED'S I.D. NUMBER** (For Program in Item 1) 6589444

2. PATIENT'S NAME (Last Name, First Name, Middle Initial)
Jones, Samantha

3. PATIENT'S BIRTH DATE MM 06 DD 11 YY 1984   **SEX** M □ F [X]

4. INSURED'S NAME (Last Name, First Name, Middle Initial)
Jones, Samantha

5. PATIENT'S ADDRESS (No., Street)
5 Glennview Drive

6. PATIENT RELATIONSHIP TO INSURED Self [X] Spouse □ Child □ Other □

7. INSURED'S ADDRESS (No., Street)
5 Glennview Drive

CITY Woodland Hills **STATE** XY

8. RESERVED FOR NUCC USE

CITY Woodland Hills **STATE** XY

ZIP CODE 123450000 **TELEPHONE (Include Area Code)** (555) 5451212

ZIP CODE 123450000 **TELEPHONE (Include Area Code)** (555) 5451212

9. OTHER INSURED'S NAME (Last Name, First Name, Middle Initial)

10. IS PATIENT'S CONDITION RELATED TO:

11. INSURED'S POLICY GROUP OR FECA NUMBER

a. OTHER INSURED'S POLICY OR GROUP NUMBER

a. EMPLOYMENT? (Current or Previous) □ YES [X] NO

a. INSURED'S DATE OF BIRTH MM 06 DD 11 YY 1984 **SEX** M □ F [X]

b. RESERVED FOR NUCC USE

b. AUTO ACCIDENT? □ YES [X] NO **PLACE (State)**

b. OTHER CLAIM ID (Designated by NUCC)

c. RESERVED FOR NUCC USE

c. OTHER ACCIDENT? □ YES [X] NO

c. INSURANCE PLAN NAME OR PROGRAM NAME Aetna

d. INSURANCE PLAN NAME OR PROGRAM NAME

10d. CLAIM CODES (Designated by NUCC)

d. IS THERE ANOTHER HEALTH BENEFIT PLAN? □ YES [X] NO *If yes*, complete items 9, 9a, and 9d.

READ BACK OF FORM BEFORE COMPLETING & SIGNING THIS FORM.
12. PATIENT'S OR AUTHORIZED PERSON'S SIGNATUREI authorize the release of any medical or other information necessary to process this claim. I also request payment of government benefits either to myself or to the party who accepts assignment below.

SIGNED *Samantha Jones*   DATE *10/1/XX*

13. INSURED'S OR AUTHORIZED PERSON'S SIGNATURE I authorize payment of medical benefits to the undersigned physician or supplier for services described below.

SIGNED *Samantha Jones*

14. DATE OF CURRENT: ILLNESS, INJURY, or PREGNANCY(LMP) MM DD YY QUAL.

15. OTHER DATE QUAL. MM DD YY

16. DATES PATIENT UNABLE TO WORK IN CURRENT OCCUPATION FROM MM DD YY TO MM DD YY

17. NAME OF REFERRING PROVIDER OR OTHER SOURCE DN Brady Coccidioides MD

17a.
17b. NPI 64211067XX

18. HOSPITALIZATION DATES RELATED TO CURRENT SERVICES FROM MM DD YY TO MM DD YY

19. ADDITIONAL CLAIM INFORMATION (Designated by NUCC)

20. OUTSIDE LAB? □ YES [X] NO **$ CHARGES**

21. DIAGNOSIS OR NATURE OF ILLNESS OR INJURY Relate A-L to service line below (24E) **ICD Ind.** 0

A. L03011 B. C. D.
E. F. G. H.
I. J. K. L.

22. RESUBMISSION CODE ORIGINAL REF. NO.

23. PRIOR AUTHORIZATION NUMBER

24. A. DATE(S) OF SERVICE						B. PLACE OF SERVICE	C. EMG	D. PROCEDURES, SERVICES, OR SUPPLIES (Explain Unusual Circumstances)		E. DIAGNOSIS POINTER	F. $ CHARGES	G. DAYS OR UNITS	H. EPSDT Family Plan	I. ID. QUAL.	J. RENDERING PROVIDER ID. #
From			To					CPT/HCPCS	MODIFIER						
MM	DD	YY	MM	DD	YY										
10	01	XX				24		11730	F6	A	120 00	1		NPI	50307117XX
														NPI	
														NPI	
														NPI	
														NPI	
														NPI	

25. FEDERAL TAX I.D. NUMBER XX12210XX **SSN** □ **EIN** [X]

26. PATIENT'S ACCOUNT NO. 098

27. ACCEPT ASSIGNMENT? (For govt. claims, see back) [X] YES □ NO

28. TOTAL CHARGE $ 120 00

29. AMOUNT PAID $

30. Rsvd for NUCC Use $

31. SIGNATURE OF PHYSICIAN OR SUPPLIER INCLUDING DEGREES OR CREDENTIALS (I certify that the statements on the reverse apply to this bill and are made a part thereof.)
Cosmo Graff MD   100320XX
SIGNED *Cosmo Graff, MD* DATE

32. SERVICE FACILITY LOCATION INFORMATION
Woodland Hills Ambulatory Center
1229 Center Street
Woodland Hills XY 123450001
a. X950513700 b.

33. BILLING PROVIDER INFO & PH # (555) 4869002
College Clinic
4567 Broad Avenue
Woodland Hills XY 123450001
a. 3664021CC b.

NUCC Instruction Manual available at: www.nucc.org   PLEASE PRINT OR TYPE   OMB APPROVAL PENDING

Fig. 13.1 Completed CMS 1500 claim form highlighting the procedure and modifier boxes.

CARRIER

PATIENT AND INSURED INFORMATION

PHYSICIAN OR SUPPLIER INFORMATION

TABLE 13.1 Level II HCPCS National Code Contents

Code Category	Contents	Code Ranges
	New/revised/deleted codes and modifiers	
Index	Alphabetically arranged	
	Table of drugs	
	Level II national modifiers	
A codes	Transportation services, including ambulance (medical and surgical supplies, administrative, and miscellaneous and investigational services and supplies)	A0000–A9999
B codes	Enteral and parenteral therapy	B4000–B9999
C codes	Temporary codes for hospital outpatient Prospective Payment System	C1000–C9999
D codes	Dental procedure codes[a]	D0000–D9999
E codes	Durable medical equipment (canes, crutches, walkers, commodes, decubitus care, bath and toilet aids, hospital beds, oxygen and related respiratory equipment, monitoring equipment, pacemakers, patient lifts, safety equipment, restraints, traction equipment, fracture frames, wheelchairs, and artificial kidney machines)	E0100–E9999
G codes	Procedures and professional services (temporary) under review before inclusion in the CPT code book	G0000–G9999
H codes	Alcohol and drug abuse treatment services	H0001–H9999
J codes	Drugs administered other than oral method (chemotherapy drugs, immunosuppressive drugs, inhalation solutions, and miscellaneous drugs and solutions)	J0100–J9999
K codes	Temporary codes (durable medical equipment and drugs)[b]	K0000–K9999
L codes	Orthotic procedures and devices (prosthetic devices, scoliosis equipment, orthopedic shoes, and prosthetic implants)	L0100–L4999
P codes	Pathology and laboratory services	P0000–P9999
Q codes	Miscellaneous temporary codes	Q0000–Q9999
R codes	Diagnostic radiology services codes	R0000–R9999
S codes	Temporary national codes (non-Medicare; replaced many of Level III (local) codes, which have been phased out)	S0009–S9999
T codes	National T codes established for state Medicaid agencies and not valid for Medicare	T1000–T9999
V codes	Vision, hearing, and speech-language pathology services	V0000–V2999

[a] Dental procedures (diagnostic, preventive, restorative, endodontic, periodontic, prosthodontic, prosthetic, orthodontic, and surgical).
Contents in HCPCS books will vary by edition. It is a good idea to compare editions to see which one is more user friendly. For example, the Professional Edition has appendices not included in the Standard Edition.
CPT, Current Procedural Terminology; HCPCS, Healthcare Common Procedure Coding System.
These codes have been removed from the official HCPCS list but remain available from and are maintained by the American Dental Association.
[b] When these codes are approved for permanent inclusion in HCPCS, they become A, E, or J codes.

EXAMPLE 13.1 Current Procedural Terminology Procedure Code Numbers

A 45-year-old woman is seen for an initial office visit for evaluation of recurrent right shoulder pain. The patient's condition warranted a detailed history and physical examination with low-complexity medical decision making. The patient complains of pain radiating down her right arm. A complete radiographic study of the right shoulder is obtained in the office and read by the physician. A corticosteroid solution is injected into the shoulder joint.

CPT Code	Description of Services
99203	Office visit, new patient (E/M service)
73030	Radiologic examination, shoulder, two views (Diagnostic service)
20610	Arthrocentesis inj.; major joint, shoulder (Therapeutic service)

! COMPLIANCE ALERT
Coding Compliance Plan

Because the government is more involved in health care, each health care organization should construct and maintain a policy and procedure manual regarding coding guidelines so that it is in compliance with state and federal guidelines. Establishing coding and billing policies and procedures helps health care organizations and their staff to address potential risk areas for fraud and abuse. A plan should include the health care organization's basic ethical philosophy, outline policies, detail coding procedures, and create an environment of confidentiality. Billing and coding specialists should sign a statement annually indicating that they have read, understood, and agreed with the health care organization's standards of conduct. The plan should provide coding specialists with the framework for correct coding and indicate that health record documentation must support the codes billed. An internal audit should be done on a regular basis, and action should be taken to correct the offense if noncompliance is discovered. Such plans must have a compliance officer or a committee that oversees the audits, monitors compliance issues, and trains employees in compliance issues.

Level I (CPT) content will be discussed in further detail in this chapter. Procedure 13.1 at the end of this chapter gives step-by-step directions on how to use a CPT code book for billing purposes.

diagnostic and therapeutic services on medical billing statements and insurance forms (Example 13.1).

The first edition of Level I (CPT) appeared in 1966. It is now updated and revised annually on January 1. Code numbers are added or deleted as new procedures are developed or existing procedures are modified. These changes are shown in each edition by the use of symbols, which are described and shown later in this chapter (Fig. 13.2). The symbols with their meanings are located at the bottom of each page of code numbers in the CPT code book.

Level II: HCPCS Codes

HCPCS Level II codes include those for the following:
- Ambulance
- Medical and surgical supplies

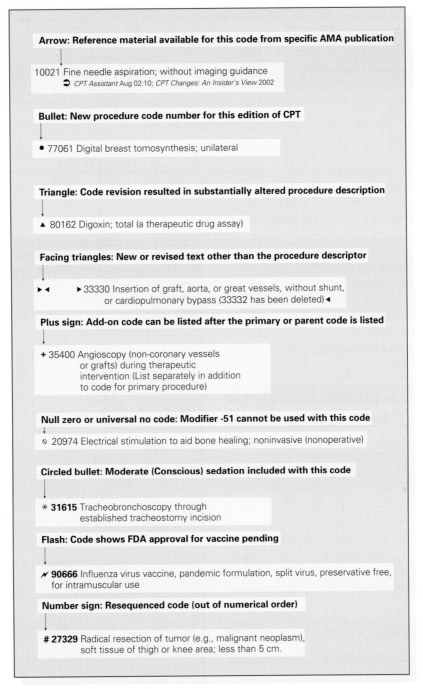

Arrow: Reference material available for this code from specific AMA publication

10021 Fine needle aspiration; without imaging guidance
　⊃ *CPT Assistant* Aug 02:10; *CPT Changes: An Insider's View* 2002

Bullet: New procedure code number for this edition of CPT

● 77061 Digital breast tomosynthesis; unilateral

Triangle: Code revision resulted in substantially altered procedure description

▲ 80162 Digoxin; total (a therapeutic drug assay)

Facing triangles: New or revised text other than the procedure descriptor

▶◀　　▶ 33330 Insertion of graft, aorta, or great vessels, without shunt,
　　　　　or cardiopulmonary bypass (33332 has been deleted)◀

Plus sign: Add-on code can be listed after the primary or parent code is listed

+ 35400 Angioscopy (non-coronary vessels
　　　or grafts) during therapeutic
　　　intervention (List separately in addition
　　　to code for primary procedure)

Null zero or universal no code: Modifier -51 cannot be used with this code

⊘ 20974 Electrical stimulation to aid bone healing; noninvasive (nonoperative)

Circled bullet: Moderate (Conscious) sedation included with this code

⊙ **31615** Tracheobronchoscopy through
　　　established tracheostomy incision

Flash: Code shows FDA approval for vaccine pending

✗ **90666** Influenza virus vaccine, pandemic formulation, split virus, preservative free,
for intramuscular use

Number sign: Resequenced code (out of numerical order)

27329 Radical resection of tumor (e.g., malignant neoplasm),
　　　soft tissue of thigh or knee area; less than 5 cm.

Fig. 13.2 Symbols that appear in the 2020 *Current Procedural Terminology (CPT)* code book and a brief explanation of what they tell the coding specialist. These symbols and their meanings appear at the bottom of each page of codes in the CPT code book. *AMA,* American Medical Association; *FDA,* Food and Drug Administration.

- Enteral and parenteral therapy
- Outpatient Prospective Payment System (PPS)
- Dental procedures
- Durable medical equipment
- Procedures/professional services
- Alcohol and drug abuse treatment services
- Drugs administered other than oral method
- Orthotic procedures
- Prosthetic procedures
- Other medical services
- Pathology and laboratory services

- Casting and splinting supplies
- Diagnostic radiology services
- Temporary non-Medicare codes
- T codes for state Medicaid agencies
- Vision and hearing services

The Level I (CPT) code should be used when both a CPT and Level II code have the same description. The Level II code should be used if the descriptions are not identical. For example, if the Level I (CPT) code narrative is generic and the HCPCS Level II code is specific, code from the HCPCS Level II.

❗ COMPLIANCE ALERT

Durable Medical Equipment

Durable medical equipment (DME) is any equipment that provides therapeutic benefits to a patient in need because of certain medical conditions and/or illnesses. Medicare covers medically necessary DME if prescribed and meets the following criteria:
• Can withstand repeated use (durable)

• Used for a medical reason
• Not usually useful to someone who isn't sick or injured
• Used in the patient's home
• Has an expected lifetime of at least 3 years

Several companies publish Level II HCPCS code books annually. Content, numbers of the appendices, color-coded coverage instructions, notes, and unlisted procedures vary between the editions. Notes or special instructions may appear in or following subsections or headings or as part of the description in a heading or code.

The Level II HCPCS is updated each January 1, with periodic updates made throughout the year as needed. In some states, the TRICARE and Medicaid programs accept HCPCS codes. Most commercial insurance companies have adopted the Level I (CPT) and Level II (HCPCS) code systems.

Procedure 13.2 at the end of this chapter gives step-by-step directions on how to use an HCPCS code book for billing purposes.

❗ COMPLIANCE ALERT

HIPAA Diagnostic and Procedural Code Guidelines

Under HIPAA, providers and medical facilities are responsible for using ICD-10-CM diagnostic codes to document why patients are seen and CPT-4 and HCPCS codes for what is done to patients during their encounter. They are also responsible for implementing the updated codes in a timely manner, using the HIPAA-mandated transaction code set codes, and deleting old or obsolete codes.

CPT, Current Procedural Terminology; HCPCS, Healthcare Common Procedure Coding System; HIPAA, Health Insurance Portability and Accountability Act; ICD-10-CM, International Classification of Diseases, Tenth Revision, Clinical Modification.

✒ 13.2 QUICK REVIEW
Question: What is a modifier?

CURRENT PROCEDURAL TERMINOLOGY CONTENT AND FORMAT

The AMA is responsible for creating and maintaining the official CPT code set. The CPT content is outlined in Table 13.2, with three categories of codes.

Category I Codes

Category I contains five-digit code numbers with no decimal (Example 13.2). It is divided into categories and subcategories according to anatomic body systems, procedure, condition, description, and specialty. Fig. 13.3A illustrates the format of the Index, and Fig. 13.3B illustrates the format of the CPT section.

EXAMPLE 13.2 Category I Codes

10060	Incision and drainage of abscess
42825	Tonsillectomy, younger than age 12

TABLE 13.2 Current Procedural Terminology Book Content Outline

Category I Codes	(99202–99607)
Evaluation and Management (E/M)	99202–99499
Anesthesia	00100–01999
Surgery	10021–69990
Radiology, Nuclear Medicine, and Diagnostic Ultrasound	70010–79999
Pathology and Laboratory	80047–89398
Medicine	90281–99607
Category II Codes	0001F–7025F
Category III Codes	0019T–0290T
Appendices	
A—Modifiers	
B—Summary of Additions, Deletions, and Revisions	
C—Clinical Examples	
D—Summary of CPT Add-On Codes	
E—Summary of CPT Codes Exempt From Modifier 51	
F—Summary of CPT Codes Exempt From Modifier 63	
G—Summary of CPT Codes That Include Moderate (Conscious) Sedation	
H—Alphabetical Clinical Topics Listing	
I—Genetic Testing Code Modifiers	
J—Electrodiagnostic Medicine Listing of Sensory, Motor, and Mixed Nerves	
K—Product Pending FDA ApprovaIL—Vascular Families	
M—Renumbered CPT Codes—Citations Cross-Walk	
N—Summary of Resequenced CPT Codes	
O—Multianalyte Assays With Algorithmic Analyses	
Index	

CPT, Current Procedural Terminology; FDA, Food and Drug Administration.

Category II: Performance Measurement Codes

Category II codes describe clinical components that typically may be included in evaluation and management (E/M) services or clinical services and do not have a relative value associated with them. They also describe results from clinical laboratory or radiology tests and other procedures, identified processes intended to address patient safety practices, or services reflecting compliance with state or federal laws. These codes are used for optional performance tracking.

Category II also have an alphanumeric identifier with a letter in the last field (e.g., 0502F, Subsequent prenatal care visit) to

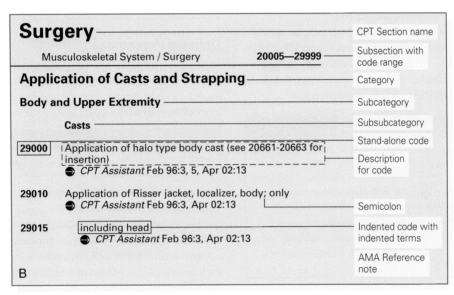

Fig. 13.3 (A) *Current Procedural Terminology* (CPT) format illustrating conventions of the Index and a section. (B) CPT format illustrating conventions of the Index and a section.

distinguish them from category I codes (Example 13.3). Four modifiers in this section are used to indicate that a service specified by a performance measure was considered but because of either medical or patient circumstance(s) documented in the health record, or as a result of system issues, the service was not provided. The modifiers are 1P, 2P, 3P, and 8P. Use of these codes is optional for correct coding.

EXAMPLE 13.3	**Category II Codes**
0500F	Initial prenatal care visit
0502F	Subsequent prenatal care visit

Category III: New and Emerging Technology Codes

Category III codes are a temporary set of tracking codes used to code emerging technologies that do not yet have any procedure code assignment in category I (Example 13.4). They are intended to expedite data collection and assessment of new services and procedures to substantiate widespread use and clinical effectiveness. A category III code may become a category I code. When it is deleted from category III and adopted as a category I

code, the CPT code book provides clear indication of this change by inserting a cross reference in place of the former category III code; for example, ▶(0051T, 0052T, 0053T have been deleted. To report, see 33927, 33928, 33929)◀. The AMA website posts updates to this category in January and July of every year.

EXAMPLE 13.4	**Category III Codes**
0329T	Monitoring of intraocular pressure for 24 h or longer, unilateral or bilateral, with interpretation and report.
0331T	Myocardial sympathetic innervation imaging, planar qualitative, and quantitative assessment.

Code Book Symbols

CPT is published each year with deletions, new codes, and description changes. Coding and billing specialists should become familiar with the new codes and any description changes or deleted codes related to codes that may exist on the health care organization's fee schedule. Fig. 13.2 shows how to identify new codes and description changes by following the symbols that are used. The symbols placed below many codes throughout the code book indicate that the AMA has published reference material on those particular codes. The reference citation is also provided. All these symbols are also located at the bottom of each page of codes in the CPT code book.

When using a new code, marked with a bullet (●), it may take as long as 6 months before a third-party payer has a mandatory value assignment; therefore, reimbursements are received in varying amounts during that time. An exception is in the Medicare program, which has a value assignment published annually each fall in the *Federal Register*.

Revised codes or revised text, marked with a triangle (▲) or (► ◄), highlight what is new or deleted. This saves time in trying to figure out what was changed and prevents using these codes incorrectly. Appendix B in the CPT code book provides a summary of code additions, deletions, and revisions.

Add-on codes, shown with a plus sign (+), indicate that the code can *only* be listed after the primary or parent code has been listed (Example 13.5). Add-on codes always reference the appropriate primary codes. Add-on codes are always exempt from using Modifier -51 to indicate an additional procedure.

EXAMPLE 13.5 **Add-On Codes**	
+49568	Implantation of mesh or other prosthesis for open incisional or ventral hernia repair or mesh for closure of debridement for necrotizing soft tissue infection (List separately in addition to code for the incisional or ventral hernia repair) (Use 49568 in conjunction with 11004–11006, 49560–49566)
+59525	Subtotal or total hysterectomy after cesarean delivery (List separately in addition to code for primary procedure) (Use 59525 in conjunction with 59510, 59514, 59515, 59618, 59620, 59622)

Modifier -51 is attached to CPT codes when multiple procedures are performed. Some CPT codes are exempt, shown with a symbol Ø which means that the modifier cannot be used with this code (Example 13.6). Codes with this symbol are not add-on codes; they can be stand-alone procedures. They are typically exempt from multiple procedure reductions in payment. These codes are listed in Appendix E.

EXAMPLE 13.6 **Modifier -51 Exempt Codes**	
Ø 20974	Electrical stimulation to aid bone healing; noninvasive (nonoperative) invasive (operative)
Ø 20975	
Ø 31500	Intubation, endotracheal, emergency procedure

A flash symbol (✗) is used to identify codes for vaccines that are pending Food and Drug Administration (FDA) approval (Example 13.7). A complete list of these appears in Appendix K in the CPT code book.

EXAMPLE 13.7 **Codes Pending FDA Approval**	
✗ 90587	Dengue vaccine, quadrivalent, live, 3 dose schedule, for subcutaneous use.
✗ 90666	Influenza virus vaccine (IIV), pandemic formulation, split virus, preservative free, for intramuscular use.

Resequenced codes that are not placed numerically are identified with the # symbol and a reference placed numerically ("Code is out of numerical sequence. See …") is a navigational alert to direct the user to the location of the out-of-sequence code (Example 13.8). A list appears in Appendix N.

EXAMPLE 13.8 **Codes That Are Out of Sequence**	
27337	Code is out of numerical sequence. See 27326–27331
27339	Code is out of numerical sequence. See 27326–27331
27326	Neurectomy, popliteal (gastrocnemius)
27327	Excision, tumor, soft tissue of thigh or knee area, subcutaneous; less than 3 cm
#27337	3 cm or greater
27328	Excision, tumor, soft tissue of thigh or knew area; subfascial (e.g., intramuscular); less than 5 cm
#27339	5 cm or greater

Unlisted Procedures

When an unusual service is rendered, an unlisted code (Example 13.9) should be used rather than guessing or using an incorrect code. Supporting documentation such as a letter and copy of operative report should be sent explaining the service.

EXAMPLE 13.9 **Unlisted Procedure Code**	
31599	Unlisted procedure, larynx

Since the development of category III codes, it is important to double check that section of the CPT code book to verify whether a code exists before using an unlisted code. Unlisted codes generally end in -99 and are found at the end of each section or subsection. A comprehensive list of unlisted codes is found at the beginning of each section. Some Medicare Administrative Contractors (MACs) do not pay for any of the special -99 adjunct or unlisted codes.

13.3 QUICK REVIEW

Question: What symbol is used to designate an add-on code? What does this mean?

EVALUATION AND MANAGEMENT SERVICES (99202–99499)

The E/M section is divided into office visits, hospital visits, consultations, and other types of patient management services. Some subcategories of codes, such as office or outpatient visits, are divided into subcategories based on whether the patient is a new or an established patient. Hospital visits also have two bold-faced subcategories: initial and subsequent. Each subcategory has levels of E/M services identified by specific codes. This classification is based on the nature of the provider's work, such as type of service, place of service, and the patient's status. Levels of service within each subcategory are typically based on the required elements for that subcategory of services. Elements could include:

- New versus established patient
- Place of service
- Extent of the service (e.g., was the exam comprehensive or problem focused.)

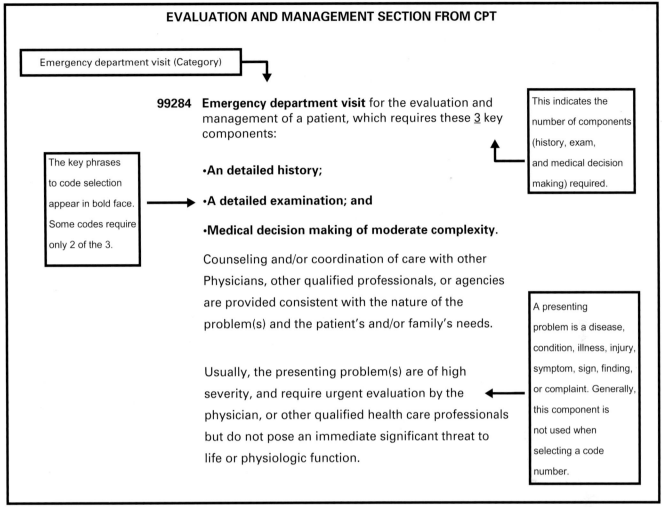

Fig. 13.4 Evaluation and management code 99284 defining the main words and phrases. This code is used for a patient seen in the emergency department setting.

- Nature of the presenting problem
- Time typically needed to provide the service (Example 13.10 defines the various types of time involved in E/M services.)

EXAMPLE 13.10 Categories of Time

1. **Face-to-face:** Office and outpatient visits (Provider meets face-to-face with the patient or family.)
2. **Floor/unit time:** Hospital observation services, inpatient hospital care, initial and follow-up hospital consultations, and nursing facility services (Provider is present on the patient's hospital floor or unit providing bedside services to the patient, such as time with patient, time working on patient's chart, and discussing patient's care with nurses.)
3. **Non–face-to-face time:** Inpatient hospital pre-encounter and post-encounter time, obtaining records and test results, talking with other health care providers, and arranging for additional services. (Provider does work related to the patient before or after face-to-face time or floor/unit time.)

To begin the coding process, the provider of service must identify the category such as office, hospital inpatient, outpatient, or consultation. Once the category of service is identified, the elements used for determining the level of service within the category must be reviewed. The code description should be read thoroughly to fully understand the required components or elements for that service. Review the sample in Fig. 13.4 illustrating an E/M code for a patient seen in the emergency department setting.

Codes in the E/M section of CPT have from three to five levels for reporting purposes. Many times, providers will refer to the E/M codes as level 5 for the most complex to level 1 for the least complex. These levels coincide with the fifth or last digit of the CPT code (e.g., 99205). It is common to hear a provider say, "Ted Brown was seen for a level 5 today." This terminology may appear on encounter forms with five-digit CPT code numbers and be referred to as levels 1 through 5 (Fig. 13.5).

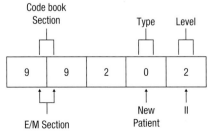

Fig. 13.5 *Current Procedural Terminology* code digit analysis.

TABLE 13.3   Levels With Code Numbers

	OFFICE VISITS		CONSULTATIONS	
	New	Established	Office	Hospital
Level 1	N/A	99211	99241	99251
Level 2	99202	99212	99242	99252
Level 3	99203	99213	99243	99253
Level 4	99204	99214	99244	99254
Level 5	99205	99215	99245	99255

Alternatively, this terminology may be seen abbreviated as L-1, L-2, and so on. The level also may be written out as level one, level two, and so on, depending on the complexity of the case. A breakdown of the E/M levels with code numbers is shown in Table 13.3.

As discussed in Chapter 11, E/M services should have the appropriate history and exam documented by the provider. All elements of medical decision making should be detailed to indicate the appropriate level of service that should be selected in the coding process. In code selection, different types of E/M services have different required elements. These elements must be supported in the documentation.

Office or Other Outpatient Services

Office or other outpatient services are divided into sections based on new or established patients. They are used to report evaluation and management services in a provider office, or an outpatient or ambulatory facility setting. There are four levels of service for new patients and five for established ones.

E/M code 99211 for established patients is often called a "nurse visit" and does not always require the presence of a physician. However, the patient must be established, and the physician must have initiated the service. To report a nurse visit, Medicare requires that the nurse must be following a plan of care that was established by the physician in a previous encounter. Medicare also requires that the patient encounter must be face to face, and the physician must be on-site in the immediate suite of offices. Telephone calls with patients do not meet the requirements for reporting 99211.

Some services that may allow reporting of this code include the following:
- Rechecking a patient for conjunctivitis
- Checking blood pressure of a patient who is being treated for high blood pressure
- Checking a wound beyond the global period
- Reading a tuberculin test result
- Recheck for issuing a return-to-work certificate

99202 (new) and 99212 (established) typically indicate a patient with 1 *self-limited or minor problem*. A self-limited or minor problem is one that runs a definite course and is not likely to create a permanent change to the patient's health. It is typically transient in nature. An example of a self-limited or minor problem would be diaper rash or the common cold.

99203 (new) and 99213 (established) typically indicate that a patient has either two or more self-limited or minor problems,

or one *stable, chronic illness*, or one *acute, uncomplicated illness or injury*. A stable, chronic illness is one with an expected duration of at least one year or longer. Whether a patient is stable or not is determined by their treatment goals. If a patient is not at the treatment goal, they are not stable, even if there has been no change in their condition. Examples of a stable, chronic illness would be well-controlled hypertension. An acute, uncomplicated illness or injury is a recent or new short-term problem with low risk of morbidity. Full recovery is expected. Examples of an acute, uncomplicated illness or injury are a sprained ankle or rhinitis.

99204 (new) or 99214 (established) are typically indicated if a patient presents with one of the following:
- One or more chronic illnesses with exacerbation, progression, or side effects of treatment
- Two or more stable chronic illnesses
- One undiagnosed new problem with uncertain prognosis
- One acute illness with systemic symptoms
- One acute, complicated injury

A *chronic illness with exacerbation, progression, or side effects of treatment* is one that is worsening, poorly controlled, or requires additional supportive care or attention to side effects. An example would be an established diabetic patient managed through diet and oral medication presenting with frequent urination, and glucose levels in the 300s. An *undiagnosed new problem with uncertain prognosis* is one that typically results in a high risk of morbidity without treatment. An example of this would be a lump in the breast. An *acute illness with systemic symptoms* is one that has a high risk of morbidity without treatment. Examples of such an illness are colitis and pneumonia. An *acute, complicated injury* is one that may require evaluation of a body system not directly linked to the injured one. It may also have multiple treatment options or an associated risk of morbidity. An example would be a head injury with loss of consciousness.

99205 (new) and 99215 (established) typically indicate that a patient has one or more *chronic illnesses with severe exacerbation, progression, or side effects of treatment*, or one *acute or chronic illness or injury that poses a threat to life or bodily function*. These patients may require hospital-level care. Examples of illness and injury that would typically require this level of service would be severe chest pain, severe respiratory distress, psychiatric illness with potential threat to self or others, or acute renal failure.

Office visits and other outpatient services base much of code selection on either time or medical decision making. Providers are able to include both face-to-face as well as non-face-to-face time if they choose to use this as the criteria for code selection. Fig. 13.6 shows a breakdown of time indicated in the CPT book for this purpose.

Observation Care

Patients are often placed in observation care as a result of an emergency room encounter. In these cases, the patient is not considered well enough to be sent home; however, they must be monitored further before a proper course of treatment may be determined. A patient held in observation status is

Evaluation and Management Time			
Outpatient-New		Outpatient-Established	
99201	DELETED	99211	Nurse
99202	15–29 minutes	99212	10–19 minutes
99203	30–44 minutes	99213	20–29 minutes
99204	45–59 minutes	99214	30–39 minutes
99205	60–74 minutes	99215	40–54 minutes
≥ 75 minutes, see prolonged services		≥ 55 minutes, see prolonged services	

Fig. 13.6 Break down of office and outpatient codes by time.

considered to be an outpatient. For example, if a patient has a possible concussion, they may be admitted to observation so that health care providers may monitor the patient for a time. If the patient's condition worsens, they would then be admitted to the hospital as an inpatient. If the patient's condition improves, they will be discharged. A patient may be placed in observation for up to 3 days before being admitted or discharged.

Codes reflect admission to observation, subsequent observation care, and discharge from observation. These codes do not distinguish between new and established patients. It is not necessary for the patient to be in a designated observation area of the hospital. An admission and a discharge may be reported on the same day. If a patient is admitted to the hospital from observation, the observation services are not coded.

Hospital Inpatient Services

The hospital inpatient service codes include subcategories for Initial Hospital Care, Subsequent Hospital Care, and Discharge Services. They do not differentiate between new and established patients. Documentation of the appropriate level of history, exam, and medical decision making (MDM) will determine the code selection. Only the admitting provider reports an Initial Hospital Care code. Any other provider seeing the patient should report initial inpatient consultation codes or subsequent care codes, as appropriate. If a patient is seen in the emergency department (ED) and is subsequently admitted to the hospital by the same provider on the same date of service as the ED visit, it is billed as initial hospital care. The provider includes the services related to the admission that he or she provided in the other hospital service departments as well as in the inpatient setting.

Discharge Services are time-based codes. These services include final examination, continuing care instructions, discharge paperwork, prescriptions, and referrals.

Consultations

As previously discussed in the documentation chapter, a consultation includes services rendered by a provider whose opinion or advice is requested by another health care provider or agency in the evaluation or treatment of a patient's illness or a suspected problem. A consulting provider must submit a written report containing their findings and opinions to the

---

BOX 13.1 HCPCS Telehealth Consultation Codes

G0425	Telehealth consultation, emergency department or initial inpatient, typically 30 min communicating with the patient via telehealth
G0426	Telehealth consultation, emergency department or initial inpatient, typically 50 min communicating with the patient via telehealth
G0427	Telehealth consultation, emergency department or initial inpatient, typically 70 min or more communicating with the patient via telehealth

requesting physician. In contrast, a referral is the transfer of the total or specific care of a patient from one provider to another for known problems.

Effective January 1, 2010, the CMS no longer reimburses consultation codes (ranges 99241 through 99245, and 99251 through 99255) for inpatient and office or outpatient settings and for various places of service. The codes are still included in CPT as other insurance carriers still reimburse for them. CMS indicates that the initial hospital care codes 99221 through 99223 should be used when billing a consultation on a hospital inpatient. The attending physician must append with HCPCS Level II modifier AI (A-eye) *principal physician of record* to the code. An exception would be for telehealth consultation (HCPCS G-codes) (see Box 13.1). For non-Medicare cases, codes for consultations are as follows:

- Office or other outpatient consultations (new or established patient): 99241 through 99245 (Example 13.11)

EXAMPLE 13.11 Outpatient Consultation

A 20-year-old woman is seen for an office consultation for cystitis. She complains of burning on urination and urinary frequency. The patient's records from the referring provider were reviewed. Urine culture confirmed a urinary tract infection, which was reported to her primary care provider for treatment. Obtained problem-focused history and examination with straightforward medical decision making.

99241	Office consultation
87086	Urine culture, bacterial

- Inpatient consultations (new or established patient): 99251 through 99255 (Example 13.12)

EXAMPLE 13.12   Inpatient Consultation

A 50-year-old man is seen for an initial inpatient consultation with a status post–left hip fracture and a history of well-controlled type 2 diabetes mellitus. Consultation is requested for surgical clearance. Reviewed medical data on the unit. Obtained a detailed history and performed a detailed examination with low-complexity medical decision making. Discussed diagnosis and treatment options with patient and completed health record documentation. Will give ongoing consultation to referring provider.

99253   Inpatient consultation

In the office setting, use the appropriate consultation code for the initial encounter; if a follow-up visit is required for additional diagnostic testing or examination, then use the appropriate established patient code. In a hospital setting, use the appropriate inpatient hospital consultation code; if a follow-up is required for additional services, then use subsequent hospital care codes. Remember the four Rs of consultations: There must be a *requesting* provider and the consultant must *render* an opinion and send a *report*. The requesting provider must document the *reason* on the health record.

Emergency Department Services

Codes 99281 through 99285 describe various levels of emergency care provided in an emergency department. An emergency department is defined as an organized hospital-based facility for the provision of unscheduled episodic services to patients who present for immediate medical attention. An ED must be open 24 hours, 7 days/week. CPT codes 99281 through 99285 should not be used to report emergency care provided in an office setting.

Code 99288 is used when advanced life support is necessary during emergency care and the provider is located in a hospital emergency or critical care department and is in two-way voice communication with ambulance or rescue personnel outside the hospital.

Miscellaneous service codes 99050 through 99058 can be used depending on the hour at which the patient is seen as an emergency either in the provider's office or if taken to the ED of a hospital (24-hours facility). Most payers, including Medicare, do not pay for these codes. Some payers might pay for these codes and require documentation from the provider to support the code. Other codes under Miscellaneous Services in the Medicine section may be applicable for a patient receiving emergency care, so these should be scrutinized carefully.

Critical Care

According to CPT guidelines, critical care is the direct delivery of medical care by a provider for a critically ill or injured patient. A critical illness or injury acutely impairs one or more vital organ systems and makes an imminent or life-threatening deterioration in the patient's condition highly probable. Critical care involves highly complex decision making to assess, manipulate, and support vital system functions to treat single or multiple vital organ system failure or prevent further life-threatening deterioration of the patient's condition. Examples of vital organ system failure include but are not limited to central nervous system

failure; circulatory failure; shock; and renal, hepatic, metabolic, or respiratory failure. Critical care may be provided on multiple days, even if no changes are made in the treatment rendered to the patient, as long as the patient's condition supports it.

Critical care is not always given in a critical care area, such as the coronary care unit, intensive care unit, pediatric intensive care unit, respiratory care unit, or emergency care facility. It could occur in the patient's room or in the ED. Also, it is important to note that a service that takes place in an intensive or critical care unit is not automatically coded as critical care. Services for a patient who is not critically ill but is in a critical care or intensive care unit are reported by use of other appropriate in-hospital E/M codes.

Critical care codes 99291 and 99292 are used to report the total duration of time spent by a provider performing critical care services to a critically ill or injured patient. For any given period spent providing critical care services, the provider must devote their full attention to the patient and therefore cannot provide services to any other patient during the same period.

Time spent with the individual patient must be recorded in the patient's record. Time spent engaged in work directly related to the individual patient's care, whether that time was spent at the immediate bedside or elsewhere on the floor or unit (even if not continuous), is reported as critical care. For example, time spent on the unit or at the nursing station on the floor reviewing test results or imaging studies, discussing the critically ill patient's care with other medical staff, or documenting critical care services in the health record is reported as critical care, even though it does not occur at the bedside.

Time spent in activities that occur outside of the unit or off the floor may not be reported as critical care because the provider is not immediately available to the patient. Time spent in activities that do not directly contribute to the treatment of the patient may not be reported as critical care, even if they are performed in the critical care unit. Time spent performing separately reportable procedures or services should not be included in the time reported as critical care time.

Code 99291 is used to report the first 30 to 74 minutes of critical care on a given date. It should be used only once per date, even if the time spent by the provider is not continuous on that date. Critical care of less than 30 minutes total duration on a given date should be reported with the appropriate E/M code. Code 99292 is used to report additional blocks of time, up to 30 minutes each, beyond the first 74 minutes. This code has a plus sign (+) and is an "add-on" code. It is never used alone.

Critical care and other E/M services may be provided to the same patient on the same date by the same provider. Some services are included in critical care codes used to report critical care when performed during the critical period by the provider performing critical care. They are not coded in addition to critical care codes. These services are as follows:

- Interpretation of cardiac output measurements (93561, 93562)
- Chest radiographs (71045, 71046)
- Pulse oximetry (94760, 94761, 94762)
- Blood gases and information data stored in computers (e.g., electrocardiograms, blood pressures, hematologic data [99090])

- Gastric intubation (43752, 43753)
- Temporary transcutaneous pacing (92953)
- Ventilator management (94002 through 94004, 94660, 94662)
- Vascular access procedures (36000, 36410, 36415, 36591, 36600)

Any services performed in excess of those listed earlier should be reported separately.

Inpatient critical care services provided to neonates and infants 29 days through 24 months of age are reported with pediatric critical care codes 99468 through 99476. The pediatric critical care codes are reported as long as the infant or young child qualifies for critical care services during the hospital stay. Inpatient critical care services provided to neonates (28 days of age or younger) are reported with the neonatal critical care codes 99468 and 99469. The neonatal critical care codes are reported as long as the neonate qualifies for critical care services through the 28th postnatal day. The reporting of the pediatric and neonatal critical care services is not based on time or on the type of unit (e.g., pediatric or neonatal critical care unit), nor is it dependent on the type of provider delivering the care. For additional instructions on reporting these services, see the section on Inpatient Neonatal and Pediatric Critical Care in the Evaluation and Management section of CPT.

There are subcategories for critical care for neonates, infants 29 days through 24 months of age, and various ages of children, as well as those subcategories for adults. A coding specialist must be sure to read the age categories carefully when choosing the appropriate subcategory of codes.

Nursing Facilities, Prolonged Services, Case Management

The Nursing Facilities subcategory is for services provided to patients in nursing facilities or psychiatric residential treatment facilities. Documentation of the appropriate level of history, exam and MDM will determine the code selection.

Preventive Medicine

Preventive medicine is composed of services provided to prevent the occurrence of illness, injury, and disease, such as vaccine immunizations, routine physical examinations, and screening programs for detection of signs of disorders. Codes 99381 through 99397 describe initial or periodic comprehensive preventive medicine examination and are based on the age of the patient. Codes 99401 through 99412 should be used for reporting counseling given at an encounter separate from the preventive medicine examination.

Sometimes a patient may have an annual checkup, but while having the examination, he or she tells the health care provider of another issue. The provider performs both preventive and problem-focused services at the same time. Both services may be billed with the modifier -25 to indicate a separately identifiable service. Medicare does not cover this range of preventive visit codes. Therefore, when this occurs with Medicare patients, only the Medicare covered screenings or services (e.g., problem-focused E/M, Papanicolaou [Pap] test, colon/rectal cancer screening, or prostate cancer screening) may be billed to

the insurance. Noncovered services must be "carved out" to be billed to the patient.

Although Medicare does not cover the preventive visit codes 99281–99397, they have developed preventive services for their beneficiaries. For those patients who have just became eligible for Medicare, there is the Initial Preventive Physical Exam (IPPE) which is also referred to as the "Welcome to Medicare" physical. The IPPE is a face-to-face visit, and services are limited to a patient during their first 12 months of Medicare enrollment. The IPPE is coded with the Level II HCPCs code G0402.

Medicare has also created the Annual Wellness Visit (AWV) for Medicare beneficiaries, which is similar to a preventive visit, although it has different elements that are required. The purpose of the AWV is to review the patient's wellness and develop a personalized prevention plan. The AWV is coded with the Level II HCPCs codes G0438 (initial AWV) and G0439 (subsequent AWV).

Prolonged Services and Standby

Codes 99354 through 99359 should be used to indicate prolonged services with direct face-to-face patient contact; for example, the provider has spent time beyond the usual amount allotted for the service. There are specific codes for services with face-to-face contact and without face-to-face contact. Prolonged service that is less than 30 minutes should not be billed using these codes because the time is included in the E/M code. Time should be documented in the health record to justify the use of these codes. Reimbursement for prolonged attendance in the hospital is higher than payment for many other types of care and reimbursement for critical care is even higher.

Physician standby services over the first 30 minutes are billed using code 99360. Some insurance programs or plans like Medicare do not pay for physician standby services, so be sure to check before billing to see whether the commercial payer will pay. The charge for this type of service is based on what the provider believes to be the value of 1 hour of their time. An example of this might be when a pediatrician is on standby during a high-risk cesarean section performed on a pregnant woman.

Other Evaluation and Management Codes

Other subcategories in this section cover home health care, case management, care plan oversight, telephone and online services, transitional care management, and advance care planning.

13.4 QUICK REVIEW
Question: What are the four Rs of consultations?

13.5 QUICK REVIEW
Question: What place of service is required to report critical care codes?

13.6 QUICK REVIEW
Question: What is preventive medicine?

ANESTHESIA SERVICES (00100–01999)

Anesthesia services are usually provided by an anesthesiologist, certified registered nurse anesthetist (CRNA), or a team of both. When a provider overseas one or more teams of CRNAs, it is required that the provider be present for specific portions of the procedure including the following:

- Providing a preanesthetic examination
- Outlining the anesthesia plan
- Participating in induction and emergence
- Monitoring at frequent intervals
- Being present and immediately available for emergencies
- Handling postanesthetic care

Anesthesia codes are grouped anatomically. Because the anesthesia code is directly related to the type of surgery a patient has, it is important for coding specialists to have a good knowledge of terminology from many different specialties.

All anesthesia codes include the following:

- Standard preoperative and postoperative visits
- Anesthesia care during the procedure
- Administration of fluids and/or blood products
- Usual monitoring services, such as electrocardiogram (ECG), temperature, blood pressure, pulse oximetry, and mass spectrometry

Anesthesia billing is made of two components: a base unit and a time unit. Anesthesia codes are assigned base units by the American Society of Anesthesiology based on the difficulty of the procedure. Time units are determined by the length of the procedure. The start time begins when the anesthesiologist prepares the patient for anesthesia. This does not include the pre-anesthesia visit and assessment. The anesthesia time ends when the patient is safely transferred to the care of the postanesthesia care unit or equivalent area.

Medicare requires that time is reported per minute. Other payers may require that a time unit be equal to 15 minutes or any increment thereof. It is important that coding and billing specialist check with each insurance payer to determine their requirements.

When multiple procedures are performed on a patient during anesthesia, the surgery that represents the most complex procedure is reported as it will have a higher base unit. The total anesthesia time for all procedures is reported.

Anesthesia codes should include a physical status (PS) modifier to indicate the health status of the patient and the potential issues with anesthesia they may pose. Some payers such as Medicare will not pay additional units for these modifiers, but some will. They are as follows:

- P1: Patient is normal and healthy (+0 units)
- P2: Patient has a mild systemic disease (+0 units)
- P3: Patient has a severe systemic disease (+1 units)
- P4: Patient has a severe systemic disease that is a constant threat to life (+2 units)
- P5: Patient is not expected to survive without the operation (+3 units)
- P6: Patient is brain dead and organs are being removed for donor purpose (+0 units)

To arrive at a fee for anesthesia, a billing specialist must understand the following formula: Base units + Time units + PS + QC = Total units. (Example 13.13)

EXAMPLE 13.13   Calculating Anesthesia Units

A 36-year-old patient receives anesthesia services by an MD for carpal tunnel surgery:
- The procedure starts at 0800 and ends at 0856.
- Code 01810 is allotted 3 base units.
- One time unit = 15 minutes or any increment thereof.
- The provider charges $100.00 per unit.

To determine the anesthesia fee:
- 3 base units (for procedure) + 4 time units = 7 total units × $100.00 per unit = $700.00

Qualifying circumstances (QC) are add-on codes for anesthesia services. They are used when a patient's age or status has a significant effect on the service provided. Although these are not paid by Medicare, many third-party payers do cover them.

- 99100, Anesthesia for patient of extreme age, younger than 1 year and older than 70 (+1 units)
- 99116, Anesthesia complicated by utilization of total body hypothermia (+5 units)
- 99135, Anesthesia complicated by utilization of controlled hypotension (+5 units)
- 99140, Anesthesia complicated by emergency conditions (must specify) (+2 units)

Anesthesia teams often provide other services such as endotracheal intubation, central venous catheters, and arterial catheterization for monitoring, as well as various nerve blocks for postoperative and chronic pain management.

Surgical anesthesia codes always include a two-letter modifier that indicates the provider who performed the service. Some examples are included here. AA indicates an anesthesiologist working solo on the case. When anesthesia is provided by a physician and CRNA team, the charge is split in half and billed with a QX to indicate the CRNA, and a QK to indicate the physician (Example 13.14). In some states, CRNAs are able to provide their own anesthesia with no physician oversight. This would be indicated with a QZ modifier.

EXAMPLE 13.14   Anesthesia Teams and Modifiers

Anesthesia for Total Knee Replacement		
Anesthesiologist working alone:	01402AA	$1000.00
Anesthesiologist and CRNA working as a team:	01402QX	$500.00
	01402QK	$500.00

13.7   QUICK REVIEW
Question: What is included in all anesthesia services?

13.8   QUICK REVIEW
Question: What is the formula for calculating anesthesia units?

SURGERY GUIDELINES

Coding From an Operative Report

It is best to obtain a copy of the patient's operative report from the hospital when coding surgery. A photocopy can be used so the coding specialist can make notes right on the document. When reviewing the report, use a ruler to read the report line by line. Highlight words that could indicate that the procedure performed may be altered by specific circumstances and to indicate that a code modifier may be necessary. Look up any unfamiliar terms using a medical dictionary or anatomic reference book and write the definitions in the margin.

Assign the code for the postoperative diagnosis shown at the beginning of the operative report. Also search for additional diagnoses in the body of the report that can be added as secondary diagnostic codes to support medical necessity, especially if the case is complex.

If the complex surgical procedure is not accurately described in the procedure code nomenclature, include an operative report and list "Attachment" in Block 19 of the insurance claim form so that the claims adjuster clearly understands the case and generates maximum payment.

Code numbers that describe a part of the body treated render higher reimbursement, depending on their location (e.g., suturing of a facial laceration pays a higher rate than suturing of an arm laceration).

Remember the rule: Not documented, not done. Code only the procedures that are actually documented in the report.

Do not code using only the name of the procedure as it is given in the heading of the operative report. Read the report thoroughly before coding to see whether additional procedures were performed and whether they were part of the main procedure, performed independently, or unrelated.

Check to see how many surgeons were involved in the operative procedure and their roles (assistant surgeon, co-surgeon, team surgeon).

Look for unusual details, such as special instruments used, unusually long or complex procedures, rare approach techniques, reoperation, or extensive scarring encountered. These conditions may need one or more modifiers appended to the code.

Surgical code descriptions may define a correct coding relationship wherein one code is part of another based on the language used in the description (Example 13.15). An explanation of how to read a description for stand-alone codes and indented codes can be found in Procedure 13.2 at the end of this chapter.

EXAMPLE 13.15 Integral Code

Partial and complete, which means the partial procedure is included in the complete procedure.
56620   Vulvectomy simple; partial
56625   complete
Partial and total, which means the partial procedure is included in the total procedure.
58940   Oophorectomy, partial or total, unilateral or bilateral
Unilateral and bilateral, which means the unilateral procedure is included in the bilateral procedure.
58900   Biopsy of ovary, unilateral or bilateral
Single and multiple, which means the single procedure is included in the multiple procedure.
49321   Laparoscopy, surgical, with biopsy (single or multiple)

Confirm that the report findings agree with the procedure codes on the claim.

Global Surgical Package

Global surgical package is a phrase commonly encountered when billing. Generally, a surgical procedure includes the standard preoperative, intraoperative, and postoperative services, with the preoperative service component depending on whether it is a minor or major surgery.

A major procedure is extensive and will typically require an overnight stay in the hospital. These procedures most often require entering a body cavity, removing an organ, or altering a patient's anatomy. Anesthesia and respiratory assistance are often required. Examples of major procedures would be a bowel resection or cardiac surgery. In contrast, a minor procedure is less invasive and does not require penetration of a body cavity. Many times the patient does not require deep sedation. Examples of minor procedures would be removal of lesions, small wound repairs, or a breast biopsy.

The majority of surgical procedures, including fracture care, are handled in this manner. Typical postoperative follow-up care includes only care that is usually a part of the surgical service. Complications, exacerbations, recurrence, or the presence of other diseases or injuries that require additional services should be reported separately. Table 13.4 lists what is and is not included in a global package.

Medicare defines the postoperative global periods of 0, 10, or 90 days, and most third-party insurance companies apply the same criteria. Procedures shown in the *Federal Register* may show one of the three-digit or three-alpha codes in the global period column. These codes are not used on the claim form.

TABLE 13.4 What Is and Is Not Included in a Global Package

Services Included in Global Package	Services Not Included in Global Package
Preoperative visits on the day before of day of a major procedure (090), and preoperative visits on the day of a minor procedure (010)	Initial evaluation, regardless of when it occurs, to decision for surgery (see modifier -57)
Intraoperative services that are a usual and necessary part of the surgical procedure	Postoperative visits unrelated to the diagnosis for which the surgical procedure was performed (see modifier -24)
Complications after surgery that do not require additional trips to the operating room (medical and surgical services)	Treatment necessary to stabilize seriously ill patients before surgery
Postoperative visits, including hospital visits, discharge, and office visits for appropriate postoperative periods (10 or 90 days)	Diagnostic tests and procedures
Writing orders	Related procedure for postoperative complications requiring a return trip to the operating room (see modifier -78)
Evaluating the patient in the recovery area	Immunosuppressive therapy after transplant surgery
Normal postoperative pain management	An additional, more extensive procedure if a less extensive procedure fails

TABLE 13.5 Global Package Status Indicators

000	No global package. Endoscopies and some minor procedures.
010	Minor procedures with expected normal follow-up in a 10-day period.
090	Major surgery with a 1-day preoperative period and a 90-day postoperative period included in the fee.
MMM	No global period. Uncomplicated maternity cases, which include prenatal care, delivery, and postnatal care.
XXX	No global period. Visits, procedures, and follow-up services may be billed separately.
YYY	The global period will be determined by the local Medicare fiscal agent because the code is for an unlisted procedure.
ZZZ	The code is part of another service and falls within that service's global period.

From Medicare and Medicaid Services: Global surgery, https://www.cms.gov/Outreach-and-Education/Medicare-Learning-Network-MLN/MLNProducts/downloads/GlobalSurgery-ICN907166.pdf.

They give information related to billing rules and regulations that indicate whether a global time period is part of a CPT code. This is particularly important when a patient comes in for a visit after surgery and helps in deciding whether the encounter can be billed or is included in the surgical fee. These codes are outlined in Table 13.5.

⚠ COMPLIANCE ALERT

HIPAA and Medicare Global Billing Guidelines

Understanding which services are included, what constitutes the global surgical period, and how to code related or unrelated services in the global surgical package for Medicare patients is critical in ensuring correct payment and meeting compliance guidelines.

Never Event

Effective January 15, 2009, Medicare no longer covers certain surgical never events, and some insurance companies have stopped payment to hospitals for never events. A never event is an occurrence related to a surgical procedure that involves the following:

- Performed on the wrong side, wrong site, wrong body part, or wrong person
- Retention of a foreign object in a patient after a procedure
- Patient death or disability associated with the use of contaminated drugs, devices, or biologics provided by the health care facility
- Patient death or serious disability associated with a medication error
- Stage 3 or 4 pressure ulcers acquired after admission to the health care facility
- Patient death or disability associated with a fall while being cared for at the health care facility

Such occurrences should never happen in a health care organization and are usually preventable. Medicare will not cover hospitalization and other services related to these noncovered procedures.

Supplies

When billing for office surgery and supplies used, checklists for the items used on the sterile tray (Fig. 13.7) should be used. These items can be charged only if the surgery required the use of additional items not normally used for this type of surgery. Medicare pays for trays with some procedure codes but not with others.

Integumentary System (10030–19499)

Procedure codes in the integumentary system involve skin, hair, nails, sebaceous glands, subcutaneous tissue, and breasts. There are codes for debridement, skin tags, and biopsies, as well as treatment of burns and pressure ulcers. The breast section includes various types of biopsies and lumpectomy and mastectomy procedures, as well as cosmetic procedures such as augmentation, lifts, and reductions.

MINOR OPERATING ROOM INSTRUMENT TRAY SUPPLY CHECKLIST

1 Adson Brown tissue forceps   _____
1 Adson tissue forceps with teeth   _____
1 long tissue forceps   _____
2 mosquito clamps   _____
1 Peck Joseph dissecting scissors   _____
1 Kahn dissecting scissors   _____
1 Reynolds dissecting scissors   _____
1 Stratte needle holder   _____
1 Webster needle holder   _____
4 small piercing towel clips   _____
2 double-skin hooks   _____
2 single-skin hooks   _____
1 knife handle   _____
1 #15 blade   _____
10 4 x 4s   _____
2 cotton-tipped applicators   _____
1 small basin   _____
3 sterile towels (drapes)   _____
1 Bovie pencil   _____
Sutures:_____ _____ _____
Dressings: 1/2-inch Steri-strips   _____

A

OFFICE SURGERY MEDICAL RECORD CHECKLIST

Patient information sheet   _____
H and P or progress note   _____
Consent form   _____
Diagnostic studies   _____
Pathology report(s)   _____
Anesthesia record   _____
Circulating nurse's note   _____
Doctor's orders   _____
Discharge note   _____
Operative report   _____
Signature/operative report   _____

B

Fig. 13.7 (A) Checklist to document supplies used when billing for office surgery. This list can be kept with the patient's health record. (B) Checklist for identifying complete and incomplete health records used for a patient receiving office surgery. As each item or document is completed, it is checked off so that the person reviewing the chart can see at a glance what needs to be finalized.

Multiple Lacerations

Surgical procedures of the integumentary system, such as repair of lacerations, are listed in the procedure code book as *simple, intermediate,* or *complex* repairs. Simple lacerations are superficial, requiring one-layer closure. Intermediate lacerations require layered closure of one or more of the deeper layers of the skin and tissues. Complex lacerations require more than layered closure and may require reconstructive surgery. Documentation should list the length in centimeters of all incisions and layers of involved tissues (subcutaneous, fascia, muscle, and grafts) so that correct procedure codes for excision of lesions and type of repair can be determined.

If multiple lacerations are repaired with the same technique and are in the same anatomic category, the insurance billing specialist should add up the total length of all lacerations and report one code to obtain maximum reimbursement. However, always read the notes and directives from the CPT manual when assigning these codes because these sites and sums can be confusing. Anatomic categories are the scalp, neck, axillae, external genitalia, trunk, extremities (hands or feet), face, ears, eyelids, nose, lips, and mucous membranes. If a patient has lacerations on both sides of the face, the lengths of all lacerations should be combined because the anatomic region is the same, and a claim should be submitted for the total length. No modifier is used and the right and left sides of the face are not billed separately (Example 13.16). Example 13.17 shows a more complicated coding situation.

EXAMPLE 13.16 Repair of Multiple Simple Lacerations

Three simple lacerations of the face totaling 8.2 cm

Incorrect Coding
12011	Repair 2.5-cm laceration of face
12013	Repair 2.7-cm laceration of face
12013	Repair 3-cm laceration of face

Correct Coding
| 12015 | Repair 8.2-cm laceration of face |

EXAMPLE 13.17 Repair of Multiple Lacerations

Simple repair of two lacerations of the face: one 5.2 cm, one 3.6 cm
Intermediate repair of one laceration of the arm totaling 6.2 cm
Complex repair of two lacerations of the left thigh: one 2.1 cm, one 5.1 cm

Incorrect Coding
12013	Simple repair 3.6 cm laceration of face
12014	Simple repair 5.2 cm laceration of face
12032	Intermediate repair 6.2 cm laceration of arm
13120	Complex repair 2.1 cm laceration of left thigh
13121	Complex repair 5.1 cm laceration of left thigh

Correct Coding
13121	Complex repair 7.2 cm laceration of left thigh
12032-59	Intermediate repair 6.2 cm laceration of arm
12015-59	Simple repair 8.8 cm laceration of face

Multiple Lesions

The descriptions for the surgical codes that relate to accessory structures (e.g., scalp, arms, and legs) and lesions found in the integumentary system (pertaining to the skin) can cause confusion. Code descriptions, including indentations, should be read completely with attention paid to terms such as *complex, complicated, extensive,* and *multiple.* Lesion excision code selection is based on the lesion's clinical diameter plus margin before excision and the character of the lesion—benign or malignant. Measurements should be taken and documented before excision because a specimen subject to pathologic examination may shrink. It is preferable not to use a pathology report because the diameter of the mass may be measured after shrinkage or fragmentation of the specimen. However, if the provider did not document the measurement, it may be necessary to refer to the pathology report. Example 13.18 is a guide to obtain appropriate reimbursement for the paring of seven corns.

EXAMPLE 13.18 Paring of Seven Corns

Incorrect Coding
11055	Paring; single lesion
11056-51	Two to four lesions
11057-51	More than four lesions
Or	
11055 × 7	Paring; single lesion (× seven corns)

Correct Coding
| 11057 | Paring; more than four lesions (seven corns) |

If possible, delay submission of the insurance claim for removal of a lesion or lesions until the pathology report is received. Usually a malignant lesion is reimbursed at a higher rate because of the more detailed nature of the procedure.

Repairs, Flaps, and Tissue Transfers

Wound repairs are divided into three types: simple, intermediate, and complex. Simple repairs require a single-layer closure and suture. Intermediate is a layered closure or a heavily contaminated single-layer closure with extensive cleaning and removal of debris. A complex repair includes extensive undermining. Wounds must be measured and reported in centimeters.

Many times, a wound repair may involve tissue transfers and rearrangements to restore appearance and maintain proper healing. Tissue transfers and flaps are coded by type, location, and size of the wound.

Flaps are another type of tissue rearrangement where the flap is formed in another area of the body and moved to the wound. They are often completed in stages.

Musculoskeletal System (20005–29999)

The Musculoskeletal System section is the longest section of the CPT book. Procedures in this section address joints, muscles, bones, ligaments, tendons, and cartilage. Codes are grouped by anatomic site with the exception of sections for casting/strapping and arthroscopies.

Fractures

One of the first distinctions that must be made in coding a fracture is whether it is open or closed treatment. Closed fracture treatment is one where no incision is made at the fracture site. Open treatment occurs when an incision is made and the bones are held together with some type of internal fixation. The type of fracture does not necessarily indicate the type of treatment. For example, a closed fracture of the elbow may require an open treatment if the elbow is shattered. The global fracture code typically includes the first cast and its later removal. It also includes standard setting and care of a closed fracture.

Arthroscopies

Arthroscopy is used to diagnose and treat joint pathologies. It is less invasive than an open surgical approach and heals faster. If a procedure begins as a diagnostic arthroscopy and turns into a surgical arthroscopy, the diagnostic portion of the procedure would be included in the surgical portion and not coded separately. If an arthroscopic procedure turns into an open procedure, it is appropriate to code both procedures and attach the appropriate modifier on the arthroscopic code.

Respiratory (30000–32999)

The respiratory anatomic sections begin with the nose and sinuses, continue through the larynx and trachea, and end in the lungs and pleura. Many types of endoscopy codes appear in this section.

Laryngoscopies and Bronchoscopies

Laryngoscopies can be either direct or indirect. It is important to determine this before choosing a code. An indirect laryngoscopy uses mirrors and lights to visualize the larynx by reflection, whereas a direct laryngoscopy examines the back of the throat and the vocal cords directly.

Bronchoscopies help a health care provider visualize the airway using an instrument called a bronchoscope. Similar to the endoscopic joint procedures, a diagnostic bronchoscopy that leads to a surgical bronchoscopy would be included in the surgical portion and not billed separately. However, if a diagnostic bronchoscopy prompts the surgeon to perform an open procedure, both may be billed.

Video-Assisted Thoracoscopic Surgery

Many procedures in the lungs may be performed with video-assisted thoracoscopic surgery (VATS). This is a minimally invasive method of treating lung diseases. Often, patients who have VATS are more likely to have less pain, quicker healing time, and shorter hospital stays than those having open procedures. VATS uses a small video camera introduced into the chest cavity. A surgical VATS code always includes the diagnostic VATS as well. If a diagnostic VATS prompts an open procedure, both may be billed, using the appropriate modifier.

Cardiovascular System (33010–37799)

Cardiovascular procedure codes encompass catheters, pacemakers, and bypass surgeries, among many others. Other procedures described in this section include, shunts, valve repairs, aneurysms, noncardiac bypass grafts, and angioplasty. Many codes in this section will require additional codes from the medicine or radiology sections as well.

Pacemakers and Cardioverter Defibrillators

A pacemaker is made up of a pulse generator (or battery) and one or more electrodes or leads. A cardioverter defibrillator is similar in that it also has a pulse generator and electrodes. However, a defibrillator uses a combination of pacing and shocks to treat ventricular tachycardia or fibrillation. There are many different procedures described in this section, so read the descriptors carefully. More than one code may be needed to fully describe the procedure. To choose the correct code, a coding specialist must know the following information:

- What type of system is it?
- Is it temporary or permanent?
- How many leads?
- Where will the electrodes be placed?
- What is being done (removal, replacement, or insertion)?

Coronary Artery Bypass Graft

A coronary artery bypass graft (CABG) is performed to redirect blood flow around a blockage in the artery or vein. Other veins and arteries in the patient's body are harvested for the grafts. Harvesting of most arteries and the saphenous vein are included in the CABG codes and not reported separately. Only endoscopic harvesting is reported separately. To accurately code a CABG, consider the following questions:

- How many grafts were performed?
- How many were from arteries? Which ones?
- How many were from veins? Which ones?
- Were the grafts harvested endoscopically or in an open procedure?
- Did the patient have a previous CABG?
- Is the whole system being worked on or just a component?

Vascular Injection Procedures

Vascular injection procedures are sometimes referred to as *interventional radiology*. Catheters are introduced through vessels for diagnostic and therapeutic purposes. Catheterization should be coded to the highest level accessed. Appendix L in the CPT book explains the vascular families and is helpful in choosing the appropriate code.

Hemic and Lymphatic Systems (38100–38999)

Codes in this section focus on bone marrow and stem cell procedures. Lymph node procedures are limited to biopsies, removal, and imaging procedures.

Digestive System (40490–49999)

Digestive system codes range from diagnostic and therapeutic procedures from the lips to the anus. It also includes the accessory organs used in digestion, the pancreas, liver, and gallbladder. Some procedures found here are gastric bypasses, appendectomies, and colon resections.

Colonoscopies and Upper Gastrointestinal Endoscopies

Endoscopic procedures of the colon and the upper gastrointestinal (GI) tract allow health care providers to visualize organs to diagnose and treat various conditions such as bleeding, infections, ulcers, and tumors. Similar to endoscopic procedures in the respiratory system, a diagnostic endoscopy that converts to a surgical endoscopy is not coded separately. More than one surgical endoscopy may be billed for the same date of service. For example, if more than one polyp is removed with more than one technique, each type of removal may be reported.

Hernias

A hernia is a protrusion of one body part into another. To choose the correct code in this section, a coding specialist must know the following:

- Site of the hernia
- Type of repair performed (laparoscopic or open)
- Age of the patient
- If the hernia is new or recurrent
- Clinical aspects of the hernia (incarcerated, strangulated, reducible)
- If mesh was used in the repair

Urinary System (50100–53899)

Codes in the Urinary System section address procedures in the kidneys, ureters, bladder, and urethra. They include incisions, excisions, endoscopies, removals, and repairs, as well as some procedures involving the prostate.

Male Genital System (54000–55899)

Procedures in the Male Genital System section include those done on the penis, testis, epididymis, scrotum, spermatic cord, and prostate. The codes describe excisions, repairs, penile implants, and prostatectomies, to name a few.

Female Reproductive System (56405–58999)

Codes in the Female Reproductive System section include not only repairs and treatments for the reproductive organs but also obstetric codes for prenatal care, delivery, and postnatal care. As with other sections, there are endoscopy procedures that aid in the diagnosis and treatment of various disease and disorders.

Endocrine System (60000–60699)

The majority of codes for the endocrine system describe excisions. In some cases, the excision is for a tumor or cyst, but many codes describe excising the endocrine gland itself.

Nervous System (61000–64999)

The nervous system codes include the skull and brain, spine and spinal cord, and nerves. When coding spinal surgery, it is important to note the approach, such as transpedicular or anterior, as well as the number of vertebral levels.

Nerve Injections

Nerve blocks are reported based on the nerve targeted. When coding nerve injections, consider the following questions:

1. What is being injected? Was it an anesthetic agent or a neurolytic agent?
2. Which nerve is being injected?
3. Is it single or multiple injections? Unilateral or bilateral?
4. What is the duration of the infusion? Was it a single injection or continuous infusion?
5. Was there imaging guidance?

Eye and Auditory Systems (65091–69979)

The Eye and Auditory Systems sections describe surgical procedures for repair and treatment of the various parts of the ocular and auditory systems. Eye examinations and services for glasses or contact lens are not in this section but may be found in the Medicine section. The same is true for hearing tests and hearing aid fittings.

 13.9 QUICK REVIEW
Question: What is a never event?

 13.10 QUICK REVIEW
Question: How are lesions measured?

 13.11 QUICK REVIEW
Question: What is the difference between a closed and open fracture treatment?

 13.12 QUICK REVIEW
Question: What information is needed to code a pacemaker?

 13.13 QUICK REVIEW
Question: What information is needed to code a hernia?

RADIOLOGY (70010–79999)

Radiology procedures can be done on any part of the body. They can be a separate procedure like a radiograph (x-ray examination) of the knee or part of another procedure such as guidance to place a nerve block. It is important to understand directional terms like those discussed in the documentation chapter, as well as the different types of radiologic procedures.

Diagnostic radiology includes radiographs, computed tomography (CT), and magnetic resonance imaging (MRI). An x-ray examination uses ionizing radiation to take a picture. It is particularly useful in imaging bones. CT produces cross-sectional pictures and are used to diagnose internal injuries and vascular disease. MRIs are useful in diagnosing cancers and various disorders of soft tissue. MRI may also be used to analyze blood vessels.

Diagnostic ultrasound uses sound waves to visualize internal structures. One of the most common uses is to visualize the fetus during pregnancy. This noninvasive test allows health care providers to measure and observe the fetus.

Breast mammography is a method of looking at breast tissue. It may be unilateral or bilateral. Screening mammography is considered to be part of preventive care and is covered by most health insurance without being applied to the deductible.

Other types of procedures found in the radiology section include bone and joint studies, radiation oncology, and nuclear medicine.

13.14 QUICK REVIEW
Question: What is the difference between an x-ray, a CT, and an MRI?

PATHOLOGY AND LABORATORY (80047–89398)

The Pathology and Laboratory section of CPT describe tests that can be performed on tissue, blood, urine, tumors and so on. It is important to understand the difference between the different types of tests.

Presumptive tests assume that there is a disease or infection. In these tests, a culture is grown to prove or disprove this. Qualitative tests determine only the presence of a virus, infection, or bacteria. Quantitative tests will determine not only the presence of a virus or bacteria but the exact amount of it present. Semiquantitative tests will determine the amount of bacteria or virus within a given range, but not the exact amount.

13.15 QUICK REVIEW
Question: What is the difference between the four types of lab tests—presumptive, qualitative, quantitative, and semi-quantitative?

MEDICINE (90281–99607)

The Medicine section contains codes describing a multitude of noninvasive or minimally invasive procedures. This section covers many areas including but not limited to the following:

- Immunizations and vaccines
- Psychiatry
- Biofeedback
- Dialysis
- Gastroenterology
- Ophthalmology
- Vestibular function and audiologic function tests
- Therapeutic cardiovascular procedures
- Allergy testing
- Noninvasive vascular diagnostic studies
- Pulmonary management and diagnostic tests
- Neurology and neuromuscular tests
- Genetic counseling
- Hydration and chemotherapy
- Physical and rehabilitative therapy
- Acupuncture, osteopathic, and chiropractic services

Drugs and Injections

Reporting of drugs and injections generally requires two codes. One code is reported for the administration of the drug. CPT codes for immunization administration for vaccines are 90460 through 90474, and for therapeutic or diagnostic injections are 96372 through 96379.

A second code is reported to identify the product being administered; either immune globulin codes 90281 through

90399, vaccine/toxoid codes 90476 through 90479, or Level II HCPCs national alphanumeric codes J0000 to J9999.

Documentation in the patient's health record must identify the name of the drug, amount of dosage, strength, and how it was administered. This information will be reported in Block 19 of the claim form. If the drug is experimental, attach a copy of the invoice to the claim form.

13.16 QUICK REVIEW
Question: How many codes are needed to report an injection?

CODE MODIFIERS

The use of a CPT code's two-digit add-on *modifier* permits the health care providers to indicate circumstances in which a procedure is performed differs in some way from that described by its usual five-digit code (Example 13.19).

> **EXAMPLE 13.19 How to Report a Modifier on a Claim Form**
>
> Add a two-digit modifier to the five-digit code number.
>
> **Single line item:**   **12345**-22 OR 1234522

It may be necessary when using a modifier to include an operative, pathology, x-ray, or special report to justify its use to a third-party payer. A modifier can indicate the following:

- A service or procedure has either a professional component or a technical component.
- A service or procedure was performed by more than one health care provider, in more than one location or in the case of anesthesia, a physician alone, or as a team with a CRNA.
- A service or procedure has been increased or reduced.
- A service or procedure was provided more than once.
- Only part of a service was performed.
- An adjunctive service was performed.
- A bilateral procedure was performed.
- Unusual events occurred.

Common *Current Procedural Terminology* Modifiers

Any modifier that fits the situation being coded may be used, except when the modifier definition restricts the use of specific codes; for example, modifier -51, Multiple Procedures, states that -51 is to be appended for "multiple procedures, other than Evaluation and Management Services…." Discussion of the most commonly used modifiers follows. A complete listing of CPT modifiers may be found in Appendix A of the CPT.

Modifier -22: Increased Procedural Services

Modifier -22 is used when the service provided is substantially greater than that typically required for the listed procedure. If modifier -22 is added, the documentation in the health record, such as operative reports and/or chart notes, must support the substantial additional work. The reasons for the use of this modifier are that the work encompasses increased intensity, time, technical difficulty of procedure, severity of the patient's condition, and physical and mental effort needed. This modifier may not be used with E/M services. Most third-party payers send an insurance claim to medical review before payment is made if modifier -22, indicating unusual services, appears on the claim. Because payments may be delayed, be cautious when using this modifier. An operative report should be submitted with the claim. If the third-party payer routinely denies the claim with modifier -22, an appeal for review should be made.

Modifier -25: Significant, Separately Identifiable Evaluation and Management Service

Modifier -25 is defined as "significant, separately identifiable evaluation and management service by the same provider on the same day of the procedure or other service." It is important to note that -25 should only be used when the patient's condition required the separate E/M service in addition to that typically included in the procedure code. This E/M service must require additional documentation for history, exam, and medical decision making above and beyond that which is typically required for the procedure. To better understand this modifier, a coding specialist should review the National Correct Coding Initiative Guidelines General Guidelines).

Modifier -26: Professional Component

Certain procedures are a combination of a professional component (PC) and a technical component (TC) and are considered a global service. Usually these involve radiology and pathology procedures. The PC is a portion of a test or procedure that the provider does, such as interpreting an ECG, reading an x-ray film, or making an observation and determination using a microscope. The TC refers to the use of the equipment, the supplies, and the operator who performs the test or procedure; such as ECG machine and technician, radiography machine and technician, and microscope and technician. The TC is billed by the entity that owns the equipment. Do not modify procedures that are either 100% technical or 100% professional or when the provider performs both the PC and the TC. Modifier -26 represents the PC only. Use of this modifier alerts the insurance company to expect a separate claim from another provider or facility for the TC.

In Example 13.20, the provider is performing only one of two services—he or she is interpreting the results of bilateral hip x-ray films.

EXAMPLE 13.20 Professional and Technical Components

73521-**26**	**Professional component** only for a radiograph of both hips. Use to bill provider's fee for interpretation of x-ray film.
73521-**TC**	**Technical component** only for a radiograph of both hips. Use to bill fee for facility that owns equipment and employs technician. Modifier -TC is at carrier's discretion.
73521	**Global service:** Radiologic examination, hips, bilateral. Minimum of two views of each hip. Use to bill complete fee when provider owns equipment, employs technician, and interprets x-ray film.

The facility where the patient had the x-ray film taken bills only for the TC by using 73521 with modifier -TC. If the provider owns the equipment and reads the x-ray film, there is no need to modify the x-ray code (73521) because both the PC and the TC were done in the office. Modifier -TC is assigned at the carrier's discretion.

Modifier -51: Multiple Procedures

Multiple procedures occur when more than one surgical service and/or related surgical service is performed on the same day or at the same surgical session by the same provider. In such cases, first report the primary service or procedure, which can be determined easily by the highest dollar value. Identify all additional services or procedures by appending codes with modifier -51 (Example 13.21).

EXAMPLE 13.21 Multiple Procedure Modifier -51

Excision of 2.0-cm benign lesion on the nose and at the same session a biopsy of the skin and subcutaneous tissue of the forearm.

Code	Description of Services
11442	Excision, other benign lesion including margins, face, ears, eyelids, nose, lips, mucous membrane; excised diameter 1.1–2.0 cm
11100-**51**	Biopsy of skin, subcutaneous tissue, or mucous membrane (including simple closure), unless otherwise listed; single lesion **(second; multiple procedure)**

The operative report should clearly state which procedures were done through separate incisions and which were done through the same incision. There are many circumstances when multiple procedures are performed. Modifier -51 may be used to identify the following:

- Multiple surgical procedures performed at the same session by the same provider
- Multiple related surgical procedures performed at the same session by the same provider
- Surgical procedures performed in combination at the same session, whether through the same or another incision or involving the same or different anatomy
- A combination of medical and surgical procedures performed at the same session by the same provider

The primary surgical procedure code must always be listed first on the claim form for full reimbursement and the secondary procedures must be listed in succession. Usually, payment by third-party payers for the primary code is 100% of the allowable charge, for the second code is 50%, for the third code is 25%, and for the fourth and remaining codes is 10%. However, under Medicare guidelines, Medicare pays 100% of the allowable charge for the primary code and 50% for two to five secondary procedures. Some computer systems can determine code order and automatically make the code adjustment.

Many carriers no longer require modifier -51 because they process claims electronically and the software program

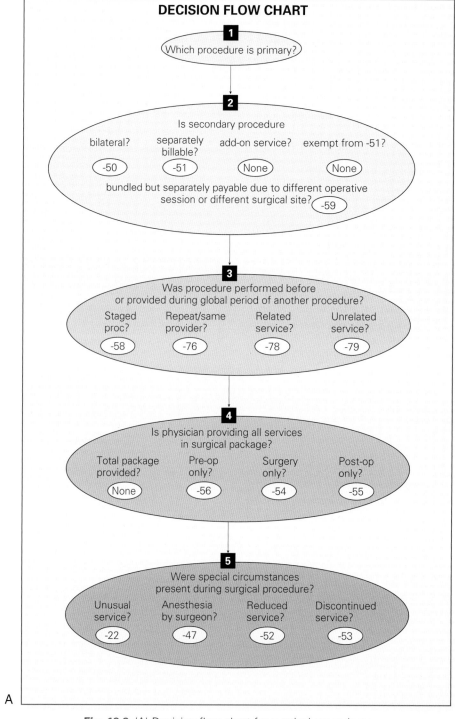

Fig. 13.8 (A) Decision flow chart for surgical procedures.

recognizes when multiple procedures are performed and automatically makes the reduction in payment. Contact insurance carriers and ask which method is preferred when reporting multiple surgical procedures. Then note this for each payer's policy to refer to for future billings. Always bill the full amount and let the third-party payer make the payment adjustments for percentage considerations. A decision flow chart is provided for reference to help simplify the modifier decision process (Fig. 13.8A and B).

Do not use the -51 modifier with add-on codes designated with a "+" (see Appendix D in CPT) or codes listed as exempt to modifier -51 (see Appendix E in CPT). Add-on codes are codes that cannot stand alone. When billing with add-on codes, first list another code referred to as the

MULTIPLE SURGICAL PROCEDURES

Multiple services must be related to:
- Same patient
- Same provider
- Same date of service

- List all procedures in order of reimbursement, highest to lowest.
- Most comprehensive service brings greatest reimbursement and is considered primary.
- Check all procedures to make sure there is no unbundling (i.e., using two codes when one code describes procedure).
- Decision making expands at this point. Follow numbered question to determine correct modifier usage.

2

-50 Bilateral procedure, not described by code
-51 Not bundled, separately billable
-59 Ordinarily bundled, separately payable due to special circumstance

3

- The term "primary procedure" can also refer to the first procedure initiating a global surgical period
-58 Current service was planned prospectively at time of first service
-76 Physician repeats procedure subsequent to original procedure
-78 Return to operating room for subsequent procedure, complication relating to original procedure
-79 Unrelated procedure performed during global period of previous surgery

4

- Surgical package means one fee covers the whole package, surgical procedure, and postoperative care.

5

-22 An extremely difficult procedure due to altered anatomy or unusual circumstances (add 10% to 30% reimbursement)
-47 When the surgeon administers regional or general anesthesia
-52 Procedure/service reduced or eliminated at the discretion of the physician
-53 Procedure is discontinued due to extenuating circumstances or because of threat to the patient

B

Fig. 13.8 (B) Guidelines and description of modifiers for multiple surgical procedures.

"parent code" to give a full description for service billed (Example 13.22).

EXAMPLE 13.22		**Add-On Code**
Parent code	11100	Biopsy of skin ... single lesion each separate/additional lesion (list separately in addition to code for primary procedure)
Add-on code	+11101	

Modifier -52: Reduced Services

Use of the modifier -52 indicates that under certain circumstances a service or procedure is partially reduced or eliminated at the provider's discretion. It is wise to provide an explanation of why the service was reduced. A cover letter or a copy of the operative report should not accompany these claims because usually they are not sent to medical review and attached documents may impede processing. Never use this modifier if the fee is reduced because of a patient's inability to pay. A good example

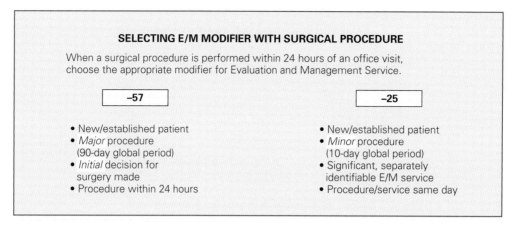

Fig. 13.9 Two selections, with criteria to evaluate them, when choosing the appropriate code or modifier for evaluation and management *(E/M)* services when a surgical procedure is performed within 24 hours of an office visit.

of when to use this modifier is a complete ophthalmological exam when the patient only has one eye.

Modifier -57: Decision for Surgery

The modifier -57 is used strictly to report an E/M service that resulted in the initial decision to perform a major surgical procedure within 24 hours of the office visit; see Example 13.23. A -57 modifier may be used for inpatient or outpatient consultations, inpatient hospital visits, and new or established patient visits that occur the day of or the day before surgery. Do not attach modifier -57 to a hospital visit code for the day before surgery or the day of surgery when a decision for a major surgical procedure was made a week before surgery. Think of -57 as telling the insurance company that the office visit is not part of the global fee.

EXAMPLE 13.23   Decision for Surgery

A new patient is seen in the office complaining of a great deal of pain. Cholangiography is done and reveals blocked bile ducts. The patient is scheduled for surgery the next day.

| 8-1-20XX | 99204-**57** | New patient office visit |
| 8-2-20XX | 47600 | Cholecystectomy |

Modifier -57 is often confused with modifier -25. Remember modifier -25 is used with minor procedures, whereas modifier -57 is used with major procedures. Consult Fig. 13.9 when making the decision about which modifier to use for a surgical procedure that is performed within 24 hours of an office visit.

Modifier -58: Staged or Related Procedure

The modifier -58 is used to indicate that the performance of a procedure or service during the postoperative period was as follows:

- Planned (staged) at the time of the original procedure
- More extensive than the original procedure
- For therapy after a surgical procedure

Such circumstances should be reported by adding modifier -58 to the staged or related procedure. The use of this

modifier requires accurate documentation of events leading up to the initial surgery and any subsequent surgery. It is only possible to modify procedures if the coding specialist has all of the relevant facts and circumstances. In Example 13.24 the fracture is considered surgery because it is in the surgery section of the CPT book. All fracture codes have 90-day postoperative periods.

EXAMPLE 13.24   Decision for Surgery

A new patient comes to the office after sustaining a fall while in-line skating. She is in distress, complaining of right wrist pain and swelling of the joint. The injury is evaluated **(1)** with an x-ray film. **(2)** It is determined that the patient has a Smith fracture and manipulation is performed. A long-arm cast is applied **(3)** using fiberglass (Hexcelite) material **(4)**.

(1)	99203-57	Initial office evaluation (detailed) with decision for surgery
(2)	73100-RT	Radiologic examination, right wrist, anteroposterior (AP) and lateral (lat) views
(3)	25605	Closed treatment of distal radial fracture (e.g., Colles or Smith type), with manipulation
(4)	99070	Supplies: Casting material (third-party payer) Medicine section code
		or
		Supplies: Hexcelite material (Medicare fiscal agent)
	A4590	HCPCS Level II code

The patient returns in 4 weeks for follow-up care **(1)**. The wrist is radiographed again **(2)**, the long-arm cast is removed **(3)**, and a short-arm cast is applied **(4)** using plaster material **(5)**.

(1)	No code	Follow-up care included in global fee
(2)	73100-RT	Radiologic examination, right wrist, AP and lateral views
(3)	No code	Cast removal included in original fracture care (25605)
(4)	29075-58	Application, plaster, elbow to finger (short arm) staged procedure
(5)	99070	Supplies: Casting material (third-party payer) Medicine section code
		or
		Supplies: Plaster material (Medicare fiscal agent)
	A4580	HCPCS Level II code

Modifiers -62, -66, -80, -81, and -82: More Than One Surgeon

If more than one surgeon is involved, the appropriate modifier will clarify who is billing the service:

- 62, Co-surgeon: Two surgeons work together as primary surgeons performing distinct parts of a procedure. Each provider reports their distinct operative work by adding this modifier.
- 66, Team surgery: A group of surgeons work together. Each participating provider adds this modifier to the basic procedure number for the service.
- 80, Assistant at surgery: Used when the surgery is not performed in a teaching hospital (Example 13.25).

EXAMPLE 13.25 Assistant at Surgery

Closure of Intestinal Cutaneous Fistula

Operating surgeon bills	44640	No modifier
Assistant surgeon bills	44640-**80**	**With modifier**

- 81, Minimum assistant surgeon.
- 82, Assistant surgeon: Used for surgeries performed in a teaching hospital when a qualified resident surgeon is not available to act as an assistant at surgery.

The assisting doctor is paid a reduced fee of 16% to 30% of the allowed fee the primary surgeon receives for performing the surgery on the basis of the patient's contract. The assisting provider uses the same surgical code as the primary surgeon and adds the -80 modifier to it. Some payers require the billed fee reflect the reduced percentage. Others prefer to have the full fee listed and make the reduction themselves. Under some insurance contracts, there may be some surgical procedures that restrict payment for an assistant surgeon.

Modifier -99: Multiple Modifiers

If a procedure requires more than one modifier code, use the two-digit modifier -99 after the usual five-digit CPT code number, all typed on one line; then list each modifier on a separate line (Example 13.26). Some insurance companies require -99 with a separate note in Block 19 of the CMS-1500 claim form or in the freeform area of electronic submissions, indicating which two or more modifiers are being used.

EXAMPLE 13.26 Multiple Modifiers

A provider sees a patient who is grossly obese. The operative report documents that a bilateral sliding-type inguinal herniorrhaphy was performed and the procedure took 2 h 15 min.

49525-**99**	Bilateral repair sliding inguinal hernia requiring 2 h 15 min
-50	
-22	

HCPCS Level II Modifiers

In addition to CPT modifiers, HCPCS Level II modifiers are used by Medicare and may be used by some commercial payers. HCPCS Level II modifiers may be two alpha digits (Example 13.27), two alphanumeric characters (Fig. 13.10), or a single alpha digit used for reporting ambulance services or results of positron emission tomography scans. A comprehensive list of HCPCs Level II modifiers can be found in an HCPCS national Level II code book.

EXAMPLE 13.27 HCPCS Modifiers

When taking x-ray films of both feet, the billing portion of the insurance claim appears as follows.

05/06/XX	73620 **RT**	Radiologic examination, foot—right
05/06/XX	73620 **LT**	Radiologic examination, foot—left

HCPCS LEVEL II ALPHANUMERIC MODIFIERS

26596-F3 Excision of Constricting Ring on Ring Finger of Left Hand

Fig. 13.10 Healthcare Common Procedural Coding System *(HCPCS)* Level II alpha modifiers (*LT* and *RT* used to identify left and right hands) and alphanumeric modifiers (*FA* through *F9*) used to identify digits (fingers) of left and right hands.

Use the two-digit HCPCS modifiers whenever they are necessary. HCPCS modifiers further describe the services provided and can increase or decrease the health care provider's fee. If not used properly, they can drastically affect the provider's fee profile by reducing future payments to the provider.

13.17 QUICK REVIEW
Question: What is the difference between modifier -25 and modifier -51?

13.18 QUICK REVIEW
Question: When should modifier -57 be used?

13.19 QUICK REVIEW
Question: When should modifier -58 be used?

CORRECT CODING EDITS AND PRACTICES

National Correct Coding Initiative Edits

In 1996, Medicare implemented a code editing system called the National Correct Coding Initiative (NCCI). Medicare's Correct Coding Initiative was implemented by the Centers for Medicare and Medicaid Services (CMS) in an attempt to eliminate unbundling or other inappropriate reporting of *Current Procedural Terminology* (CPT) codes. By using the editing system, coding conflicts are easily identified and claims are reviewed, suspended, or denied when conflicts occur. NCCI edits are updated quarterly. CMS has a free resource for the NCCI at https://www.cms.gov/Medicare/Coding/NationalCorrectCodInitEd.

Software is available to give providers, private insurance companies, and billing services access to the same government database used in auditing providers for improper use of CPT codes. It is currently available on the CMS website at no charge. This software system is sometimes referred to as *code editing* or *code screening*.

Some code pairs in the NCCI edits are followed by a 0 and others by a 1. If the superscript 0 appears with a code pair, it means that Medicare never allows a modifier to be used with the codes, so the code pair could never be reported together. The superscript 1 means that a modifier may be used under certain circumstances with appropriate documentation to have both codes reimbursed.

Because every health care organization has billing problems and questions unique to its specialty, coding and billing specialists must become detectives and discover how to obtain maximum reimbursements in the appropriate specialty. The best way is to telephone the third-party payer to inquire about new coding options and to note improvements in reimbursement. Coding requires expertise. It is an art, not an exact science. The following explanations of various ways of coding claims assist in obtaining maximum reimbursement for each service rendered and avoiding denials, lowered reimbursement, and possible audit.

Comprehensive and Component Edits

A comprehensive code is a single code that describes or covers two or more component codes that are bundled together as one

unit. A component code is a lesser procedure and is considered part of the major procedure. Each component code represents a portion of the service described in the comprehensive code and should be used only if a portion of the comprehensive service was performed (Example 13.28).

EXAMPLE 13.28 Comprehensive and Component Codes

Comprehensive code	93015	Cardiovascular stress test
Component codes	93016, 93017, 93018	
93015		Cardiovascular stress test using maximal or submaximal treadmill or bicycle exercise, continuous electrocardiographic monitoring, or pharmacologic stress; with physician supervision, with interpretation and report
93016		Physician supervision only, without interpretation and report
93017		Tracing only, without interpretation and report
93018		Interpretation and report only

Under the Medicare program, NCCI component code edits involve procedures that meet any of the following criteria:
1. Code combinations that are specified as "separate procedures" by CPT
2. Codes that are included as part of a more extensive procedure
3. Code combinations that are restricted by the guidelines outlined in CPT
4. Component codes that are used incorrectly with the comprehensive code

If any one of these restricted code combinations is billed, Medicare allows payment for only the procedure with the highest relative value (Example 13.29).

EXAMPLE 13.29 Separate Procedure

Inguinal hernia repair with lesion excised from spermatic cord
   Comprehensive code: 49505 Repair initial hernia age 5 years or older; reducible
   Component code: 55520 Excision of lesion of spermatic cord (separate procedure)

For example, when performing an inguinal hernia repair, the surgeon makes an incision in the groin and dissects tissue to expose the hernia sac, internal oblique muscle, and spermatic cord. If a lesion is excised from the spermatic cord, it is considered a component of the comprehensive hernia repair procedure and is not separately billable. Medicare will deny code 55520 (lesion excision) as a component of procedure code 49505 (hernia repair) when performed during the same operative session.

Mutually Exclusive Code Edits

Mutually exclusive code edits relate to procedures that meet any of the following criteria:
1. Code combinations that are restricted by the guidelines outlined in CPT
2. Procedures that represent two methods of performing the same service

3. Procedures that cannot reasonably be done during the same session
4. Procedures that represent medically impossible or improbable code combinations

In Example 13.30, if one were to submit codes 47605 and 47563, both these procedures are different methods of accomplishing the same result (removal of the gallbladder with cholangiography). They represent a duplication of effort and an overlap of services; therefore, Medicare would deny code 47563 (laparoscopy) as mutually exclusive to code 47605 (the excision).

EXAMPLE 13.30 Mutually Exclusive

47605	Excision, cholecystectomy; with cholangiography
47563	Laparoscopy, surgical; cholecystectomy with cholangiography

Note: These are different methods of accomplishing the same procedure.

Bundling

For insurance claim purposes, bundled codes means to group related codes together. To completely understand bundled codes, one must have a thorough knowledge of the service or procedure that is being provided or use an unbundling book as a reference guide.

Example 13.31 illustrates one type of bundling found in the CPT code book. Because code 19272 (excision of chest wall tumor with plastic reconstruction; with mediastinal lymphadenectomy) includes mediastinal lymphadenectomy, a separate code for mediastinal lymphadenectomy (38746) should not be billed in addition to it on the same date of service.

EXAMPLE 13.31 Bundled Code

Component code	19271	Excision of chest wall tumor involving ribs, with plastic reconstruction; without mediastinal lymphadenectomy
Comprehensive code	19272	with mediastinal lymphadenectomy

In the Medicare program, a number of services may be affected because CMS considers the services to be bundled. Because many commercial third-party payers may follow Medicare guidelines, an understanding of this bundling concept is necessary. When dealing with private insurance, an explanation of benefits (EOB) document may print out with the statement "Benefits have been combined," which means the same thing as bundling.

For example, when listing a sterile tray for an in-office surgical procedure, the tray is bundled with the procedure unless supplies are necessary in addition to those usually used. CPT code 99070 (supplies and materials) is not reimbursed by Medicare; however, HCPCS level II alphanumeric codes may be used in such cases. The cost of some services and supplies is bundled in E/M codes. For example, telephone services and reading of test results are not separately billable. However, Medicare pays for slings, splints, rib belts, cast supplies, Hexcelite and light casts, pneumatic ankle-control splints, and prosthetics, but a supplier number is necessary to bill for take-home surgical supplies and DME.

Some coding reference books also include a comprehensive list of codes that CMS considers bundled for the Medicare program. When appealing a claim, a great deal of time may be spent on paperwork only to discover that the code is bundled and denial is imminent. When in doubt about whether or not services are combined, contact the third-party payer and ask.

Unbundling

Unbundling is coding and billing numerous CPT codes to identify procedures that usually are described by a single code. It is also known as *exploding* or *a la carte* medicine.

Some health care organizations do this unwittingly, but it is considered fraud if it is done intentionally to gain increased reimbursement. Unbundling can lead to downward payment adjustments and possible audit of claims.

Types of unbundling are as follows:
- Fragmenting one service into component parts and coding each component part as if it were a separate service (Example 13.32)

EXAMPLE 13.32 Unbundled Code

Incorrect Coding

12011	Simple repair of superficial wounds of face, ears, eyelids, nose, lips and/or mucous membranes 2.5 cm or less.
12014	5.1–7.5 cm

Correct Coding

12015	7.6–12.5 cm

- Reporting separate codes for related services when one comprehensive code includes all related services (Example 13.33)

EXAMPLE 13.33 Unbundling (Comprehensive Code)

Unbundled Claim

58150	Total abdominal hysterectomy (corpus and cervix) with removal of tubes and with removal of ovary ($1200)
58700	Salpingectomy ($650)
58940	Oophorectomy ($685)
	Total Charge: $2535

Claim Coded Correctly

58150	Comprehensive code for all three services
	Total Charge: $1200

- Coding bilateral (both sides of the body) procedures as two codes when one code is proper (Example 13.34)

EXAMPLE 13.34 Unbundling (Bilateral)

Incorrect Coding

77065-RT	Right mammography
77065-LT	Left mammography

Correct Coding

77066	Mammography, bilateral

- Separating a surgical approach from a major surgical service that includes the same approach (Example 13.35)

EXAMPLE 13.35 Bundling (Surgical Approach)

Incorrect Coding
49000   Exploratory laparotomy
44150   Colectomy, total, abdominal

Correct Coding
44150   Colectomy, total, abdominal (correct because it includes exploration of the surgical field)

To avoid this problem, always use a current CPT code book. The use of outdated codes often inadvertently results in unbundling. A new technology or technique may have its own code when it is developed but may be bundled with another code as it becomes commonplace. If the health care organization uses a billing service, request in writing that the service's computer system include no unbundling programming.

⚠ COMPLIANCE ALERT
HIPAA and Procedural Coding Guideline

Always submit current *Current Procedural Terminology* (CPT) codes. If outdated codes are used, this could red flag a provider with Medicare as being in noncompliance.

Downcoding

Downcoding at the health care organization level typically occurs when there is not enough documentation to support the correct code or to code the diagnosis to the optimal level of specificity. It may also occur because a provider mistakenly hopes to avoid audits by staying within a lower payment range.

This also occurs at the payer level when the coding system used on a claim submitted to a third-party payer does not match the coding system used by the company receiving the claim. The computer system converts the code submitted to the closest code in use, which is usually down one level from the submitted code. Therefore, the payment that is generated is usually less.

In many states it is illegal for an insurance company to downcode a claim. Insurance commissioners have published bulletins warning payers to cease this claims adjudication practice. When a payer receives a claim, the payer is allowed to pay or deny the claim. If additional information is necessary to adjudicate the claim, it should be requested from the patient or provider. The payer is limited by the number of days it has to review the claim. At completion of the review, the payer must pay or deny the claim (Example 13.36).

EXAMPLE 13.36 Downcoding

Document states: Excision of bone tumor from anterior tibial shaft.
Pathology report states: Tibia bone tumor; benign

Incorrect Coding
11400   Excision of benign lesion including margins except skin tag, trunk, arms or legs; excised diameter 0.5 cm or less

Correct Coding
27635   Excision of bone tumor of tibia, benign

⚠ COMPLIANCE ALERT
HIPAA Documentation Guideline

Make sure that the documentation from the provider supports the code that is being submitted to prevent downcoding.

Upcoding

The term *upcoding* is used to describe deliberate manipulation of CPT codes for increased payment. This practice can be spotted by Medicare fiscal agents and third-party payers using prepayment and postpayment screens or "stop alerts," which are built into most computer coding software programs. An example of intentional upcoding might be a provider who selects one level of service code for all visits with the theory that the costs even out, such as always using code 99213. This opens the door to audits and in the end may cost the health care organization money. Upcoding may occur unintentionally if the coding specialist is ill informed or does not keep current.

Code Monitoring

Monitoring of CPT codes is done to maximize reimbursement from all third-party payers. First, determine which codes are used most often in the health care organization. Many computer programs can generate a list of codes, ranking them according to frequency of use. If the health care organization does not have a computer, take a sampling of the charge slips to determine the prevalent codes. Once the high-volume codes are known, focus on coding strategies for the best possible reimbursement.

Monitor every remittance advice (RA) and EOB that comes in directly or via patients. Every private insurance, Medicare, Medicaid, and TRICARE payment received should be checked for accuracy to see whether it is consistently the same or if coding changes have occurred. Incorrect payments should be investigated and appealed. Examine all payments made for codes that do not match those submitted. Be sure to appeal every payment that is less than half of what the health care provider bills.

13.20   QUICK REVIEW
Question: What types of codes fall under the NCCI?

13.21   QUICK REVIEW
Question: What are four ways to unbundle a procedure?

13.22   QUICK REVIEW
Question: What is upcoding and downcoding?

METHODS OF PAYMENT

Most methods of payments are based on individual procedure codes. Private insurance companies, as well as federal and state programs, adopt different methods for establishing payment rates for outpatient services: (1) fee schedules; (2) usual, customary, and reasonable; and (3) relative value scales. Additional reimbursement methods for hospital claims are discussed in Chapters 18 and 19.

Fee Schedule

A fee schedule is simply a listing of accepted charges or established allowances for specific medical procedures. A health care organization can have more than one fee schedule unless specific state laws restrict this practice. Charges should be related consistently to the cost of the services and uniformly applied to all patients whether inpatient or outpatient. The following situations can occur:

1. Health care organizations *participating* in the Medicare program typically would be paid by the fee schedule set annually by Medicare. Health care organizations *not participating* in the Medicare program would be paid a limited charge set forth by Medicare and based on the fee schedule set annually be Medicare.
2. Health care providers who treat Medicaid patients cannot bill the patient for any balance after the Medicaid payment is received. Those balances must be adjusted off.
3. Health care organizations *participating* with TRICARE would be paid by TRICARE at the TRICARE rate.
4. Health care organizations *not participating* with TRICARE are able to charge 115% of the TRICARE allowed charge. The patient may be billed for the difference between the 115% and the amount TRICARE paid.
5. Health care organizations having a contractual arrangement with an insurance carrier would be paid on the basis of the negotiated contract.
6. Health care organizations rendering services to those who have sustained industrial injuries would be paid based on that state's workers' compensation fee schedule.

Section 1128(b) of the Social Security Act states that a provider may risk exclusion or suspension from the Medicare program if their Medicare charges are in excess of its usual charges. To prevent a possible violation of Section 1128(b) of the Social Security Act, the provider should assign one fee for each procedure code when establishing a fee schedule. This fee should be billed to all third-party payers and to self-pay patients. By establishing one fee for each procedure instead of multiple fees for each procedure, the provider helps establish the usual and customary fee for their geographic area. It is equally important to monitor third-party payer adjustments to determine how much revenue is lost because of poor contracts and to monitor employee theft.

The fees should be above the maximums paid by the third-party payers to whom the health care organization generally bills. A health care organization may wish to evaluate the fee schedules annually to decide whether fees should be raised for certain procedures or services.

Because mistakes can be costly in terms of lost revenue and possible violations, one fee schedule for all patients, with provisions for financial hardship cases, is usually the safest course for health care providers.

Usual, Customary, and Reasonable

Usual, customary, and reasonable (UCR) is a complex system in which three fees are considered in calculating payment. This is an older payment methodology that was introduced in the Social Security Act of 1965. Although most carriers have stopped using it, it is still a concept that billing specialists should be familiar with. UCR is used mostly in reference to fee-for-service reimbursement. The usual fee is the fee that a health care provider usually charges for a given service to a private patient. A customary fee is one that is charged by providers of similar training and experience in a geographic area. A reasonable fee is the fee that is, in the opinion of the medical review committee, justifiable considering the special circumstances of the case. Fig. 13.11 illustrates how a surgeon's payment is determined under this method.

PARTICIPATING SURGEON UCR CALCULATION

Four Example Cases

Surgeon's bill	Usual fee	compared to	Customary fee		Payment
1) $400	$350	→	$350 →	declared reasonable (extenuating circumstances)	$400
2) $400	$350	→	$350 →	declared customary (no unusual circumstances)	$350
3) $375	$350	→	$400 →	declared customary (does not exceed customary level)	$375
4) $350	$350	→	$400 →	declared customary (falls within customary range)	$350

Usual Fee—usual submitted fee for a given service to patient.

Customary Fee—in the range of usual fees charged by providers of similar training and experience in a geographical area (i.e., the history of charges for a given service).

Reasonable Fee—meets the aforementioned criteria or is, in the opinion of the medical review committee, justifiable considering the special circumstances of the case.

Payment—based on the lower of usual and customary fees.

Fig. 13.11 Usual, customary, and reasonable *(UCR)* calculation for four participating surgeons' cases.

Reimbursement is based on the lower of the usual or customary fee and determines the approved or allowed amount. In a UCR system, payment can be extremely low for a rarely performed but highly complex procedure because there may be no history of billed charges from other health care providers on which to base payment. Some private health insurance plans use this method and pay a provider's full charge if it does not exceed UCR charges.

Depending on the policies of each insurance company, the UCR system is periodically updated. UCR is a method chosen by third-party payers and not the provider. If the health care provider has a UCR that is significantly lower than those of other health care organizations in their area, document this and ask the third-party payer for a review and possible adjustment. Most plans have discontinued the UCR system and are adopting the Medicare resource-based relative value scale method for provider reimbursement.

Relative Value Studies

In 1956, the California Medical Association Committee on Fees published the first edition of the *California Relative Value Studies* (CRVS). RVS, referred to as either relative value studies or scale, is a coded listing of procedure codes with unit values that indicate the relative value of the various services performed, taking into account the time, skill, and overhead cost necessary for each service (Example 13.37).

EXAMPLE 13.37 Relative Value Scale

Procedure Code	Description	Units
10060	Incision & drainage of cyst	0.8

Using a hypothetical conversion factor of $153/unit, this procedure is valued at $122.40.

Math: $153.00 × 0.8 = $122.40

Units in RVS are based on the median charges of all providers during the period in which the RVS was published. A conversion factor is used to translate the abstract units in the scale to dollar fees for each service.

The RVS is a sophisticated system for coding and billing of professional services. After the successful use of the California RVS, many state and medical specialty associations adopted the CRVS method. In 1975, the Federal Trade Commission (FTC) challenged the legality of using the RVS as a fee schedule, stating that it could be interpreted as a form of price fixing in violation of antitrust laws. Since that time, many medical societies and medical specialty associations issued new publications that omitted unit values for the procedures listed but retained the procedure code portion of RVS.

Some states passed legislation mandating the use of RVS codes for procedures and the unit values as the schedule of fees for workers' compensation claims. In these states the conversion factor to be used in applying the units is also stated in the law. The third-party payer pays a specific dollar amount for each unit listed for each procedure in the RVS code book.

An insurer or other third party could devise an RVS on the basis of its own data. This type of RVS would not be created by providers in an effort to regulate fees and therefore would be acceptable on the basis of FTC guidelines. An example is *Optum's Relative Values for Physicians (RVP)*, which is based on survey data from Relative Value Studies, Inc. Additionally, a national RVS developed under a government contract may be acceptable and would not be in violation of antitrust laws.

Resource-Based Relative Value Scale

The resource-based relative value scale (RBRVS) is an RVS developed for CMS by William Hsiao and associates at the Harvard School of Public Health. CMS used it to devise the Medicare fee schedule that was phased in from 1992 through 1996. This approach to fees was developed to redistribute Medicare dollars more equitably among providers and to control escalating fees that were out of control using the UCR system. This became the basis for providers' payments nationwide.

This system consists of a fee schedule based on relative value units (RVUs) (Box 13.2). The formula for obtaining RVUs is somewhat complex and involves a bit of mathematics in computing three components: an RVU for the service, a geographic adjustment factor (GAF), and a monetary conversion factor (CF).

Box 13.2 RVU Formula. RVUs are based on the physician work RVU, the practice expense RVU, and the malpractice insurance RVU. To bring the fees in line for the region where the physician practices and to adjust for regional overhead and malpractice costs, each of the RVUs is adjusted for each Medicare local fiscal agent by geographic pricing cost indices (GPCIs). A geographic pricing cost index is an adjustment added to reimbursement rates to take into consideration differences in cost of living and running a practice in various geographic areas. There are different GPCIs for cost of living, malpractice, and practice expenses.

A CF is used to convert a geographically adjusted relative value into a payment amount. This CF is updated to a new amount each year. Fig. 13.12 provides an example of calculating payment for one procedure code.

BOX 13.2 RVU Formula

Relative Value Unit (RVU) Formula

(RVU physician work × GCPI physician work)
+ (RVU practice expense × GPCI practice expense)
+ (RVU malpractice cost × GCPI malpractice cost)

RVU TOTAL

RVU TOTAL × CF = Medicare $ for service

HCPCS/CPT CODE	WORK RVUs	PRACTICE EXPENSE RVUs	MALPRACTICE RVUs	
44360 RVUs	2.49	1.38	0.27	
GPCI*	× 1.000	× 0.952	× 0.673	= Total adjusted
	2.49	1.31	0.170	RVUs, 3.97

For 2020, the conversion factor for nonsurgical care is
$36.0896 × 3.97 = Allowed amount $143.28

*The geographical practice cost indices (GPCI) for the medical practice whose location in the example is Syracuse, New York.

Fig. 13.12 Formula used to calculate the fee for a specific procedure using the resource-based relative value scale system. *RVU,* Relative value unit.

The figures to work out this formula in the chart for each service are published annually in the *Federal Register*.

RVUs help when determining cost accounting because they take into account the practice expense, malpractice expense, work effort, and cost of living. They are also helpful when negotiating the best contract available with managed care plans. A crosswalk is an effective way to see how the practice may be affected by an RBRVS contract (Table 13.6).

Many health care providers and organizations use RBRVS to establish their own fee schedule. Health care fees can be adjusted if they are too high or too low. It is legal to use an RVS guide for setting, realigning, or evaluating fees as long as the provider does not enter into any price-fixing agreements.

Medicare Fee Schedule

Medicare fee schedules are based on RBRVS and are published every year, listing three columns of figures: participating amount, nonparticipating amount, and limiting charge for each procedure code number (Table 13.7). Currently, fee schedules may be accessed online at each local MAC's website.

13.23 QUICK REVIEW
Question: What is UCR?

13.24 QUICK REVIEW
Question: What is the RBRVS formula?

DISCUSSION POINT
Discuss various ways in which coding errors can increase or decrease payment. Why is it important for an insurance billing specialist to become proficient in CPT coding?

TABLE 13.6 Resource-Based Relative Value Scale Crosswalk

A	B	C	D	E	F	G	H
Code	Code Description	RBRVS/RVU	Conversion Factor	FEE	Contract Conversion Factor	Contract FEE	% Contract Payment
99212	Office Visit	0.68	72.06	$49	64.71	$44.00	90%

RBRVS, Resource-based relative value scale; *RVU*, relative value unit.

TABLE 13.7 Mock Medicare Fee Schedule

CPT	Description	Participating	Nonparticipating	Limiting Charge	Global Package
99202	New OV, expanded problem focused	47.52	45.14	51.91	
99203	New OV, detailed	64.92	61.67	70.92	
99204	New OV, comprehensive, level 4	97.13	92.27	106.11	
99205	New OV, comprehensive, level 5	121.08	115.03	132.28	
99211	Nurse visit	14.70	13.97	16.07	
99212	Est OV, problem focused	26.14	24.83	28.55	
99213	Est OV, expanded prob focused	36.80	34.96	40.20	
99214	Est OV, detailed	56.31	53.79	61.51	
99215	Est OV, comprehensive	88.76	84.32	96.97	
11720	Debridement of nails, 1–5	29.82	28.33	32.58	0
11721	Debridement of nails, 6 or more	29.82	28.33	32.58	0
11750	Exc nail or nail matrix	177.07	168.22	193.45	10
11765	Wedge exc of nail fold	53.04	50.39	57.95	10
19100	Bx breast, needle	88.03	83.63	96.17	0
19101	Bx breast, incisional	257.67	244.79	281.51	10
21330	Nasal fracture, open, complicated	548.71	521.27	599.46	90
27455	Osteotomy, proximal tibia	1142.36	1085.24	1248.03	90
45380	Colonoscopy with biopsy	349.98	332.48	382.35	0

Bx, Biopsy; *CPT*, Current Procedural Terminology; *est*, established; *exc*, excision; *OV*, office visit.

PROCEDURE 13.1   Choose Correct Procedural Codes for Professional Services

Objective
Accurately locate and select procedural codes for professional services

Equipment/Supplies
Current Procedural Terminology (CPT) code book and medical dictionary

Directions
Follow these step-by-step procedures, which include rationales, to practice this job skill. Fig. 13.13 will explain how to search and choose correct CPT codes for a procedure, eponym, and acronym.
1. Read the patient's health record and identify the main term by asking what is wrong with the patient.
2. Always read the Introduction section at the beginning of the code book, which may change annually with each edition.
3. Use the Index at the back of the book to locate a specific item by generalized code numbers, not by page numbers. Never code from the Index. Listings may be looked up according to names of procedures or services, organs, conditions, synonyms, eponyms, and abbreviations; for example, some primary entries might be as follows:
   • Procedure or service (e.g., anastomosis, endoscopy, splint)
   • Organ or other anatomic site (e.g., salivary gland, tibia, colon)
   • Condition (e.g., abscess, entropion, tetralogy of Fallot)
   • Synonyms, eponyms, and abbreviations (e.g., electroencephalogram [EEG], Bricker operation, Clagett procedure)If the procedure performed is not listed, check for the organ involved. If the procedure or organ is difficult to find, look up the condition. Keywords, such as synonyms or eponyms, and abbreviations, will help to find the appropriate code.
4. Locate the code number in the code section for the code range given in the Index.
5. Turn to the beginning of the section for the code range given in the Index and read the Guidelines at the beginning of the section. This gives general information and instructions on coding certain procedures within the section, defines commonly used terms, explains classifications within the section, and gives instructions specific to the section.
6. Turn to the correct section, subsection, category, or subcategory and read through the narrative description to locate the most appropriate code to apply to the patient's procedure. Some code books have color-coded titles, making this determination easier. In the surgery section, each subsection is further divided into categories based on anatomic site. Within each category are subcategories listed by type of procedure (e.g., excision, repair, destruction, graft) or condition (burn, fracture). Read the notes and special subsection information throughout the section.

7. Notice punctuation and indenting. Descriptions for standalone codes begin at the left margin and have a full description. No matter how many indented codes are listed, always go back to the standalone code to begin reading the description. A semicolon (;) separates common portions from subordinate designations; subterms are indented (Fig. 13.14A). Any terminology after the semicolon has a dependent status, as do the subsequent indented entries. Fig. 13.14 B shows the placement of the CPT code and any modifiers on the CMS-1500. This patient who has had seven skin tags removed.
8. When trying to locate an evaluation and management (E/M) code, identify the place or type of service rendered. Then identify whether the patient is new or established and locate the category or subcategory. Review any guidelines or instructions pertaining to the category or subcategory. Read the descriptors of the levels of E/M service. Identify the requirements necessary for code assignment. Ensure that the components necessary were performed by the provider and documented in the chart for the assigned E/M code. Commercial templates are available to aid in E/M code selection and help tremendously when verifying a code that has been selected by the provider.
9. For a code that has been assigned, note the following:
   • Parentheses, ( ), further define the code and tell where other services are located (Fig. 13.15).
   • Measurements throughout the code book are based on the metric system (Fig. 13.16).
   • All anesthesia services are reported by use of the five-digit anesthesia code plus a physical status modifier. Physical status modifiers describe the overall health of the patient by referencing patients who are healthy or those who have mild or severe systemic diseases. Example: Patient is a healthy 23-year-old Caucasian woman. Anesthesia is given for a vaginal delivery. The procedure code with modifier is 01960-P1. The P-1 identifies the patients as "a normal healthy patient."
   • The Surgery section is the largest segment of the code book. It has many subsections and subheadings. Learn to break down a procedure and identify various terms that will aid in choosing the correct code. Blocks 24A through 24J of the revised CMS-1500 insurance claim form show placement of the code on Line 2 (see Example 13.38).
10. Determine whether one or more modifiers are necessary to give a more accurate description of the services rendered or the circumstances in which they were performed.
11. Enter the five-digit code number and modifier to the proper field on the insurance claim form exactly as given for each procedure or service rendered. Be careful not to transpose code numbers.

PROCEDURE 13.2   Locate Correct Level II HCPCS Codes for Professional Services

Objective
Accurately locate and select Level II Healthcare Common Procedural Coding System (HCPCS) codes for professional services

Equipment/Supplies
HCPCS code book and medical dictionary

Directions
Follow these step-by-step procedures, which include rationales, to practice this job skill.
1. Read the patient's health record for items or services that might be covered under Level II HCPCS codes.

2. Go to the Index that is arranged alphabetically and locate the name of the supply, drug, or service. This will point to the proper code. Never code from the Index.
3. Turn to the code number in the section and verify that it is the proper code for the item or service the provider supplied to the patient.
4. Select the code.
5. Determine whether a modifier is necessary to give a more accurate description of the service or item.
6. Enter the code number and modifier (if needed) to the proper field on the insurance claim form exactly as given for each service or item. Be careful not to transpose code numbers.

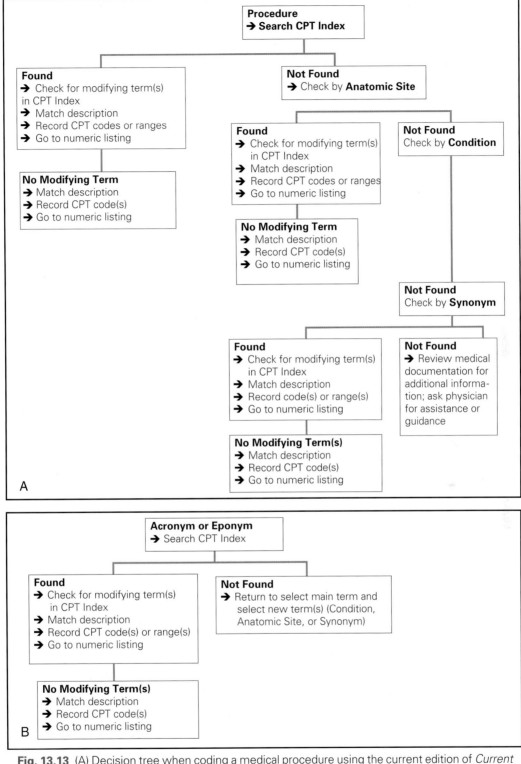

Fig. 13.13 (A) Decision tree when coding a medical procedure using the current edition of *Current Procedural Terminology (CPT)* published by the American Medical Association (AMA). (B) Decision tree when coding a medical procedure using an acronym or eponym and using the current edition of CPT published by the AMA.

Paring or Cutting

11055   Paring or cutting of benign hyperkeratotic lesion (e.g., corn or callus); single lesion

11056   two to four lesions

11057   more than four lesions

A

24. A. DATE(S) OF SERVICE From / To MM DD YY MM DD YY	B. PLACE OF SERVICE	C. EMG	D. PROCEDURES, SERVICES, OR SUPPLIES (Explain Unusual Circumstances) CPT/HCPCS | MODIFIER	E. DIAGNOSIS POINTER	F. $ CHARGES	G. DAYS OR UNITS	H. EPSDT Family Plan	I. ID. QUAL.	J. RENDERING PROVIDER ID. #
05 11 20XX	11		99203	A	120 00	1		NPI	4627889700
05 11 20XX	11		11200	A	100 00	1		NPI	4627889700
								NPI	
								NPI	
								NPI	
								NPI	

B

Fig. 13.14 (A) Procedure codes from the Surgery section of the *Current Procedural Terminology (CPT)* code book. (B) Blocks 24A through 24J of the revised CMS-1500 (02-12) insurance claim form showing placement of the code on Line 2.

Use of parentheses

Further defining →

15780   Dermabrasion; total face (eg. for acne scarring fine wrinkling, rhytids, general keratosis)

15781   segmental, face

15782   regional, other than face

15783   superficial, any site (eg. tattoo removal)

or

Location of other services→

67810   Incisional biopsy of eyelid skin including lid margin (For biopsy of skin of the eyelid, see 11102, 11103, 11104, 11105, 11106, 11107)

Fig. 13.15 Use of parentheses in the Surgery section of the *Current Procedural Terminology* code book.

13151   Repair, complex, eyelids, nose, ears, and/or lips; 1.1 cm to 2.5 cm

13152   2.6 cm to 7.5 cm

+13153   each additional 5 cm or less

Fig. 13.16 Metric measurements in the Surgery section of the *Current Procedural Terminology* code book.

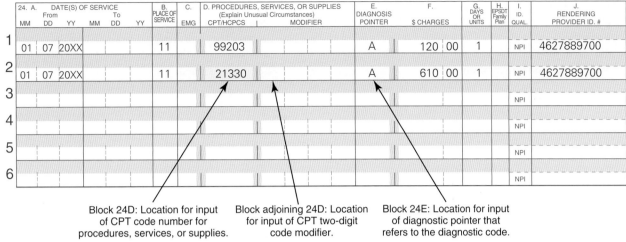

Block 24D: Location for input of CPT code number for procedures, services, or supplies.

Block adjoining 24D: Location for input of CPT two-digit code modifier.

Block 24E: Location for input of diagnostic pointer that refers to the diagnostic code.

Fig. 13.17 The billing portion of a completed claim form for closed reduction of a nasal fracture.

EXAMPLE 13.38   Blocks 24A Through 24J of the CMS-1500 Claim Form

Open Treatment of Nasal Fracture, Complicated

Section:	Surgery, Musculoskeletal System
Anatomic subheading:	Head
Condition:	Fracture or Dislocation
Code:	21330

Thus, when completing an insurance claim form for open treatment of nasal fracture, complicated, the billing portion appears as follows (Fig. 13.17).

KEY POINTS

This is a brief chapter review of the key issues presented. To further enhance your knowledge of the technical subject matter, review the key terms and key abbreviations for this chapter by locating the meaning for each in the Glossary at the end of this text, which appears in a section before the Index.

1. *Current Procedural Terminology* (CPT) codes are a standardized five-digit numeric method used to precisely describe each service and procedure performed by providers and allied healthcare professionals.

2. The Healthcare Common Procedure Coding System (HCPCS) has two levels: Level I, the American Medical Association's CPT codes and modifiers, and Level II, Centers for Medicare and Medicaid Services (CMS)–designated codes and alpha modifiers. HCPCS national codes are used to bill for ambulance, medical and surgical supplies, durable medical equipment, drugs administered other than via the oral method, and so on.

3. Each year when a new CPT code book is published, become familiar with code deletions, new codes, and description changes and observe the symbols and their interpretation in relation to the codes.

4. In CPT coding, *surgical package* is a term used to describe a surgical procedure code that includes the operation; local infiltration, digital block, or topical anesthesia; and normal, uncomplicated postoperative care all included in one fee. Code edits are performed on submitted insurance claims

to detect unbundling, splitting of codes, and other types of improper code submissions.

5. Ensure that the documentation from the provider supports the code submitted to prevent downcoding by the third-party payer.

6. Use two-digit add-on CPT modifiers to indicate circumstances in which a procedure performed differs in some way from that described by its usual five-digit code.

7. A fee schedule is a listing in an insurance policy of procedure code numbers with charges or preestablished allowances for specific medical services and procedures. The Medicare fee schedule is published annually and shows the maximum dollar amounts that Medicare will allow for each service rendered for a beneficiary.

8. The various methods of payment by insurance companies and state and federal programs are (1) fee schedules; (2) usual, customary, and reasonable (UCR); and (3) relative value studies or scale (RVS).

9. In final summary, the seven steps to accurate coding are as follows:
   a. Read the patient's encounter form completely and any notes made by the health care provider.
   b. Highlight words important to the selection of diagnostic and procedural codes.
   c. Ask the provider to clarify any inconsistent or missing information and code only from actual documentation. Do not assume or guess.

d. Code each confirmed diagnosis and accompanying signs or symptoms using the highest level of specificity.

e. Code each medical service, procedure, and treatment provided in the documentation.

f. Verify medical necessity by associating each procedure code to the diagnostic code.

g. Recheck the codes selected by rereading the code descriptions and match them with the provider's notes to confirm the codes assigned.

INTERNET RESOURCES

- National Correct Coding Initiative: https://www.cms.gov/Medicare/Coding/NationalCorrectCodInitEd/index.html?redirect=/nationalcorrectcodinited/

- Medicare RVU file: https://www.cms.gov/Medicare/Medicare-Fee-for-Service-Payment/PhysicianFeeSched/PFS-Relative-Value-Files

STUDENT ASSIGNMENT

- Study Chapter 13.
- Complete all assignments in the *Workbook* to reinforce the theory learned in this chapter.

- Turn to the Glossary at the end of this text for a further understanding of the key terms and key abbreviations used in this chapter.

Claims Submission in the Medical Office

14

The Paper Claim CMS-1500

Linda M. Smith

OBJECTIVES

After reading this chapter, you should be able to:

1. Identify the circumstances in which paper claims continue to be used.
2. Explain the role of the National Uniform Claim Committee (NUCC).
3. Discuss the history of the Health Insurance Claim Form (CMS-1500).
4. Define and discuss the two types of claims submissions.
5. Explain the difference between clean, pending, rejected, incomplete, and invalid claims, and discuss specific terms used to describe Medicare claims.
6. List the elements typically abstracted from the health record that are included in a cover letter accompanying an insurance claim.
7. Describe basic guidelines for submitting insurance claims.
8. Explain how the diagnostic fields of the CMS-1500 claim form would be completed.
9. Explain National Provider Identifier (NPI) numbers.
10. Discuss claim signatures, as well as the importance of proofreading every paper claim and supporting documentation for claims.
11. List common reasons why claims are rejected.
12. Identify claim submission errors and discuss the solutions to correct those errors.
13. Demonstrate the ability to complete the CMS-1500 claim form accurately for federal, state, and private payer insurance contracts using current basic guidelines.

KEY TERMS

Administrative Simplification Compliance Act
clean claim
deleted claim
dirty claim
durable medical equipment number
electronic claim
employer identification number
facility provider number

group National Provider Identifier
Health Insurance Claim Form
incomplete claim
intelligent character recognition
invalid claim
National Provider Identifier
National Uniform Claim Committee
optical character recognition
paper claim

pending claim
physically clean claim
purchased service provider
rejected claim
Social Security number
state license number
suspended claim
taxonomy code

KEY ABBREVIATIONS

ASCA	EIN	LMP	NUCC
CMS-1500	EMG	MSP	OCR
DME	EPSDT	NA, N/A	SOF
DNA	ICR	NPI	SSN

Deb H.: Credentials: LPN, CPC, CPC-I, CPC-H, CMRS, CMBS

I started in health care over 40 years ago as a licensed practical nurse (LPN). Eventually, I moved over to medical billing and coding. I have obtained various coding credentials and continue to work as a certified biller, a certified coder, and a coding instructor. I remind my students that one of the challenges of medical billing is that, although we strive for consistency in guidelines, every insurance will want something different. It is important to follow the National Uniform Claim Committee (NUCC) claim form instructions, which are published on the NUCC website. This should be used as a basis for paper claim form completion and modified as required by individual payers.

THE PAPER CLAIM CMS-1500

This chapter will focus on the submission of paper claims for *professional* services. Further instructions on paper claims submissions for *facility* services will be covered in Chapter 19.

The Health Insurance Claim Form (CMS-1500) is the standard paper claim form used by health care professionals and suppliers to bill insurance carriers for services provided to patients. The claim form has gone through many transitions throughout the years. The most recent version of the CMS-1500 claim form (02-12) was made mandatory as of April 1, 2014 (Fig. 14.1).

Fig. 14.1 CMS-1500 standard paper claim form. This is the most recent version of the CMS-1500 claim form (02-12).

Paper claims were once used as our sole method of reporting health insurance claims, but as a result of the Administrative Simplification Compliance Act (ASCA), most health care organizations now send most of their claims to insurance carriers electronically. The ASCA was enacted by Congress to improve administration of the Medicare program by increasing efficiencies gained through electronic claims submission. Effective Oct. 16, 2003, the ASCA required that all claims sent to the Medicare program be submitted electronically. With limited exceptions, the ASCA prohibits payment of services or supplies not submitted to Medicare electronically.

Despite the transition to electronic claims submission, the paper claim continues to be an important part of the claims process that the insurance billing specialist must learn as a basic skill set. There are still circumstances under which the paper claim continues to be used, such as the following:

1. The ASCA provides an exception to the Medicare electronic claims submission requirements to small health care organizations. The ASCA defines a small health care organization or supplier as a provider of services with fewer than 25 full-time equivalent employees or a service provider, health care organization, facility, or supplier (other than a provider of services) with fewer than 10 full-time equivalent employees.

2. The ASCA also allows an exemption to any health care organization who may be in an area that has disruptions in electricity and communication connections beyond control and expected to last more than 2 business days. Those health care organizations may report claims to Medicare on paper.

3. The ASCA does not preclude health care organizations from submitting paper claims to other health plans. Other payers may allow or require submission of claims on paper.

4. There may be occasions whereby the health care organization's software program experiences technical downtime and the organization is unable to submit claims electronically for a period.

5. Paper claims often are used when reporting special services or require special processing because of unusual circumstances.

6. Paper claims are often used when resubmitting a claim for review after initial denial of the claim.

7. Paper claims can be provided to patients who have insurance coverage with which the organization does not participate. The patient can then forward the paper claim to the insurance carrier for processing.

8. The paper claim may also be used to report patient encounter data to federal, state, and other public health agencies.

9. Claim-editing software programs frequently present data in the CMS-1500 claim format.

Essentially the paper claim is the basis for electronic claim submission, and many software and hardware systems depend on the CMS-1500 claim form. Because of this and because paper claims are still part of the claims process in many circumstances, it is essential for the insurance billing specialist to fully understand the basic guidelines for submitting paper claims and how to properly complete the claim form.

It is recommended that the insurance billing specialist also become familiar with the reverse side of the CMS-1500 claim form, which provides additional instructions for government programs. The reverse side of the claim form provides a notice to all involved in completion of the claim form which states: *"Any person who knowingly files a statement of claim containing any misrepresentation or any false, incomplete or misleading information may be guilty of a criminal act punishable under law and may be subject to civil penalties."*

National Uniform Claim Committee

The CMS-1500 claim form was developed by the National Uniform Claim Committee (NUCC). The NUCC is a voluntary organization co-chaired by the American Medical Association (AMA) and Centers for Medicare and Medicaid Services (CMS). The committee is made up of health care industry stakeholders representing providers, payers, designated standards maintenance organizations, public health organizations, and vendors.

The NUCC was formally named in the administrative simplification of the Health Insurance Portability and Accountability Act of 1996 (HIPAA) as the authoritative voice regarding national standard content. The committee is responsible for maintaining the integrity of the data sets and physical layout of the CMS-1500 claim form. It is further charged with the task of standardizing national instructions for completion of the claim form to be used by all payers. This may result in even more changes to the CMS-1500 claim form in the future.

History of the Paper Claim CMS-1500

The paper claim has origins as far back as 1958, when the Health Insurance Association of America (HIAA) and the American Medical Association (AMA) attempted to standardize the insurance claim form. Over the years, standardization has been the driving force to even further changes (Table 14.1). The current version of the claim form is referred to as the CMS-1500.

Widespread use of the CMS-1500 has saved time and simplified processing of claims for both health care organizations and insurance carriers. It has eliminated the need to complete the many different insurance forms previously brought into the office by patients.

Insurance carriers with various computer programs and equipment may have instructions on completion of the form that vary by locality and program. Local representatives of insurance carriers should always be contacted to find out their specific claim form instructions for completion. Quantities of the CMS-1500 can be purchased from many medical office supply companies or from the AMA by calling the toll free number: 800-621-8335. Per Medicare guidelines, the red ink versions of the

TABLE 14.1 History of the Paper Claim CMS-1500

Year	Description
1958	The Health Insurance Association of America (HIAA) and the American Medical Association (AMA) attempted to create a standardized insurance claim form that eventually became known as *COMB-1*, or *Attending Physician's Statement*.
1975	The AMA approved a "universal claim form," called the *Health Insurance Claim Form*, referred to as the *HCFA-1500*, which was an abbreviation for the *Health Care Financing Administration*. The AMA joined forces with the Centers for Medicare and Medicaid Services (CMS) and many other payer organizations, known as the *Uniform Claim Form Task Force*, to standardize and promote the use of their universal health claim form.
1990	The HCFA-1500 (12-90) was revised and printed in red ink to allow optical scanning of claims. All services for Medicare patients from health care organizations, service providers, and suppliers (except for ambulance services) reported after May 1, 1992, had to be billed on the scannable HCFA-1500 (12-90) form.
Mid-1990s	The Uniform Claim Form Task Force was replaced by the National Uniform Claim Committee (NUCC). The committee's goal was to develop the NUCC Data Set (NUCC-DS), a standardized data set for use in an electronic environment but applicable to and consistent with evolving paper claim form standards.
2001	The HCFA-1500 became known as the CMS-1500 when the Health Care Finance Administration was retitled the Centers for Medicare and Medicaid Services (CMS).
2005	It became necessary to change the CMS-1500 (12-90) so that it could accommodate reporting of the National Provider Identifier (NPI) for providers; this form was referred to as the CMS-1500 (08-05).
2009	The NUCC began revision of the 1500 Claim Form to accommodate the updated Electronic Claims Submission (Version 5010 837P) changes and implementation of the new diagnosis coding system, ICD-10.
2012	The NUCC released the revised version of the 1500 Health Insurance Claim Form (version 02-12), which accommodated changes needed for implementation of ICD-10.
January 6, 2014	Effective January 6, 2014, health plans, clearinghouses, and other information support vendors were required to handle and accept the newly revised (02-12) form. Providers were allowed to use either the 08-05 or the revised (02-12) 1500 Claim Form until March 31, 2014.
April 1, 2014	The 1500 Claim Form (08-05) was discontinued, and only revised claims (02-12) will be accepted for processing.

CMS-1500 claim form cannot be duplicated. Therefore, the claim forms must be originals and not photocopies or they will not be processed.

14.1 QUICK REVIEW

Question: What is the National Uniform Claim Committee (NUCC) responsible for?

TYPES OF SUBMITTED CLAIMS

A paper claim is one that is printed on a paper form and is sent to the payer through the mail. In contrast, an electronic claim is one that is generated by computer software and transmitted electronically over telephone or computer connection to a health insurer or other third-party payer for processing and payment. Electronic claims are digital files that are not printed on paper claim forms and reduce the administrative burden and expense generally associated with manual claims processing and submission.

! COMPLIANCE ALERT

Compliance and Insurance Claim Forms

HIPAA federal laws affect insurance claim submission. The provider rendering the service or procedure must be properly identified with the correct provider number. Claims must show only services rendered that have been properly documented and are medically necessary without evidence of fraud or abuse issues. HIPAA mandates the use of electronic standards for automated transfer of certain health care data among payers, plans, and health care organizations. The National Provider Identifier (NPI) system for health care providers became effective on May 27, 2007, in connection with the electronic transactions identified in HIPAA.

Claim Status

Paper or electronic claims can be designated as clean, rejected, or pending/suspended.

A clean claim is a claim that was submitted within a third-party payer's time limit and contains all the necessary information so that it can be processed and paid promptly. A physically clean claim is one that has no staples or highlighted areas and on which the bar code area has not been deformed.

A rejected claim has not been processed or cannot be processed for various reasons. For example, a claim cannot be processed if the patient is not identified in the payer system, the provider is not active in the third-party payer records, or the claim was not submitted in a timely manner. A rejected claim is one that requires investigation, further clarification, and possibly answers to some questions. Such a claim should be resubmitted after proper corrections are made.

A pending or suspended claim is an insurance claim that is held for review or other reason by the third-party payer. The amount of time a claim is pended varies from carrier to carrier and from claim to claim. Some claims may take only an additional 9 to 10 days to process, whereas others may take more time and may be dependent on additional information requests sent to the health care organization. The insurance billing specialist should handle all additional information requests promptly to eliminate the long-term pending of claims. All pended claims should be monitored and followed up on if they are not promptly cleared for payment or denied.

Medicare Claim Status

In the Medicare program, specific terms are used to describe various claim processing situations. These terms may or may not be used by other insurance programs.

A *clean claim* means the following:

1. The claim has no deficiencies and passes all electronic edits.
2. The carrier does not need to investigate outside of the carrier's operation before paying the claim.
3. The claim is investigated on a postpayment basis, meaning that a claim is not delayed before payment and may be paid. After investigation, payments may be reconsidered and deemed not due. A refund may be requested from the health care organization.
4. The claim is subject to medical review with attached information or forwarded simultaneously with electronic medical claim (EMC) records.

Medicare claims not considered "clean" claims, which require investigation or development on a prepayment basis, are known as *other claims*. Health care organizations that participate in the Medicare program can expect electronic claim submissions to be processed within approximately 14 days of receipt. Health care organizations that are participating in the Medicare program and send paper submissions will not have claims processed until at least 27 days after receipt, and health care organizations that do not participate with the Medicare program will not have claims processed until at least 27 days after receipt.

An incomplete claim is any Medicare claim missing required information. It is identified to the health care organization so that it can be resubmitted as a new claim.

An invalid claim is any Medicare claim that contains complete, necessary information but is illogical or incorrect. For example, a claim listing an incorrect provider number for a referring physician is invalid. An invalid claim is identified to the health care organization and may be resubmitted.

A dirty claim is a claim submitted with errors, one requiring manual processing for resolving problems, or one rejected for payment. Pending or suspended claims are placed in this category because something is holding the claim back from payment.

A deleted claim is a claim canceled, deleted, or voided by a Medicare fiscal intermediary for the following reasons:

- CMS-1500 form is not used
- Itemized charges are not provided
- More than six line items are submitted on the CMS-1500 claim form
- Patient's address is missing
- Internal clerical error was made
- Certificate of Medical Necessity (CMN) for durable medical equipment was not with the Part B claim or was incomplete or invalid
- Name of the store is not on the receipt that includes the price of the durable medical equipment item

The Omnibus Budget Reconciliation Act (OBRA) requires Medicare administrative contractors to pay the prompt payment interest rate on all clean claims not paid in a timely manner. The government updates the interest rate on January 1 and July 1 each year on the United States Treasury Bureau of Fiscal Services page (https://www.fiscal.treasury.gov/fsservices/gov/pmt/promptPayment/rates.htm).

 14.2 QUICK REVIEW

Question: What are the two types of claims submitted for health care services?

ABSTRACTING FROM MEDICAL RECORDS

The insurance billing specialist must be skilled at abstracting information from medical records. Abstraction of technical and clinical information from patient records may be necessary for claims processing. Insurance carriers often request additional information to process the claim or to support medical necessity before payment of a claim (Fig. 14.2A and B).

Cover Letter Accompanying Insurance Claims

When requesting a review of a denied claim, the insurance billing specialist is required to send a cover letter with the claim. A letter accompanying insurance claims will generally require abstraction of information from the medical record and should include the following:

- Patient's name
- Subscriber's name (if different from that of the patient)
- Subscriber identification number
- Date and type of service
- Total amount of the claim
- A short history
- A clear but concise explanation of the medical necessity, difficulty or complexity, or unusual circumstance (e.g., an emergency)

The letter and insurance claim should be sent to the attention of the claims supervisor so that it may be directed to the appropriate person for processing.

 14.3 QUICK REVIEW

Question: List the information that is generally required when abstracting information from the medical record into a letter that will accompany an insurance claim.

BASIC GUIDELINES FOR SUBMITTING A HEALTH INSURANCE CLAIM FORM (CMS-1500)

The CMS-1500 claim form is accepted by nearly all Medicare, Medicaid, and private third-party payers, as well as by TRICARE and workers' compensation (WC). A claim form should be completed and submitted as required by payer rules on behalf of a patient who is covered by third-party insurance.

Individual Insurance

In very rare cases, the patient may bring in a form from a private insurance plan that is not a CMS-1500 claim form. This occurs less often today than in the past. The patient should sign the CMS-1500 claim form in Block 13 (Assignment of Benefits). If the health care organization has a signed assignment of benefits form in the patient's health record, it can state "signature on file" on the CMS-1500 claim form. The patient's portion of the private insurance form should be checked to ensure that

A

Block 24A Dates of service

Block 24D Documentation of professional services rendered

Block 14 Date of last menstrual period

Block 21 Primary and secondary diagnoses

DATE	PROGRESS
2-10-20XX	This 35-year-old Hispanic female recently moved to this city. She is employed as a legal secretary. She began having labor pains and was admitted to College Hospital on 2/10/20XX. LMP 5-5-20XX. Primiparous. Healthy 6 lb 4 oz baby girl was delivered vaginally.
	mtf Bertha Caesar, MD
2-11-20XX	Hospital visit. Normal postpartum. Patient resting comfortably.
	mtf Bertha Caesar, MD
2-12-20XX	Hospital visit.
2-13-20XX	mtf Bertha Caesar, MD
	Discharged from hospital. Patient has been off work since Jan. 25, 2 weeks before delivery and will return to work March 29, 6 weeks after delivery. Patient to be seen in the office for 2-week check up.
	mtf Bertha Caesar, MD

Block 18 Dates of hospitalization

Block 16 Dates of disability

B

Fig. 14.2 **(A)** Example of a chart note illustrating important information to read through and abstract for insurance claim completion. **(B)** The location of the abstracted information placed in the blocks on a CMS-1500 insurance claim form in optical character recognition (OCR) format.

it is complete and accurate. The forms should then be mailed together to the insurance carrier. It is not recommended to let patients direct their own forms to insurance companies or employers. Patients have been known to lose forms or alter data on documents before mailing, to forget to send the forms, or to mail them to an incorrect address.

Group Insurance

When a patient has group insurance through an employer, ensure that all information about the employer is complete and correct. If the employer's section is complete, both the CMS-1500 and the group insurance forms should be sent directly to the insurance carrier after the service provider's portion is completed.

Secondary Insurance

When two insurance policies are involved, one is considered primary and the other secondary (Example 14.1). This is sometimes called *dual coverage* or *duplication of coverage*. The patient's signature should always be acquired for assignment of benefits for both insurance companies.

If the patient is insured by two companies, the primary carrier should be determined and the claim should be submitted to that carrier first. After the primary insurance carrier has paid out, a claim should be submitted to the secondary carrier with a copy of the primary carrier's explanation of benefits (EOB) document attached.

Completion of Insurance Claim Forms

It is recommended that the CMS-1500 claim form be completed following the NUCC's Reference Instruction Manual, unless the individual payer has advised otherwise and provided their own guidelines for completion of the form. The NUCC's guidelines provide block-by-block instructions for completion. Those blocks that are conditional will be noted in the instructions. If any questions are unanswerable, do not use the abbreviations

DNA (does not apply), NA (not applicable), or N/A (not applicable), but leave the space blank.

Diagnosis

In Block 21, the diagnosis field of the CMS-1500 claim form, all accurate diagnostic codes that affect the patient's condition should be inserted, with the primary diagnosis code listed first, followed by any secondary or tertiary diagnosis codes. The CMS-1500 claim form has the ability to report 12 diagnostic codes.

A diagnosis should never be submitted without supporting documentation in the medical record. The diagnosis must support the medical necessity of the treatment and services rendered. If there is no formal diagnosis at the conclusion of an encounter, the code(s) for the patient's symptom(s) should be submitted.

It is best to list only one illness or injury and its treatment per form, unless there are concurrent conditions, to avoid confusing services with multiple medical conditions. A concurrent condition is a disorder that coexists with the primary condition, complicating the treatment and management of the primary disorder. It may alter the course of treatment required or lengthen the expected recovery time of the primary condition. It also is referred to as comorbidity.

Service Dates

Dates of service must be entered with no spaces using a 6-digit or 8-digit format; for example, January 2, 20XX, should appear as either 0102XX or 010220XX. The appropriate date of service format to be used is noted in the NUCC's instructions section of each Item Number on the CMS-1500 claim form. Do not use ditto marks (") to indicate repetition of dates for services performed on subsequent lines. Charges for services rendered in different years should not be submitted on the same claim form. This type of situation can occur when claims processing is affected by deductible and eligibility factors, thereby delaying reimbursement.

Consecutive Dates

Some carriers allow medical services, hospital services, or office encounters to be grouped if each visit is consecutive, occurs in the same month, uses the same procedure code, or results in the same fee. The total fee for the procedures should be listed in Block 24F and the number of times the procedure was performed or service supplied should be listed in Block 24G, as illustrated in the following graphic (Example: $80.00 \times 5 = 400.00).

24. A. DATE(S) OF SERVICE						B. PLACE OF SERVICE	C. EMG	D. PROCEDURES, SERVICES, OR SUPPLIES (Explain Unusual Circumstances)		E. DIAGNOSIS POINTER	F. $ CHARGES		G. DAYS OR UNITS	H. EPSDT Family Plan	I. ID. QUAL.	J. RENDERING PROVIDER ID. #
From			To					CPT/HCPCS	MODIFIER							
MM	DD	YY	MM	DD	YY											
1																
10	04	XX	10	08	XX	21		99232		A	80	00	5		NPI	32783127XX
2															NPI	

However, some private insurance carriers require a single fee listed in Block 24F, rather than the total fee for the procedures. If there is a difference in the procedure code or fee for several

encounters listed on the claim, each separately coded hospital or office encounter must be itemized and each procedure or service code and charge entered on a separate line.

No Charge

Insurance claims should not be submitted for services that have no charge, such as global or surgical package postoperative visits, unless the patient requests that it be sent. These services should only appear documented in the patient's health and financial records.

Physician's or Service Provider's Identification Numbers

Insurance companies and federal and state programs require certain identification numbers on claim forms to be submitted from health care organizations and service providers. This can be confusing to the beginner, as well as to someone experienced in insurance billing procedures, because there are so many different numbers.

- *State license number.* To practice within a state, each physician or service provider must obtain a state license number. Sometimes this number is requested on forms and is used as a provider number.
- *Employer identification number.* In a health care organization, many service providers may file taxes as a group and thus be under the same employer identification number (EIN) or tax identification number (TIN). This is issued by the Internal Revenue Service for income tax purposes. Some organizations may opt to separate finances and require separate TINs for each provider.

25. FEDERAL TAX I.D. NUMBER		SSN	EIN
74 10640XX		☐	☒

- *Social Security number.* Each service provider has a Social Security number (SSN) for other personal use and use this as an EIN in a solo practice.
- An SSN is not typically used on the claim form unless the provider does not have an EIN, in which case the SSN may be required.

25. FEDERAL TAX I.D. NUMBER		SSN	EIN
082 XX 1707		☒	☐

- *National Provider Identifiers.* The National Provider Identifier (NPI) is a HIPAA administrative simplification standard. Covered health care providers, health care organizations, all health plans, and health care clearinghouses must use the unique 10-digit NPIs in the administrative and financial transactions adopted under HIPAA. The NPI is a lifetime 10-digit number that replaces all other numbers assigned by various health plans. A health care provider is assigned only one NPI, which is retained for a lifetime, even if the provider moves to another state. Under HIPAA, providers are required to share their NPIs with other providers, organizations, health plans, clearinghouses, and any entity that may need it for their own billing purposes. The Centers for Medicare & Medicaid Services (CMS) provides access to all active NPI records through the NPI Registry Public Search. This will provide the insurance billing specialist the ability to search for a health care provider by name and practice address and it will identify the specialty (taxonomy) and NPI number for billing purposes. An internet link has been provided to access the NPI Registry Public Search at the end of this chapter, under *Internet Resources.*

NPI root
check digit
locator code

Claims may require several NPI numbers: one for the referring health care provider, one for the ordering provider, one for the performing provider, and one for the billing entity. It is possible that the ordering provider and performing provider are the same. On rare occasions, the number may be the same for all three, but more commonly, different numbers are required, depending on the circumstances of the case. For placement of the NPI number on the CMS-1500 claim form, refer to the block-by-block instructions for Blocks 17a, 17b, and 24J. Keep in mind what the role of the health care provider, as well as their number, represents in relation to the provider listed in Block 33. The following examples of blocks from the CMS-1500 insurance claim form show where these numbers are commonly placed. Insurance billing manuals from major insurers give specific directions.

When a non-physician practitioner (NPP) bills incident-to a physician in the same group but that physician is out of the office on a day the NPP sees the patient, another physician in the same group can provide direct supervision to meet the incident-to requirements. When the ordering and supervising provider are different individuals, the ordering provider's name goes in Block 17 and their NPI goes in Block 17b. The NPI of the supervising provider goes in Block 24J and the supervising provider signs the form in Block 31. The group's NPI goes in Block 33a.

To assist with claims completion, a reference list of provider numbers should be compiled for all ordering and referring health care providers. For Medicare claims, the health care provider's numbers can be obtained by calling the provider's offices, contacting the Medicare carrier, or searching the NPI Registry on the internet. For license numbers, search the state licensing board on the internet.

Group National Provider Identifier (group NPI). The group NPI is used instead of the individual NPI for the performing provider who is a member of a group practice that submits claims to insurance companies under the group name.

33. BILLING PROVIDER INFO & PH #	(555) 4869002
College Clinic 4567 Broad Avenue Woodland Hills XY 123450001	
a. 3664021CC	b.

- *Durable medical equipment number.* Health care organizations that charge patients a fee for supplies and equipment such as crutches, urinary catheters, ostomy supplies, surgical dressings, and so forth must bill insurance carriers using a durable medical equipment (DME) number.

33. BILLING PROVIDER INFO & PH #	(555) 4869002
College Clinic	
4567 Broad Avenue	
Woodland Hills XY 123450001	
a. 34007600XX	b.

DME #

- **Facility provider number.** Each facility (e.g., hospital, laboratory, radiology office, skilled nursing facility) is issued a facility provider number to be used by the performing health care provider and to report services done at the location.

32. SERVICE FACILITY LOCATION INFORMATION	
College Hospital	
4500 Broad Avenue	
Woodland Hills XY 123450001	
a. X9507310XX	b.

- **Taxonomy code.** A taxonomy code is assigned to each health care provider based on education and training. It is used to define specialty. When applying for an NPI number, a health care provider must select the Health Care Provider Taxonomy code or code description that identifies the health care provider's type, classification, or specialization and report that in the NPI application. Some payers may either assign a provider identifier or prefer that the taxonomy code be inserted on CMS-1500 claim forms. Depending on issues of each case, provider taxonomy codes may or may not be required on the form. When needed, the blocks affected are Blocks 17a, 19, 24I, 24J, 32b, or 33b (Example 14.2).

Physician or Service Provider's Signature

The physician or service provider should sign the insurance claim form above or under their typed or preprinted name. In the computerized office environment, the health care organization's billing system will generate a paper CMS-1500 form. In general, the participating contract with the third-party payer allows the service provider's name to simply be printed in the signature block. This is an acceptable method for the provider's signature.

EXAMPLE 14.2 Service Provider Specialty and Taxonomy Codes

Medicare Specialty Code	Medicare Provider/ Supplier Type Description	Provider Taxonomy Code	Provider Taxonomy Description: Type, Classification, Specialization
33	Physician/Thoracic Surgery	208G00000X	Allopathic and Osteopathic Physicians/ Thoracic Surgery
34	Physician/Urology	208800000X	Allopathic and Osteopathic Physicians/Urology
34	Physician/Urology	2088P0231X	Allopathic and Osteopathic Physicians/Urology, Pediatric Urology

Insurance Billing Specialist's Initials

If more than one person is assigned to complete insurance paper claims, then the insurance billing specialist should place his or her initials in the bottom left or top right corner of the claim form. Placement of this reference should be consistent. The following are three good reasons to adopt this habit:

- To identify who in the office is responsible for the insurance form
- To decrease errors
- To avoid being accused of someone else's error, especially if another biller submitted a fraudulent claim

Proofread

Ideally, every paper claim should be proofread for transposition of numbers (group, policy, health care provider's ID, procedure, and diagnostic codes), misspelled name, missing date of birth, blanks, and attachments. Larger, more complex claims require special attention because they involve greater sums of money and may be more difficult to complete. Ensure that the bill is for the right patient by checking the address and date of birth to verify the correct individual. Review the encounter form to charge for the correct tests and number of tests so that the patient is not charged more than once for the same service.

Review the bill for the correct number of units when reporting time-based services. For example, a patient seen for 16 minutes should show a billing for one 15-minute session. Check for any overcoding. For example, do not bill for a longer office encounter that included paperwork time when only actual face-to-face time should have been charged. Double-check to ensure that codes are not unbundled. It is fraudulent to bill for charges that should be included in the cost of something else, or codes that are included in another code. Proofreading data prevents subsequent denials and avoids time-consuming responses to questions.

Supporting Documentation

Occasionally, claims need supporting documents to further explain services billed and to obtain appropriate reimbursement. The following information should be included in case the attachment is separated from the claim during processing.

- The patient's name
- Subscriber's name (if different from that of the patient)
- Date of service
- Insurance identification number

This same information should be placed on each page of the document, front and back if two-sided. If a medication is expensive or experimental, a copy of the invoice received from the supply house or pharmacy should be sent.

When a procedure is complicated, takes additional time to perform, or falls outside of the manner in which the procedure is typically performed, it is reasonable for the health care organization to request additional reimbursement. In those cases, a copy of all pertinent reports (operative, radiology, laboratory, pathology, and discharge summary) should be included with the claim. For a treatment not listed in the procedure code book, a special detailed report should be sent that gives the nature, extent, and need for the services, along with the time, effort, supplies, and equipment required. The correct code number should be used for unlisted services or procedures (Example 14.3).

EXAMPLE 14.3 Unlisted Procedure

95199	Unlisted allergy/clinical immunologic service or procedure

Office Pending File

The office copy of the insurance form should be filed in a separate alpha file for insurance claim copies unless the computer system maintains files. This file should be reviewed for follow-up every 30 days. The health care organization's billing system will keep an accurate record of all patients and activity on their accounts.

 14.4 QUICK REVIEW

Question: What set of guidelines should be used when completing a CMS-1500 claim form?

COMMON REASONS WHY CLAIM FORMS ARE DELAYED OR REJECTED

It is wise to be aware of common billing errors and know how to correct them to reduce the number of appeals and to get claims paid faster. This also may help to avoid additional administrative burdens, such as telephone calls, resubmission of claims, and appeal letters. Table 14.2 contains some reasons why claims are rejected or delayed and suggested solutions when completing the CMS-1500 insurance claim form blocks.

ADDITIONAL CLAIM SUBMISSION ERRORS

PROBLEM: Carolyn, the insurance billing specialist, telephoned the insurance company and discovered there was no record of the claim at the third-party payer.

SOLUTION: Always keep copies of paper claims. Send claims with large dollar amounts by certified mail with return receipt requested. Another option is to request that the customer service representative search the insurance carrier's imaging file for the period beginning on the date of service and ending on the date you are calling. Sometimes the claim was received and scanned but was never crossed over to the processing unit.

PROBLEM: Claire is in a hurry and submits a claim form that is illegible.

SOLUTION: Never handwrite a claim form. Check printer ink or toner and replace when necessary.

PROBLEM: Untimely or lack of response to claim development letters is discovered.

SOLUTION: Pay close attention to the due date and reply to third-party payer's requests for additional information as soon as possible. Send a copy of the claim with the letter and appropriate medical documentation listing the claim control number, if assigned.

PROBLEM: Noncovered service occurs because a routine screening procedure is performed in conjunction with a routine examination.

SOLUTION: Determine whether it is a diagnostic or preventive service and if the code is correct. Use the GY modifier when submitting a statutory-excluded service for payment by the secondary insurance carrier.

PROBLEM: Payment is adjusted because the care may be covered by another insurance plan per coordination of benefits.

SOLUTION: Always check all patients' insurance coverage.

PROBLEM: Payment is adjusted because the medical service is not paid separately as it is a global surgery or a National Correct Coding Initiative (NCCI) denial.

SOLUTION: Determine the global period for the surgical procedure. Use a modifier to report an unrelated or exception service within a global period. Check the NCCI edits to see if the code selected has been deleted or is a bundled service.

PROBLEM: Irene submits a claim with missing, incomplete, or invalid information regarding where the medical services were performed.

SOLUTION: Include the zip code of where the service was performed.

 14.5 QUICK REVIEW

Question: What steps should be taken if services are being performed within a global surgical period?

CLAIM COMPLETION GUIDELINES

The CMS-1500 claim form was designed using red ink to allow scanning through optical character recognition (OCR), less commonly referred to as intelligent character recognition (ICR) or *image copy recognition (ICR)*. This technology has been used across the nation in processing insurance claims to enable greater speed and efficiency. A scanner can transfer printed or typed text and bar codes to the insurance company's computer memory. Scanners read at such a fast speed that they reduce data entry cost and decrease processing time. More control is gained over data input using OCR. It improves accuracy, thus reducing coding errors because the claim is entered exactly as coded by the insurance billing specialist. Medicare and most other carriers require that paper claims be submitted on the OCR-compliant claim form in red ink; photocopies are not processable.

Do's and Don'ts for Claim Completion

Basic do's and don'ts for completing claims follow.

Do: Use original claim forms printed in red ink; photocopies and forms generated from ink jet or laser printers cannot be scanned. Laser jet printing is preferable for computer-generated claims.

Do: Computer-generate or type all information in black ink.

Don't: Handwrite information on the document. Handwriting is accepted only for signatures. Handwritten claims require manual processing.

Don't: Use script, slant, mini-font, or italicized fonts or expanded, compressed, or bold print. Use fonts that have the same width for each character.

TABLE 14.2 The Paper Claim: Problem Solving

Block Number(s)	Problem	Solution
1	When submitting a paper claim, the wrong block is checked (that is, claim submitted to the secondary insurer instead of the primary insurer).	Obtain data from the patient during the first encounter as to which company is the primary insurer, depending on illness, injury, or accident. Submit the claim to the primary carrier and then send in a claim with a copy of the primary carrier's EOB to the secondary carrier.
1–13	Information missing on patient portion of the claim form.	Obtain a complete patient registration form from which information can be extracted. If patients are filling out their portion, educate patients on data requirements at the time of their first encounter to the health care organization. Be sure to ask if there have been any changes on subsequent office encounters.
1a	Patient's insurance number is incorrect or transposed (especially in Medicare and Medicaid cases).	Proofread numbers carefully from source documents. Always photocopy front and back sides of insurance identification cards.
2	Patient's name and insured's name are entered as the same when the patient is a dependent. A common error is that the patient is listed as the insured when he or she is not the insured (for example, spouse or child). Block 4 is used for listing the insured's name.	Verify the insured party and check for Sr., Jr., and correct birth date.
2	Patient name is missing, illegible, or incorrect.	Patient's name must be entered exactly as it appears on the patient's ID card.
3	Incorrect gender identification, resulting in a diagnosis or procedure code that is inconsistent with patient's gender.	Proofread the claim before mailing and review the patient's medical record to locate gender, especially if the patient's first name could be male or female.
5	Patient address is missing or illegible.	Enter the patient's complete address. Do not puncture the address. When entering a 9-digit zip code, do not include the hyphen.
9a–9d	Incomplete entry for other insurance coverage.	Accurately abstract data from the patient's registration form and input it to the computer database. Telephone the patient if information is incomplete.
10	Failure to indicate whether patient's condition is related to employment or an "other" type of accident.	Review patient's medical history to find out details of injury or illness and proofread claim before mailing. Telephone the employer to see if permission was given to treat the patient as a workers' compensation case.
14	Date of injury, date of LMP, or dates of onset of illness are omitted. This information is important for determining whether accident benefits apply, patient is eligible for maternity benefits, or there was a preexisting condition.	Do not list unless dates are clearly documented in the patient's medical record. Read the patient's medical history and call the patient to obtain the date of accident or LMP. Compose an addendum to the record if necessary. Always proofread a paper claim before mailing, in case data are missing.
17, 17a, 17b	Incorrect or missing name or NPI of referring health care provider on claim for consultation or other services requiring this information.	Check the patient registration form and the chart note for reference to the referring health care provider. Develop a list of NPI numbers for all health care providers in the area.
21	The diagnostic code is missing, incomplete, invalid, or not in standard nomenclature (for example, missing fourth or fifth digit); it includes a written description or does not correspond to the treatment (procedure code) rendered by the health care provider.	Verify and submit correct diagnostic codes by referring to an updated diagnostic code book and reviewing the patient record. Check with the provider if the diagnosis code listed does not go with the procedure code shown. Do not include decimal point.
24A	Omitted, incorrect, overlapping, or duplicate dates of service.	Verify against the encounter form or medical record that all dates of service are listed, are accurate, and appear on individual lines on paper claims. Date spans for multiple services must be adequate for the number and types of services provided. Each month should be on a separate line and each year should be on a separate claim.
24B	Missing or incorrect place of service code. If a provider sees a patient in a skilled nursing facility (SNF) that is in the same building as a domicile rest home or a hospice, it is possible to incorrectly document the SNF as the site for each patient.	Verify the place of service from the encounter form or medical record and list the correct code for place of service and submitted procedure.
24D	Procedure codes are incorrect, invalid, or missing.	Verify the coding system used by the third-party payer and submit correct procedure code(s) by referring to a current procedure codebook. For Medicare patients and certain private insurance plans, check the Healthcare Common Procedure Coding System (HCPCS) manual for CMS national and local procedure codes.

TABLE 14.2 The Paper Claim: Problem Solving—cont'd

Block Number(s)	Problem	Solution
24D	Incorrect or missing modifier(s).	Verify usage of modifiers by referring to a current procedure codebook and HCPCS manual. Submit valid modifiers with the correct procedure codes
24E	Diagnosis pointer is required.	Enter the associated diagnosis by referencing the pointers (A to L) listed in Block 21 that relate to the date of service and the procedures performed. Diagnosis codes must be valid ICD-10 codes for the date of service.
24F	Omitted or incorrect amount billed.	Be certain that the fee column is filled in. Check the amounts charged with the appropriate fee schedule.
24G	Days/units are required on claim forms.	Enter quantity. Value entered must be greater than zero. (Field allows up to three digits.)
24G	Reasons for multiple visits made in 1 day are not stated on an attachment sheet.	Depending on insurance guidelines, submit documentation explaining reason for multiple visits. Use appropriate modifiers or upcode evaluation and management services to include all visits.
24G	Incorrect quantity billed.	Verify charge amounts. Ensure that the number of units listed is equal to the date span when more than one date of service is billed (for example, hospital encounters).
24J	Provider's identification number is missing.	Verify and insert the required provider's number in this block.
24A–24J, Line 6	More than six lines entered on a paper claim.	Insert service date and corresponding procedure on Lines 1 to 6 only. Complete an additional paper claim if more services should be billed.
27	Assignment acceptance must be indicated on the claim.	"Yes" or "No" must be checked.
28	Total amounts do not equal itemized charges.	Total charges for each claim and verify amounts with patient account. If number of units listed in Block 24G is more than one, multiply the units by the fee listed in Block 24F and add to all other charges listed.
31	Health care provider's signature is missing.	Have the health care provider or their representative sign the claim or key in "SOF" or "signature on file".
32	Information is not centered in block as required when submitting a paper claim.	Enter data centered in block.
33	Provider's address, NPI, or group number is missing.	The billing provider's name and address are required. A physical location must be entered; P.O. boxes are not acceptable. Obtain provider's data from a list that contains all providers' professional information.

CMS, Centers for Medicare and Medicaid Services; *EOB,* explanation of benefits; *HCPCS,* Health Care Common Procedure Coding System; *LMP,* last menstrual period; *NPI,* National Provider Identifier; *SNF,* skilled nursing facility.

Do: Place characters within the borders of each field. Use Pica 10 Pitch, Arial, or 10-, 11-, or 12-point type.

Do: Align the printer correctly so that characters appear exactly in the proper fields. Enter all information within designated fields.

Don't: Allow characters to touch lines

Correct

Incorrect

Do: Complete a new form for additional services if the case has more than six lines of service.

Correct

Correct

Incorrect

Don't: Use highlighter pens or colored ink on claims.

Don't: Use decimals in Block 21 or dollar signs ($) in the money column.

Correct

Incorrect

Don't: Use narrative descriptions of procedures, modifiers, or diagnoses; code numbers are sufficient.

Correct

Incorrect

Don't: Use N/A or DNA when information is not applicable. Leave the space blank.

Correct

Incorrect

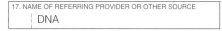

Don't: Use paper clips, cellophane tape, stickers, rubber stamps, or staples.

Do: Enter 6-digit or 8-digit date formats: 0601XX, 060120XX, or 06-01-20XX, depending on the block instructions.

Correct

Correct

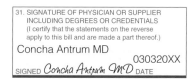

Do: Keep signature within signature block.

Correct

Incorrect

Do: Keep claim form clean and free from stains, tear-off pad glue, notations, circles, scribbles, strikeovers, crossed-out information, or white-out.

Don't: Fold or spindle forms when mailing.

Don't: Send claim attachments smaller than 8½ × 11.

> 📌 **14.6   QUICK REVIEW**
>
> Question: Explain why Medicare and most other carriers require that paper claims be submitted on the OCR-compliant claim form in red ink.

INSTRUCTIONS FOR COMPLETING THE HEALTH INSURANCE CLAIM FORM (CMS-1500)

The NUCC has developed a general instruction guide for completing the CMS-1500 claim form, which is referred to as the *NUCC Reference Instruction Manual.** Updated versions of the instruction manual are released each July.

The NUCC's instructions align with the specifications created by the Accredited Standards Committee (ASC) and are approved by the Department of Health and Human Services (HHS) for filing of HIPAA-compliant electronic transactions. Throughout the NUCC's instructions, reference is made to the Health Care Claim Professional 837 and 5010A1.

- The 837 is the HIPAA-compliant standard format used by health care professionals and suppliers to transmit claims electronically.
- Version 5010A1 is the most recent update of the HIPAA-compliant standard format for electronic transactions for health care professionals and suppliers.

*Content from the NUCC's 1500 Health Insurance Claim Form Reference Instruction Manual is reprinted by permission of the American Medical Association.

The NUCC Reference Instruction Manual is not specific to any applicable public or private payer. However, most insurance carriers have adopted the NUCC guidelines for completion of the CMS-1500 claim form. It is recommended that claims be processed using NUCC guidelines unless carriers advise otherwise. NUCC guidelines provide instructions and examples that demonstrate how to enter the data in every field of the CMS-1500 claim form. The instructions on the following pages can be used to complete claims. Blocks should be completed for all carriers as indicated in the "Instructions" unless a more specific guideline for the carrier is indicated.

! COMPLIANCE ALERT

HIPAA Transactions and Code Sets Standards

Question

Do the HIPAA transactions and code sets standards apply to paper claims and other nonelectronic transactions?

Answer

No. The HIPAA transactions and code sets standards only apply to electronic transactions conducted by covered entities. Other entities such as employers or casualty insurance plans may decide to use them voluntarily but are not required to do so.

For paper transactions, health plans are free to set their own data requirements. Other federal or state laws may require plans or health care organizations to use specific code sets for certain paper transactions. However, all covered health plans and organizations must be able to use the HIPAA standards for electronic transactions. Health plans may choose to require that paper claims include the same data elements, codes, and identifiers that are required by the HIPAA regulations for electronic transactions.

HIPAA, Health Insurance Portability and Accountability Act.

Block-By-Block Instructions for Completion of the CMS-1500

DRAFT - NOT FOR OFFICIAL USE

ABC Insurance Company
Suite 600
52 Insurance Lane
Oakland IL 605000120

HEALTH INSURANCE CLAIM FORM

APPROVED BY NATIONAL UNIFOR MCLAIM COMMITTEE (NUCC) 02/12

| | PICA | | | | | | | PICA | |

| 1. MEDICARE (Medicare#) | MEDICAID (Medicaid#) | TRICARE (ID#DoD#) | CHAMPVA (Member ID#) | GROUP HEALTH PLAN [X] (ID#) | FECA BLK LUNG (ID#) | OTHER (ID#) | 1a. INSURED'S I.D. NUMBER (For Program in Item 1) 111704521 |
| 2. PATIENT'S NAME (Last Name, First Name, Middle Initial) Forehand, Harry, N | | 3. PATIENT'S BIRTH DATE MM 01 DD 06 YY 1946 SEX M [X] F [ ] | | 4. INSURED'S NAME (Last Name, First Name, Middle Initial) Forehand, Harry, N |

Carrier Block

The carrier block can be found in the upper right corner of the CMS-1500 form. In the upper left corner of the form, a Quick Response (QR) code symbol and the date approved by the NUCC can be located. The payer is the carrier, health plan, third-party administrator, or other payer that will handle the claim. This information directs the claim to the appropriate payer. Note: Some carriers may prefer that this area of the claim be left blank because identifying data are printed during the initial insurance claims processing stage.

Instructions: Enter in the white, open carrier area the name and address of the payer to whom the claim is being sent. Information should be entered in the following format:

- 1st line: Name of insurance carrier
- 2nd line: First line of address
- 3rd line: Second line of address (if necessary) (If address only has three lines, leave blank.)
- 4th line: City, state (two-character state code), and zip code (Examples 14.4 and 14.5)

Do not use punctuation (that is, commas and periods) or other symbols in the address (for example, 123 N Main Street 101 instead of 123 N. Main St, #101). When entering a 9-digit zip code, do not include the hyphen.

EXAMPLE 14.4   Four-Line Address

Worldwide Health Insurance Company
Suite 101
123 Main Street
Anytown, IL 60605

EXAMPLE 14.5   Three-Line Address

Worldwide Health Insurance Company
123 Main Street
Anytown, IL 60605

PICA								PICA

1. MEDICARE	MEDICAID	TRICARE	CHAMPVA	GROUP HEALTH PLAN	FECA BLK LUNG	OTHER	1a. INSURED'S I.D. NUMBER	(For Program in Item 1)
☐ (Medicare#)	☐ (Medicaid#)	☐ (ID#DoD#)	☐ (Member ID#)	☒ (ID#)	☐ (ID#)	☐ (ID#)	111704521	

2. PATIENT'S NAME (Last Name, First Name, Middle Initial)	3. PATIENT'S BIRTH DATE SEX	4. INSURED'S NAME (Last Name, First Name, Middle Initial)
Forehand, Harry, N	MM 01	DD 06	YY 1946 M ☒ F ☐	Forehand, Harry, N

Block 1: Medicare, Medicaid, TRICARE, CHAMPVA, Group Health Plan, FECA, Black Lung, Other This block is used to identify the insurance type to whom the claim is being submitted and may establish primary liability.

Instructions: Indicate the type of health insurance coverage applicable to this claim by placing an "X" in the appropriate box. Only one box can be marked. If the patient has group contract insurance with a private payer, Group Health Plan is selected. "Other" indicates individual health insurance coverage, including health maintenance organizations (HMOs), commercial insurance, automobile accident, liability, WC. *Note: When completing the* Workbook *assignments for private payer cases or Medicare/Medigap cases, if the insured is employed, assume that the insurance is through the employer and is "group" insurance; otherwise, assume that it is an individual policy and enter "Other."*

PICA								PICA

1. MEDICARE	MEDICAID	TRICARE	CHAMPVA	GROUP HEALTH PLAN	FECA BLK LUNG	OTHER	1a. INSURED'S I.D. NUMBER	(For Program in Item 1)
☐ (Medicare#)	☐ (Medicaid#)	☐ (ID#DoD#)	☐ (Member ID#)	☒ (ID#)	☐ (ID#)	☐ (ID#)	111704521	

2. PATIENT'S NAME (Last Name, First Name, Middle Initial)	3. PATIENT'S BIRTH DATE SEX	4. INSURED'S NAME (Last Name, First Name, Middle Initial)
Forehand, Harry, N	MM 01	DD 06	YY 1946 M ☒ F ☐	Forehand, Harry, N

Block 1a: Insured's ID Number The "Insured's ID Number" is the identification number of the insured and identifies the insured to the payer.

Instructions: Enter the "Insured's ID Number" as shown on the insured's ID card for the payer to which the claim is being submitted. If the patient has a unique member identification number assigned by the payer, enter that number in this field.

✚ TRICARE CLAIMS

Enter the sponsor's Department of Defense (DoD) benefits number from the back of the ID card. This is an 11-digit number.

▶ CHAMPVA CLAIMS

Enter the sponsor's SSN or Veterans Affairs (VA) file number.

⚡ WORKERS' COMPENSATION CLAIMS

Enter the employee ID or WC claim number. If none is assigned, enter the employer's policy number.

PROPERTY AND CASUALTY CLAIMS

Enter the appropriate identifier of the injured person or entity.

PICA								PICA

1. MEDICARE	MEDICAID	TRICARE	CHAMPVA	GROUP HEALTH PLAN	FECA BLK LUNG	OTHER	1a. INSURED'S I.D. NUMBER	(For Program in Item 1)
☐ (Medicare#)	☐ (Medicaid#)	☐ (ID#DoD#)	☐ (Member ID#)	☒ (ID#)	☐ (ID#)	☐ (ID#)	111704521	

2. PATIENT'S NAME (Last Name, First Name, Middle Initial)	3. PATIENT'S BIRTH DATE SEX	4. INSURED'S NAME (Last Name, First Name, Middle Initial)
Forehand, Harry, N	MM 01	DD 06	YY 1946 M ☒ F ☐	Forehand, Harry, N

Block 2: Patient's Name The "Patient's Name" is the name of the person who received the treatment or supplies.

Instructions: Enter the patient's full last name, first name, and middle initial. If the patient uses a last name suffix (for example, Jr., Sr.), enter it after the last name and before the first name. Titles (for example, Sister, Capt., Dr.) and professional suffixes (for example, PhD, MD, Esq.) should not be included with the name. Use commas to separate the last name, first name, and middle initial. A hyphen can be used for hyphenated names. Do not use periods within the name (Example 14.6). If the patient is the insured, it is not necessary to report the patient's name.

EXAMPLE 14.6 Surname Format

Hyphenated name: Smith-White = Smith-White

Prefixed name: MacIverson = MacIverson

Seniority name with numeric suffix: John R. Ellis, III = Ellis III, John, R

								1a. INSURED'S I.D. NUMBER	(For Program in Item 1)
PICA									PICA
1. MEDICARE	MEDICAID	TRICARE	CHAMPVA	GROUP HEALTH PLAN	FECA BLK LUNG	OTHER		111704521	
(Medicare#)	(Medicaid#)	(ID#DoD#)	(Member ID#)	X (ID#)	(ID#)	(ID#)			

2. PATIENT'S NAME (Last Name, First Name, Middle Initial)	3. PATIENT'S BIRTH DATE SEX	4. INSURED'S NAME (Last Name, First Name, Middle Initial)
Forehand, Harry, N	MM 01 | DD 06 | YY 1946 M X F	Forehand, Harry, N

Block 3: Patient's Birth Date, Sex The patient's birth date and gender are pieces of information that will identify the patient and distinguish persons with similar names.

Instructions: Enter the patient's 8-digit birth date (MM/DD/YYYY). Enter an "X" in the correct box to indicate the sex of the patient. Only one box can be marked. If gender is unknown, leave blank. The patient's age must be as follows to correlate with the diagnosis in Block 21:

- Birth: Newborn diagnosis
- Birth to 17 Years: Pediatric diagnosis
- 12 to 55 years: Maternity diagnosis
- 15 to 124 years: Adult diagnosis

								1a. INSURED'S I.D. NUMBER	(For Program in Item 1)
PICA									PICA
1. MEDICARE	MEDICAID	TRICARE	CHAMPVA	GROUP HEALTH PLAN	FECA BLK LUNG	OTHER		111704521	
(Medicare#)	(Medicaid#)	(ID#DoD#)	(Member ID#)	X (ID#)	(ID#)	(ID#)			

2. PATIENT'S NAME (Last Name, First Name, Middle Initial)	3. PATIENT'S BIRTH DATE SEX	4. INSURED'S NAME (Last Name, First Name, Middle Initial)
Forehand, Harry, N	MM 01 | DD 06 | YY 1946 M X F	Forehand, Harry, N

Block 4: Insured's Name The "Insured's Name" identifies the person who holds the policy, which would be the employee for employer-provided health insurance.

Instructions: Enter the insured's full last name, first name, and middle initial. If the insured uses a last name suffix (for example, Jr., Sr.), enter it after the last name and before the first name. Titles (for example, Sister, Capt., Dr.) and professional suffixes (for example, PhD, MD, Esq.) should not be included with the name. Use commas to separate the last name, first name, and middle initial. A hyphen can be used for hyphenated names. Do not use periods within the name.

⚡ WORKERS' COMPENSATION CLAIMS

Enter the name of the employer.

◩ PROPERTY AND CASUALTY CLAIMS

Enter the name of the insured person or entity.

5. PATIENT'S ADDRESS (No., Street)	6. PATIENT RELATIONSHIP TO INSURED	7. INSURED'S ADDRESS (No., Street)	
1456 Main Street	Self X Spouse Child Other		
CITY	STATE	8. RESERVED FOR NUCC USE	CITY	STATE
Woodland Hills	XY			
ZIP CODE	TELEPHONE (Include Area Code)		ZIP CODE	TELEPHONE (Include Area Code)
123450000	( )		( )

Block 5: Patient's Address The patient's address is the patient's permanent residence. A temporary address or school address should not be used.

Instructions: Enter the patient's mailing address. The first line is for the street address; the second line is for the city and two-character state code; the third line is for the zip code. Enter the 9-digit zip code without the hyphen. If reporting a foreign address, contact payer for specific reporting instructions. If the patient is the insured, it is not necessary to report the patient's address. "Patient's Telephone" does not exist in 5010A1. The NUCC recommends that the phone number not be reported.

⚡ WORKERS' COMPENSATION CLAIMS

If required by a payer to report a telephone number, do not use a hyphen or space as a separator within the telephone number.

🔀 PROPERTY AND CASUALTY CLAIMS

If required by a payer to report a telephone number, do not use a hyphen or space as a separator within the telephone number.

5. PATIENT'S ADDRESS (No., Street)	6. PATIENT RELATIONSHIP TO INSURED	7. INSURED'S ADDRESS (No., Street)	
1456 Main Street	Self [X] Spouse [ ] Child [ ] Other [ ]		
CITY Woodland Hills STATE XY	8. RESERVED FOR NUCC USE	CITY	STATE
ZIP CODE 123450000 TELEPHONE (Include Area Code) ( )		ZIP CODE	TELEPHONE (Include Area Code) ( )

Block 6: Patient Relationship to Insured The "Patient Relationship to Insured" indicates how the patient is related to the insured. "Self" would indicate that the insured is the patient. "Spouse" would indicate that the patient is the husband of the wife or qualified partner as defined by the insured's plan. "Child" would indicate that the patient is a minor dependent as defined by the insured's plan. "Other" would indicate that the patient is other than the self, spouse, or child, which may include employee, ward, or dependent as defined by the insured's plan.

Instructions: Enter an "X" in the correct box to indicate the patient's relationship to the insured when Block 4 is completed. Only one box should be marked.

⚡ WORKERS' COMPENSATION CLAIMS

Check "Other."

🔀 PROPERTY AND CASUALTY CLAIMS

Check "Other."

5. PATIENT'S ADDRESS (No., Street)	6. PATIENT RELATIONSHIP TO INSURED	7. INSURED'S ADDRESS (No., Street)	
1456 Main Street	Self [X] Spouse [ ] Child [ ] Other [ ]		
CITY Woodland Hills STATE XY	8. RESERVED FOR NUCC USE	CITY	STATE
ZIP CODE 123450000 TELEPHONE (Include Area Code) ( )		ZIP CODE	TELEPHONE (Include Area Code) ( )

Block 7: Insured's Address The "Insured's Address" is the insured's permanent residence, which may be different from the patient's address in Block 5.

Instructions: Enter the insured's address and telephone number. Complete this item only when item 4 is completed. The first line is for the street address; the second line is for the city and state; the third line is for the zip code. Do not use punctuation or other symbols in the address. For example, use 123 N Main Street 101 instead of 123 N. Main Street, #101. When entering a 9-digit zip code, do not include the hyphen. If reporting a foreign address, contact payer for specific reporting instructions. "Insured's Telephone" does not exist in 5010A1. The NUCC recommends that the phone number not be reported.

⚡ WORKERS' COMPENSATION CLAIMS

Enter the employer's address. If required by a payer to report a telephone number, do not use a hyphen or space as a separator within the telephone number.

🔀 PROPERTY AND CASUALTY CLAIMS

Enter the address of the insured noted in Item Number 4. If required by a payer to report a telephone number, do not use a hyphen or space as a separator within the telephone number.

5. PATIENT'S ADDRESS (No., Street)	6. PATIENT RELATIONSHIP TO INSURED	7. INSURED'S ADDRESS (No., Street)		
1456 Main Street	Self [X] Spouse [ ] Child [ ] Other [ ]			
CITY STATE	8. RESERVED FOR NUCC USE	CITY		STATE
Woodland Hills XY				
ZIP CODE TELEPHONE (Include Area Code)		ZIP CODE TELEPHONE (Include Area Code)		
123450000 ( )		( )		

Block 8: Reserved for NUCC Use This field is reserved for NUCC use. The NUCC will provide instructions for any use of this field.

Instructions: This field was previously used to report "Patient Status." "Patient Status" does not exist in 5010A1, so this field has been eliminated.

2. PATIENT'S NAME (Last Name, First Name, Middle Initial)	3. PATIENT'S BIRTH DATE SEX	4. INSURED'S NAME (Last Name, First Name, Middle Initial)	
Forehand, Harry, N	MM DD YY	Forehand, Harry, N	
	01 06 1946 M[X] F[ ]		
5. PATIENT'S ADDRESS (No., Street)	6. PATIENT RELATIONSHIP TO INSURED	7. INSURED'S ADDRESS (No., Street)	
1456 Main Street	Self [X] Spouse [ ] Child [ ] Other [ ]	1456 Main Street	
CITY STATE	8. RESERVED FOR NUCC USE	CITY	STATE
Woodland Hills XY		Woodland Hills	XY
ZIP CODE TELEPHONE (Include Area Code)		ZIP CODE TELEPHONE (Include Area Code)	
123450000 ( )		123450000 ( )	
9. OTHER INSURED'S NAME (Last Name, First Name, Middle Initial)	10. IS PATIENT'S CONDITION RELATED TO:	11. INSURED'S POLICY GROUP OR FECA NUMBER	
Forehand, Susan		A482	
a. OTHER INSURED'S POLICY OR GROUP NUMBER	a. EMPLOYMENT? (Current or Previous)	a. INSURED'S DATE OF BIRTH SEX	
124897777	YES [ ] [X] NO	MM DD YY	
		01 06 1946 M[X] F[ ]	
b. RESERVED FOR NUCC USE	b. AUTO ACCIDENT? PLACE (State)	b. OTHER CLAIM ID (Designated by NUCC)	
	YES [ ] [X] NO		
c. RESERVED FOR NUCC USE	c. OTHER ACCIDENT?	c. INSURANCE PLAN NAME OR PROGRAM NAME	
	YES [ ] [X] NO	ABC Insurance Company	
d. INSURANCE PLAN NAME OR PROGRAM NAME	10d. CLAIM CODES (Designated by NUCC)	d. IS THERE ANOTHER HEALTH BENEFIT PLAN?	
Blue Shield		[X] YES [ ] NO *If yes,* complete items 9, 9a, and 9d.	

Block 9: Other Insured's Name The "Other Insured's Name" indicates that there is a holder of another (additional) policy that may cover the patient.

Instructions: If Block 11d is marked YES, complete fields 9, 9a, and 9d; otherwise, leave fields 9, 9a, and 9d blank. When additional group health coverage exists, enter other insured's full last name, first name, and middle initial of the enrollee in another health plan if it is different from that shown in Block 2. If the insured uses a last name suffix (for example, Jr., Sr.), enter it after the last name and before the first name. Titles (for example, Sister, Capt., Dr.) and professional suffixes (for example, PhD, MD, Esq.) should not be included with the name. Use commas to separate the last name, first name, and middle initial. A hyphen can be used for hyphenated names. Do not use periods within the name.

Block 9a: Other Insured's Policy or Group Number The "Other Insured's Policy or Group Number" identifies the policy or group number for coverage of the insured as indicated in Block 9.

Instructions: Enter the policy or group number of the other or secondary insured. Do not use a hyphen or space as a separator within the policy or group number.

Block 9b: Reserved for NUCC Use This field is reserved for NUCC use. NUCC will provide instructions for any use of this field.

Instructions: This field was previously used to report "Other Insured's Date of Birth, Sex." "Other Insured's Date of Birth, Sex" does not exist in 5010A1, so this field has been eliminated.

Block 9c: Reserved for NUCC Use This field is reserved for NUCC use. NUCC will provide instructions for any use of this field.

Instructions: This field was previously used to report "Employer's Name or School Name." "Employer's Name or School Name" does not exist in 5010A1, so this field has been eliminated.

Block 9d: Insurance Plan Name or Program Name The "Insurance Plan Name or Program Name" identifies the name of the additional plan or program of the other insured as indicated in Block 9.

Instructions: Enter the other or secondary insured's insurance plan or program name.

◎ MEDICARE/MEDIGAP CLAIMS

To ensure the crossover of Medicare/Medigap claims, complete Blocks 9 through 9d and list the payer identification (PAYRID) number of the Medigap (MG) plan in Block 9d. The PAYRID for MG plans is referred to as Other Carrier Name and Address (OCNA) number and is published in the Medicare newsletter. If automatic crossover capabilities are not offered in one's state, attach the Medicare Remittance Advice (RA) to the claim form and submit to the MG plan separately.

9. OTHER INSURED'S NAME (Last Name, First Name, Middle Initial)	10. IS PATIENT'S CONDITION RELATED TO:	11. INSURED'S POLICY GROUP OR FECA NUMBER
		A482
a. OTHER INSURED'S POLICY OR GROUP NUMBER	a. EMPLOYMENT? (Current or Previous) [ ]YES [X]NO	a. INSURED'S DATE OF BIRTH MM 01 DD 16 YY 1946 SEX M[X] F[ ]
b. RESERVED FOR NUCC USE	b. AUTO ACCIDENT? [ ]YES [X]NO PLACE (State)	b. OTHER CLAIM ID (Designated by NUCC)
c. RESERVED FOR NUCC USE	c. OTHER ACCIDENT? [ ]YES [X]NO	c. INSURANCE PLAN NAME OR PROGRAM NAME ABC Insurance Company
d. INSURANCE PLAN NAME OR PROGRAM NAME	10d. CLAIM CODES (Designated by NUCC)	d. IS THERE ANOTHER HEALTH BENEFIT PLAN? [ ]YES [X]NO If yes, complete items 9, 9a, and 9d.

Block 10a to 10c: Is Patient's Condition Related To "Is patient's condition related to" indicates whether the patient's illness or injury is related to employment, auto accident, or other accident.

"Employment (current or previous)" indicates that the condition is related to the patient's job or workplace. "Auto accident" indicates that the condition is the result of an automobile accident. "Other accident" indicates that the condition is the result of any other type of accident.

Instructions: When appropriate, enter an "X" in the correct box to indicate whether one or more of the services described in Block 24 are for a condition or injury that occurred on the job or as a result of an automobile or other accident. Only one box on each line should be marked.

The state postal code where the accident occurred must be reported if "YES" is marked in 10b for "Auto accident." Any item marked "YES" indicates that there may be other applicable insurance coverage that would be primary, such as automobile liability insurance. Primary insurance information must then be shown in Block 11.

9. OTHER INSURED'S NAME (Last Name, First Name, Middle Initial)	10. IS PATIENT'S CONDITION RELATED TO:	11. INSURED'S POLICY GROUP OR FECA NUMBER
		A482
a. OTHER INSURED'S POLICY OR GROUP NUMBER	a. EMPLOYMENT? (Current or Previous) [ ]YES [X]NO	a. INSURED'S DATE OF BIRTH MM 01 DD 16 YY 1946 SEX M[X] F[ ]
b. RESERVED FOR NUCC USE	b. AUTO ACCIDENT? [ ]YES [X]NO PLACE (State)	b. OTHER CLAIM ID (Designated by NUCC)
c. RESERVED FOR NUCC USE	c. OTHER ACCIDENT? [ ]YES [X]NO	c. INSURANCE PLAN NAME OR PROGRAM NAME ABC Insurance Company
d. INSURANCE PLAN NAME OR PROGRAM NAME	10d. CLAIM CODES (Designated by NUCC)	d. IS THERE ANOTHER HEALTH BENEFIT PLAN? [ ]YES [X]NO If yes, complete items 9, 9a, and 9d.

Block 10d: Claim Codes (Designated by the NUCC) The "Claim Codes" identify additional information about the patient's condition or the claim.

Instructions: When applicable, use the report "Claim Codes." Applicable claim codes are designated by the NUCC. Refer to the most current instructions from the public or private payer regarding the need to report claim codes.

When required by payers to provide the subset of condition codes approved by the NUCC, enter the "Condition Code" in this field. The condition codes approved for use on the 1500 Claim Form are available at www.nucc.org, under Code Sets.

⚡ WORKERS' COMPENSATION CLAIMS

A condition code is required when submitting a bill that is a duplicate (W2) or an appeal (W3 = Level 1, W4 = Level 2, W5 = Level 3). The original reference number must be entered in Block 22 for these conditions. *Note:* Do not use condition codes when submitting a revised or corrected bill.

9. OTHER INSURED'S NAME (Last Name, First Name, Middle Initial)	10. IS PATIENT'S CONDITION RELATED TO:	11. INSURED'S POLICY GROUP OR FECA NUMBER A482
a. OTHER INSURED'S POLICY OR GROUP NUMBER	a. EMPLOYMENT? (Current or Previous) ☐ YES ☒ NO	a. INSURED'S DATE OF BIRTH SEX MM ¦ DD ¦ YY 01 ¦ 16 ¦ 1946 M ☒ F ☐
b. RESERVED FOR NUCC USE	b. AUTO ACCIDENT? PLACE (State) ☐ YES ☒ NO	b. OTHER CLAIM ID (Designated by NUCC)
c. RESERVED FOR NUCC USE	c. OTHER ACCIDENT? ☐ YES ☒ NO	c. INSURANCE PLAN NAME OR PROGRAM NAME ABC Insurance Company
d. INSURANCE PLAN NAME OR PROGRAM NAME	10d. CLAIM CODES (Designated by NUCC)	d. IS THERE ANOTHER HEALTH BENEFIT PLAN? ☐ YES ☒ NO *If yes*, complete items 9, 9a, and 9d.

Block 11: Insured's Policy, Group, or FECA Number The "Insured's Policy, Group, or FECA Number" is the alphanumeric identifier for the health, auto, or other insurance plan coverage.

The FECA number is the 9-digit alphanumeric identifier assigned to a patient claiming work-related condition(s) under the Federal Employees' Compensation Act 5 USC 8101.

Instructions: Enter the insured's policy or group number as it appears on the insured's health care identification card. If Block 4 is completed, this field should be completed. Do not use a hyphen or space as a separator within the policy or group number.

Block 11a: Insured's Date of Birth, Sex The "Insured's Date of Birth, Sex" (gender) is the birth date and gender of the insured as indicated in Block 1a.

Instructions: Enter the 8-digit date of birth (MM/DD/YYYY) of the insured and an "X" to indicate the sex of the insured. Only one box should be marked. If gender is unknown, leave blank.

Block 11b: Other Claim ID (Designated by the NUCC) The "Other Claim ID" is another identifier applicable to the claim.

Instructions: Enter the "Other Claim ID." Applicable claim identifiers are designated by the NUCC.

WORKERS' COMPENSATION CLAIMS

The claim qualifier Y4 (Agency Claim Number) should be entered to the left of the vertical dotted line. Enter the claim ID number to the right of the vertical, dotted line (if known). The claim number is assigned by the payer.

PROPERTY AND CASUALTY CLAIMS

The claim qualifier Y4 (Agency Claim Number) should be entered to the left of the vertical dotted line. Enter the claim ID number to the right of the vertical dotted line (if known). The claim number is assigned by the payer.

Block 11c: Insurance Plan Name or Program Name The "Insurance Plan Name or Program Name" is the name of the plan or program of the insured as indicated in Block 1a.

Instructions: Enter the "Insurance Plan Name or Program Name" of the insured. Some payers require an identification number of the primary insurer rather than the name in this field.

Block 11d: Is There Another Health Benefit Plan? This block indicates that the patient has insurance coverage other than the plan indicated in Block 1.

Instructions: When appropriate, enter an "X" in the correct box. If marked "YES," complete Blocks 9, 9a, and 9d. Only one box can be marked.

READ BACK OF FORM BEFORE COMPLETING & SIGNING THIS FORM.

12. PATIENT'S OR AUTHORIZED PERSON'S SIGNATUREI authorize the release of any medical or other information necessary to process this claim. I also request payment of government benefits either to myself or to the party who accepts assignment below.

SIGNED *Harry N. Forehand*   DATE *March 3, 20XX*

13. INSURED'S OR AUTHORIZED PERSON'S SIGNATURE I authorize payment of medical benefits to the undersigned physician or supplier for services described below.

SIGNED *Harry N. Forehand*

A

READ BACK OF FORM BEFORE COMPLETING & SIGNING THIS FORM.

12. PATIENT'S OR AUTHORIZED PERSON'S SIGNATUREI authorize the release of any medical or other information necessary to process this claim. I also request payment of government benefits either to myself or to the party who accepts assignment below.

SIGNED ___ SIGNATURE ON FILE ___   DATE ___

13. INSURED'S OR AUTHORIZED PERSON'S SIGNATURE I authorize payment of medical benefits to the undersigned physician or supplier for services described below.

SIGNED ___ SIGNATURE ON FILE

B

Block 12: Patient's or Authorized Person's Signature This block indicates that there is an authorization on file for the release of any medical or other information necessary to process and adjudicate the claim. This block should be signed regardless of whether the health care organization is participating or nonparticipating. A form created by the health care organization may be used to keep the patient's signature on file in the office. This can be used instead of having a patient sign the CMS-1500. The signed authorization should be kept on file in the patient's medical record for an episode of care or for a designated time frame such as 1 year.

Instructions: Enter "Signature on File," "**SOF**," or legal signature. When legal signature is entered, enter the date signed in 6-digit (MMDDYY) or 8-digit (MMDDYYYY) format. If there is no signature on file, leave blank or enter "No Signature on File."

SOF situations that may occur in a health care organization are as follows:

Illiterate or physically handicapped. When an illiterate or physically handicapped enrollee signs by mark (X), a witness should sign his or her name and address next to the mark. If the claim is filed for the patient by another person, that person should enter the patient's name and write "By," sign his or her own name and address, indicate relationship to the patient, and state why the patient cannot sign.

Note: When completing the Workbook assignments, enter "Signature on File," not "SOF," in this block.

READ BACK OF FORM BEFORE COMPLETING & SIGNING THIS FORM.

12. PATIENT'S OR AUTHORIZED PERSON'S SIGNATUREI authorize the release of any medical or other information necessary to process this claim. I also request payment of government benefits either to myself or to the party who accepts assignment below.

SIGNED *Harry N. Forehand*   DATE *March 3, 20XX*

13. INSURED'S OR AUTHORIZED PERSON'S SIGNATURE I authorize payment of medical benefits to the undersigned physician or supplier for services described below.

SIGNED *Harry N. Forehand*

A

READ BACK OF FORM BEFORE COMPLETING & SIGNING THIS FORM.

12. PATIENT'S OR AUTHORIZED PERSON'S SIGNATUREI authorize the release of any medical or other information necessary to process this claim. I also request payment of government benefits either to myself or to the party who accepts assignment below.

SIGNED ___ SIGNATURE ON FILE ___   DATE ___

13. INSURED'S OR AUTHORIZED PERSON'S SIGNATURE I authorize payment of medical benefits to the undersigned physician or supplier for services described below.

SIGNED ___ SIGNATURE ON FILE

B

Block 13: Insured's or Authorized Person's Signature This block indicates that there is a signature on file authorizing payment of medical benefits.

Instructions: Enter "Signature on File," "SOF," or legal signature. If there is no signature on file, leave blank or enter "No Signature on File."

Note: When completing the Workbook assignments, enter "Signature on File," not "SOF," in this block.

14. DATE OF CURRENT: ILLNESS, INJURY, or PREGNANCY(LMP)   MM 03 DD 01 YY 20XX   QUAL. 431

15. OTHER DATE   QUAL.   MM DD YY

16. DATES PATIENT UNABLE TO WORK IN CURRENT OCCUPATION   FROM MM DD YY   TO MM DD YY

17. NAME OF REFERRING PROVIDER OR OTHER SOURCE   DN Perry Cardi MD

17a.
17b. NPI 67805027XX

18. HOSPITALIZATION DATES RELATED TO CURRENT SERVICES   FROM MM DD YY   TO MM DD YY

19. ADDITIONAL CLAIM INFORMATION (Designated by NUCC)

20. OUTSIDE LAB?   [ ] YES [X] NO $ CHARGES

Block 14: Date of Current Illness, Injury, or Pregnancy (LMP) This block identifies the first date of onset of illness, the actual date of injury, or the last menstrual period (LMP) for pregnancy.

Instructions: Enter the 6-digit (MMDDYY) or 8-digit (MMDDYYYY) date of the first date of the present illness, injury, or pregnancy. For pregnancy, use the date of the LMP as the first date.

Enter the applicable qualifier to the right of the vertical, dotted line to identify which date is being reported:

- 431: Onset of Current Symptoms or Illness
- 484: Last Menstrual Period

14. DATE OF CURRENT: ILLNESS, INJURY, or PREGNANCY(LMP)			15. OTHER DATE				16. DATES PATIENT UNABLE TO WORK IN CURRENT OCCUPATION					
MM	DD	YY	QUAL.	MM	DD	YY		MM	DD	YY	MM	DD	YY
03	01	20XX QUAL. 431					FROM				TO		

Block 15: Other Date The "Other Date" identifies additional date information about the patient's condition or treatment.

Instructions: Enter an "Other Date" related to the patient's condition or treatment. Enter the date in the 6-digit (MMDDYY) or 8-digit (MMDDYYYY) format. Previous pregnancies are not a similar illness. Leave blank if unknown.

Enter the applicable qualifier between the vertical, dotted lines to identify which date is being reported.

- 454: Initial Treatment
- 304: Latest Visit or Consultation
- 453: Acute Manifestation of a Chronic Condition
- 439: Accident
- 455: Last x-ray
- 471: Prescription
- 090: Report Star (assumed care date)
- 444: Fist Visit or Consultation

14. DATE OF CURRENT: ILLNESS, INJURY, or PREGNANCY(LMP)			15. OTHER DATE				16. DATES PATIENT UNABLE TO WORK IN CURRENT OCCUPATION					
MM	DD	YY	QUAL.	MM	DD	YY		MM	DD	YY	MM	DD	YY
03	01	20XX QUAL. 431					FROM 03	04	20XX	TO 03	04	20XX	

Block 16: Dates Patient Unable to Work in Current Occupation Block 16 indicates the time span the patient is or was unable to work.

Instructions: If the patient is employed and is unable to work in current occupation, a 6-digit (MMDDYY) or 8-digit (MMDDYYYY) date must be shown for the "from-to" dates that the patient is unable to work. An entry in this field may indicate employment-related insurance coverage.

Note: When completing the Workbook assignments, enter information when it is documented in the medical record.

17. NAME OF REFERRING PROVIDER OR OTHER SOURCE	17a.	G2	ABC1234567890	18. HOSPITALIZATION DATES RELATED TO CURRENT SERVICES					
DN Perry Cardi MD	17b.	NPI	67805027XX	MM	DD	YY	MM	DD	YY
				FROM			TO		
19. ADDITIONAL CLAIM INFORMATION (Designated by NUCC)				20. OUTSIDE LAB? ☐ YES ☒ NO			$ CHARGES		

Block 17: Name of Referring Provider or Other Source The name entered is the referring provider, ordering provider, or supervising provider who referred, ordered, or supervised the service(s) or supply(ies) on the claim. The qualifier indicates the role of the provider being reported.

Instructions: Enter the name (first name, middle initial, last name) and credentials of the professional who referred, ordered, or supervised the service(s) or supply(ies) on the claim.

If multiple providers are involved, enter one provider using the following priority order:

1. Referring provider
2. Ordering provider
3. Supervising provider

Do not use periods or commas within the name. A hyphen can be used for hyphenated names.

Enter the applicable qualifier to the left of the vertical, dotted line to identify which provider is being reported.

- DN Referring provider
- DK Ordering provider
- DQ Supervising provider

Block 17a: Other ID Number The non-NPI ID number of the referring, ordering, or supervising provider is the unique identifier of the professional or provider designated taxonomy code.

Instructions: The "Other ID Number" of the referring, ordering, or supervising provider is reported in 17a, the shaded area. The qualifier indicating what the number represents is reported in the qualifier field to the immediate right of 17a.

The NUCC defines the following qualifiers used in 5010A1:

- 0B State License Number
- 1G Provider UPIN Number
- G2 Provider Commercial Number
- LU Location Number (This qualifier is used for supervising provider only.)

Block 17b: NPI The NPI number refers to the HIPAA NPI number.

Instructions: Enter the 10-digit NPI number of the referring, ordering, or supervising provider in Block 17b.

17. NAME OF REFERRING PROVIDER OR OTHER SOURCE	17a.		18. HOSPITALIZATION DATES RELATED TO CURRENT SERVICES
DN Perry Cardi MD	17b. NPI	67805027XX	MM DD YY MM DD YY FROM 03 01 20XX TO 03 03 20XX

Block 18: Hospitalization Dates Related to Current Services Information in this field refers to an inpatient hospital stay and indicates the admission and discharge dates associated with the service(s) on the claim.

Instructions: Enter the inpatient 6-digit (MMDDYY) or 8-digit (MMDDYYYY) hospital admission date followed by the discharge date (if discharge has occurred). If not discharged, leave discharge date blank. This date is when a medical service is furnished as a result of or subsequent to a related hospitalization.

19. ADDITIONAL CLAIM INFORMATION (Designated by NUCC)	20. OUTSIDE LAB?	$ CHARGES
NTEADDSurgery was unusually long due to scarring	☐ YES ☒ NO	

A

19. ADDITIONAL CLAIM INFORMATION (Designated by NUCC)	20. OUTSIDE LAB?	$ CHARGES
REFG21234567890	☐ YES ☒ NO	

B

19. ADDITIONAL CLAIM INFORMATION (Designated by NUCC)	20. OUTSIDE LAB?	$ CHARGES
PWK03AA12363545465	☐ YES ☒ NO	

C

19. ADDITIONAL CLAIM INFORMATION (Designated by NUCC)	20. OUTSIDE LAB?	$ CHARGES
NTEADDSurgery was unusually long due to scarring PWKOBBM1213141	☐ YES ☒ NO	

D

Block 19: Additional Claim Information (Designated by the NUCC) Block 19 identifies additional information about the patient's condition or the claim.

Instructions: Refer to the most current instructions from the public or private payer regarding use of this field. Some payers ask for certain identifiers in this field. Do not enter a space, hyphen, or other separator between the qualifier code and the number.

When reporting a second item of data, enter three blank spaces and then the next qualifier and number/code/information.

For additional claim information, the NUCC defines the following qualifiers, used in 5010A1:
- ADD: Additional Information
- CER: Certification Narrative
- DCP: Goals, Rehabilitation Potential, or Discharge Plans
- DGN: Diagnosis Description
- TPO: Third Party Organization Notes

When using the qualifiers listed above, enter the qualifier "NTE," followed by the appropriate qualifier, then the information. Do not enter spaces between the qualifier and the first word of the information. After the qualifier, use spaces to separate any words. Example: "NTEADDSurgery was unusually long due to abdominal scarring."

⚡ WORKERS' COMPENSATION CLAIMS

Additional claim information is required based on jurisdictional WC guidelines.

19. ADDITIONAL CLAIM INFORMATION (Designated by NUCC)	20. OUTSIDE LAB?	$ CHARGES
	[X] YES [ ] NO	125 | 00

Block 20: Outside Lab? $Charges A **purchased service provider** is an individual or entity that performs a service on a contractual basis for a separate provider who is billing for the service. For example, a health care organization may purchase processing of a lab specimen from an outside lab; however, the health care organization bills for the service and reimburses the outside lab for its services under a contract.

Instructions: A "NO" is checked to indicate that there was no purchased service included on the claim. A "YES" is checked to indicate that there is, in fact, a purchased service included on the claim. If a "YES" is annotated, enter the purchase price under "$Charges" and complete Block 32. Each purchased service must be reported on a separate claim form because only one charge can be entered.

When entering the charge amount, enter the amount in the field to the left of the vertical line. The entered number should be right-justified to the left of the vertical line. Enter "00" for cents if the amount is a whole number. Do not use dollar signs, commas, or a decimal point when reporting amounts. Negative dollar amounts are not allowed. Leave the right field blank.

21. DIAGNOSIS OR NATURE OF ILLNESS OR INJURY Relate A-L to service line below (24E) ICD Ind. 0	22. RESUBMISSION CODE | ORIGINAL REF. NO.
A. H66009 B. C. D. E. F. G. H. I. J. K. L.	23. PRIOR AUTHORIZATION NUMBER

Block 21: Diagnosis or Nature of Illness or Injury The "ICD indicator" identifies the version of the International Classification of Diseases (ICD) code set being reported. The "Diagnosis or Nature of Illness or Injury" is the sign, symptom, complaint, or condition of the patient relating to the service(s) on the claim.

Instructions: Enter the applicable ICD indicator to identify which version of ICD codes is being reported.
- 9 ICD-9-CM
- 0 ICD-10-CM
- Enter the indicator between the vertical, dotted lines.

Enter the patient's diagnosis and/or condition codes. Do not include the decimal point in the diagnosis code; it is implied. List no more than 12 ICD-9-CM or ICD-10-CM diagnosis codes. Relate lines A to L to the lines of service in Block 24E by the letter of the line. Use the highest level of specificity. This block specifically links medical necessity to the billing claim.

21. DIAGNOSIS OR NATURE OF ILLNESS OR INJURY Relate A-L to service line below (24E) ICD Ind. 0	22. RESUBMISSION CODE | ORIGINAL REF. NO. 7 | ABC123456888
A. H66009 B. C. D. E. F. G. H. I. J. K. L.	23. PRIOR AUTHORIZATION NUMBER

Block 22: Resubmission and/or Original Reference Number "Resubmission" means the code and original reference number assigned by the destination payer or receiver to indicate a previously submitted claim or encounter.

Instructions: List the original reference number for resubmitted claims. Refer to the most current instructions from the public or private payer regarding use of this field (that is, code).

When resubmitting a claim, enter the appropriate bill frequency code so that it is left-justified in the left side of the field.
- 7 Replacement of prior claim
- 8 Void/cancel of prior claim

This block is not intended for use of original claim submissions.

21. DIAGNOSIS OR NATURE OF ILLNESS OR INJURY Relate A-L to service line below (24E) ICD Ind. 0	22. RESUBMISSION CODE | ORIGINAL REF. NO.
A. H66009 B. C. D. E. F. G. H. I. J. K. L.	23. PRIOR AUTHORIZATION NUMBER 12345679090A

Block 23: Prior Authorization Number This block identifies the payer-assigned number authorizing the service(s).

Instructions: Enter any of the following: prior authorization number, referral number, mammography precertification number, or Clinical Laboratory Improvement Amendments (CLIA) number, as assigned by the payer for the current service.

Do not enter hyphens or spaces within the number.

◎ MEDICARE CLAIMS

When laboratory services are performed in the health care office, the 10-digit CLIA certificate number should be entered in Block 23. Health care providers who are billing patients for outside lab work are not held to CLIA standards but may charge the patient only what the laboratory charges, plus any additional services the health care organization provides, such as drawing, shipping, and handling.

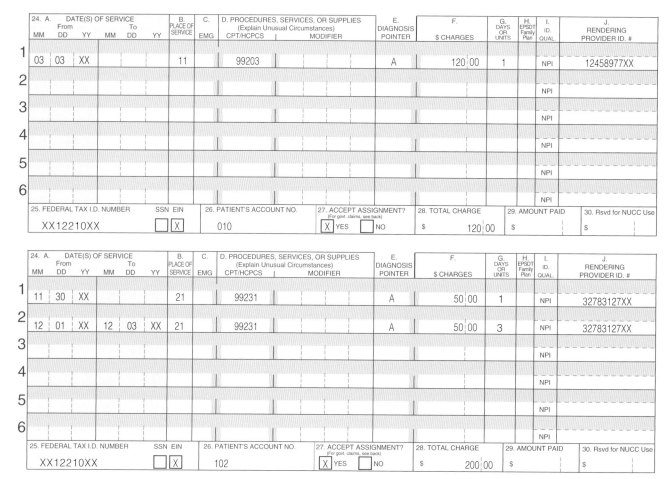

Block 24A: Date(s) of Service (Lines 1 to 6) Block 24A indicates the actual month, day, and year the service(s) was provided. Grouping services refers to a charge for a series of identical services without listing each date of service.

Instructions: Enter date(s) of service, both the "From" and "To" dates. If there is only one date of service, enter that date under "From." Leave "To" blank or re-enter the "From" date. If grouping services, the place of service, procedure code, charges, and individual provider for each line must be identical for that service. Grouping is allowed only for services on consecutive days. The number of days must correspond to the number of units in Block 24G.

When required by payers to provide additional anesthesia services information (e.g, anesthesia begin and end times), narrative description of an unspecified code, National Drug Code (NDC), contract rate, or tooth numbers and areas of the oral cavity, enter the applicable qualifier and number/code/information, starting with the first space in the shaded line of this field. Do not enter a space, hyphen, or other separator between the qualifier and the number/code/information. The information may extend to Block 24G.

Block 24B: Place of Service (Lines 1 to 6) This block identifies the location where the service was rendered.

Instructions: In Block 24B, enter the appropriate two-digit code from the Place of Service Code list for each item used or service performed. The Place of Service Codes can be referenced in Table 14.3 and are available at www.cms.gov/Medicare/Coding/place-of-service-codes/Place_of_Service_Code_set.html.

TABLE 14.3 Place of Service Codes

BLOCK 24B	
Place of Service CODES	**Place of Service Description**
01	Pharmacy
02	Telehealth
03	School
04	Homeless shelter
05	Indian health services free-standing facility
06	Indian health services provider-based facility
07	Tribal 638 free-standing facility
08	Tribal 638 provider-based facility
09	Prison/correctional facility
10	Unassigned
11	Office
12	Patient's home
13	Assisted living facility
14	Group home
15	Mobile unit
16	Temporary lodging
17	Walk-in retail health clinic
18	Place of employment—worksite
19	Off campus—outpatient hospital
20	Urgent care facility
21	Inpatient hospital
22	On campus—outpatient hospital
23	Emergency department—hospital
24	Ambulatory surgical center
25	Birthing center
26	Military treatment facility/uniformed service treatment facility
27–30	Unassigned
31	Skilled nursing facility (swing bed visits)
32	Nursing facility (intermediate/long-term care facilities)
33	Custodial care facility (domiciliary or rest home services)
34	Hospice (domiciliary or rest home services)
35–40	Unassigned
41	Ambulance—land
42	Ambulance—air or water
43–48	Unassigned
49	Independent clinic
50	Federally qualified health center
51	Inpatient psychiatric facility
52	Psychiatric facility—partial hospitalization
53	Community mental health care (outpatient, 24-hours-a-day services, admission screening, consultation, and educational services)
54	Intermediate care facility/individuals with intellectual disabilities
55	Residential substance abuse treatment facility
56	Psychiatric residential treatment facility
57	Nonresidential substance abuse treatment facility
58	Non-residential Opioid Treatment Facility
59	Unassigned
60	Mass immunization center
61	Comprehensive inpatient rehabilitation facility
62	Comprehensive outpatient rehabilitation facility
63–64	Unassigned
65	End-stage renal disease treatment facility
66–70	Unassigned
71	State or local public health clinic
72	Rural health clinic
73–80	Unassigned
81	Independent laboratory
82–90	Unassigned
99	Other place of service not identified above

24. A. DATE(S) OF SERVICE From / To MM DD YY / MM DD YY	B. PLACE OF SERVICE	C. EMG	D. PROCEDURES, SERVICES, OR SUPPLIES CPT/HCPCS | MODIFIER	E. DIAGNOSIS POINTER	F. $ CHARGES	G. DAYS OR UNITS	H. EPSDT Family Plan	I. ID. QUAL.	J. RENDERING PROVIDER ID. #
1 03 03 XX	11		99203	A	120 00	1		NPI	12458977XX
2								NPI	
3								NPI	
4								NPI	
5								NPI	
6								NPI	

25. FEDERAL TAX I.D. NUMBER XX12210XX SSN EIN [X] | 26. PATIENT'S ACCOUNT NO. 010 | 27. ACCEPT ASSIGNMENT? [X] YES [ ] NO | 28. TOTAL CHARGE $ 120 00 | 29. AMOUNT PAID $ | 30. Rsvd for NUCC Use $

Block 24C: EMG (Lines 1 to 6) "EMG" identifies whether the service was an emergency.

Instructions: Check with the payer to determine whether this element is necessary. If required, enter "Y" for "YES," or leave blank if "NO" in the bottom, unshaded area of the field. The definition of an emergency would be defined by federal or state regulations, programs or payer contract, or would be as defined in 5010A1.

24. A. DATE(S) OF SERVICE From / To MM DD YY / MM DD YY	B. PLACE OF SERVICE	C. EMG	D. PROCEDURES, SERVICES, OR SUPPLIES CPT/HCPCS | MODIFIER	E. DIAGNOSIS POINTER	F. $ CHARGES	G. DAYS OR UNITS	H. EPSDT Family Plan	I. ID. QUAL.	J. RENDERING PROVIDER ID. #
1 03 03 XX	11		99203 | 25	A	120 00	1		NPI	12458977XX
2 03 03 XX	11		10060 | 25	B	130 00	1		NPI	12458977XX
3								NPI	
4								NPI	
5								NPI	
6								NPI	

25. FEDERAL TAX I.D. NUMBER XX12210XX SSN EIN [X] | 26. PATIENT'S ACCOUNT NO. 010 | 27. ACCEPT ASSIGNMENT? [X] YES [ ] NO | 28. TOTAL CHARGE $ 250 00 | 29. AMOUNT PAID $ | 30. Rsvd for NUCC Use $

Block 24D: Procedures, Services, or Supplies (Lines 1 to 6) This block identifies the medical services and procedures provided to the patient.

Instructions: Enter the Current Procedural Terminology (CPT) or Health care Common Procedure Coding System (HCPCS) code(s) and modifier(s) (if applicable) from the appropriate code set in effect on the date of service. This field accommodates the entry of up to four two-digit modifiers. The specific procedure code(s) must be shown without a narrative description.

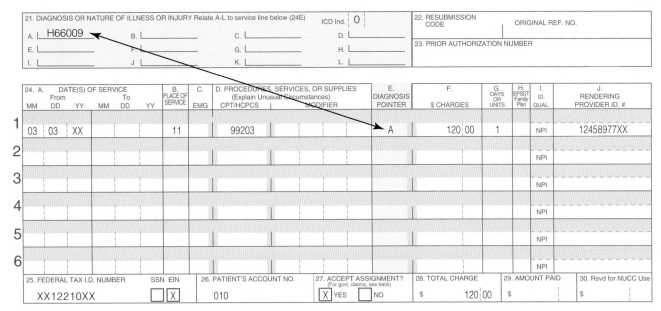

Block 24E: Diagnosis Pointer (Lines 1 to 6) The "Diagnosis Pointer" is the line letter from Block 21 that relates to the reason the service(s) was performed.

Instructions: In Block 24E, enter the diagnosis code reference letter (pointer) as shown in Block 21 to relate the date of service and the procedures performed to the primary diagnosis. When multiple services are performed, the primary reference number for each service should be listed first and other applicable services should follow. The reference letter(s) should be A to L or multiple letters as applicable. ICD-9-CM or ICD-10-CM diagnosis codes must be entered in Block 21 only. Do not enter them in Block 24E.

Enter numbers left-justified in the field. Do not use commas between the numbers.

Block 24F: $Charges (Lines 1 to 6) This block indicates the total billed amount for each service line.

Instructions: Enter the charge for each listed service.

Enter numbers right-justified in the dollar area of the field. Do not use commas when reporting dollar amounts. Negative dollar amounts are not allowed. Dollar signs should not be entered. Enter "00" in the cents area if the amount is a whole number.

24. A. DATE(S) OF SERVICE						B. PLACE OF SERVICE	C. EMG	D. PROCEDURES, SERVICES, OR SUPPLIES (Explain Unusual Circumstances)		E. DIAGNOSIS POINTER	F. $ CHARGES	G. DAYS OR UNITS	H. EPSDT Family Plan	I. ID. QUAL.	J. RENDERING PROVIDER ID. #
	From			To				CPT/HCPCS	MODIFIER						
MM	DD	YY	MM	DD	YY										
1	03	03	XX				11		99203		A	120 00	1		NPI	12458977XX
2															NPI	
3															NPI	
4															NPI	
5															NPI	
6															NPI	

25. FEDERAL TAX I.D. NUMBER	SSN EIN	26. PATIENT'S ACCOUNT NO.	27. ACCEPT ASSIGNMENT? (For govt. claims, see back)	28. TOTAL CHARGE	29. AMOUNT PAID	30. Rsvd for NUCC Use
XX12210XX	☐ ☒	010	☒ YES ☐ NO	$ 120 00	$	$

Block 24G: Days or Units (Lines 1 to 6) This block indicates the number of days corresponding to the dates entered in Block 24A or units as defined in CPT or HCPCS coding manual(s).

Instructions: Enter the number of days or units. This block is most commonly used for multiple visits, units of supplies, anesthesia units or minutes, or oxygen volume. If only one service is performed, the numeral "1" must be entered.

Enter numbers left-justified in this block. No leading zeros are required. If reporting a fraction of a unit, use the decimal point.

Anesthesia services must be reported as minutes. Units may only be reported for anesthesia services when the codes description includes a time period, such as "daily management."

24. A. DATE(S) OF SERVICE						B. PLACE OF SERVICE	C. EMG	D. PROCEDURES, SERVICES, OR SUPPLIES (Explain Unusual Circumstances)		E. DIAGNOSIS POINTER	F. $ CHARGES	G. DAYS OR UNITS	H. EPSDT Family Plan	I. ID. QUAL.	J. RENDERING PROVIDER ID. #
	From			To				CPT/HCPCS	MODIFIER						
MM	DD	YY	MM	DD	YY										
1	03	03	XX				11		99203		A	120 00	1		NPI	12458977XX
2															NPI	
3															NPI	
4															NPI	
5															NPI	
6															NPI	

25. FEDERAL TAX I.D. NUMBER	SSN EIN	26. PATIENT'S ACCOUNT NO.	27. ACCEPT ASSIGNMENT? (For govt. claims, see back)	28. TOTAL CHARGE	29. AMOUNT PAID	30. Rsvd for NUCC Use
XX12210XX	☐ ☒	010	☒ YES ☐ NO	$ 120 00	$	$

Block 24H: EPSDT/Family Plan (Lines 1 to 6) The "EPSDT/Family Plan" identifies certain services that may be covered under some state Medicaid plans.

Instructions: For Early and Periodic Screening, Diagnosis, and Treatment (**EPSDT**)-related services, enter the response in the shaded portion of the field as follows.

If there is a requirement to report a reason code for EPDST, enter the appropriate reason code as noted below. (A "Y" or "N" response is not entered with the code.) The two-character code is right-justified in the shaded area of the field.

The following codes for EPSDT are used in 5010A1:
- AV Available—Not Used (Patient refused referral.)
- S2 Under Treatment (Patient is currently under treatment for referred diagnostic or corrective treatment or is scheduled for another appointment with screening provider for diagnostic or corrective treatment for at least one health problem identified during an initial or periodic screening service, not including dental referrals.)
- ST New Service Requested (Referral to another provider for diagnostic or corrective treatment/scheduled for another appointment with screening provider for diagnostic or corrective treatment for at least one health problem identified during an initial or periodic screening service, not including dental referrals.)
- NU—Not Used (Used when no EPSDT patient referral was given.)
- If the service is Family Planning, enter "Y" ("YES") or "N" ("NO") in the bottom, unshaded area of the field.

When there is no requirement to report that this is a Family Planning Service, leave the field blank.

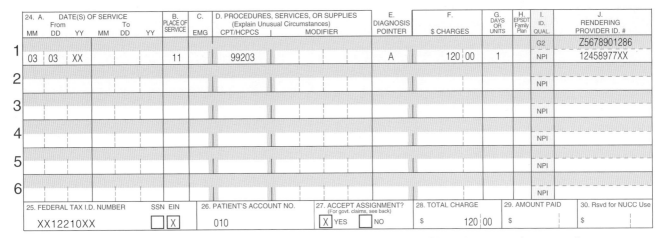

Block 24I: ID Qualifier (Lines 1 to 6) If the provider does not have an NPI number, enter the appropriate qualifier and non-NPI identifying number in the shaded area.

The qualifiers will indicate the non-NPI number being reported.

Instructions: Enter in the shaded area of Block 24I the qualifier, identifying if the number is a non-NPI. The other ID number of the rendering provider should be reported in Block 24J in the shaded area.

The NUCC defines the following qualifiers used in 5010A1:

- 0B State License Number
- 1G Provider UPIN Number
- G2 Provider Commercial Number
- LU Location Number
- ZZ Provider Taxonomy (The qualifier in the 5010A1 for Provider Taxonomy is PXC, but ZZ remains the qualifier for the 1500 Claim Form.)

The above list contains both provider identifiers and the provider taxonomy code. The provider identifiers are assigned to the provider either by a specific payer or by a third party to uniquely identify the provider. The taxonomy code is designated by the provider in order to identify the provider type, classification, and area of specialization. Both provider identifiers and provider taxonomy may be used in this field.

The rendering provider is the person or company (laboratory or other facility) that rendered or supervised the care. In the case where a substitute provider (locum tenens) was used, enter that provider's information here. Report the identification number in Blocks 24I and 24J only when different from data recorded in Blocks 33a and 33b.

Block 24J: Rendering Provider ID. # (Lines 1 to 6) The individual performing or rendering the service should be reported in Block 24J and the qualifier indicating if the number is a non-NPI goes in Block 24I. The non-NPI ID number of the rendering provider refers to the payer-assigned unique identifier of the professional.

Instructions: The individual rendering the service should be reported in Block 24J. Enter the non-NPI ID number in the shaded area of the field. Enter the NPI number in the unshaded area of the field.

The rendering provider is the person or company (laboratory or other facility) that rendered or supervised the care. In the case where a substitute provider (locum tenens) was used, enter that provider's information here. Report the identification number in Blocks 24I and 24J only when different from data recorded in Blocks 33a and 33b. Enter numbers so that they are left-justified in the block.

INSTRUCTIONS AND EXAMPLES OF SUPPLEMENTAL INFORMATION IN BLOCK 24

The following are types of supplemental information that can be entered in the shaded areas of Block 24:

- Narrative descriptions of unspecified codes
- National Drug Codes (NDC) for drugs
- Device Identifier of the Unique Device Identifier for supplies
- Contract rate
- Tooth numbers and areas of the oral cavity

The following qualifiers are to be used when reporting these services:

- ZZ Narrative Description of Unspecified Code
- N4 National Drug Codes (NDC)
- DI Device Identifier of the Unique Device Identifier (UDI)
- CTR Contract Rate
- JP Universal/National Tooth Designation System
- JO ANSI/ADA/ISO Specification No. 3950-1984 Dentistry Designation System for Tooth and Areas of the Oral Cavity

If required to report other supplemental information not listed above, follow payer instructions for the use of a qualifier for the information being reported. When reporting a service that does not have a qualifier, enter two blank spaces before entering the information.

To enter supplemental information, begin at Block 24A by entering the qualifier and then the information. Do not enter a space between the qualifier and the number/code/information. Do not enter hyphens or spaces with the number/code.

More than one supplemental item can be reported in the shaded lines of Block 24. Enter the first qualifier and number/code/information at Block 24A. After the first item, enter three blank spaces and then the next qualifier and number/code/information.

When reporting dollar amounts in the shaded area, always enter the dollar amount, a decimal point, and cents. Use "00" for the cents if the amount is a whole number. Do not use commas. Do not enter dollar signs.

Additional Information for Reporting NDC

When entering supplemental information for NDC, add in the following order: qualifier, NDC code, one space, unit/basis of measurement qualifier, quantity. The number of digits for the quantity is limited to eight digits before the decimal and three digits after the decimal. If entering a whole number, do not use a decimal. Do not use commas.

When a dollar amount is being reported, enter the following after the quantity: one space, dollar amount. Do not enter a dollar sign.

The following qualifiers are to be used when reporting NDC unit/basis of measurement:

- F2 International Unit
- ME Milligram
- ML Milliliter
- GR Gram
- UN Unit

Additional Information for Reporting Tooth Numbers and Areas of the Oral Cavity

When reporting tooth numbers, add in the following order: qualifier, tooth number (for example, JP16). When reporting an area of the oral cavity, enter in the following order: qualifier, area of oral cavity code (for example, J010).

When reporting multiple tooth numbers for one procedure, add in the following order: qualifier, tooth number, blank space, tooth number, blank space, tooth number, and so on (for example, JP1 16 17 32).

When reporting multiple tooth numbers for one procedure, the number of units reported in Block 24G is the number of teeth involved in the procedure.

When reporting multiple areas of the oral cavity for one procedure, add in the following order: qualifier, oral cavity code, blank space, oral cavity code, and so on (for example, J010 20).

When reporting multiple areas of the oral cavity for one procedure, the number of units reported in Block 24G is the number of areas of the oral cavity involved in the procedure.

The following are the codes for tooth numbers, reported with the JP qualifier:

- 1-32 Permanent dentition
- 51-82 Permanent supernumerary dentition
- A-T Primary dentition
- AS-TS Primary supernumerary dentition

The following are the codes for areas of the oral cavity, reported with the JO qualifier:

- 00 Entire oral cavity
- 01 Maxillary arch
- 02 Mandibular arch
- 10 Upper right quadrant
- 20 Upper left quadrant
- 30 Lower left quadrant
- 40 Lower right quadrant

For further information on these codes, refer to the Current Dental Terminology (CDT) Manual available from the American Dental Association.

25. FEDERAL TAX I.D. NUMBER	SSN EIN	26. PATIENT'S ACCOUNT NO.	27. ACCEPT ASSIGNMENT? (For govt. claims, see back)	28. TOTAL CHARGE	29. AMOUNT PAID	30. Rsvd for NUCC Use
XX12210XX	☐ ☒	010	☒ YES ☐ NO	$ 120 ¦ 00	$	$

Block 25: Federal Tax ID Number The "Federal Tax ID Number" is the unique identifier assigned by a federal or state agency.

Instructions: Enter the "Federal Tax ID Number" (EIN or SSN) of the billing provider identified in Block 33. This is the tax ID number intended to be used for 1099 reporting purposes. Enter an "X" in the appropriate box to indicate which number is being reported. Only one box can be marked.

Do not enter hyphens with numbers. Enter numbers so that they are left-justified in the field.

When completing the Workbook assignments, enter the group's federal tax ID number and check the appropriate box except in Medicare/Medigap cases.

25. FEDERAL TAX I.D. NUMBER	SSN EIN	26. PATIENT'S ACCOUNT NO.	27. ACCEPT ASSIGNMENT? (For govt. claims, see back)	28. TOTAL CHARGE	29. AMOUNT PAID	30. Rsvd for NUCC Use
XX12210XX	☐ ☒	010	☒ YES ☐ NO	$ 120 00	$	$

Block 26: Patient's Account No. The "Patient's Account No." is the identifier assigned by the health care organization.

Instructions: Enter the patient's account number assigned by the service provider's or supplier's accounting system.

Do not enter hyphens with numbers. Enter numbers so that they are left-justified in the field.

Note: When completing the Workbook *assignments, list the patient account number when provided.*

25. FEDERAL TAX I.D. NUMBER	SSN EIN	26. PATIENT'S ACCOUNT NO.	27. ACCEPT ASSIGNMENT? (For govt. claims, see back)	28. TOTAL CHARGE	29. AMOUNT PAID	30. Rsvd for NUCC Use
XX12210XX	☐ ☒	010	☒ YES ☐ NO	$ 120 00	$	$

Block 27: Accept Assignment? "Accept Assignment?" indicates that the health care organization agrees to accept assignment under the terms of the payer's program.

Instructions: Enter an "X" in the correct box. Only one box can be marked.

Report "Accept Assignment?" for all payers.

⊚ MEDICARE/MEDICAID CLAIMS

For Medi-Medi claims, check "Yes" for assignment in Block 27. If the provider does not accept assignment, then payment will go to the patient and Medicaid will not pick up the residual.

25. FEDERAL TAX I.D. NUMBER	SSN EIN	26. PATIENT'S ACCOUNT NO.	27. ACCEPT ASSIGNMENT? (For govt. claims, see back)	28. TOTAL CHARGE	29. AMOUNT PAID	30. Rsvd for NUCC Use
XX12210XX	☐ ☒	010	☒ YES ☐ NO	$ 120 00	$	$

Block 28: Total Charge This block indicates the total billed amount for all services entered in Block 24F (Lines 1 to 6).

Instructions: Enter the total charges for the services (that is, total of all charges in Block 24F).

Enter the amount so that it is right-justified in the dollar area of the field. Do not use commas. Negative dollar amounts are not allowed. Dollar signs should not be entered. Enter "00" in the cents area if the amount is a whole number.

25. FEDERAL TAX I.D. NUMBER	SSN EIN	26. PATIENT'S ACCOUNT NO.	27. ACCEPT ASSIGNMENT? (For govt. claims, see back)	28. TOTAL CHARGE	29. AMOUNT PAID	30. Rsvd for NUCC Use
XX12210XX	☐ ☒	010	☒ YES ☐ NO	$ 120 00	$	$

Block 29: Amount Paid This block indicates payment received from the patient or other payers.

Instructions: Enter the total amount that the patient and/or other payers paid on the covered services only.

Enter the number so that it is right-justified in the dollar area of the field. Do not use commas when reporting dollar amounts. Negative dollar amounts are not allowed. Dollar signs should not be entered. Enter "00" in the cents area if the amount is a whole number.

25. FEDERAL TAX I.D. NUMBER	SSN EIN	26. PATIENT'S ACCOUNT NO.	27. ACCEPT ASSIGNMENT? (For govt. claims, see back)	28. TOTAL CHARGE	29. AMOUNT PAID	30. Rsvd for NUCC Use
XX12210XX	☐ ☒	010	☒ YES ☐ NO	$ 120 00	$	$

Block 30: Reserved for NUCC Use This field is reserved for NUCC use. The NUCC will provide instructions for any use of this field.

Instructions: This field was previously used to report "Balance Due." "Balance Due" does not exist in 5010A1, so this field has been eliminated.

31. SIGNATURE OF PHYSICIAN OR SUPPLIER INCLUDING DEGREES OR CREDENTIALS (I certify that the statements on the reverse apply to this bill and are made a part thereof.)	32. SERVICE FACILITY LOCATION INFORMATION		33. BILLING PROVIDER INFO & PH # (555) 4869002
Concha Antrum MD 030320XX			College Clinic 4567 Broad Avenue Woodland Hills XY 123450001
SIGNED *Concha Antrum MD* DATE	a. NPI	b.	a. 3664021CC	b.

Block 31: Signature of Physician or Supplier Including Degrees or Credentials This block refers to the authorized or accountable person and the degree, credentials, or title.

Instructions: "Signature of Physician or Supplier Including Degrees or Credentials" does not exist in 5010A1.

Enter the legal signature of the practitioner or supplier, signature of the practitioner or supplier representative, "Signature on File," or "SOF." Enter either the 6-digit date (MM/DD/YY), 8-digit date (MM/DD/YYYY), or alphanumeric date (for example, January 1, 2003) on which the form was signed.

31. SIGNATURE OF PHYSICIAN OR SUPPLIER INCLUDING DEGREES OR CREDENTIALS (I certify that the statements on the reverse apply to this bill and are made a part thereof.)	32. SERVICE FACILITY LOCATION INFORMATION		33. BILLING PROVIDER INFO & PH # (555) 4869002
Concha Antrum MD 030320XX	College Hospital 4500 Broad Avenue Woodland Hills XY 123450001		College Clinic 4567 Broad Avenue Woodland Hills XY 123450001
SIGNED *Concha Antrum MD* DATE	a. X950731067	b. G2A1234567890	a. 3664021CC	b.

Block 32: Service Facility Location Information The name and address of the facility where services were rendered identifies the site where services were provided.

Instructions: Enter the name, address, city, state, and zip code of the location where the services were rendered. Providers of service must identify the supplier's name, address, zip code, and NPI number when billing for purchased diagnostic tests. When more than one supplier is used, a separate 1500 Claim Form should be used to bill for each supplier.

Enter the name and address information in the following format: Do not use punctuation (that is, commas and periods) or other symbols in the address (for example, use 123 N Main Street 101 instead of 123 N. Main Street, #101). Enter a space between the town name and state code; do not include a comma. When reporting a 9-digit zip code, do not include the hyphen.

If reporting a foreign address, contact payer for specific reporting instructions.

Block 32a: NPI# The NPI number refers to the HIPAA NPI number.

Instructions: If a service facility is entered in Block 32, enter the NPI number of the service facility location in Block 32a.

Only report a Service Facility Location NPI when the NPI is different from the Billing Provider NPI.

Block 32b: Other ID# The non-NPI ID number of the service facility is the payer-assigned unique identifier of the facility.

Instructions: Enter the two-digit qualifier identifying the non-NPI number, followed by the ID number. Do not enter a space, hyphen, or other separator between the qualifier and number.

The NUCC defines the following qualifiers, since they are the same as those used in 5010A1:

- 0B State License Number
- G2 Provider Commercial Number
- LU Location Number

31. SIGNATURE OF PHYSICIAN OR SUPPLIER INCLUDING DEGREES OR CREDENTIALS (I certify that the statements on the reverse apply to this bill and are made a part thereof.)	32. SERVICE FACILITY LOCATION INFORMATION	33. BILLING PROVIDER INFO & PH # (555) 4869002
Concha Antrum MD 030320XX		College Clinic 4567 Broad Avenue Woodland Hills XY 123450001
SIGNED *Concha Antrum MD* DATE	a. NPI b.	a. 3664021CC b. G2Z5678901234

Block 33: Billing Provider Info & Ph# The billing provider's or supplier's billing name, address, zip code, and phone number are the billing office location and telephone number of the provider and supplier.

Instructions: Enter the provider's or supplier's billing name, address, zip code, and phone number. The phone number is entered in the area to the right of the field title. Enter the name and address information in the following format: Block 33 identifies the provider that is requesting to be paid for the service rendered and should always be completed. Do not use punctuation (that is, commas and periods) or other symbols in the address (for example, use 123 N Main Street 101 instead of 123 N. Main Street, #101). Enter a space between the town name and two-character state code; do not include a comma. When reporting a 9-digit zip code, do not include the hyphen. Do not use a hyphen or space as a separator within the telephone number.

If reporting a foreign address, contact the payer for specific reporting instructions. 5010A1 requires the "Billing Provider Address" to be a street address or physical location. The NUCC recommends that the same requirements be applied here.

Block 33a: NPI# The NPI number refers to the HIPAA NPI number.
Instructions: Enter the NPI number of the billing provider in Block 33a.
Block 33b: Other ID# The non-NPI number of the billing provider refers to the payer-assigned unique identifier of the professional.
Instructions: Enter the two-digit qualifier identifying the non-NPI number, followed by the ID number. Do not enter a space, hyphen, or other separator between the qualifier and number.
The NUCC defines the following qualifiers used in 5010A1:
- 0B State License Number
- G2 Provider Commercial Number
- ZZ Provider Taxonomy (The qualifier in the 5010A1 for provider taxonomy is PXC, but ZZ remains the qualifier for the 1500 claim form.)

The list above contains both provider identifiers and the provider taxonomy code. The provider identifiers are assigned to the provider either by a specific payer or by a third party in order to uniquely identify the provider. The taxonomy code is designated by the provider in order to identify the provider type, classification, and area of specialization. Both provider identifiers and provider taxonomy may be used in this field.

INSURANCE PROGRAM TEMPLATES

The following pages show the completed CMS-1500 insurance claim forms and templates for the most common insurance programs encountered in a health care organization. Add a tab at the page margin for ease in flipping to this reference section when completing the *Workbook* assignments. The following examples illustrate entries for basic cases:
- Fig. 14.3 Private payer.
- Fig. 14.4 Medicaid.
- Fig. 14.5 Medicare.
- Fig. 14.6 Medicaid/Medicare—a crossover claim.
- Fig. 14.7 Medicare/Medigap—a crossover claim.
- Fig. 14.8 **MSP**—(Medicare Secondary Payer) other insurance primary and Medicare secondary.
- Fig. 14.9 TRICARE—standard.
- Fig. 14.10 CHAMPVA.
- Fig. 14.11 Workers' compensation.

PRIVATE PAYER
NO SECONDARY COVERAGE

DRAFT - NOT FOR OFFICIAL USE

HEALTH INSURANCE CLAIM FORM

APPROVED BY NATIONAL UNIFOR MCLAIM COMMITTEE (NUCC) 02/12

| | PICA | | | | | | | PICA | |

1. MEDICARE (Medicare#) ☐   MEDICAID (Medicaid#) ☐   TRICARE (ID#DoD#) ☐   CHAMPVA (Member ID#) ☐   GROUP HEALTH PLAN (ID#) ☒   FECA BLK LUNG (ID#) ☐   OTHER (ID#) ☐

1a. INSURED'S I.D. NUMBER (For Program in Item 1)
111704521

2. PATIENT'S NAME (Last Name, First Name, Middle Initial)
Forehand, Harry, N

3. PATIENT'S BIRTH DATE MM 01 | DD 06 | YY 1946   **SEX** M ☒ F ☐

4. INSURED'S NAME (Last Name, First Name, Middle Initial)
Forehand, Harry, N

5. PATIENT'S ADDRESS (No., Street)
1456 Main Street

6. PATIENT RELATIONSHIP TO INSURED
Self ☒   Spouse ☐   Child ☐   Other ☐

7. INSURED'S ADDRESS (No., Street)

CITY Woodland Hills   STATE XY

8. RESERVED FOR NUCC USE

CITY   STATE

ZIP CODE 123450000   TELEPHONE (Include Area Code) ( )

ZIP CODE   TELEPHONE (Include Area Code) ( )

9. OTHER INSURED'S NAME (Last Name, First Name, Middle Initial)

10. IS PATIENT'S CONDITION RELATED TO:

11. INSURED'S POLICY GROUP OR FECA NUMBER
A482

a. OTHER INSURED'S POLICY OR GROUP NUMBER

a. EMPLOYMENT? (Current or Previous) YES ☐ NO ☒

a. INSURED'S DATE OF BIRTH MM | DD | YY   **SEX** M ☐ F ☐

b. RESERVED FOR NUCC USE

b. AUTO ACCIDENT? YES ☐ NO ☒   PLACE (State)

b. OTHER CLAIM ID (Designated by NUCC)

c. RESERVED FOR NUCC USE

c. OTHER ACCIDENT? YES ☐ NO ☒

c. INSURANCE PLAN NAME OR PROGRAM NAME
ABC Insurance Company

d. INSURANCE PLAN NAME OR PROGRAM NAME

10d. CLAIM CODES (Designated by NUCC)

d. IS THERE ANOTHER HEALTH BENEFIT PLAN?
YES ☐ NO ☒   *If yes,* complete items 9, 9a, and 9d.

READ BACK OF FORM BEFORE COMPLETING & SIGNING THIS FORM.

12. PATIENT'S OR AUTHORIZED PERSON'S SIGNATURE I authorize the release of any medical or other information necessary to process this claim. I also request payment of government benefits either to myself or to the party who accepts assignment below.

SIGNED *Harry N. Forehand*   DATE *March 3, 20XX*

13. INSURED'S OR AUTHORIZED PERSON'S SIGNATURE I authorize payment of medical benefits to the undersigned physician or supplier for services described below.

SIGNED *Harry N. Forehand*

14. DATE OF CURRENT: ILLNESS, INJURY, or PREGNANCY(LMP) MM 03 | DD 01 | YY 20XX   QUAL. 431

15. OTHER DATE QUAL.   MM | DD | YY

16. DATES PATIENT UNABLE TO WORK IN CURRENT OCCUPATION FROM MM | DD | YY   TO MM | DD | YY

17. NAME OF REFERRING PROVIDER OR OTHER SOURCE
DN   Perry Cardi MD

17a.
17b. NPI 67805027XX

18. HOSPITALIZATION DATES RELATED TO CURRENT SERVICES FROM MM | DD | YY   TO MM | DD | YY

19. ADDITIONAL CLAIM INFORMATION (Designated by NUCC)

20. OUTSIDE LAB? YES ☐ NO ☒ $ CHARGES

21. DIAGNOSIS OR NATURE OF ILLNESS OR INJURY Relate A-L to service line below (24E)   ICD Ind. 0

A. H66009   B.   C.   D.
E.   F.   G.   H.
I.   J.   K.   L.

22. RESUBMISSION CODE   ORIGINAL REF. NO.

23. PRIOR AUTHORIZATION NUMBER

24. A. DATE(S) OF SERVICE From MM DD YY	To MM DD YY	B. PLACE OF SERVICE	C. EMG	D. PROCEDURES, SERVICES, OR SUPPLIES (Explain Unusual Circumstances) CPT/HCPCS MODIFIER	E. DIAGNOSIS POINTER	F. $ CHARGES	G. DAYS OR UNITS	H. EPSDT Family Plan	I. ID. QUAL.	J. RENDERING PROVIDER ID. #
1 03 03 XX		11		99203	A	120 00	1		NPI	1245897700
2									NPI	
3									NPI	
4									NPI	
5									NPI	
6									NPI	

25. FEDERAL TAX I.D. NUMBER   SSN EIN
XX12210XX   ☐ ☒

26. PATIENT'S ACCOUNT NO.
010

27. ACCEPT ASSIGNMENT? (For govt. claims, see back)
YES ☒ NO ☐

28. TOTAL CHARGE
$ 120 00

29. AMOUNT PAID
$

30. Rsvd for NUCC Use
$

31. SIGNATURE OF PHYSICIAN OR SUPPLIER INCLUDING DEGREES OR CREDENTIALS (I certify that the statements on the reverse apply to this bill and are made a part thereof.)
Concha Antrum MD   030320XX
SIGNED *Concha Antrum MD* DATE

32. SERVICE FACILITY LOCATION INFORMATION

a. NPI   b.

33. BILLING PROVIDER INFO & PH # (555) 4869002
College Clinic
4567 Broad Avenue
Woodland Hills XY 123450001

a. 3664021CC   b.

NUCC Instruction Manual available at: www.nucc.org   PLEASE PRINT OR TYPE   OMB APPROVAL PENDING

Fig. 14.3 Front side of the scannable Health Insurance Claim Form approved by the American Medical Association's (AMA's) Council on Medical Service. This form is also known as the CMS-1500 and is shown illustrating completion to a private third-party payer with no secondary coverage. Third-party payer, state, and local guidelines vary and may not always follow the visual guide presented here.

DRAFT - NOT FOR OFFICIAL USE

CARRIER

HEALTH INSURANCE CLAIM FORM

APPROVED BY NATIONAL UNIFOR MCLAIM COMMITTEE (NUCC) 02/12

| | PICA | | | | | | | PICA | | |

1. MEDICARE	MEDICAID	TRICARE	CHAMPVA	GROUP HEALTH PLAN	FECA BLK LUNG	OTHER	1a. INSURED'S I.D. NUMBER (For Program in Item 1)
(Medicare#)	[X] (Medicaid#)	(ID#DoD#)	(Member ID#)	(ID#)	(ID#)	(ID#)	276835090

2. PATIENT'S NAME (Last Name, First Name, Middle Initial)	3. PATIENT'S BIRTH DATE	SEX	4. INSURED'S NAME (Last Name, First Name, Middle Initial)
Abramson, Adam	MM 02 DD 12 YY 1995 M [X] F		Abramson, Adam

5. PATIENT'S ADDRESS (No., Street)	6. PATIENT RELATIONSHIP TO INSURED	7. INSURED'S ADDRESS (No., Street)
760 Finch Street	Self [X] Spouse Child Other	

CITY	STATE	8. RESERVED FOR NUCC USE	CITY	STATE
Woodland Hills	XY			

ZIP CODE	TELEPHONE (Include Area Code)	ZIP CODE	TELEPHONE (Include Area Code)
12345	( )		( )

9. OTHER INSURED'S NAME (Last Name, First Name, Middle Initial)	10. IS PATIENT'S CONDITION RELATED TO:	11. INSURED'S POLICY GROUP OR FECA NUMBER
a. OTHER INSURED'S POLICY OR GROUP NUMBER	a. EMPLOYMENT? (Current or Previous) YES [X] NO	a. INSURED'S DATE OF BIRTH MM DD YY SEX M F
b. RESERVED FOR NUCC USE	b. AUTO ACCIDENT? YES [X] NO PLACE (State)	b. OTHER CLAIM ID (Designated by NUCC)
c. RESERVED FOR NUCC USE	c. OTHER ACCIDENT? [X] YES NO	c. INSURANCE PLAN NAME OR PROGRAM NAME Medicaid
d. INSURANCE PLAN NAME OR PROGRAM NAME	10d. CLAIM CODES (Designated by NUCC)	d. IS THERE ANOTHER HEALTH BENEFIT PLAN? YES [X] NO If yes, complete items 9, 9a, and 9d.

READ BACK OF FORM BEFORE COMPLETING & SIGNING THIS FORM.

12. PATIENT'S OR AUTHORIZED PERSON'S SIGNATURE I authorize the release of any medical or other information necessary to process this claim. I also request payment of government benefits either to myself or to the party who accepts assignment below.

SIGNED *Adam Abramson*   DATE 7/14/XX

13. INSURED'S OR AUTHORIZED PERSON'S SIGNATURE I authorize payment of medical benefits to the undersigned physician or supplier for services described below.

SIGNED *Adam Abramson*

14. DATE OF CURRENT: ILLNESS, INJURY, or PREGNANCY(LMP) MM DD YY QUAL.	15. OTHER DATE QUAL. MM DD YY	16. DATES PATIENT UNABLE TO WORK IN CURRENT OCCUPATION FROM MM DD YY TO MM DD YY
17. NAME OF REFERRING PROVIDER OR OTHER SOURCE	17a. 17b. NPI	18. HOSPITALIZATION DATES RELATED TO CURRENT SERVICES FROM MM DD YY TO MM DD YY
19. ADDITIONAL CLAIM INFORMATION (Designated by NUCC)		20. OUTSIDE LAB? YES [X] NO $ CHARGES

21. DIAGNOSIS OR NATURE OF ILLNESS OR INJURY Relate A-L to service line below (24E)   ICD Ind. 0

A. T169xxA	B.	C.	D.
E.	F.	G.	H.
I.	J.	K.	L.

22. RESUBMISSION CODE	ORIGINAL REF. NO.
23. PRIOR AUTHORIZATION NUMBER	

24. A. DATE(S) OF SERVICE From MM DD YY	To MM DD YY	B. PLACE OF SERVICE	C. EMG	D. PROCEDURES, SERVICES, OR SUPPLIES (Explain Unusual Circumstances) CPT/HCPCS	MODIFIER	E. DIAGNOSIS POINTER	F. $ CHARGES	G. DAYS OR UNITS	H. EPSDT Family Plan	I. ID. QUAL.	J. RENDERING PROVIDER ID. #
1	07 14 XX		23	Y	99282	25	A	50 00	1		NPI	37640017XX
2	07 14 XX		23	Y	69200		A	120 00	1		NPI	37640017XX
3											NPI	
4											NPI	
5											NPI	
6											NPI	

25. FEDERAL TAX I.D. NUMBER SSN EIN	26. PATIENT'S ACCOUNT NO.	27. ACCEPT ASSIGNMENT? (For govt. claims, see back)	28. TOTAL CHARGE	29. AMOUNT PAID	30. Rsvd for NUCC Use
XX12210XX [X]	030	[X] YES NO	$ 170 00	$	$

31. SIGNATURE OF PHYSICIAN OR SUPPLIER INCLUDING DEGREES OR CREDENTIALS (I certify that the statements on the reverse apply to this bill and are made a part thereof.) Pedro Atrics MD SIGNED *Pedro Atrics MD* DATE 071420XX	32. SERVICE FACILITY LOCATION INFORMATION College Hospital 4500 Broad Avenue Woodland Hills XY 123450001 a. X950731067 b.	33. BILLING PROVIDER INFO & PH # (555) 4869002 College Clinic 4567 Broad Avenue Woodland Hills XY 123450001 a. 3664021CC b.

NUCC Instruction Manual available at: www.nucc.org   PLEASE PRINT OR TYPE   OMB APPROVAL PENDING

PATIENT AND INSURED INFORMATION

PHYSICIAN OR SUPPLIER INFORMATION

Fig. 14.4 A Medicaid case with no secondary coverage, emphasizing basic elements.

MEDICARE
NO SECONDARY COVERAGE

CARRIER

HEALTH INSURANCE CLAIM FORM

APPROVED BY NATIONAL UNIFOR MCLAIM COMMITTEE (NUCC) 02/12

	PICA									PICA		

1. MEDICARE	MEDICAID	TRICARE	CHAMPVA	GROUP HEALTH PLAN	FECA BLK LUNG	OTHER	1a. INSURED'S I.D. NUMBER (For Program in Item 1)
[X] (Medicare#)	(Medicaid#)	(ID#DoD#)	(Member ID#)	(ID#)	(ID#)	(ID#)	123 XX 6789A

2. PATIENT'S NAME (Last Name, First Name, Middle Initial)	3. PATIENT'S BIRTH DATE	SEX	4. INSURED'S NAME (Last Name, First Name, Middle Initial)
Hutch, Bill	MM 05 DD 07 YY 1910 M [X] F [ ]		Hutch, Bill

5. PATIENT'S ADDRESS (No., Street)	6. PATIENT RELATIONSHIP TO INSURED	7. INSURED'S ADDRESS (No., Street)
8888 Main Street	Self [X] Spouse [ ] Child [ ] Other [ ]	

CITY	STATE	8. RESERVED FOR NUCC USE	CITY	STATE
Woodland Hills	XY			

ZIP CODE	TELEPHONE (Include Area Code)	ZIP CODE	TELEPHONE (Include Area Code)
12345	( )		( )

9. OTHER INSURED'S NAME (Last Name, First Name, Middle Initial)	10. IS PATIENT'S CONDITION RELATED TO:	11. INSURED'S POLICY GROUP OR FECA NUMBER

a. OTHER INSURED'S POLICY OR GROUP NUMBER	a. EMPLOYMENT? (Current or Previous) [ ] YES [X] NO	a. INSURED'S DATE OF BIRTH MM DD YY SEX M [ ] F [ ]

b. RESERVED FOR NUCC USE	b. AUTO ACCIDENT? [ ] YES [X] NO PLACE (State)	b. OTHER CLAIM ID (Designated by NUCC)

c. RESERVED FOR NUCC USE	c. OTHER ACCIDENT? [ ] YES [X] NO	c. INSURANCE PLAN NAME OR PROGRAM NAME Medicare

d. INSURANCE PLAN NAME OR PROGRAM NAME	10d. CLAIM CODES (Designated by NUCC)	d. IS THERE ANOTHER HEALTH BENEFIT PLAN? [ ] YES [X] NO If yes, complete items 9, 9a, and 9d.

READ BACK OF FORM BEFORE COMPLETING & SIGNING THIS FORM.

12. PATIENT'S OR AUTHORIZED PERSON'S SIGNATUREI authorize the release of any medical or other information necessary to process this claim. I also request payment of government benefits either to myself or to the party who accepts assignment below.

SIGNED ___Signature on file___   DATE _____

13. INSURED'S OR AUTHORIZED PERSON'S SIGNATURE I authorize payment of medical benefits to the undersigned physician or supplier for services described below.

SIGNED _____

14. DATE OF CURRENT: ILLNESS, INJURY, or PREGNANCY(LMP) MM 03 DD 07 YY XX QUAL. 431	15. OTHER DATE QUAL. MM DD YY	16. DATES PATIENT UNABLE TO WORK IN CURRENT OCCUPATION FROM MM DD YY TO MM DD YY

17. NAME OF REFERRING PROVIDER OR OTHER SOURCE DN Gerald Practon MD	17a. 17b. NPI 46278897XX	18. HOSPITALIZATION DATES RELATED TO CURRENT SERVICES FROM MM DD YY TO MM DD YY

19. ADDITIONAL CLAIM INFORMATION (Designated by NUCC)	20. OUTSIDE LAB? [ ] YES [X] NO $ CHARGES

21. DIAGNOSIS OR NATURE OF ILLNESS OR INJURY Relate A-L to service line below (24E) ICD Ind. 0	22. RESUBMISSION CODE ORIGINAL REF. NO.
A. J129 B. ___ C. ___ D. ___ E. ___ F. ___ G. ___ H. ___ I. ___ J. ___ K. ___ L. ___	23. PRIOR AUTHORIZATION NUMBER

24. A. DATE(S) OF SERVICE						B. PLACE OF SERVICE	C. EMG	D. PROCEDURES, SERVICES, OR SUPPLIES (Explain Unusual Circumstances)		E. DIAGNOSIS POINTER	F. $ CHARGES	G. DAYS OR UNITS	H. EPSDT Family Plan	I. ID. QUAL.	J. RENDERING PROVIDER ID. #
	From			To				CPT/HCPCS	MODIFIER						
	MM DD YY		MM DD YY												
1	03 10 XX					11		99205		A	230 00	1		NPI	64211067XX
2														NPI	
3														NPI	
4														NPI	
5														NPI	
6														NPI	

25. FEDERAL TAX I.D. NUMBER SSN EIN XX12210XX [X]	26. PATIENT'S ACCOUNT NO. 040	27. ACCEPT ASSIGNMENT? (For govt. claims, see back) [X] YES [ ] NO	28. TOTAL CHARGE $ 230 00	29. AMOUNT PAID $	30. Rsvd for NUCC Use $

31. SIGNATURE OF PHYSICIAN OR SUPPLIER INCLUDING DEGREES OR CREDENTIALS (I certify that the statements on the reverse apply to this bill and are made a part thereof.) Brady Coccidioides 031020XX SIGNED *Brady Coccidioides MD* DATE	32. SERVICE FACILITY LOCATION INFORMATION a. NPI b.	33. BILLING PROVIDER INFO & PH # (555)4869002 College Clinic 4567 Broad Avenue Woodland Hills XY 123450001 a. 3664021CC b.

NUCC Instruction Manual available at: www.nucc.org   *PLEASE PRINT OR TYPE*   OMB APPROVAL PENDING

PHYSICIAN OR SUPPLIER INFORMATION / PATIENT AND INSURED INFORMATION

Fig. 14.5 Example of a completed CMS-1500 Health Insurance Claim Form for a basic Medicare case with no other insurance coverage. The provider has accepted assignment. Screened blocks should not be completed for a Medicare case with no other insurance.(Beik, Health Insurance Today, 6th edition, p. 23)

MEDICARE/MEDICAID
(primary)   (secondary)
CROSSOVER CLAIM

CARRIER

DRAFT - NOT FOR OFFICIAL USE

HEALTH INSURANCE CLAIM FORM
APPROVED BY NATIONAL UNIFOR MCLAIM COMMITTEE (NUCC) 02/12

| | PICA | | | | | | | | PICA | | |

1. MEDICARE	MEDICAID	TRICARE	CHAMPVA	GROUP HEALTH PLAN	FECA BLK LUNG	OTHER	1a. INSURED'S I.D. NUMBER (For Program in Item 1)
[X] (Medicare#)	[X] (Medicaid#)	[ ] (ID#/DoD#)	[ ] (Member ID#)	[ ] (ID#)	[ ] (ID#)	[ ] (ID#)	660 XX 2715A

2. PATIENT'S NAME (Last Name, First Name, Middle Initial)	3. PATIENT'S BIRTH DATE / SEX	4. INSURED'S NAME (Last Name, First Name, Middle Initial)
Johnson, Kathryn	MM 09 DD 07 YY 1937 M [ ] F [X]	Johnson, Kathryn

5. PATIENT'S ADDRESS (No., Street)	6. PATIENT RELATIONSHIP TO INSURED	7. INSURED'S ADDRESS (No., Street)
218 Vega Drive	Self [X] Spouse [ ] Child [ ] Other [ ]	
CITY: Woodland Hills STATE: XY	8. RESERVED FOR NUCC USE	CITY STATE
ZIP CODE: 123450000 TELEPHONE ( )		ZIP CODE TELEPHONE ( )

9. OTHER INSURED'S NAME (Last Name, First Name, Middle Initial)	10. IS PATIENT'S CONDITION RELATED TO:	11. INSURED'S POLICY GROUP OR FECA NUMBER
Johnson, Kathryn		
a. OTHER INSURED'S POLICY OR GROUP NUMBER: MCD016745289	a. EMPLOYMENT? (Current or Previous) [ ] YES [X] NO	a. INSURED'S DATE OF BIRTH MM DD YY SEX M [ ] F [ ]
b. RESERVED FOR NUCC USE	b. AUTO ACCIDENT? [ ] YES [X] NO PLACE (State)	b. OTHER CLAIM ID (Designated by NUCC)
c. RESERVED FOR NUCC USE	c. OTHER ACCIDENT? [ ] YES [X] NO	c. INSURANCE PLAN NAME OR PROGRAM NAME: Medicare
d. INSURANCE PLAN NAME OR PROGRAM NAME: Medicaid	10d. CLAIM CODES (Designated by NUCC)	d. IS THERE ANOTHER HEALTH BENEFIT PLAN? [X] YES [ ] NO If yes, complete items 9, 9a, and 9d.

READ BACK OF FORM BEFORE COMPLETING & SIGNING THIS FORM.

12. PATIENT'S OR AUTHORIZED PERSON'S SIGNATURE I authorize the release of any medical or other information necessary to process this claim. I also request payment of government benefits either to myself or to the party who accepts assignment below.

SIGNED *Kathryn Johnson*   DATE 10/1/XX

13. INSURED'S OR AUTHORIZED PERSON'S SIGNATURE I authorize payment of medical benefits to the undersigned physician or supplier for services described below.

SIGNED *Kathryn Johnson*

PATIENT AND INSURED INFORMATION

14. DATE OF CURRENT: ILLNESS, INJURY, or PREGNANCY(LMP) MM DD YY QUAL.	15. OTHER DATE QUAL. MM DD YY	16. DATES PATIENT UNABLE TO WORK IN CURRENT OCCUPATION FROM MM DD YY TO MM DD YY
17. NAME OF REFERRING PROVIDER OR OTHER SOURCE DN Brady Coccidioides MD	17a. 17b. NPI 64211067XX	18. HOSPITALIZATION DATES RELATED TO CURRENT SERVICES FROM MM DD YY TO MM DD YY
19. ADDITIONAL CLAIM INFORMATION (Designated by NUCC)		20. OUTSIDE LAB? [ ] YES [X] NO $ CHARGES

21. DIAGNOSIS OR NATURE OF ILLNESS OR INJURY Relate A-L to service line below (24E) ICD Ind. 0	22. RESUBMISSION CODE ORIGINAL REF. NO.
A. C4370 B. C. D. E. F. G. H. I. J. K. L.	23. PRIOR AUTHORIZATION NUMBER 7680560012

24. A. DATE(S) OF SERVICE From MM DD YY To MM DD YY	B. PLACE OF SERVICE	C. EMG	D. PROCEDURES, SERVICES, OR SUPPLIES (Explain Unusual Circumstances) CPT/HCPCS MODIFIER	E. DIAGNOSIS POINTER	F. $ CHARGES	G. DAYS OR UNITS	H. EPSDT Family Plan	I. ID. QUAL.	J. RENDERING PROVIDER ID. #
1	10 01 XX	24		11600	A	200 00	1		NPI	50307117XX
2									NPI	
3									NPI	
4									NPI	
5									NPI	
6									NPI	

25. FEDERAL TAX I.D. NUMBER SSN EIN	26. PATIENT'S ACCOUNT NO.	27. ACCEPT ASSIGNMENT? (For govt. claims, see back)	28. TOTAL CHARGE	29. AMOUNT PAID	30. Rsvd for NUCC Use
XX12210XX [ ] [X]	050	[X] YES [ ] NO	$ 200 00	$	$

31. SIGNATURE OF PHYSICIAN OR SUPPLIER INCLUDING DEGREES OR CREDENTIALS (I certify that the statements on the reverse apply to this bill and are made a part thereof.) Cosmo Graff MD 100320XX SIGNED *Cosmo Graff, MD* DATE	32. SERVICE FACILITY LOCATION INFORMATION Woodland Hills Ambulatory Center 1229 Center Street Woodland Hills XY 123450001 a. X950513700 b.	33. BILLING PROVIDER INFO & PH # (555) 4869002 College Clinic 4567 Broad Avenue Woodland Hills XY 123450001 a. 3664021CC b.

NUCC Instruction Manual available at: www.nucc.org   PLEASE PRINT OR TYPE   OMB APPROVAL PENDING

PHYSICIAN OR SUPPLIER INFORMATION

Fig. 14.6 Example of a Medicare/Medicaid crossover claim. The CMS-1500 claim form is sent to Medicare (primary payer) and then processed automatically by Medicaid (secondary payer).

MEDICARE/MEDIGAP
(primary)   (secondary)
CROSSOVER CLAIM

DRAFT - NOT FOR OFFICIAL USE

HEALTH INSURANCE CLAIM FORM
APPROVED BY NATIONAL UNIFOR MCLAIM COMMITTEE (NUCC) 02/12

| | PICA | | | | | | | | | PICA | |

1. MEDICARE	MEDICAID	TRICARE	CHAMPVA	GROUP HEALTH PLAN	FECA BLK LUNG	OTHER	1a. INSURED'S I.D. NUMBER (For Program in Item 1)
[X] (Medicare#)	[ ] (Medicaid#)	[ ] (ID#DoD#)	[ ] (Member ID#)	[X] (ID#)	[ ] (ID#)	[ ] (ID#)	419 XX 7272A

2. PATIENT'S NAME (Last Name, First Name, Middle Initial)
Barnes, Agusta, E

3. PATIENT'S BIRTH DATE   08 29 1917   SEX M [X] F [ ]

4. INSURED'S NAME (Last Name, First Name, Middle Initial)
Barnes, Agusta, E

5. PATIENT'S ADDRESS (No., Street)
356 Encina Avenue

6. PATIENT RELATIONSHIP TO INSURED
Self [X] Spouse [ ] Child [ ] Other [ ]

7. INSURED'S ADDRESS (No., Street)

CITY   Woodland Hills   STATE XY

8. RESERVED FOR NUCC USE

CITY   STATE

ZIP CODE 123450000   TELEPHONE (Include Area Code) (   )

ZIP CODE   TELEPHONE (Include Area Code) (   )

9. OTHER INSURED'S NAME (Last Name, First Name, Middle Initial)
Barnes, Agusta, E

10. IS PATIENT'S CONDITION RELATED TO:

11. INSURED'S POLICY GROUP OR FECA NUMBER

a. OTHER INSURED'S POLICY OR GROUP NUMBER
MEDIGAP 419167272

a. EMPLOYMENT? (Current or Previous) YES [ ] NO [X]

a. INSURED'S DATE OF BIRTH   MM DD YY   SEX M [ ] F [ ]

b. RESERVED FOR NUCC USE

b. AUTO ACCIDENT? YES [ ] NO [X]   PLACE (State)

b. OTHER CLAIM ID (Designated by NUCC)

c. RESERVED FOR NUCC USE

c. OTHER ACCIDENT? YES [ ] NO [X]

c. INSURANCE PLAN NAME OR PROGRAM NAME
Medicare

d. INSURANCE PLAN NAME OR PROGRAM NAME
CALFCA002

10d. CLAIM CODES (Designated by NUCC)

d. IS THERE ANOTHER HEALTH BENEFIT PLAN? [X] YES [ ] NO   If yes, complete items 9, 9a, and 9d.

READ BACK OF FORM BEFORE COMPLETING & SIGNING THIS FORM.
12. PATIENT'S OR AUTHORIZED PERSON'S SIGNATURE I authorize the release of any medical or other information necessary to process this claim. I also request payment of government benefits either to myself or to the party who accepts assignment below.

SIGNED *Agusta E. Barnes*   DATE *11/21/XX*

13. INSURED'S OR AUTHORIZED PERSON'S SIGNATURE I authorize payment of medical benefits to the undersigned physician or supplier for services described below.

SIGNED *Agusta E. Barnes*

14. DATE OF CURRENT: ILLNESS, INJURY, or PREGNANCY(LMP)   MM DD YY   QUAL.

15. OTHER DATE QUAL.   MM DD YY

16. DATES PATIENT UNABLE TO WORK IN CURRENT OCCUPATION   FROM MM DD YY   TO MM DD YY

17. NAME OF REFERRING PROVIDER OR OTHER SOURCE
DN Gaston Input MD

17a.
17b. NPI 32783127XX

18. HOSPITALIZATION DATES RELATED TO CURRENT SERVICES   FROM MM DD YY   TO MM DD YY

19. ADDITIONAL CLAIM INFORMATION (Designated by NUCC)

20. OUTSIDE LAB? YES [ ] NO [X] $ CHARGES

21. DIAGNOSIS OR NATURE OF ILLNESS OR INJURY Relate A-L to service line below (24E)   ICD Ind. 0

A. R0789   B.   C.   D.
E.   F.   G.   H.
I.   J.   K.   L.

22. RESUBMISSION CODE   ORIGINAL REF. NO.

23. PRIOR AUTHORIZATION NUMBER

24. A. DATE(S) OF SERVICE From MM DD YY	To MM DD YY	B. PLACE OF SERVICE	C. EMG	D. PROCEDURES, SERVICES, OR SUPPLIES (Explain Unusual Circumstances) CPT/HCPCS MODIFIER	E. DIAGNOSIS POINTER	F. $ CHARGES	G. DAYS OR UNITS	H. EPSDT Family Plan	I. ID. QUAL.	J. RENDERING PROVIDER ID. #
1	11 21 XX		11		93350	A	190 00	1		NPI	67805027XX
2	11 21 XX		11		93017	A	70 00	1		NPI	67805027XX
3										NPI	
4										NPI	
5										NPI	
6										NPI	

25. FEDERAL TAX I.D. NUMBER   SSN [ ] EIN [ ]

26. PATIENT'S ACCOUNT NO.
060

27. ACCEPT ASSIGNMENT? (For govt. claims, see back) YES [X] NO [ ]

28. TOTAL CHARGE $ 260 00

29. AMOUNT PAID $

30. Rsvd for NUCC Use

31. SIGNATURE OF PHYSICIAN OR SUPPLIER INCLUDING DEGREES OR CREDENTIALS (I certify that the statements on the reverse apply to this bill and are made a part thereof.)
Perry Cardi MD   112220XX
SIGNED *Perry Cardi, MD*   DATE

32. SERVICE FACILITY LOCATION INFORMATION

a. NPI   b.

33. BILLING PROVIDER INFO & PH # (555) 4869002
College Clinic
4567 Broad Avenue
Woodland Hills XY 123450001

a. 3664021CC   b.

Fig. 14.7 Example of a completed CMS-1500 Health Insurance Claim Form for a Medicare (primary) and Medigap (secondary) crossover claim.

OTHER INSURANCE/MEDICARE-MSP
(primary)   (secondary)

DRAFT - NOT FOR OFFICIAL USE

HEALTH INSURANCE CLAIM FORM
APPROVED BY NATIONAL UNIFOR MCLAIM COMMITTEE (NUCC) 02/12

☐☐ PICA   PICA ☐☐

1. MEDICARE	MEDICAID	TRICARE	CHAMPVA	GROUP HEALTH PLAN	FECA BLK LUNG	OTHER	1a. INSURED'S I.D. NUMBER (For Program in Item 1)
[X] (Medicare#)	☐ (Medicaid#)	☐ (ID#DoD#)	☐ (Member ID#)	[X] (ID#)	☐ (ID#)	☐ (ID#)	609 XX 5523

2. PATIENT'S NAME (Last Name, First Name, Middle Initial)
Blair, Gwendolyn

3. PATIENT'S BIRTH DATE   SEX
MM 09 | DD 01 | YY 1931   M☐   F[X]

4. INSURED'S NAME (Last Name, First Name, Middle Initial)
Blair, Gwendolyn

5. PATIENT'S ADDRESS (No., Street)
416 Richmond Street

6. PATIENT RELATIONSHIP TO INSURED
Self [X]   Spouse ☐   Child ☐   Other ☐

7. INSURED'S ADDRESS (No., Street)

CITY **Woodland Hills**   STATE **XY**

8. RESERVED FOR NUCC USE

CITY   STATE

ZIP CODE **123450000**   TELEPHONE (Include Area Code) ( )

ZIP CODE   TELEPHONE (Include Area Code) ( )

9. OTHER INSURED'S NAME (Last Name, First Name, Middle Initial)
Blair, Gwendolyn

10. IS PATIENT'S CONDITION RELATED TO:

11. INSURED'S POLICY GROUP OR FECA NUMBER
7845931Q

a. OTHER INSURED'S POLICY OR GROUP NUMBER
609 XX 5523A

a. EMPLOYMENT? (Current or Previous)
YES ☐   NO [X]

a. INSURED'S DATE OF BIRTH   SEX
MM | DD | YY   M☐   F☐

b. RESERVED FOR NUCC USE

b. AUTO ACCIDENT?   PLACE (State)
YES ☐   NO [X] ☐

b. OTHER CLAIM ID (Designated by NUCC)

c. RESERVED FOR NUCC USE

c. OTHER ACCIDENT?
YES ☐   NO [X]

c. INSURANCE PLAN NAME OR PROGRAM NAME
ABC Insurance Company

d. INSURANCE PLAN NAME OR PROGRAM NAME
Medicare

10d. CLAIM CODES (Designated by NUCC)

d. IS THERE ANOTHER HEALTH BENEFIT PLAN?
[X] YES   ☐ NO   *If yes*, complete items 9, 9a, and 9d.

READ BACK OF FORM BEFORE COMPLETING & SIGNING THIS FORM.
12. PATIENT'S OR AUTHORIZED PERSON'S SIGNATURE I authorize the release of any medical or other information necessary to process this claim. I also request payment of government benefits either to myself or to the party who accepts assignment below.

SIGNED **Signature on file**   DATE _____

13. INSURED'S OR AUTHORIZED PERSON'S SIGNATURE I authorize payment of medical benefits to the undersigned physician or supplier for services described below.

SIGNED **Signature on file**

14. DATE OF CURRENT: ILLNESS, INJURY, or PREGNANCY(LMP)
MM | DD | YY   QUAL.

15. OTHER DATE
QUAL.   MM | DD | YY

16. DATES PATIENT UNABLE TO WORK IN CURRENT OCCUPATION
FROM MM | DD | YY   TO MM | DD | YY

17. NAME OF REFERRING PROVIDER OR OTHER SOURCE
DN **Gerald Practon MD**
17a.
17b. NPI **46278897XX**

18. HOSPITALIZATION DATES RELATED TO CURRENT SERVICES
FROM MM | DD | YY   TO MM | DD | YY

19. ADDITIONAL CLAIM INFORMATION (Designated by NUCC)

20. OUTSIDE LAB? $ CHARGES
☐ YES   [X] NO

21. DIAGNOSIS OR NATURE OF ILLNESS OR INJURY Relate A-L to service line below (24E)   ICD Ind. **0**

A. **B351**   B. _____   C. _____   D. _____
E. _____   F. _____   G. _____   H. _____
I. _____   J. _____   K. _____   L. _____

22. RESUBMISSION CODE   ORIGINAL REF. NO.

23. PRIOR AUTHORIZATION NUMBER

24. A. DATE(S) OF SERVICE From MM DD YY	To MM DD YY	B. PLACE OF SERVICE	C. EMG	D. PROCEDURES, SERVICES, OR SUPPLIES (Explain Unusual Circumstances) CPT/HCPCS	MODIFIER	E. DIAGNOSIS POINTER	F. $ CHARGES	G. DAYS OR UNITS	H. EPSDT Family Plan	I. ID. QUAL.	J. RENDERING PROVIDER ID. #
1	03 15 XX		11		99243	25	A	110 00	1		NPI	54022287XX
2	03 15 XX		11		11750		A	170 00	1		NPI	54022287XX
3											NPI	
4											NPI	
5											NPI	
6											NPI	

25. FEDERAL TAX I.D. NUMBER   SSN EIN
XX12210XX   ☐ [X]

26. PATIENT'S ACCOUNT NO.
070

27. ACCEPT ASSIGNMENT? (For govt. claims, see back)
[X] YES   ☐ NO

28. TOTAL CHARGE
$ **280 00**

29. AMOUNT PAID
$ **100 00**

30. Rsvd for NUCC Use
$

31. SIGNATURE OF PHYSICIAN OR SUPPLIER INCLUDING DEGREES OR CREDENTIALS (I certify that the statements on the reverse apply to this bill and are made a part thereof.)
Nick Pedro DPM   031620XX
SIGNED *Nick Pedro, DPM* DATE

32. SERVICE FACILITY LOCATION INFORMATION
a. NPI   b.

33. BILLING PROVIDER INFO & PH # (**555**) **4869002**
College Clinic
4567 Broad Avenue
Woodland Hills XY 123450001
a. **3664021CC**   b.

Fig. 14.8 Template for a case in which another insurance carrier is the primary payer and Medicare is the secondary payer (MSP).

DRAFT - NOT FOR OFFICIAL USE

TRICARE
NO SECONDARY COVERAGE

HEALTH INSURANCE CLAIM FORM

APPROVED BY NATIONAL UNIFOR MCLAIM COMMITTEE (NUCC) 02/12

CARRIER

| | PICA | | | | | | | | | | PICA | | |

1. | MEDICARE | MEDICAID | TRICARE | CHAMPVA | GROUP HEALTH PLAN | FECA BLK LUNG | OTHER | 1a. INSURED'S I.D. NUMBER (For Program in Item 1)
(Medicare#) | (Medicaid#) | [X] (ID#DoD#) | (Member ID#) | (ID#) | (ID#) | (ID#) | 581147211

2. PATIENT'S NAME (Last Name, First Name, Middle Initial)
Smith, Susan, J

3. PATIENT'S BIRTH DATE
MM 03 DD 16 YY 1976   SEX M [ ] F [X]

4. INSURED'S NAME (Last Name, First Name, Middle Initial)
Smith, William D

5. PATIENT'S ADDRESS (No., Street)
420 Maple Street

6. PATIENT RELATIONSHIP TO INSURED
Self [ ] Spouse [X] Child [ ] Other [ ]

7. INSURED'S ADDRESS (No., Street)
420 Maple Street

CITY
Woodland Hills   STATE XY

8. RESERVED FOR NUCC USE

CITY
Woodland Hills   STATE XY

ZIP CODE
123450000   TELEPHONE (Include Area Code)
(   )

ZIP CODE
123450000   TELEPHONE (Include Area Code)
(   )

9. OTHER INSURED'S NAME (Last Name, First Name, Middle Initial)

10. IS PATIENT'S CONDITION RELATED TO:

11. INSURED'S POLICY GROUP OR FECA NUMBER

a. OTHER INSURED'S POLICY OR GROUP NUMBER

a. EMPLOYMENT? (Current or Previous)
YES [ ] NO [X]

a. INSURED'S DATE OF BIRTH
MM 06 DD 12 YY 1974   SEX M [X] F [ ]

b. RESERVED FOR NUCC USE

b. AUTO ACCIDENT?   PLACE (State)
YES [ ] NO [X]

b. OTHER CLAIM ID (Designated by NUCC)

c. RESERVED FOR NUCC USE

c. OTHER ACCIDENT?
YES [ ] NO [X]

c. INSURANCE PLAN NAME OR PROGRAM NAME
TRICARE

d. INSURANCE PLAN NAME OR PROGRAM NAME

10d. CLAIM CODES (Designated by NUCC)

d. IS THERE ANOTHER HEALTH BENEFIT PLAN?
YES [ ] NO [X] *If yes*, complete items 9, 9a, and 9d.

READ BACK OF FORM BEFORE COMPLETING & SIGNING THIS FORM.
12. PATIENT'S OR AUTHORIZED PERSON'S SIGNATUREI authorize the release of any medical or other information necessary to process this claim. I also request payment of government benefits either to myself or to the party who accepts assignment below.

SIGNED Signature on file   DATE

13. INSURED'S OR AUTHORIZED PERSON'S SIGNATURE I authorize payment of medical benefits to the undersigned physician or supplier for services described below.

SIGNED Signature on file

PATIENT AND INSURED INFORMATION

14. DATE OF CURRENT: ILLNESS, INJURY, or PREGNANCY(LMP)
MM 10 DD 28 YY 20XX QUAL. 484

15. OTHER DATE
QUAL.   MM DD YY

16. DATES PATIENT UNABLE TO WORK IN CURRENT OCCUPATION
FROM MM 07 DD 21 YY 20XX TO MM 09 DD 17 YY 20XX

17. NAME OF REFERRING PROVIDER OR OTHER SOURCE
DN Adam Langerhans MD

17a.
17b. NPI 47680657XX

18. HOSPITALIZATION DATES RELATED TO CURRENT SERVICES
FROM MM 08 DD 06 YY 20XX TO MM 08 DD 08 YY 20XX

19. ADDITIONAL CLAIM INFORMATION (Designated by NUCC)

20. OUTSIDE LAB? $ CHARGES
YES [ ] NO [X]

21. DIAGNOSIS OR NATURE OF ILLNESS OR INJURY Relate A-L to service line below (24E)   ICD Ind. 0
A. O80   B. _____   C. _____   D. _____
E. _____   F. _____   G. _____   H. _____
I. _____   J. _____   K. _____   L. _____

22. RESUBMISSION CODE   ORIGINAL REF. NO.

23. PRIOR AUTHORIZATION NUMBER

24. A. DATE(S) OF SERVICE						B. PLACE OF SERVICE	C. EMG	D. PROCEDURES, SERVICES, OR SUPPLIES (Explain Unusual Circumstances)		E. DIAGNOSIS POINTER	F. $ CHARGES	G. DAYS OR UNITS	H. EPSDT Family Plan	I. ID. QUAL.	J. RENDERING PROVIDER ID. #
From MM	DD	YY	To MM	DD	YY			CPT/HCPCS	MODIFIER						
1 08	06	XX				21		59400		A	2290 00	1		NPI	43056757XX
2														NPI	
3														NPI	
4														NPI	
5														NPI	
6														NPI	

25. FEDERAL TAX I.D. NUMBER   SSN EIN
XX12210XX   [ ] [X]

26. PATIENT'S ACCOUNT NO.
080

27. ACCEPT ASSIGNMENT? (For govt. claims, see back)
YES [X] NO [ ]

28. TOTAL CHARGE
$ 2290 00

29. AMOUNT PAID
$

30. Rsvd for NUCC Use
$

31. SIGNATURE OF PHYSICIAN OR SUPPLIER INCLUDING DEGREES OR CREDENTIALS
(I certify that the statements on the reverse apply to this bill and are made a part thereof.)
Bertha Caesar MD   081020XX
SIGNED *Bertha Caesar, MD* DATE

32. SERVICE FACILITY LOCATION INFORMATION
College Hospital
4500 Broad Avenue
Woodland Hills XY 123450001
a. X950731067   b.

33. BILLING PROVIDER INFO & PH # (555) 4869002
College Clinic
4567 Broad Avenue
Woodland Hills XY 123450001
a. 3664021CC   b.

PHYSICIAN OR SUPPLIER INFORMATION

NUCC Instruction Manual available at: www.nucc.org   PLEASE PRINT OR TYPE   OMB APPROVAL PENDING

Fig. 14.9 Example of a completed CMS-1500 claim form used when billing for professional services rendered in a TRICARE standard case.

CHAMPVA
NO SECONDARY COVERAGE

DRAFT - NOT FOR OFFICIAL USE

HEALTH INSURANCE CLAIM FORM

APPROVED BY NATIONAL UNIFOR MCLAIM COMMITTEE (NUCC) 02/12

| | PICA | | | | | | | | | PICA | | |

1. MEDICARE (Medicare#) □ MEDICAID (Medicaid#) □ TRICARE (ID#DoD#) □ CHAMPVA (Member ID#) [X] GROUP HEALTH PLAN (ID#) □ FECA BLK LUNG (ID#) □ OTHER (ID#) □

1a. INSURED'S I.D. NUMBER (For Program in Item 1)
560 XX 4444

2. PATIENT'S NAME (Last Name, First Name, Middle Initial)
Dexter, Bruce, R

3. PATIENT'S BIRTH DATE MM 03 DD 13 YY 1934 SEX M [X] F □

4. INSURED'S NAME (Last Name, First Name, Middle Initial)
Dexter, Bruce, R

5. PATIENT'S ADDRESS (No., Street)
226 Irwin Road

6. PATIENT RELATIONSHIP TO INSURED
Self [X] Spouse □ Child □ Other □

7. INSURED'S ADDRESS (No., Street)

CITY Woodland Hills STATE XY

8. RESERVED FOR NUCC USE

CITY STATE

ZIP CODE 12345 TELEPHONE (Include Area Code) ( )

ZIP CODE TELEPHONE (Include Area Code) ( )

9. OTHER INSURED'S NAME (Last Name, First Name, Middle Initial)

10. IS PATIENT'S CONDITION RELATED TO:

11. INSURED'S POLICY GROUP OR FECA NUMBER
023

a. OTHER INSURED'S POLICY OR GROUP NUMBER

a. EMPLOYMENT? (Current or Previous) [X] YES □ NO

a. INSURED'S DATE OF BIRTH MM DD YY SEX M □ F □

b. RESERVED FOR NUCC USE

b. AUTO ACCIDENT? □ YES [X] NO PLACE (State)

b. OTHER CLAIM ID (Designated by NUCC)

c. RESERVED FOR NUCC USE

c. OTHER ACCIDENT? □ YES [X] NO

c. INSURANCE PLAN NAME OR PROGRAM NAME
CHAMPVA

d. INSURANCE PLAN NAME OR PROGRAM NAME

10d. CLAIM CODES (Designated by NUCC)

d. IS THERE ANOTHER HEALTH BENEFIT PLAN?
□ YES [X] NO **If yes**, complete items 9, 9a, and 9d.

READ BACK OF FORM BEFORE COMPLETING & SIGNING THIS FORM.
12. PATIENT'S OR AUTHORIZED PERSON'S SIGNATURE I authorize the release of any medical or other information necessary to process this claim. I also request payment of government benefits either to myself or to the party who accepts assignment below.

SIGNED Signature on file DATE

13. INSURED'S OR AUTHORIZED PERSON'S SIGNATURE I authorize payment of medical benefits to the undersigned physician or supplier for services described below.

SIGNED Signature on file

14. DATE OF CURRENT: ILLNESS, INJURY, or PREGNANCY(LMP) MM DD YY QUAL.

15. OTHER DATE QUAL. MM DD YY

16. DATES PATIENT UNABLE TO WORK IN CURRENT OCCUPATION FROM MM DD YY TO MM DD YY

17. NAME OF REFERRING PROVIDER OR OTHER SOURCE
DN Gerald Practon MD

17a.
17b. NPI 46278897XX

18. HOSPITALIZATION DATES RELATED TO CURRENT SERVICES FROM MM 07 DD 29 YY 20XX TO MM 07 DD 31 YY 20XX

19. ADDITIONAL CLAIM INFORMATION (Designated by NUCC)

20. OUTSIDE LAB? □ YES [X] NO $ CHARGES

21. DIAGNOSIS OR NATURE OF ILLNESS OR INJURY Relate A-L to service line below (24E) ICD Ind. 0

A. N400 B. C. D.
E. F. G. H.
I. J. K. L.

22. RESUBMISSION CODE ORIGINAL REF. NO.

23. PRIOR AUTHORIZATION NUMBER

24. A. DATE(S) OF SERVICE From MM DD YY	To MM DD YY	B. PLACE OF SERVICE	C. EMG	D. PROCEDURES, SERVICES, OR SUPPLIES (Explain Unusual Circumstances) CPT/HCPCS	MODIFIER	E. DIAGNOSIS POINTER	F. $ CHARGES	G. DAYS OR UNITS	H. EPSDT Family Plan	I. ID. QUAL.	J. RENDERING PROVIDER ID. #
1	07 29 XX		21		52601		A	800 00	1		NPI	25678831XX
2											NPI	
3											NPI	
4											NPI	
5											NPI	
6											NPI	

25. FEDERAL TAX I.D. NUMBER SSN EIN
XX12210XX □ [X]

26. PATIENT'S ACCOUNT NO.
090

27. ACCEPT ASSIGNMENT? (For govt. claims, see back)
[X] YES □ NO

28. TOTAL CHARGE
$ 800 00

29. AMOUNT PAID
$

30. Rsvd for NUCC Use
$

31. SIGNATURE OF PHYSICIAN OR SUPPLIER INCLUDING DEGREES OR CREDENTIALS (I certify that the statements on the reverse apply to this bill and are made a part thereof.)
Gene Ulibarri MD 073020XX
SIGNED Gene Ulibarri MD DATE

32. SERVICE FACILITY LOCATION INFORMATION
College Hospital
4500 Broad Avenue
Woodland Hills XY 123450001
a. X950731067 b.

33. BILLING PROVIDER INFO & PH # (555) 4869002
College Clinic
4567 Broad Avenue
Woodland Hills XY 123450001
a. 3664021CC b.

NUCC Instruction Manual available at: www.nucc.org   PLEASE PRINT OR TYPE   OMB APPROVAL PENDING

Fig. 14.10 An example of a completed CMS-1500 Health Insurance Claim Form for a CHAMPVA case with no secondary coverage.

WORKERS' COMPENSATION

DRAFT - NOT FOR OFFICIAL USE

HEALTH INSURANCE CLAIM FORM

APPROVED BY NATIONAL UNIFOR MCLAIM COMMITTEE (NUCC) 02/12

| | PICA | | | | | | | | | PICA | |

1. MEDICARE ☐ (Medicare#) MEDICAID ☐ (Medicaid#) TRICARE ☐ (ID#/DoD#) CHAMPVA ☐ (Member ID#) GROUP HEALTH PLAN ☐ (ID#) FECA BLK LUNG ☐ (ID#) OTHER ☒ (ID#)

1a. INSURED'S I.D. NUMBER   (For Program in Item 1)
667289

2. PATIENT'S NAME (Last Name, First Name, Middle Initial)
Barton, Peter, A

3. PATIENT'S BIRTH DATE
MM 11 | DD 14 | YY 1976   SEX M ☒ F ☐

4. INSURED'S NAME (Last Name, First Name, Middle Initial)
D F Construction

5. PATIENT'S ADDRESS (No., Street)
14890 Daisy Avenue

6. PATIENT RELATIONSHIP TO INSURED
Self ☐ Spouse ☐ Child ☐ Other ☒

7. INSURED'S ADDRESS (No., Street)
1212 Hardrock Place

CITY
Woodland Hills   STATE XY

8. RESERVED FOR NUCC USE

CITY
Woodland Hills   STATE XY

ZIP CODE
123450000

TELEPHONE (Include Area Code)
(   )

ZIP CODE
123450000

TELEPHONE (Include Area Code)
(555) 4278200

9. OTHER INSURED'S NAME (Last Name, First Name, Middle Initial)

10. IS PATIENT'S CONDITION RELATED TO:

11. INSURED'S POLICY GROUP OR FECA NUMBER

a. OTHER INSURED'S POLICY OR GROUP NUMBER

a. EMPLOYMENT? (Current or Previous)
☒ YES   ☐ NO

a. INSURED'S DATE OF BIRTH
MM | DD | YY   SEX M ☐ F ☐

b. RESERVED FOR NUCC USE

b. AUTO ACCIDENT?
☐ YES   ☒ NO   PLACE (State)

b. OTHER CLAIM ID (Designated by NUCC)
Y4 | DFC186

c. RESERVED FOR NUCC USE

c. OTHER ACCIDENT?
☐ YES   ☒ NO

c. INSURANCE PLAN NAME OR PROGRAM NAME
State Insurance Fund

d. INSURANCE PLAN NAME OR PROGRAM NAME

10d. CLAIM CODES (Designated by NUCC)

d. IS THERE ANOTHER HEALTH BENEFIT PLAN?
☐ YES   ☐ NO   **If yes**, complete items 9, 9a, and 9d.

READ BACK OF FORM BEFORE COMPLETING & SIGNING THIS FORM.
12. PATIENT'S OR AUTHORIZED PERSON'S SIGNATURE I authorize the release of any medical or other information necessary to process this claim. I also request payment of government benefits either to myself or to the party who accepts assignment below.

SIGNED   Signature on file   DATE

13. INSURED'S OR AUTHORIZED PERSON'S SIGNATURE I authorize payment of medical benefits to the undersigned physician or supplier for services described below.

SIGNED

14. DATE OF CURRENT: ILLNESS, INJURY, or PREGNANCY(LMP)
MM 01 | DD 04 | YY 20XX QUAL. 431

15. OTHER DATE
QUAL.   MM | DD | YY

16. DATES PATIENT UNABLE TO WORK IN CURRENT OCCUPATION
FROM MM 01 | DD 04 | YY 20XX   TO MM 03 | DD 27 | YY 20XX

17. NAME OF REFERRING PROVIDER OR OTHER SOURCE

17a.
17b. NPI

18. HOSPITALIZATION DATES RELATED TO CURRENT SERVICES
FROM MM | DD | YY   TO MM | DD | YY

19. ADDITIONAL CLAIM INFORMATION (Designated by NUCC)

20. OUTSIDE LAB? $ CHARGES
☐ YES   ☐ NO

21. DIAGNOSIS OR NATURE OF ILLNESS OR INJURY Relate A-L to service line below (24E)   ICD Ind. 0
A. M24419   B. _____   C. _____   D. _____
E. _____   F. _____   G. _____   H. _____
I. _____   J. _____   K. _____   L. _____

22. RESUBMISSION CODE   ORIGINAL REF. NO.

23. PRIOR AUTHORIZATION NUMBER

24. A. DATE(S) OF SERVICE From MM DD YY To MM DD YY	B. PLACE OF SERVICE	C. EMG	D. PROCEDURES, SERVICES, OR SUPPLIES (Explain Unusual Circumstances) CPT/HCPCS	MODIFIER	E. DIAGNOSIS POINTER	F. $ CHARGES	G. DAYS OR UNITS	H. EPSDT Family Plan	I. ID. QUAL.	J. RENDERING PROVIDER ID. #
1 02 27 XX	11		29055		A	570 00	1		NPI	12678547XX
2									NPI	
3									NPI	
4									NPI	
5									NPI	
6									NPI	

25. FEDERAL TAX I.D. NUMBER   SSN EIN
XX12210XX   ☐ ☒

26. PATIENT'S ACCOUNT NO.
100

27. ACCEPT ASSIGNMENT? (For govt. claims, see back)
☐ YES   ☐ NO

28. TOTAL CHARGE
$ 570 00

29. AMOUNT PAID
$

30. Rsvd for NUCC Use
$

31. SIGNATURE OF PHYSICIAN OR SUPPLIER INCLUDING DEGREES OR CREDENTIALS (I certify that the statements on the reverse apply to this bill and are made a part thereof.)
Raymond Skelton MD
SIGNED Raymond Skelton, MD   DATE 022820XX

32. SERVICE FACILITY LOCATION INFORMATION

a. NPI   b.

33. BILLING PROVIDER INFO & PH # (555) 4869002
College Clinic
4567 Broad Avenue
Woodland Hills XY 123450001

a. 3664021CC   b.

NUCC Instruction Manual available at: www.nucc.org   PLEASE PRINT OR TYPE   OMB APPROVAL PENDING

CARRIER / PATIENT AND INSURED INFORMATION / PHYSICIAN OR SUPPLIER INFORMATION

Fig. 14.11 An example of a completed CMS-1500 Health Insurance Claim Form for a workers' compensation case.

14.7 QUICK REVIEW

Question: Explain the importance of verifying block 21. Block 24D and 24E.

DISCUSSION POINT

Most claims for health care services are filed electronically. Explain why it is important for the insurance billing specialist to learn how to complete paper claim forms.

PROCEDURE 14.1 CMS-1500 Claim Form-Identification of Block and Source Documents

Objective: There are 33 blocks on the CMS-1500 Paper Claim Form. To become most efficient in completing claim forms, it is essential that the insurance billing specialist understand each block number and title. Additionally, the insurance billing specialist should understand the source documents that would be used to abstract information accurately.

Step 1: Create a table with a heading, 3 columns, and 33 rows. Label the column headings as:

- Block #:
- Block Title
- Source Document

Step 2: Complete the table by identifying the block title and the source document that would be used to abstract information for completion of the block. There should be 33 block numbers in total. An example is provided below.

EXAMPLE

Block #	Block Title	Source Document
1	Medicare, Medicaid, TRICARE, CHAMPVA, Group Health Plan, FECA, Black Lung, Other	Patient's insurance card
1.a	Insured's ID Number	Patient's insurance card

KEY POINTS

This is a brief chapter review of the key issues presented.

1. There are two types of claims submitted to insurance companies for payment: *paper claims* and *electronic claims.*
2. A *clean claim* is one that was submitted to the third-party payer within the time limit, had the necessary information for processing, and was paid promptly. Under the Medicare program, a clean claim is one that has passed all electronic edits and is routed for payment.
3. Other types of claims are called *dirty,* when a claim is submitted with errors; *incomplete,* when missing required information; *invalid,* when illogical or incorrect; *pending,* when held in suspense for review; *rejected,* when the claim needs investigation and answers to some questions; or *deleted,* when the Medicare fiscal intermediary cancels, deletes, or voids a claim.
4. When two insurance policies are involved (*dual coverage* or *duplication of coverage*), one is considered primary and the other secondary. First, an insurance claim is submitted to the primary plan; after payment, the secondary carrier is billed with a copy of the explanation of benefits (EOB) from the primary carrier.
5. A diagnosis should never be submitted on an insurance claim without supporting documentation in the medical record.
6. Every insurance claim should be proofread for completeness and accuracy of content before it is submitted to the insurance carrier.
7. Be aware of common billing errors and learn how to correct them for quicker claim settlements and to reduce the number of appeals.
8. HIPAA transactions and code sets standards only apply to electronic transactions conducted by covered entities.
9. Copies of submitted insurance claim forms should be filed in a tickler file and reviewed for follow-up every 30 days unless the computer system maintains the files.
10. Ensure that the correct NPI is shown on the claim for the health care provider rendering the medical service to the patient.

INTERNET RESOURCES

National Uniform Claims Committee
- www.NUCC.org

NPI Registry Public Search
- https://npiregistry.cms.hhs.gov/

The Place of Service Codes
- www.cms.gov/Medicare/Coding/place-of-service-codes/Place_of_Service_Code_set.html

United States Treasury Bureau of Fiscal Services
- https://www.fiscal.treasury.gov/fsservices/gov/pmt/prompt-Payment/rates.htm

STUDENT ASSIGNMENT

- Study Chapter 14.
- Complete all exercises in the *Workbook* to reinforce the theories learned in this chapter.
- Turn to the Glossary at the end of this text for a further understanding of the key terms and key abbreviations used in this chapter.

15

The Electronic Claim

Linda M. Smith

OBJECTIVES

After reading this chapter, you should be able to:

1. Describe an electronic claim.
2. Define and discuss electronic data interchange.
3. Describe necessary components when adopting an accounts receivable management or computerized medical billing system.
4. Explain the difference between carrier-direct and clearinghouse electronically transmitted insurance claims.
5. Summarize the advantages of electronic claim submission.
6. Identify the transactions and code sets to use for insurance claims transmission.
7. Discuss the difference between insurance claim data elements which are required or situational for the 837P standard transaction format.
8. Define a claim attachment and discuss claim attachments standards.
9. Compare and contrast standard unique provider identifiers, health plan identifiers, and patient identifiers.
10. Name and discuss some methods of interactive computer transactions for transmitting insurance claims.
11. Discuss interactive transactions and relate the electronic funds transfer process and mandated requirements under the Affordable Care Act (ACA).
12. Define an electronic remittance advice and identify the ASC X12 Health Care Claim Payment/Advice (835).
13. Identify transmission reports generated to track the electronic claims process.
14. List computer transmission problems that can occur.

KEY TERMS

Accredited Standards Committee X12 (ASCX12)
ASCX12 Version 5010
Administrative Simplification Enforcement Tool
American National Standards Institute
application service provider
audit trail
batch
cable modem
carrier-direct system

claim attachments
clearinghouse
code sets
covered entity
data elements
digital subscriber line
direct data entry
electronic data interchange
electronic funds transfer
electronic remittance advice
encoder
encryption

HIPAA Transaction and Code Sets (TCS) rule
National Standard Format
real time
standard transactions
syntax error
T-1
taxonomy codes
trading partner

KEY ABBREVIATIONS

ANSI	DDE	EHR	IRS
ASC X12	DHHS	EMC	MAC
ASET	DSL	EOMB	NDC
ASP	EDI	ERA	NSF
ATM	EFT	HPID	TCS rule

THE ELECTRONIC CLAIM

This chapter will focus on the submission of electronic claims for *professional* services. Further instructions on electronic claims submission for *facility* services will be covered in Chapter 19.

An electronic claim is a *paperless* claim submitted to an insurance carrier as a request for payment of health care services provided to a patient. The electronic claim is generated by computer software and then transmitted electronically through a computer system rather than the US Postal Service or paper fax transmission.

Since the 1960s and early 1970s, claims processing has transitioned from paper claims to electronic claims submission. The federal government has implemented policies through the Administrative Simplification Compliance Act (ASCA) that require providers to submit claims electronically unless they have a waiver on file with their Medicare Administrative Contractor (MAC). Third-party payers have followed this lead, offering and encouraging the use of electronic claims submission. Today, most health care providers submit electronic claims for reimbursement.

Electronic Data Interchange

The exchange of data through computer systems is referred to as **electronic data interchange** (EDI). Using EDI, health insurance claims are exchanged between health care organizations and insurance carriers. This is a process by which understandable data are sent back and forth in a standardized format via computer linkages between entities, or **trading partners**, who function alternately as sender and receiver. Technology and the use of EDI have made processing of transactions more efficient, reducing administrative overhead costs in health care and many other industries (Fig. 15.1).

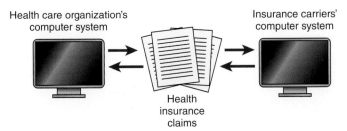

Health care organization's computer system — Insurance carriers' computer system

Health insurance claims

Fig 15.1 The process of sending data back and forth between the health care facility and the trading partner using EDI interchange.

For security purposes, electronic transmissions are encrypted by the sender so that they cannot be opened and read if received by an unauthorized individual. **Encryption** is used to assign a "secret code" to represent data, which makes data unintelligible to unauthorized parties. In encrypted versions, the data appears as gibberish to unauthorized users and must be *decrypted* to use or read.

In electronically secure environments, the sending computer system encrypts or encodes the data being sent and the receiving computer decodes the data to make them understandable. Therefore, both computers must speak the same "language." Standardizing transaction and code sets is required to use EDI effectively. To achieve this, the Health Insurance Portability and Accountability Act (HIPAA) implemented standard formats, procedures, and data content.

Accounts Receivable Management System

Health care organizations use accounts receivable management systems, or computerized billing systems, to manage their billing and cash flow processes. The accounts receivable management system is the tool used to build the insurance claim itself. This system must be able to prepare, process, and send HIPAA-compliant electronic claims efficiently and accurately. Health care organizations that do not have an accounts receivable management system capable of sending electronic claims will often use a clearinghouse to convert data into HIPAA-standard transactions.

It is important for health care organizations to find an accounts receivable management system vendor that understands their needs and the HIPAA Privacy and Security Rules. An accounts receivable management system can help with administrative burdens, such as tracking the receipt of the Notice of Privacy Practices (NPP), noting a patient's consent for treatment, or authorization, and mapping disclosures. A HIPAA-ready accounts receivable management system should do the following:

- Set security access to patient files in the software
- Indicate date of receipt and signature of NPP
- Insert date of patient's authorization
- Maintain files of the health care organization's authorization and notification forms
- Track requests for amendments, requests for restrictions on use and disclosure of protected health information (PHI), and indications of whether the service provider agreed to or denied the request
- Track expiration dates

When assessing the accounts receivable management system's functionality in accounts receivable management, consider the ability to perform the following:

- Set up all of the organization's providers as individuals to bill using correct and appropriate identifiers for each and every health care provider
- Key in all patient demographics and insurance information
- Perform electronic claim submission, by payer, either direct-to-payer or through a clearinghouse

Note that some accounts receivable management systems offer an "add-on" module to go directly to some carriers, such as Medicare, Medicaid, and Blue Cross Blue Shield.

Application Service Providers

Some health care organizations may not have an on-site accounts receivable management system. Instead, they may contract with an application service provider (ASP). An ASP is a business that contracts with a health care organization to supply software applications and services for use over the internet. Essentially, the ASP company is renting an accounts receivable management system to the health care organization over the internet. All data is housed on the server of the ASP, but the accounts are managed by the health care provider's staff. Claims are grouped together by insurance type and submitted as though the software were stored on the desktop at the health care organization.

Transmission of Electronic Claims

Whether using an on-site accounts receivable management system or an ASP, the electronic claim is generated by the health care organization and then transmitted to the insurance carrier. Claims are typically transmitted directly to the carrier or through a clearinghouse. The method for transmission that the health care organization chooses may vary according to the accounts receivable management system's or ASP's capabilities, insurance requirements, or the health care organization's preferred procedures.

Clearinghouse

A clearinghouse is a private company that serves as a middleman and provides connectivity between the health care organization and the insurance carriers. The clearinghouse receives the EDI from the health care organization's office and translates it into a standard format prescribed by HIPAA regulations. Claims are sent to the clearinghouse in batches, or groups of claims, for different patients sent at the same time from one health care organization. Once the clearinghouse receives a batch, it separates the claims by carrier, performs software edits on each claim to check for errors, and transmits claims electronically to the correct insurance payer (Fig. 15.2).

After receiving the claims transmission, a typical clearinghouse process is as follows:

- Claims are checked electronically (scrubbed) for missing or incorrect information using an elaborate editing process.
- Claims that are rejected during the editing process are not sent to the insurance carrier. Instead, they are sent back to the health care organization electronically along with a report that lists the required corrections.
- Batches of claims that pass all edits are then sent to each separate insurance payer. Several claims can be submitted to various insurance payers in a single-batch electronic transmission.

Using a clearinghouse offers the following advantages:
- Translation of various formats to the HIPAA-compliant standard format

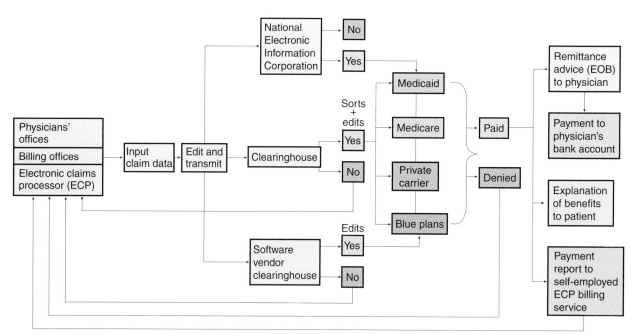

Fig. 15.2 Flow sheet of electronic transmission systems showing path for claim payment via the National Electronic Information Corporation (NEIC), clearinghouse, and independent software vendor. This system also indicates when a payment is made to the health care organization and depicts where claims may not pass an edit or are denied. *EOB,* Explanation of benefits.

- Reduction in time of claims preparation
- Cost-effective method through loss prevention
- Fewer claim rejections
- Fewer delays in processing and quicker response time
- More accurate coding with claims edits
- Consistent reimbursement

Carrier-Direct Claims Submissions

Other health care organizations may choose to transmit claims directly to the insurance companies. Fiscal agents for Medicaid, Medicare, TRICARE, and many third-party private payers use the carrier-direct system for submission of claims. With this system, the data are transmitted electronically directly from the health care organization to the payer's system, without the need for a clearinghouse.

Insurance carriers may also offer direct data entry (DDE). For example, the Centers for Medicare and Medicaid Services (CMS) allows health care organizations to submit claims electronically to a MAC if they are using a computer with software that meets electronic filing requirements as established under HIPAA claim standards. Institutional claims can be submitted to CMS MACs via direct data entry screens. The system called electronic medical claims (EMCs) is used for nearly all Medicare transactions, including claims submission, payment, direct deposit, online eligibility verification, coordination of benefits, and claims status.

Methods of Sending Claims

The methods for getting claims submitted to either the payer or the clearinghouse vary according to the office system in place. Methods can include data transmission via cable modem, digital subscriber line (DSL), or T-1.

- *Cable modem.* A modem used to connect a computer to a cable television system that offers online services.
- *DSL.* A high-speed connection through a telephone line jack and usually a means of accessing the internet.
- *T-1.* A T-carrier channel that can transmit voice or data channels quickly.

Advantages of Electronic Claim Submission

Electronic claim submission offers many advantages to health care organizations. Unlike paper claims, electronic transactions require no signature or stamp, no search for a third-party payer's address, no postage fees or trips to the post office, and no storage of claim forms in a file cabinet. Generally, electronic claim submissions result in improved cash flow and less time spent processing claims, thereby freeing staff for other duties. Information goes from one computer to another, which reduces overhead by decreasing labor costs and potential for human error. EDI claims processing is also faster. After electronic submission of claims, payment can be received in 2 weeks or less. In comparison, when claims are completed manually and sent by mail, payment may take 4 to 6 weeks on average. Electronic transactions build an audit trail, which is a chronological record of submitted data that can be traced to the source, or place of origin. The audit trail confirms if the insurance carrier received the claim, thus eliminating the potential for insurance payers to make the excuse that the claim was never received and therefore not processed.

Another important advantage of electronic claims submission is the online error-edit process that may be incorporated into the software in the health care organization's office, clearinghouse, or insurance company. This feature immediately alerts the person processing the claim to any errors so that a correction can be made before transmission of the claim.

Both paper and electronic claims begin with gathering data before, during, and after the service is rendered. Collecting thorough and accurate information is key to successful submission of both paper and electronic claims.

15.1 QUICK REVIEW

Question: Define the term "encryption" and explain why it is an important concept related to electronic claims submission.

TRANSACTION AND CODE SETS REGULATIONS: STREAMLINING ELECTRONIC DATA INTERCHANGE

Under HIPAA Title II Administrative Simplification, the Secretary of the U.S. Department of Health and Human Services (DHHS) is required to adopt standards to support the electronic exchange of health care transactions between health care providers and plans. The purposes and objectives of this component of HIPAA were to achieve a higher quality of care and reduce administrative costs by streamlining the processing of routine administrative and financial transactions. As a result, the HIPAA Transaction and Code Sets (TCS) rule was developed to introduce efficiencies into the health care system. The DHHS estimated that by implementing TCS, almost $30 billion would be saved over the course of 10 years.

The intent of implementing TCS requirements is to achieve a single, uniform standard. A code-set is any set of codes and their descriptions used to encode data elements, such as a table of terms, medical concepts, medical diagnostic codes, or medical procedure codes. Before HIPAA, there were more than 400 versions of a National Standard Format (NSF) that existed to submit a claim for payment. The TCS regulation, which took effect October 16, 2003, required the implementation of specific standards for transactions and code sets so health care organizations could submit to all carriers in the same format.

HIPAA standardization actions are similar to using a bank's automatic teller machine (ATM) or a grocery store's self-checkout. The magnetic strip on a bank card or the bar code on a grocery item can be swiped across a scanning device, allowing customers to process a transaction more quickly than with traditional, analogue methods. As these methods are adapted, benefits to both the end user and the business providing the technology increase (Table 15.1). Health care organizations benefit from having less paperwork, while the standardization of data results in more accurate information and a more efficient organization.

TABLE 15.1	**Recognized Benefits of Transaction and Code Sets and Electronic Data Interchange**
Benefit	**Result**
More reliable and timely processing—quicker reimbursement from payer	Fast eligibility evaluation; reduced time in claim life cycle; industry averages for claim turnarounds are 9–15 days for electronic versus 30–45 days for paper claims, improving cash flow
Improved accuracy of data	Decreases processing time, increases data quality, and leads to better reporting
Easier and more efficient access to information	Improves patient support
Better tracking of transactions	Assists tracking of transactions (that is, when sent and received), allowing for monitoring (for example, prompt payments)
Reduction of data entry/manual labor	Electronic transactions assist automated processes (for example, automatic payment posting)
Reduction in office expenses	Lowers office supplies, postage, and telephone expenses

Data from Hipaadocs Corporation, Columbia, MD.

As discussed earlier, HIPAA governs how a covered entity is required to handle health information. A covered entity is any health plan, health care provider, or health care clearinghouse that transmits health information in electronic form (Fig. 15.3). Under HIPAA, the following circumstances would likely make the provider a covered entity, therefore, requiring HIPAA compliance:

- If the provider submits electronic transactions to any payer, the provider is considered a covered entity.

If the provider submits paper claims to Medicare and has 10 or more employees, the provider was required to convert to electronic transactions no later than October 16, 2003.

A provider is *not* considered a covered entity under HIPAA in the following circumstances:

- If the provider has fewer than 10 employees and submits claims only on paper to Medicare. The provider may continue to submit on paper and therefore is not required to comply with HIPAA guidelines.
- If the provider submitted only paper claims until and after April 14, 2003, and does not send claims to Medicare, the provider is not required to comply with sending electronic claims.

Fig. 15.3 Decision flow chart of who is subject to the HIPAA Transaction and Code Sets rule.

Transaction and Code Sets Standards

TCS standards have been adopted for health care transactions. HIPAA standard transactions are the specific electronic file formats in which medical data are compiled to be used throughout the health care industry.

In general, code-sets are the allowable sets of codes used to enter information into a specific field on a form. All health care organizations using electronic transactions have to use and accept the code sets systems required under HIPAA that document specific health care data elements. These data elements include medical diagnoses and procedures, drugs, physician services, and medical suppliers. These codes have been in common use throughout the industry for some time, and should have helped ease the transition to the new transaction requirements. What was a standard in the health care industry and recognized by most payers has now been *mandated* under HIPAA.

HIPAA standard codes are used in conjunction with the standard electronic transactions. This standardization eliminates uncertainty when processing transactions. In turn, it improves the quality of data submitted for processing and improves the reimbursement cycle. *Medical code sets* are data elements used uniformly to document why patients are seen (that is, diagnosis, *International Classification of Diseases, Tenth Revision, Clinical Modification* [ICD-10-CM]) and what is done to them during their encounter (that is, procedure, *Current Procedural Terminology, Fourth Edition* [CPT-4], and *Healthcare Common Procedure Coding System* [HCPCS]). Each covered entity organization is responsible for implementing the updated codes in a timely manner as well as deleting old or obsolete codes (Table 15.2). Because of this, health care organizations may opt to utilize coding software or data files that have frequent updates, which include new, updated, and deleted codes. Generally, once codes are deleted, they become *obsolete* for future reporting. However, they are not *removed* from the medical billing system because they were used when billing past accounts and remain active in the system.

Data Requirements

It is essential that the insurance billing specialist understands which data elements are required to construct a HIPAA standard transaction for a paper CMS-1500 form or an electronic claim.

The health care organization's billing software system produces the required HIPAA-standard electronic formats. If the software is not capable of producing such formats, a clearinghouses' can be used to translate data to the HIPAA-standard format.

TABLE 15.2   HIPAA Medical Code Sets and Elements

Standard Code Sets	Medical Data Elements
Healthcare Common Procedure Coding System (HCPCS)	Items and supplies and nonphysician services not covered by the American Medical Association's (AMA's) CPT-4 codes
Current Procedure Terminology (CPT) codes	Medical procedures and health care professional services
International Classification of Diseases, Tenth Revision, Clinical Modification (ICD-10-CM)	Diseases, injuries, impairments, and other health-related problems and their manifestations
International Classification of Diseases, Tenth Revision, Procedural Coding System (ICD-10-PCS)	Procedures or other actions taken for diseases, injuries, and impairments on hospital inpatients reported by hospitals, including prevention, diagnosis, treatment, and management
National Drug Code (NDC)	Pharmaceuticals and biologics
Code on Dental Procedures and Nomenclature, Current Dental Terminology (CDT)	Dental services
Place of service (POS) codes	Indicates the setting in which services are provided

Required and Situational

In addition to the major code sets (ICD-10 and CPT/HCPCS), several *supporting code sets* encompass both medical and nonmedical data. When constructing a claim, the supporting code sets are made up of "required" and "situational" data elements, similar to those on the CMS-1500 paper form. These supporting code sets are embedded in the data elements identified by the HIPAA standard electronic formats. The insurance billing specialist does not need to know all of these specific codes, but it is helpful to know that they exist. When reviewing reports from the clearinghouse or the insurance payer, the insurance billing specialist may have to correct claims that were rejected for not having correct data elements.

Required refers to data elements that *must* be used in order to be considered *in compliance* with a HIPAA-standard transaction. Conversely, *situational* means that the item *may* be required, depending on the data content or context (Examples 15.1 and 15.2).

EXAMPLE 15.1   Required Data

Patient's birth date.
Patient's gender.

EXAMPLE 15.2   Situational Data

Baby's birth weight when an infant is delivered.
Last menstrual period (LMP) when a woman is pregnant.

In addition to other data elements required under HIPAA TCS standards, examples include the following:

Taxonomy Codes: Taxonomy is defined as the science of classification. Taxonomy codes are alphanumeric provider specialty codes (10 characters in length) that classify each health care provider. The taxonomy codes are self-selected by the provider, organized based on education and training, and used to define specialty, not specific services that are rendered. Common taxonomy codes include "general practice 208D0000X," "family practice 207Q00000X," and "nurse practitioner 363L00000X." Beginning January 2, 2007, CMS required providers submitting claims to include a taxonomy code. Taxonomy codes are necessary because some institutional providers may choose not to apply for a unique national provider number for each of its subparts (for example, psychiatric unit or rehabilitation unit). Taxonomy codes are maintained by the National Uniform Claim Committee (NUCC). A link to the NUCC's listing of taxonomy codes is provided at the end of this chapter under *Internet Resources.*

Patient Account Number: To be assigned to every claim.

Relationship to Patient: Expanded to 25 different relationships, including indicators such as "grandson," "adopted child," "mother," and "life partner."

Facility Code Value: Facility-related element that identifies the place of service with at least 29 locations to choose from, including "office," "ambulance air or water," and "end-stage renal disease treatment facility."

 15.2   QUICK REVIEW

Question: Under what circumstances, is a health care provider required to submit claims electronically to Medicare?

ELECTRONIC STANDARD HIPAA 837P

The American National Standards Institute (ANSI) formed the Accredited Standards Committee X12 (ASCX12). ASC X12 is a standards organization that develops, publishes, and maintains electronic data interchange standards for the health

care industry. The ASC X12 was charged with development of standards to complete the following health care related transactions:

- Obtain authorization to refer to a specialist
- Submit a claim for reimbursement
- Request and respond to additional information needed to process a claim
- Record health care claims or equivalent encounter information
- Provide health care payment and remittance advice
- Provide coordination of benefits
- Determine health care claim status
- Enroll and disenroll in a health plan
- Determine eligibility for a health insurance plan
- Make health plan premium payments
- Provide referral certification and authorization
- Make first report of injury
- Add health claims attachments
- Other transactions that DHHS may prescribe by regulation

Each of these standard transactions is identified by a three-digit number preceded by "ASC X12N" (Table 15.3). However, the transactions are referred to in the health care setting using only the three-digit number (for example, 837 or 837P [Professional]). The 837P replaces the paper CMS-1500 form and more than 400 versions of the electronic NSF.

Levels of Information for 837P Standard Transaction Format

Because the 837P is an electronic claims transmittal format, data collected to construct and submit a claim are grouped by levels. It is important for claims processing staff to know the language when following up on claims. Insurance billing specialists do not need to know exactly how these are grouped; however, if the clearinghouse or payer states that there is an invalid item at the "high level," the billing specialist will need to understand that it could be incomplete or erroneous information pertaining to the provider, subscriber, or payer (Table 15.4).

An easier way to understand this new stream-of-data format is to show a crosswalk between the legacy CMS-1500 paper claim and the 837P (Table 15.5).

Accredited Standards Committee X12 Version 5010

The programs for transmission of insurance claims data must be upgraded periodically due to continual changes to policies and regulations for payment of claims. Implementation of ICD-10-CM/PCS in 2015 resulted in the need to upgrade to HIPAA transaction standard ASCX12 Version 5010 for electronic claim submission. Providers, payers, and clearinghouses were required to implement the standard and begin using it on January 1, 2012. Version 5010 allows providers and payers to transmit either ICD-9 or ICD-10 data. Version 5010 also requires health insurers to specify when they received the claim from a health care organization, which allows organizations to calculate interest due on untimely payments. There have been many additional improvements to the system, such as returning claims that need

TABLE 15.3 HIPAA Transaction Functions and Formats

Standard Transaction Function	Industry Format Name
Official Title: Health Care Eligibility Benefit Inquiry and Response **Purpose:** Eligibility verification/response • When obtaining issues regarding benefits and coverage, this standard is used from a health care provider to a health plan or between two health plans. • The 270 is the "inquiry for eligibility verification." • The 271 is the "response."	ASC X12N 270/271
Official Title: Health Care Claim Status Request and Response **Purpose:** Health claim status inquiry/response • The 276 is the "inquiry" to determine the status of a claim. • The 277 is the "response."	ASC X12N 276/277
Official Title: Health Care Services Review—Request for Review and Response **Purpose:** Referral certification and authorization for patient health care services	ASC X12N 278
Official Title: Payroll Deducted and Other Group Premium Payment for Insurance Products **Purpose:** Health plan premium payments, including payroll deductions	ASC X12N 820
Official Title: Benefit Enrollment and Maintenance **Purpose:** Transmission of subscriber enrollment information to a health plan to establish coverage or terminate the policy	ASC X12N 834
Official Title: Payment and Remittance Advice **Purpose:** Transmission indicating the explanation of benefits or remittance advice from a health plan payer to the health care provider • This also may be data sent from a health plan directly to the provider's financial institution (bank) and may include payment and information about the processing of the claim.	ASC X12N 835
Official Title: Health Care Claim or Equivalent Encounter **Purpose:** To obtain payment for the transmitted health services encounter information • The 837P (Professional) replaces the paper CMS-1500 form and the electronic National Standard Format (NSF). • The 837I (Institutional) replaces the paper UB-04 often used in hospitals. • The 837D (Dental) is used for dentistry. • Additionally, the coordination of benefits (COB) for claims and payment will be transmitted through the 837 format.	ASC X12N 837 includes: A. 837P—Health Care Claim, Professional B. 837I—Health Care Claim, Institutional C. 837D—Health Care Claim, Dental
Proposed Official Title: First Report of Illness, Injury, or Incident **Potential Purpose:** This standard will be used to report information on a claim pertaining to factors such as date of onset of illness or date of accident.	PROPOSED ASC X12N 148

TABLE 15.3 HIPAA Transaction Functions and Formats—cont'd

Standard Transaction Function	Industry Format Name
Proposed Official Title: Health Claims Attachment **Potential Purpose:** Transmit additional information to claim 1. This means no more photocopied attachments stapled to paper claims or additional information mailed after the claim is initially received.	PROPOSED ASC X12 275 and HL7

TABLE 15.4 Data Grouping in 837P Standard Transaction Format

Level	Information
High-level information: Applies to the entire claim and reflects data pertaining to the billing provider, subscriber, and patient	• Billing/pay to provider information • Subscriber/patient information • Payer information
Claim-level information: Applies to the entire claim and all service lines and is applicable to most claims	Claim information
Specialty claim–level information: Applies to specific claim types	Specialty
Service line–level information: Applies to specific procedure or service that is rendered and is applicable to most claims	Service line information
Specialty service line–level information: Applies to specific claim types; required data are required only for the specific claim type	Specialty service line information
Other information	• Coordination of benefits • Repriced claim/line • Credit/debit information • Clearinghouse/value added network tracking

corrections to the provider sooner, assignment of claim numbers closer to the time received by the payer, and more consistency of claims editing and error handling. Going forward, insurance billing specialists can expect ongoing upgrades. A newer electronic transaction standard, the Version 6020, was tabled in 2015, and Version 7030 is under development.

Claim Attachments Standards

Claim attachments are supplemental documents providing additional medical information to the claims processor that cannot be accommodated within the claim format. Common attachments are Certificates of Medical Necessity (CMNs), lab reports, discharge summaries, and operative reports. Accounts receivable management and claims software include a data field that can be used to indicate that a paper claims attachment is included with the claim.

HIPAA identified a health claim attachment as one of the transactions for which electronic standards were to be adopted.

TABLE 15.5   Comparison of CMS-1500 and 837P v5010A1

| | 1500 FORM LOCATOR | ANSI 837P VERSION 5010 | | |
Block Number	Block Title	Loop ID	Segment/ Data Element	837P Title
N/A	Carrier Block	2010BB	NM103 N301 N302 N401 N402 N403	
1	Medicare, Medicaid, TRICARE, CHAMPUS, CHAMPVA, Group Health Plan, FECA, Black Lung, Other	2000B	SBR09	Claim Filing Indicator
1a	Insured's ID Number	2010BA	NM109	Subscriber Primary Identifier
2	Patient's Name	2010CA or 2010BA	NM103 NM104 NM105 NM107	Subscriber last, first and middle name.
3	Patient's Birth Date, Sex	2010CA or 2010BA	DMG02 DMG03	Birth Date/Gender
4	Insured's Name	2010BA	NM103 NM104 NM105 NM107	Subscriber
5	Patient's Address	2010CA	N302 N401 N402 N403	Patient Address
6	Patient Relationship to Insured	2000B2000C	SBR02 PAT01	Individual Relationship Code
7	Insured's Address	2010BA	N301 N302 N401 N402 N403	Subscriber Address
8	Reserved for NUCC use.	Leave blank.	N/A	Does not exist in the 837P
9	Other Insured's Name	2330A	NM103 NM104 NM105 NM107	Other Subscriber Name
9a	Other Insured's Policy or Group Number	2320	SBR03	Insured Group or Policy Number
9b	Reserved for NUCC use.	Leave blank.	N/A	Does not exist in 837P.
9c	Reserved for NUCC use.	Leave blank	N/A	Does not exist in 837P.
9d	Insurance Plan Name or Program Name	2320	SBR04	Other Group Name
10a,10b, 10c	Is Patient's Condition Related to: Employment?Auto accident?Other accident?	2300	CLM11	Related Causes Code
10d	Reserved for local use	2300	HI	Other condition codes.
11	Insured's Policy, Group, or FECA Number	2000B	SBR03	Subscriber Group or Policy Number.
11a	Insured's Date of Birth, Sex	2010BA	DMG02 DMG03	Subscriber Birth Date and Subscriber Gender Code.
11b	Other Claim ID (Designated by NUCC)	2010BA.	REF01 REF02	Other Claim ID.
11c	Insurance Plan Name or Program Name	2000B	SBR04	Subscriber Group Name.
11d	Is there another Health Benefit Plan?	2320		
12	Patient's or Authorized Person's Signature	2300	CLM09	Release of Information Code.
13	Insured's or Authorized Person's Signature	2300	CLM08	Benefits Assignment Certification Indicator
14	Date of Current Illness, Injury, Pregnancy	2300	DTP01 DTP03	Date of Onset of Current Illness or Symptom Date of Last Menstrual Period

TABLE 15.5 Comparison of CMS-1500 and 837P v5010A1—cont'd

| | 1500 FORM LOCATOR | ANSI 837P VERSION 5010 | | |
Block Number	Block Title	Loop ID	Segment/ Data Element	837P Title
15	Other Date	2300	DTP01 DTP03	Dates for initial treatment, last seen date, acute manifestation, accident, last x-ray date, hearing and vision prescription date, assumed and relinquished care, property and casualty date of first contact.
16	Dates Patient Unable to Work in Current Occupation	2300	DTP03	Disability Form Date and Work Return Date.
17	Name of Referring Provider or Other Source	2310A (referring) 2310D (supervising) 2420E (ordering)	NM101 NM103 NM104 NM105 NM107	Referring Providerapplicable.
17a	Other ID#	2310A (referring) 2310D (supervising) 2420 (ordering)	REF01 REF02	Referring Provider Secondary Identifier, Supervising Provider Secondary Identifier and Ordering Provider Secondary Identifier.
17b	NPI#	2310A (referring) 2310D (supervising) 2420E (ordering)	NM109	Referring Provider Identifier, Supervising Provider Identifier and Ordering Provider Identifier.
18	Hospitalization Dates Related to Current Services	2300	DTP03	Related Hospitalization Admission Date and Related Hospitalization Discharge Date.
19	Additional Claim Information Reserved for local use	2300 2310A (referring) 2310B (rendering) 2310C (service facility) 2310D (supervising)	NTE PWK REF01 REF102	Do not use in 837P.
20	Outside Lab Charges	2400	PS102	Purchased Service Charge Amount.
21	Diagnosis or Nature of Illness or Injury	2300	HI01-2 HI02-2 HI03-2 HI04-2 HI05-2 HI06-2 HI07-2 HI08-2 HI09-2 HI10-2 HI11-2 HI12-2	Diagnosis Codes 1 through 12.
22	Resubmission and/or Original Reference Number	2300	CLM05-3	Claim Frequency Code
		2300	REF02	Payer Claim Control Number.
23	Prior Authorization Number	2300	REF02	Prior Authorization Number
		2300	REF02	Referral Number
		2300	REF02	Clinical Laboratory Improvement Amendment Number
		2300	REF02	Mammography Certification Number
24A	Date(s) of Service	2400	DTP03	Service Date
24B	Place of Service	2300	CLM05-1	Facility Code Value
		2400	SV105	Place of Service Code
24C	EMG	2400	SV109	Emergency Indicator
24D	Procedures, Services, or Supplies	2400	SV101-2 SV101-3 SV101-4 SV101-5 SV101-6	Procedure/Service ID and Procedure Modifier.
24E	Diagnosis Pointer	2400	SV107-1 SV107-2 SV107-3 SV107-4	Diagnosis Code Pointer.

TABLE 15.5   Comparison of CMS-1500 and 837P v5010A1—cont'd

Block Number	Block Title	Loop ID	Segment/ Data Element	837P Title
	1500 FORM LOCATOR		**ANSI 837P VERSION 5010**	
24F	$Charges	2400	SV102	Line Item Charge Amount
24G	Days or Units	2400	SV104	Service Unit Count
24H	EPSDT/Family Plan	2400	SV111 SV112	EPSDT Indicator and Family Planning Indicator
24I Shaded Line	ID Qualifier	2310B	PRV02 REF01	Reference Identification Qualifier
		2420A	PRV02 REF01	Reference Identification Qualifier
24J Shaded line	Rendering Provider ID#	2310B 2420A	PRV03 REF02	Provider Taxonomy Code and Rendering Provider Secondary Identifier
24J	Rendering Provider ID#	2310B2420A	NM109	Provider Taxonomy Code and Rendering Provider Secondary Identifier
25	Federal Tax ID Number	2010AA	REF01 REF02	Reference Identification Qualifier and Billing Provider Tax Identification Number
26	Patient's Account No.	2300	CLM01	Patient Control Number
27	Accept Assignment?	2300	CLM07	Assignment or Plan Participation Code
28	Total Charge	2300	CLM02	Total Claim Charge Amount
29	Amount Paid	23002320	AMT02	Payer Paid Amount
30	Reserved for NUCC Use.	Leave blank.	N/A	Does not exist in 837P.
31	Signature of Health care Provider or Supplier Including Degrees or Credentials	2300	CLM06	Provider or Supplier Signature Indicator
32	Service Facility Location Information	2310C	NM103 N301 N401 N402 N403	Laboratory or Facility Information
32a	NPI#	2310C	NM109	Laboratory or Facility Primary Identifier
32b	Other ID#	2310C	REF01 REF02	Reference Identification Qualifier and Laboratory or Facility Secondary Identifier.
33	Billing Provider Info & Ph #	2010AA	NM103 NM104 NM105 NM107 N301 N401 N402 N403 PER04	Billing Provider or Organization Name and Address.
33a	NPI#	2010AA	NM109	Billing Provider Identifier
33b	Other ID#	2000A 2010AA	PRV03 REF01 REF02	Provider Taxonomy Code. Reference Identification Qualifier and Billing Provider Additional Identifier.

Source: NUCC 02/12 1500 Claim Form Map to the X12 Health Care Claim: Professional (837).

However, the final rule was never adopted. The Affordable Care Act (ACA), mandatory compliance date of January 1, 2016, has come and gone. Despite this, various organizations have continued to research and develop the electronic attachment issue. It is hoped that it will be addressed in the upcoming Version 7030 standard for electronic claims submission.

15.3   QUICK REVIEW

Question: What are the six levels of data grouping used for information in the 837P standard transmission standards?

STANDARD UNIQUE IDENTIFIERS

Standard Unique Identifiers are used to identify the specific entities associated with the electronic claims process; entities include employers, providers, and health plans.

Standard Unique Employer Identifier

The employer identification number (EIN) is assigned by the Internal Revenue Service (IRS) and used to identify employers for tax purposes. HIPAA requires that the EIN be used to identify employers rather than inputting the name of the company when submitting claims. Employers use their EINs to identify themselves in transactions involving premium payments to health plans on behalf of their employees or to identify themselves or other employers as the source or receiver of information about eligibility. Employers also will use EINs to identify themselves in transactions when enrolling or disenrolling employees in a health plan.

Standard Unique Health Care Provider Identifier

In the past, health insurance plans have assigned an identifying number to each provider with whom they conduct business. This resulted in providers having many different identifier numbers when submitting claims to several different payers.

Under HIPAA, all providers were required to obtain a National Provider Identifier (NPI) that is assigned to each provider for use in transactions with all health plans. The NPI is completely numeric, is 10 characters in length, and became a requirement on all claims effective May 23, 2007.

According to CMS, NPI is a lasting identifier. It will not change with changes to a health care provider's name, address, ownership, membership in health plans, or Healthcare Provider Taxonomy classification. A link to the NPI database has been provided at the end of this chapter under *Internet Resources.*

Standard Unique Health Plan Identifier

Previously, health plans were identified in electronic transactions by multiple identifiers that differed in length, format, and meaning. The current versions of the adopted standards (ASC X12N) allow health plans to use these various identifiers in standard transactions that result in inconsistent use of identifiers for health plans.

The ACA required implementation of standard unique health plan identifiers (HPIDs). The standard unique HPID rule assigned a standard identifier to identify health plans that process and pay certain electronic health care transactions. On October 4, 2012, a corrected and final rule was posted in the *Federal Register,* which stated that health plans (with the exception of small health plans) were required to obtain an HPID by November 5, 2014. Small health plans had to obtain an HPID by November 5, 2015. Covered entities were required to use HPIDs in the standard transactions on or after November 7, 2016.

The adoption of the HPID increased standardization within HIPAA standard transactions and provided a platform for other regulatory initiatives. The use of HPIDs brought a higher level of automation to health care organizations as they process billing and perform other insurance-related tasks, such as verification of patient eligibility and processing of remittance advices.

Standard Unique Patient Identifier

In addition to standardization of a unique *provider identifier* and a unique HPID, both HIPAA and the ACA support the creation of a unique patient identifier system. However, privacy and security concerns have stalled efforts to implement the proposal. The intention to create a standard for a uniform patient identifier has also prompted protest among public interest groups who consider a universal identifier to be a civil liberties threat. Therefore, the issue of a universal patient identifier is "on hold."

15.4 QUICK REVIEW
Question: What is an NPI and explain how it can be identified?

BUILDING THE ELECTRONIC CLAIM

Claims are built with data collected from the patient, from the provider and as required by billing guidelines. Electronic claims are built in the medical billing system.

Keying Insurance Data for Claim Transmission

Data are entered into the computer system by the health care organization's staff. Information must be entered cautiously and accurately to ensure development of a "clean claim." When entering patient data into a software program, a prompt appears on the screen and the data are entered in reply to the prompt. For example, under patient name/address, the staff will be prompted to type the patient's last name, first name, and middle name (Fig. 15.4).

Reusable data are entered initially in a file and identified by a number. Each treating or referring health care provider, patient, and third-party payer has an assigned computer code number. Notice in Figs. 15.5 and 15.6 that a patient, Charles Weber, is input as account number WEBCH000; Star Insurance is STA00; and the provider is keyed as DIW, the initials of the provider. This information is stored in the database and is the same as that necessary for completing a claim manually. It is automatically

Fig. 15.4 Patient entry screen using accounts receivable management software. (Screenshot used by permission of MCKESSON Corporation. All rights reserved. ©MCKESSON Corporation 2012.)

Fig. 15.5 Insurance information using accounts receivable management software. Notice that the code for the payer is "STA00." (Screenshot used by permission of MCKESSON Corporation. All rights reserved. ©MCKESSON Corporation 2012.)

retrieved by the system when a computer code number is keyed in and used to generate a computerized claim or electronic claim.

Because there are computer code numbers and prompts for each item, the chances of error or omission of mandatory information is reduced. The program checks that data are complete and in proper format.

Some general "do's and don'ts" for keying in data and billing electronic claims follow.

Do: Use the patient account numbers to differentiate between patients with similar names.

Do: Use correct numeric locations of service code and current valid CPT, or HCPCS procedure codes.

Do: Print an insurance billing worksheet or perform a front-end edit (online error checking) to look for and correct all errors before the claim is transmitted to the third-party payer.

Do: Request electronic error reports from the third-party payer to make corrections to the system.

Do: Obtain and cross-check the electronic status report against all claims transmitted.

After input is complete, the information is stored in memory and a claim may be transmitted individually or in batches. Batched claims can be divided according to insurance type or date(s) of service and are ideally sent during low-volume times.

Because the health care provider is responsible for submitting an accurate bill, the insurance billing specialist must accurately input the codes. Medicare and other third-party payer's claims examiners are forbidden to recode a claim. During the edit and error process, software code editors identify invalid codes, age conflicts, gender conflicts, procedural and diagnostic code conflicts, and other data points before issuing payment. If certain information, such as a patient's name or insurance identification number, is submitted incorrectly, the claim is rejected and must be resubmitted with corrected data. Incorrect coding may be a keying error, or it may be a deliberate attempt to obtain fraudulent payment. The edit check allows immediate feedback about the status of an electronically transmitted claim. The service provider may revise coding on the medical record and on the claim to reflect the services more accurately until such time as the claim is transmitted for payment.

Encoder

An **encoder** is coding software that can be added to a medical billing or accounts-receivable management system. Encoders can greatly reduce the time it takes to build or review a claim before batching and can improve overall coding accuracy

Fig. 15.6 Entering patient information in an electronic encounter form. Notice that the provider's initials are DIW. (Screenshot used by permission of MCKESSON Corporation. All rights reserved. ©MCKESSON Corporation 2012.)

by utilizing this software. The insurance billing specialist is prompted with a series of questions or choices, leading to, or affecting a specific code assignment by displaying code-specific edits. Using an encoder can enhance a health care organization's compliance program when it comes to accuracy in its billing procedures. Used as an audit tool, the encoder can also be helpful in performance improvement by identifying problem areas in the billing process.

However, there are instances when an encoder does not accurately assign codes; therefore, one must never be completely dependent on code-assist software. For example, if a patient has three thorns incised and extracted (removed), the CPT code 10120 "incision and removal of foreign body, subcutaneous tissue; simple (integumentary system)," might be generated by the encoder. However, if internally audited, the case may warrant CPT code 27372 "removal of foreign body, deep, thigh region in knee area (musculoskeletal system)." Thus, one learns that not all procedures involving the skin are found in the integumentary system and, if deeper skin layers are affected, a more appropriate code may be found in another system.

Signature Requirements

The final considerations in building a claim are the signature requirements for both the patient and the service provider.

Service Provider

The service provider's signature on the agreement or contract with the third-party payer is a substitute for their signature on the claim form.

Patient

For assignment of benefits, each patient's signature must be obtained and retained in the office records because there are no handwritten signatures on electronic claims (Fig. 15.7). A clause on the patient registration form, or an authorization and assignment release document may be designed specifically to obtain signatures for transmitting electronic claims and acceptance of financial responsibility by the patient. The CMS-1500 Health Insurance Claim Form also may be used for this purpose and the patient should sign in Block 12 or 13 for a specific date of service. Most medical billing and accounts receivable management systems ask whether the patient's signature is on file and require a "yes" or "no" answer to complete the required field when the claim is submitted. When a service provider sees a patient in the hospital who has never been to the office, the authorizations obtained by the hospital apply to that provider's filing of a claim.

Clean Electronic Claims Submission

Because a denied claim can delay payment for 30 to 100 days or more, clean claims are the key to a healthy revenue cycle. By ensuring that clean claims are submitted initially, the chances of getting paid promptly are increased. According to industry experts, 90% of claim denials are preventable. The following is a review of some methods used to ensure clean electronic claims:

PATIENT'S MEDICARE ELECTRONIC SIGNATURE MONTHLY AUTHORIZATION FORM

I authorize any holder of medical or other information about me to release to the Social Security Administration and Centers for Medicare and Medicaid Services or its intermediaries or carriers any information needed for this or a related Medicare claim. I permit a copy of this authorization to be used in place of the original, and request payment of medical insurance benefits either to myself or to the party who accepts assignment.

_____   _____
Signature of Patient   Date

A

PATIENT'S MEDICARE ELECTRONIC SIGNATURE ONE-TIME AUTHORIZATION FORM

I request that payment of authorized Medicare benefits be made either to me or on my behalf to _____ for services furnished me by that physician or supplier. I permit a copy of this authorization to be used in place of the original and authorize any holder of medical information about me to release to the Centers for Medicare and Medicaid Services or its agents any information needed to determine these benefits or the benefits payable for related services.

_____   _____
Signature of Patient   Date

B

Fig. 15.7 Examples of patients' Medicare electronic signature authorization forms. (A) Monthly form. (B) One-time form.

- Incorporate claim scrubber software (prebill/edit processing) to identify errors and correct them on initial submission.
- Verify, file, and keep all transmission reports.
- Track clearinghouse claims to ensure successful transmission.
- Ensure that computer software is consistent with the claims rules.
- Verify that computer software correctly prints the CMS-1500 claim form.
- Use encoder software.
- Use an electronic clearinghouse.
- Perform single and batch claims review.

15.5 QUICK REVIEW

Question: Explain the signature requirement for health care providers on electronic claims?

FOLLOW-UP OF ELECTRONIC CLAIMS PROCESSING

After successful submission of the electronic claim, the insurance billing specialist will be required to continue their oversight and follow-up of the claims, until payment has been received or the claim has been denied and redirected.

Interactive Transactions

Continued oversight and follow-up of electronic claims submission includes communicating with the insurance carrier.

Interactive transactions involve back-and-forth communication between two computer systems. One requests information and the other provides information during what is referred to as *online real time*. Real time allows for instant information. An inquiry is made and an answer received within seconds. It can involve eligibility verification, deductible status, claim inquiries, status of claims, and other insurance claim data. Other information, such as fee schedules, allowables, procedure codes, and postoperative days for specific procedures, also may be accessed. Many insurance companies, provide access to information on assigned pending and paid claims. Additional information that may be determined includes whether the individual has other coverage and which third-party payer should be billed as primary.

Electronic Remittance Advice

Upon successful processing of the electronic claim, the insurance carrier will issue an electronic remittance advice. An electronic remittance advice (ERA) is a notice of payments and adjustments sent to providers, billers, and suppliers. The ERA may serve as a companion to a claim payment or as an explanation when there is no payment. The ERA explains reimbursement decisions, including the reasons for payments and adjustments of processed claims. The ERA is similar to the remittance advice (RA) for paper claims, except that the ERA offers additional information and administrative efficiencies.

If the health care organization elects to set the software system to automatically post the information to patients' accounts, then data entry is not required. The computer tests the claims computer data against various guidelines or parameters known as *screens*. If the services billed on the claim exceed the screens, the claim is denied, returned to the service provider for more information, or sent for review. If a claim is denied or rejected, the insurance billing specialist receives a printout stating the reason. The missing, miscoded, or incomplete information should be added or corrected, and the claim resubmitted. This process is more efficient than remaining on a telephone, on hold, or resubmitting a claim via standard mail.

Electronic Funds Transfer

Many third-party payers deposit payments in the health care organization's bank account automatically via electronic funds transfer (EFT). EFT is a paperless computerized system that enables funds to be debited, credited, or transferred and eliminates the need for personal handling of checks. A deposit-only bank account, sometimes called *zero-balance account (ZBA)*, provides protection against cyber-thieves. This account has blocks and filters so that it accepts only deposits. However, if the health plan's EFT agreement allows it to recoup overpayments from the provider's bank account, this restriction would have to be removed.

Under the ACA, the federal government has established a uniform procedure for electronically transferring funds as part of HIPAA Title II Administrative Simplification. Health care providers and others were required to comply with CMS's EFT

rules by January 1, 2014. The benefits to a health care organization for using EFT include the following:

- Reduction in the amount of paper in the office
- Time savings for staff
- Avoiding the hassles associated with depositing checks at the bank
- Elimination of the risk of paper checks being lost or stolen in the mail
- Faster access to funds
- Easier reconciliation of payments with bank statements

> **15.6   QUICK REVIEW**
> Question: Define electronic funds transfer and explain the benefits.

TRANSMISSION REPORTS

Whether claims are submitted carrier-direct or through a clearinghouse, reports are generated to track each function of the claims process. Examples are as follows:

- **Send and Receive File Reports:** Shows that a file is received by the clearinghouse and/or payer and notifies the billing specialist when a file has been sent to the service provider's account for review (Fig. 15.8).
- **Batch Claim Report Billed Summary:** Lists each patient's name, total charges for medical services, batch number, billing number, name of insurance company billed, and chronologic date on which the claim was transmitted (Fig. 15.9).
- **Scrubber Report:** Indicates the total number of claims, the charges, and the dollar amounts that were received by the clearinghouse and scrubbed for claims submitted to a specific insurance plan (Fig. 15.10). The insurance billing specialist reviews the scrubber report for each insurance payer when claims have been transmitted through the clearinghouse.
- **Transaction Transmission Summary:** Shows how many claims were originally received by the clearinghouse and/or payer and how many claims were rejected automatically (Fig. 15.11).
- **Rejection Analysis Report:** Identifies the most common reasons that claims are rejected and indicates what claims were not included for processing Corrections must be made by the insurance billing specialist and the claims need to be refiled.
- **Electronic Inquiry or Claims Status Review:** Lists files received from the provider's office and indicates the progress of the claim. For example, if a claim is sent to a clearinghouse and forwarded to a payer, the clearinghouse can indicate that the status is confirmed received by the payer.

Electronic Processing Problems

Some problems can occur in electronic claims submission. Usually a status report of claims is received electronically from the third-party payer. It consists of an acknowledgment report and indicates assigned and unassigned claims, crossed over and not

```
                          Raw 837
                          =========

                     ElectronicTechnologiesInc.
                     ==========================


ISA*00* *00*
*ZZ*1234*ZZ*VB6786786*041110*0310*U*00401*123456789*0*P*:~GS*HC*12
34*VB6786786*20041110*0310*123456789*X*004010X098A1~S *837*0001~B
HT*0019*00*1*20041110*0310*CH~REF*87*004010X098A1~NM1*41*2*GERI
ATRIC ASSOCIAS LC    *****46*1234~PER*IC*JIM
JONES*TE*8005551212~NM1*40*2*MASSACHUSETTS INS
PLAN*****46*XYZ1~HL*1*20*1~NM1*85*2*ALABAMA MEDICA
ASSOC*****24*54-5555555~N3*PO BOX
123456~N4*BOSTON *MA*12345~REF*1D*123456789~HL*2*1*22*0~SBR*P*1
8*******MC~NM1*IL*1*JONES*DEBRA  K**MI*123456789123~N *11
JEFFERS POND
ROAD~N4*BOSTON *MA*12345~DMG*D8*19640812*F~NM1 *PR*2*VMAP
FHSCFA*****PI*DMAS~N3*PO BO
123~N4*BOSTON *MA*12345~CLM*123456*150**11::1*Y*A*Y*Y*B~REF*X
4*1242522DD~HI*BK6110~NM1 *DN*1*JACKSON *DONALD~REF*1D*12345
6789~NM1*82*1*ROWLAND DAVID   ****24*54-
5555555~PRV *PE*ZZ*207ZP0102X~REF*1D*123456789~NM1*77*2*NORTH
OFFICE*****24*54-5555555~N3*123 LIPPLE
AVENUE~N4*BOSTON *MA*12345~LX*1~SV1*HC:88305:26*150*UN*1***1~
DTP *472*D8*20041028~REF*6R*11265594~
  .
  .
  .
  .
  .
SE*160*0001~GE *1*123456789~IEA*1*123456789~
```

A

```
                     Human-Readable 837
                     ==================
                   Electronic Technologies, Inc.
                     ==================
```

INTERCHANGE HEADER - Production File	Account Number: 123456
	Claim Amount: $150
Authorization: none Password: none	Facility: Office
SubmitterID: 1234 ReceiverID: VB6786786	This Claim is ORIGINAL
Date: 11.10.20XX Time: 0310	Provider Signature: On File Assignment Code: Assigned
Run #: 003 Control #: 123456789	Assignment of Benefits Indicator: Y
Request Acknowledgement: No Sub-element Separator: :	Release of Information: Yes, Provider Has a Signed Statement
	Permitting Release of Medical Billing
FUNCTIONAL GROUP HEADER - HC	Data Related to a Claim
	CLIA Number: 1242522DD
Submitter ID: 1234 ReceiverID: VB6786786	Principal Diagnosis Code: 6110
Date: 11.10.20XX Time: 0310 Control #: 123456789	
ANSI X10 Version: 004010X098A1	Referring Prov. - Person

TRANSACTION SET HEADER- 837	JACKSON, DONALD
	MA Provider Number: 123456789
Control #: 0001	
Structure Code: 0019 Purpose Code: 00	Rendering Prov. - Person
Reference ID: 1 Type: CH	---------------
Date: 11.10.20XX Time: 0310	ROWLAND, DAVID (Employer ID Number,54-5555555)
Functional Category: 004010X098A1	Provider Taxonomy Code: 207ZP0102X
	MA Provider Number: 123456789
Submitter - Non-Person	
---------	Service Location - Non-Person
GERIATRIC ASSOCIATES LLC (Electronic Transmitter ID #,1234)	---------------
Contact: JIM JONES	NORTH OFFICE (Employer ID Number,54-5555555)
Phone Number: 800.555.1212	123 LIPPLE AVENUE
	BOSTON, MA 12345
Receiver - Non-Person	
--------	Service Line # 1
MASSACHUSETTS INS PLAN (Electronic Transmitter ID #,XYZ1)	---------------
	Service Code: 88305
BATCH #1	Modifier: 26
	Amount: $150 Measurement: Unit Quantity: 1
Billing Provider - Non-Person	Diagnosis Pointer: 1
---------------	Date of Service: 20041028
ALABAMA MEDICAL ASSOC (Employer ID Number,54-5555555)	Prov. Control #: 11265594
PO BOX 123456	
BOSTON, MA 12345	**PATIENT #2**
Provider Number: 123456789	
	.
PATIENT #1	.
	.
Primary Insurance	.

Patient Relationship: Self	**TRANSACTION SET TRAILER**
Subscriber - Person	Included Segments: 160
	Control #: 0001
JONES, DEBRA K (Member ID Number,123456789123)	
11 JEFFERS POND ROAD	**FUNCTIONAL GROUP TRAILER**
BOSTON, MA 12345	
	Transaction Sets Included: 1
Date of Birth: 19640812 Gender Code: F	Group Control #: 123456789
Payer - Non-Person	**INTERCHANGE TRAILER**

VMAP FHSC FA (Payer ID Number,DMAS)	Included Functional Groups: 1
PO BOX 123	Control #: 123456789
BOSTON, MA 12345	

B

Fig. 15.8 (A) Raw 837 clearinghouse transmission report. A printed 837 electronic claims transmission file will look similar to this; however, the report becomes readable after it comes back from the clearinghouse showing the patients' claims that were submitted. (B) Readable 837 clearinghouse transmission report. (Reports supplied by Electronic Technologies, Inc., Delmar, NY.)

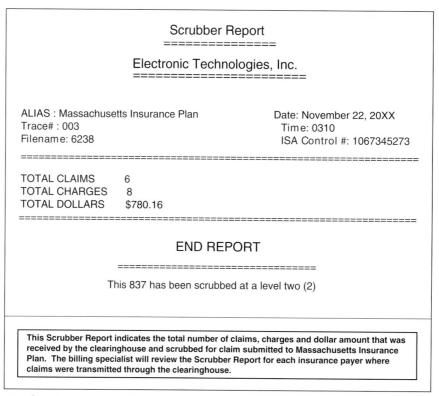

BATCH CLAIM REPORT Billed Summary

Patient code	Total charges	Batch #	Billing #	Insurance co. billed	Date sent
BORTOLUSSI	465.00	2	1005	ABCI000001	05/25/20XX
BLACKWOOD	16.07	3	1006	TRICARE	05/25/20XX
HELMS	33.25	4	1007	MDCR	05/25/20XX
JAMESON	41.07	5	1008	ROYAL	05/25/20XX
KELSEY	66.23	8	1010	XYZI000001	06/09/20XX
	621.62				

Fig. 15.9 Batch Claim Report Billed Summary by chronologic date.

Scrubber Report
================

Electronic Technologies, Inc.
=========================

ALIAS : Massachusetts Insurance Plan
Trace# : 003
Filename: 6238

Date: November 22, 20XX
Time: 0310
ISA Control #: 1067345273

TOTAL CLAIMS	6
TOTAL CHARGES	8
TOTAL DOLLARS	$780.16

END REPORT

This 837 has been scrubbed at a level two (2)

This Scrubber Report indicates the total number of claims, charges and dollar amount that was received by the clearinghouse and scrubbed for claim submitted to Massachusetts Insurance Plan. The billing specialist will review the Scrubber Report for each insurance payer where claims were transmitted through the clearinghouse.

Fig. 15.10 Clearinghouse scrubber report. (Report supplied by Electronic Technologies, Inc., Delmar, NY.)

crossed over claims, claims accepted with errors, and rejected claims (Fig. 15.12). Data transmission problems arise periodically because of hardware or software problems.

Changes to the standard electronic claims submission process can also result in errors. The upgrade to HIPAA transaction standard ASC X12 Version 5010 resulted in these common errors:

Billing Provider Address: The 5010 guidelines require providers to enter the physical address; post office boxes or lock box addresses cannot be used as a health care organization's address.

Zip Code: The 5010 guidelines require a nine-digit zip code when reporting billing provider and service facility locations.

Anesthesia Minutes: The 5010 guidelines require that anesthesia services be reported in actual minutes rather than units.

Primary Identification Code Qualifiers: The 5010 guidelines allow only an NPI as a primary identifier. EINs or Social Security numbers cannot be used as a primary identifier.

Billing Provider NPI Number: The 5010 guidelines require that a consistent NPI number be reported with all payers.

National Drug Code (NDC): The 5010 guidelines require that a drug quantity and unit of measure be reported on the claim form when an NDC is used.

Most billing software bundles claims into a batch and then the claims are transmitted together. If one claim in the batch

HIPAA Standard Transaction "Functional Acknowledgment" (ASC X12 997)

The 997 indicates whether the claim file was accepted or rejected.

Fig. 15.11 Clearinghouse 997 report that shows which 837 claim files were accepted and rejected. (Report supplied by Electronic Technologies, Inc., Delmar, NY.)

contains an error, such as, missing a patient name or missing a diagnosis code, the third-party payer may reject the entire batch and return all claims to the provider.

Some batches contain errors that occur in every transaction in the batch. These are called syntax errors. Syntax errors are inaccuracies that violate the HIPAA standard transaction format, such as incorrect sequence of patient information or incorrect batch header. Such errors make it difficult for the third-party payer's software to read the transactions in a batch.

There are other errors in which only one transaction in the batch has a syntax error or one of the batch's transactions has a data content error. In these instances, it would be inappropriate for a third-party payer to reject the entire batch. Usually the payer returns any noncompliant claims and processes the remaining claims in the batch. To avoid these types of rejections, it is important to use software that will separate out noncompliant transactions so that those can be removed from the batch and fixed before submission.

Solutions to Electronic Processing Problems

1. Review claims filed electronically by validating and confirming that claims were processed by the clearinghouse and received by the insurance carrier. Check for error messages from the clearinghouse and payer. Immediately respond to rejected claims.

2. Produce monthly aging of accounts and check the large amounts not paid in the 60-day aging column. Look at service dates of claims and the amounts. If there are many outstanding claims with the same service dates, it is possible that these claims did not reach the payer. Immediately confirm with the payer whether the claims were received and refile if appropriate.

3. File claims within the time limits because many payers have a 90-day filing deadline. Payers will not reimburse a time delinquent claim unless the health care organization can prove that the payer received the claim. Electronic confirmation that a claim reached the clearinghouse is not sufficient.

4. Double check that the correct code for place of service is shown, especially if the service provider does procedures in different locations. The payment amount may be more or less, depending on the location.

5. Be accurate in linking the correct diagnosis codes to the procedure codes. Usually payers use the first diagnosis codes to process claims. Additional diagnostic codes may be used only for informational purposes or not considered at all.

```
              ALIAS: Massachusetts Insurance Plan 997 Report
              =========================================
                     CLAIMS 997 ACKNOWLEDGMENT FILE



Trace#: 941                              ID: 114120941
SUBMISSION DATE: 11.22.20XX              997 DATE: 11.23.20XX
TIME SUBMITTED: 0112                     997 TIME: 111346
===============    =========================================

ERROR CODE          PATIENT ACCT #        LINE# / CHARGE#
251:NM1:9           628263478             2893

DESCRIPTION:        Payer Name
Segment Has Data Element Errors
DETAIL: Subscriber Identifier - (Mandatory data element missing)
SUBMITTED:


ERROR CODE          PATIENT ACCT #        LINE# / CHARGE#
251:NM1:10          123456                5454545
DESCRIPTION:        Payer Name
Segment Has Data Element Errors
DETAIL: (Invalid character in data element)
SUBMITTED:


ERROR CODE          PATIENT ACCT #        LINE# / CHARGE#
251:NM1:8           4515485               3157654
DESCRIPTION:        Payer Name
Segment Has Data Element Errors
DETAIL: Identification Qualifier (Conditional required data element
missing)
SUBMITTED:


This transaction was :            Rejected
Rejection Reason :                One or More Segments in Error
This Functional Group was :       Rejected
Transaction Sets Included :       1
Transaction Sets Received :       1
Transaction Sets Accepted :       0
```

Fig. 15.12 Clearinghouse 997 report showing the claims acknowledgment file. This report shows error codes and details the types of errors made. It also shows patient account numbers and names of the payers. (Report supplied by Electronic Technologies, Inc., Delmar, NY.)

Billing and Account Management Schedule

Maintaining a schedule will help with EDI transmissions, which will enable better cash flow. Table 15.6 suggests guidelines and procedures that can be tailored to the needs of the billing office.

Administrative Simplification Enforcement Tool

To address issues of noncompliance with the HIPAA TCS rule, the federal government has implemented the use of a web-based tool to assist health care providers, payers, clearinghouses, and others to submit complaints. This online tool, the Administrative Simplification Enforcement Tool (ASET), enables individuals or organizations to file a complaint online against a covered entity "that fails to adopt and follow the HIPAA rules for transactions and code sets". Failure to implement these standards can result in civil monetary penalties.

 15.7 QUICK REVIEW

Question: Explain what will happen if a batch of claims is transmitted electronically and one claim in the batch contains an error.

 DISCUSSION POINT

Most claims for health care services are filed electronically. Explain why it is important for the insurance billing specialist to develop a method of tracking all EDI transmissions. Explain how a tracking system could be developed.

TABLE 15.6 Daily, Weekly, and End-of-Month Guidelines and Protocols

Daily	Weekly	End of Month
Post charges in accounts receivable management system.	Batch, scrub, edit, and transmit claims (daily or weekly).	Run month-end aging reports.
Post payments in accounts receivable management system.	Analyze previous week's rejected and resubmitted claims.	Review all claim rejection reports (clearinghouse and payer), ensuring all problems are resolved and claims accepted.
Batch, scrub, edit, and transmit claims (daily or weekly); retrieve transmission reports.	Note any problematic claims and resolve outstanding files.	Update accounts receivable management system with payer information, such as EIN and NPI.
Run day sheet.	Research unpaid claims.	Run patient statements in office or through clearinghouse.
Review clearinghouse/payer transmission confirmation reports.	Make follow-up calls to resolve reasons for rejections, such as incorrect NPI, missing patient ID, incomplete data elements, and wrong format.	
Audit claims batched and transmitted with confirmation reports.		
Correct rejections and resubmit claims.		

EIN, Employer identification number; ID, identification; NPI, National Provider Identifier.

PROCEDURE 15.1 Cross-Walking Insurance Claims Data From Electronic Format 837P to the CMS 1500 Paper Claim

Objective: To become proficient at using an insurance claim crosswalk that maps from electronic format 837P to the CMS 1500 paper claim.

Step 1: Challenge a classmate. Identify approximately 10 data elements from the 837P and have a classmate crosswalk to the CMS 1500 form.

Step 2: Access the National Uniform Claim Committee's 1500 paper claim crosswalk map to the 837 electronic claim. Source: https://www.nucc.org/images/stories/PDF/1500_claim_form_map_to_837P_v3-3_2012_02.pdf

Step 3: Create a table, with a heading, 3 columns and approximately 10 rows. Label the column headings as:
- Loop ID:
- Segment/Data Element
- CMS Claim Form Block

Step 4: Using the NUCC's claim form map (crosswalk), provide the loop ID and segment/data element from the 837P. Ask your classmate to complete the 3rd column by using the crosswalk and mapping the data element to the appropriate 1500 form locator (block).

EXAMPLE

Loop ID	Segment/Data Element	CMS Claim Form Block
2000B	SBR09	1
2010CA	N302	5
	N401	
	N402	
	N403	

KEY POINTS

This is a brief chapter review of the key issues presented. To further enhance your knowledge of the technical subject matter, review the key terms and key abbreviations for this chapter by locating the meaning for each in the Glossary at the end of this book, which appears in a section before the Index.

1. Today most health care providers submit electronic claims for reimbursement.
2. The federal government has taken steps through the Administrative Simplification Compliance Act (ASCA) that require providers to submit claims electronically unless they have a waiver on file with their Medicare Administrative Contractor (MAC). Third-party payers have followed this lead, offering and encouraging electronic claims submission.
3. Health care organizations use accounts receivable management systems or computerized medical billing systems to prepare, send, and process HIPAA compliant electronic claims efficiently and accurately.
4. The method for transmission of electronic claims that the health care organization chooses may vary according to the accounts receivable management system's capabilities, insurance requirements or the health care organization's preferred procedures.
5. The American National Standards Institute (ANSI) formed the Accredited Standards Committee X12 (ASC X12). ASC X12 is a standards organization who developed, publish and maintain electronic data interchange standards for the health care industry.

6. Through HIPAA regulations, standardized transaction and code sets have been implemented to use electronic data interchange effectively.

7. Under HIPAA rules, a provider who sends Medicare claims is considered a covered entity that has 10 or more employees and must transmit claims electronically. Health care organizations with fewer than 10 employees are not considered covered entities and are not required to submit Medicare claims electronically.

8. Accounts receivable management software is used to input data, which helps generate a variety of documents including the 837P (Professional) in electronic National Standard Format (NSF), formerly the CMS-1500 paper form.

9. When constructing an insurance claim, the supporting code sets are made up of "required" and "situational" data elements identified by the HIPAA standard electronic formats.

10. Ten-character, alphanumeric provider-specialty taxonomy codes are assigned and classify each health care provider. These codes are used when transmitting electronic insurance claims.

11. Employers use their employer identification numbers (EINs) to identify themselves in transactions involving premium payments to health plans on behalf of their employees or to identify themselves to other employers as the source or receiver of information about eligibility. Employers use EINs to identify themselves in transactions when enrolling or disenrolling employees in health plans.

12. HIPAA requires that a National Provider Identifier (NPI), a 10-character numeric identifier, be assigned to each provider to be used in transactions with all health plans.

13. An encoder is helpful because it can reduce the time it takes to build or review a claim and help to improve coding accuracy before batching and transmitting to a third-party payer.

14. An electronic remittance advice (ERA) is the equivalent of a paper summarized statement called an *explanation of benefits (EOB),* which gives the status of insurance claims with payment details for one or more beneficiaries. It is referred to as *ANSI 835* or *Health Care Claim Payment/ Advice (835).*

15. Whether claims are submitted carrier-direct or through a clearinghouse, reports should be generated to track each function of the claims process.

INTERNET RESOURCES

NUCC's Taxonomy Codes

- https://www.nucc.org/images/stories/PDF/Taxonomy_20_0 .pdf

National Uniform Claim Committee's 1500 paper claim crosswalk map to the 837 electronic claim

- https://www.nucc.org/images/stories/PDF/1500_claim_ form_map_to_837P_v3-3_2012_02.pdf

NPI Database

- https://npidb.org/npi-lookup/

STUDENT ASSIGNMENT

- Study Chapter 15.
- Complete all exercises in the *Workbook* to reinforce the theory learned in this chapter.

- Turn to the Glossary at the end of this book for a further understanding of the key terms and key abbreviations used in this chapter.

Revenue Cycle Management

Receiving Payments and Insurance Problem Solving

Linda M. Smith

OBJECTIVES

After reading this chapter, you should be able to:

1. Identify and discuss the claim adjudication, determination, and appeal processes.
2. Assess reimbursement payment time frames for all submitted claims.
3. Identify the components of an explanation of benefits document and interpret and post an explanation of benefits document to a patient's account.
4. Discuss secondary insurance and guidelines to billing secondary insurance.
5. List and describe three health insurance claim management techniques.
6. Explain reasons for claim inquiries and identify strategies to discover why payments are delayed.
7. Define terminology pertinent to problem claims and discuss types of problems as well as find solutions.
8. Identify specific reasons for rebilling a claim.
9. Describe situations for filing appeals and discuss the review and appeals process.
10. Review Medicare's five levels in the redetermination (appeal) process and determine which forms to use for each level.
11. Review and discuss the TRICARE review and appeal process, including expedited and non-expedited appeals, as well as reconsideration.
12. List four objectives of state insurance commissioners.
13. Mention seven problems to submit to insurance commissioners.
14. Discuss the type of information necessary to include in an insurance commission request.
15. Explain the importance of claim denial management.

KEY TERMS

adjudication
administrative law judge
aging report
appeal
claim denial management
delinquent claim
denied claim
determination
explanation of benefits
inquiry

insurance payment poster
insurance payment posting
lost claim
medical necessity
overpayment
peer review
Qualified Independent Contractor
reassess
rebill (resubmit)
reimbursement

rejected claim
remittance advice
revenue cycle management
review
state insurance commissioner
suspended claim
suspense
tracer

KEY ABBREVIATIONS

ALJ	EOB	NPI	RA
CMS	HIPAA	QIC	RCM

REVENUE CYCLE MANAGEMENT

Revenue cycle management (RCM) is the process that health care organizations use to track services provided and patient care episodes, from registration and appointment scheduling to the final payment of the associated fees. As discussed in Chapter 1, an insurance billing specialist's primary goal is to assist in management of the revenue cycle. The insurance billing specialist will help to obtain maximum insurance benefits for services provided and ensure cash flow to the health care organization they are employed by. Revenue is the total income produced by a health care organization, and the cycle is the regularly repeating set of events for producing it.

Everything outlined in the preceding chapters has led to submission of the claim to the insurance carrier. After the medical claim is submitted, the insurance carrier goes through a series of steps to determine their financial responsibility for payment of the claim. This process is referred to as adjudication. The insurance carrier will then make a payment determination, which is a decision as to whether they will pay the claim in full, deny the claim, or reduce the amount they will pay.

Now that the claim has been successfully submitted to the insurance carrier, the next step in the revenue cycle is for the insurance billing specialist to track the claim during the adjudication process.

Response From a Submitted Claim

An insurance company can accept responsibility to pay the claim and reimburse the health care organization, they can suspend the claim to investigate the details of the claim further, or they can deny the claim for a variety of reasons. Delay in reimbursements, or payments to the health care organization, can also occur when health insurance companies state that they did not receive the claim at all. At times, the insurance company may reimburse claims lower than expected, after which an appeal can be filed. An appeal is a documented request to the insurance company to review (reassess) a claim and reconsider for payment.

This chapter begins with the claim policy guidelines, and further explains how contracts, fee schedules, and reimbursement timelines all affect reimbursement. The chapter will also demonstrate how to interpret the document that accompanies

payment and how to manage and organize financial records. Numerous potential problems are presented, along with suggested solutions to improve cash flow. Finally, the review and appeal processes for various programs are discussed.

The management of the reimbursement process and insurance company denials is often referred to as claim follow-up. By developing proficient skills and experience in following up on claims, an insurance billing specialist can become a valuable asset to their employer and bring in revenue that might otherwise be lost to the health care organization.

16.1 QUICK REVIEW

Question: Define "Revenue Cycle Management."

CLAIM POLICY GUIDELINES

A patient who seeks medical care with a health insurance card is presenting the contract that they have with the insurance company. In other words, the insurance company issued the card to the patient as evidence that it takes responsibility to pay the health care organization for the services the patient receives. In order for the health care organization to get paid for these services, insurance companies require it to submit a claim form. The insurance company dictates the guidelines for claims submission, such as which services are covered, the reimbursement rates, and the time limits for claim submission and payment.

Insured

A patient's insurance card does not specify the detailed benefits and coverages. However, before rendering services to the patient, it is in the health care providers' best interest to be aware of their patients' insurance benefits and coverages. For example, maternity care is an optional benefit; therefore, a health care provider should be aware that, by providing maternity care to a patient with no coverage, the provider risks not being reimbursed. Another example is that there may be a provision that the claimant has an obligation to notify the insurance company of a loss (injury, illness, or accident) within a certain period or the insurer has the right to deny benefits for that loss.

In some policies, if the insured disagrees with the insurer for settlement of a claim, a suit must begin within 3 years after the claim is submitted. Another provision might state that an insured person cannot bring legal action against an insurance company until 60 days after a claim is submitted.

Contracts and Fee Schedules

A fee schedule is included when a health care provider signs a contract with an insurance company or group to become a participating provider with the insurance plan. The participating health care provider agrees to the fee schedule, which is typically less than the provider's standard fee for service, and agrees not to charge the patient for the difference.

Reimbursement Time Frames

All health insurance companies are obligated to reimburse health care organizations for services rendered promptly. However, time limits vary in this provision from one third-party payer to another. Specific time limits will be stated in either the insurance contract or the payer's manual. It is reasonable to expect payment within 4 to 12 weeks if claims are submitted on paper, or in as little as 7 days when they are transmitted electronically.

Many states have implemented prompt payment laws to set standards for the prompt, fair, and equitable settlements of patient claims and provider services. For example, New York requires insurers to pay undisputed claims within 30 days after receipt of an electronic submission, or within 45 days for claims submitted by other means. Furthermore, the law requires the insurance carrier to make an interest payment on any claim that is not paid within the specified time frame written in the prompt payment law. It is important that the insurance billing specialist research to see if there are prompt pay laws in the state they are filing claims in.

If a payment delay occurs and the insurance company is slow or ignores, denies, or exceeds time limits to pay a claim, then it is prudent to contact the insurance company in writing. The letter should state the contracted time limit and seek the reason the claim has not been paid. A copy should be retained for the office files.

 16.2 QUICK REVIEW

Question: What is the standard time limit that an insurance company is required to reimburse health care organization for services rendered by them?

EXPLANATION OF BENEFITS

An **explanation of benefits (EOBs)** is a document the insurance carrier issues to both the health care provider filing the claim and the patient. The document details the outcome of the claims processing for services provided by the health care organization. It explains the allowed amount for the services provided, the paid amount, the amount that must be written off, and any financial responsibility of the patient. The EOB also provides details about claims that are denied and provides the reasons why. A **denied claim** is the refusal of an insurance carrier to honor a request to pay for health care services. Sometimes EOBs will provide details on specific claims that need to be refunded and the reasons why. Finally, if a payment is explained in the EOB, a check will be attached or evidence of an electronic transfer of funds will be evident.

Medicare and other payers may refer to the EOB as a **remittance advice (RA)**. The elements within the RA document are the same as an EOB document. A **suspended claim** is one that is processed by a third-party payer but is held in an indeterminate (pending) state. The claim is usually suspended because of an error or the need for additional information from the provider of service or the patient. The EOB also states the allowed amount for the service provided based on the contracted fee schedule by the third-party payer, as shown in Fig. 16.1. The allowed amount is the maximum dollar value that the insurance company assigns to each medical service. If the health care provider is contracted with the health insurance company, the provider will receive a copy of the EOB along with payment. If

the provider is not participating with the insurance company, payment can be sent to the patient, in which case the patient should be billed.

Components of an Explanation of Benefits

Unfortunately, there is no standard format for EOB forms from one carrier to the next, but the information contained in each one is usually the same. At first glance, the EOB may seem difficult to understand; however, the description and calculations for each patient may be understood easily if read one line at a time. The EOB breaks down how payment was determined and contains the following information in categories or columns:

1. Insurance company's name and address
2. Provider of services
3. Dates of services
4. Service or procedure (*Current Procedural Terminology* [CPT]) code
5. Amounts billed by the health care provider
6. Reduction or denial codes: comment codes (reasons, remarks, or notes) indicating reasons that payments were denied or reduced, asking for more information to determine coverage and benefits, or stating amounts of adjustment because of payments by other insurance companies (coordination of benefits)
7. Claim control number
8. Subscriber's and patient's names and policy numbers
9. Analysis of patient's total payment responsibility (allowed amount, copayment amount, deductible, coinsurance, other insurance payment, and patient's total responsibility)
10. Copayment amount(s) due from the patient
11. Deductible amounts subtracted from billed amounts
12. Total amount paid by the insurance carrier

Interpreting an Explanation of Benefits

Reading and interpreting an EOB may be overwhelming initially, so take time to read the document carefully. If several patients' claims are submitted to a third-party payer, the EOB may reflect the status of all of those claims and one check voucher may be issued. The EOB shown in Fig. 16.1 should be read line by line to interpret the meanings under each category or column, and the numbered explanations should be referred to when necessary. A helpful way to separate patients and their corresponding payments is to use a highlighter or ruler to underline the entire row across the EOB. This helps reduce errors when posting payments.

Posting an Explanation of Benefits

Insurance payment posting is the process of applying payments to the patient's account while writing off all adjustments. Posting of insurance payments is done by line item. In Fig. 16.1, each line item, or coded service, is explained separately. The **insurance payment poster**, the individual responsible for posting payments in patient accounts, must be careful to review lines that are posted and lines that are denied. Denials should be presented to the insurance billing specialist's attention as soon as possible; many denials or pending claims have a small window of time in which additional information can be forwarded to process the claim.

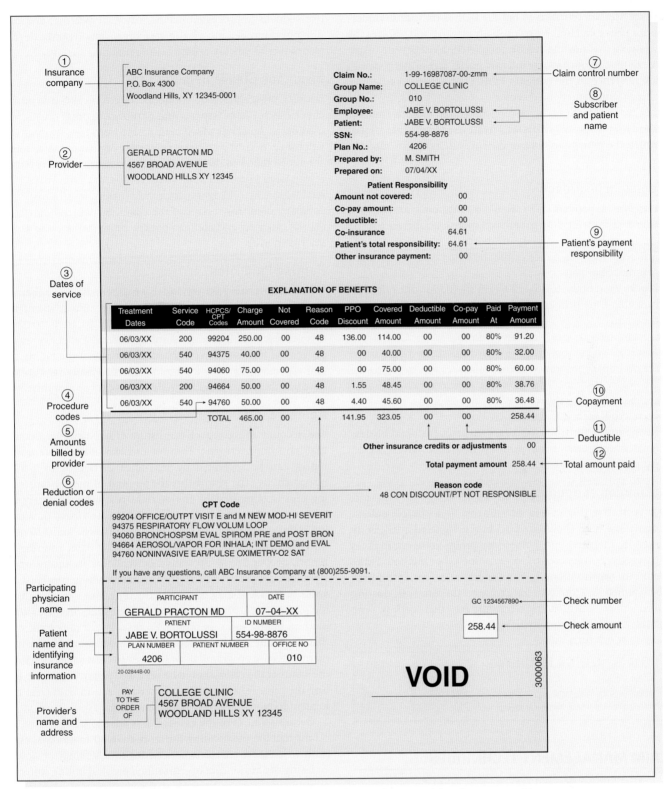

Fig. 16.1 An example of an explanation of benefits remittance advice document with accompanying check that the provider received from a private third-party payer. These payment voucher documents vary among insurance companies.

If there are any remaining balances after posting of the payment, the insurance billing specialist must determine the appropriate course of action. If the patient has secondary insurance, the secondary insurance should be billed at this time. If there is a remaining balance and the patient has no secondary insurance, the patient should be billed for the balance. It is during the posting process that payments are evaluated for correctness according to the insurance company contracted requirements.

If services are reimbursed but the EOB is difficult to understand, a phone call to the payer usually clarifies and resolves the problem so that posting can be completed. Most private insurance companies offer secure internet portal access that provides quick reference to the patient's EOB, contracted fee schedule, pending claims, and denied claims.

Claims paid with no errors are designated closed. The best method to store posted EOBs is to create a scanned e-file cabinet in which the patient account in the software program contains a link to the EOB.

Secondary Insurance

In some cases, patients carry secondary insurance to cover the coinsurance for which the patient is responsible. There are some guidelines to billing secondary insurance:

1. The secondary insurance cannot be billed until the primary insurance has paid.
2. Blocks 9a–d of the CMS-1500 form should include information about the primary insurance that paid the first part of the claim.
3. Depending on the Medicare Administrative Contractor, Medicare will automatically forward the claim it paid on to the secondary insurance. If the claim was forwarded to the secondary insurance, the EOB will state to which insurance company it was forwarded. When this happens, there is no need to bill secondary insurance.
4. Reimbursements from secondary insurances should be designated separately from primary insurance payments on patient account statements.

Explanation of Benefits Management

After posting payments and adjustments to applicable patient accounts, the EOB should be filed in a designated area clearly marked in a folder. Some offices may group these remittances by payer, by month received, or by some other method. Some health care organizations' billing systems allow for EOB forms to be scanned into the software, and some do automatic posting of payment by downloading electronic files that work in sync with the format of the remittances.

 16.3 QUICK REVIEW

Question: When an insurance billing specialist is posting payments from an Explanation of Benefits, what is the process they should follow if there is any remaining balance for the service provided?

CLAIM MANAGEMENT TECHNIQUES

In medical billing, the goal is to submit claims for patients to insurance carriers and have the claims paid within the reimbursement time frame and according to the fee schedule outlined in the contract with the insurance carrier. However, many claims do not meet this goal. Claims often can go back and forth between insurance carriers and providers for months until all issues have been resolved and the claim is closed. Therefore, health care organizations need to manage the back-end office tasks associated with claims reimbursement. This involves close

oversight of unprocessed claims, payment posting, and handling of claim denials. Health care organizations must develop techniques to quickly resolve claim reimbursement issues.

Insurance Claims Register

Because most claims are submitted electronically, it is vital to check Batch Claim Reports and Scrubber Reports on a scheduled basis. An acknowledgment report from the clearinghouse will list each insurance claim submitted per patient. This report should be followed up on each week to ensure that every claim is processed to prevent delinquent claims, or claims that are not paid within 30 to 45 days of the service date. Once the insurance company confirms receipt of the claim, insurance billing specialists can view and confirm patient claim status using secure internet portals.

Purging Paid Files

When claims are paid off and have a zero balance, they are purged, or removed in bulk, from the insurance claim file. Some medical offices remove files when EOBs are posted, but this process can be time consuming. The most effective way to purge paid files is to have a scheduled time that the billing system automatically runs a purge program. Many organizations schedule the purge program to be run weekly or monthly.

Aging Reports

The account aging report is a listing of outstanding accounts that have not been paid. In most medical billing systems, the report can be separated by insurance carrier or by patient responsibility. The report lists the amount of money outstanding and is organized by the amount of time the money has been owed (Fig. 16.2). The aging report categorizes outstanding claims as current, 30 days, 60 days, 90 days, and 120 days. The report should be generated each month. After running the report, proper follow-up should be made by inquiring why a claim has not yet been paid. The insurance billing specialist can write notes on the aging report documenting phone calls to the payer or adjustments made or include notes in the patient's medical billing software profile. For example, a note indicating that the claim is to be corrected and rebilled would be helpful; many software programs allow the user to create alerts for when the status of the claim should be reviewed again. The key to getting the most reimbursements is prompt action with clear and regular documentation of the action taken.

Because time is of the essence, it is wise to be aggressive on claims that are outstanding for more than 30 to 45 days, especially when there are issues concerning timely filing.

Using the health care organization's medical billing software, monthly reports can be generated and are useful when tracking the payment history of insurance companies. This is an easy method to discover which companies pay slowly or pay less on certain services. Billing and accounts receivable reports help illustrate trends in the financial operations of the health care office, as well as prepare for negotiations of future insurance contracts.

An insurance company payment history system can help to avoid potential problems and pinpoint requirements that

AETNA									
Patient Name	Acct #	Primary Insurance	Secondary Insurance	Aging Analysis					Total Balance
				0–30	31–60	61–90	91–120	over 120	
Bassett, Eleanor	75846	AETNA		$145.00	$0.00	$0.00	$0.00	$0.00	$145.00
Herron, John	83029	AETNA		$0.00	$42.41	$0.00	$0.00	$0.00	$42.41
Holt, Maxine	64739	AETNA	BLUE SHIELD	$145.00	$0.00	$0.00	$0.00	$0.00	$145.00
Kellog, Keenan	24537	AETNA		$0.00	$0.00	$145.00	$0.00	$0.00	$145.00
Lincoln, Frank	85940	AETNA		$0.00	$15.00	$0.00	$0.00	$0.00	$15.00
Markham, Melanie	14263	AETNA	MEDICARE	$0.00	$0.00	$0.00	$260.00	$0.00	$260.00
McDonald, Lydia	56374	AETNA		$260.00	$0.00	$0.00	$0.00	$0.00	$260.00
McLean, Mary	24395	AETNA		$0.00	$0.00	$0.00	$0.00	$260.00	$260.00
Aetna Aging Total :				$550.00	$57.41	$145.00	$260.00	$260.00	$1,272.41

Fig. 16.2 The aging report shows patient account balances according to the number of days after the date of service.

must be met to secure additional payment on a reduced or denied claim.

16.4   QUICK REVIEW
Question: After an aging report has been generated and given to the insurance billing specialist to follow up on unpaid claims, what steps should they take?

CLAIM INQUIRIES

When reviewing an aging report, unpaid claims that are more than 30 to 45 days old require an inquiry on claim status to be made to the health insurance company. These claims could be delayed because they may not have been received by the insurance company, or for other reasons relating to the member's health plan. Different types of claim inquiries can focus on denial codes on the EOB or can be related to patient coinsurance or deductible responsibilities. To reduce the number of phone calls to insurance companies, many private insurance organizations have set up online web portals that allow insurance billing specialists to review patient claim status and benefit information. If more information about the claim is needed beyond the scope of the online portal, insurance benefit specialists can be reached by calling the member services number on the back of the patient's ID card. The following are reasons for making inquiries:

- There was no response to a submitted claim within 30 to 45 days.
- Payment was not received within the time limit for the plan or program.
- Payment was received but the amount is incorrect.
- Payment was received but the amount allowed and the patient's responsibility was not defined.
- A duplicate payment or overpayment was made.
- Payment received was for a patient not seen by the provider. It is possible to receive a payment check made out to a payee's name that is different from the patient's name. Making a call may quickly clarify for whom the payment is being made.

In addition to nonpayment or reduced payment, there are other reasons for inquiries to an insurance company, including the following:

- EOB shows that a professional or diagnostic code was changed from what was submitted.

- EOB shows that the service was disallowed when it was a benefit.
- EOB shows that additional information was needed and it was sent in a timely manner but payment has not been sent.
- EOB shows claim denial and explanation of denial is insufficient or inaccurate.
- There is an error on the EOB.

Inquire about the claim if any of these situations occurs. Although there are many online web portals for private insurance claim inquiry, sometimes government health plans do not offer the same online tools. For this reason, government health plans have their own inquiry or tracer forms available online, which need to be submitted in writing along with a copy of the claim. If a claim must be reviewed after payment has been rendered, send a letter similar to the one shown in Fig. 16.3. Remember that effective follow-up centers around effective documentation, so document the name of the person spoken to, the date and time of call, the department or extension of the person, and an outline of the conversation. Save these notes in the patient account.

Problem Claims

Problems in claims filing will delay the reimbursement process. Determining the most appropriate amount of time to follow up on a claim after it has been submitted will vary from insurance carrier to insurance carrier. Many types of problem claims (e.g., delinquent, in suspense [pending], lost, rejected, denied, downcoded, partial payment, payment lost in the mail, payment made to patient, and overpayment) exist.

To keep accounting accurate and up to date, these problems require some type of follow-up action. The claim status may be indicated on an EOB. However, sometimes a claim is submitted and no status is reported. As mentioned earlier, visiting the insurance carrier's online web portal is the most efficient way to view claim status. If the insurance carrier does not have a web portal, calling to confirm claim status is the most efficient step.

The individual working at the front desk must collect insurance information accurately and update patient demographic information (e.g., insurance identification number and address) at every office visit or medical encounter. The person posting to accounts must be certain to post to the correct patient account and ensure that secondary insurances are billed after

COLLEGE CLINIC
4567 Broad Avenue
Woodland Hills, XY
12345-0001
Telephone 555/486-9002
Fax (555) 487-8976

Committee on Physician's Services

Re: Underpayment
Identification No.: _____ M18876782 _____
Patient: _____ Peaches Melba _____
Type of Service: Plastic & Reconstructive Surgery
Date of Service: _____ 1 - 3 - XX _____
Amount Paid: _____ $ 75.00 _____
My Fees: _____ $ 180.00 _____

Dear Sirs:

Herewith a request for a committee review of the above-named case, since I consider the allowance paid very low having in mind the location, the extent, the type, and the necessary surgical procedure performed: The skin graft, one inch in diameter, included the lateral third of eyebrow and was full thickness to preserve hair follicles.

Operative report for the surgery has been sent to you with the claim.

Considering these points I hope that you will authorize additional payment in order to bring the total fee to within reasonable and customary charges.

Sincerely,

Cosmo Graff, M.D.

Cosmo Graff, M.D.

mf
enclosure

Fig. 16.3 A letter signed by the health care provider appealing a fee reduction. This letter lists information specific to the patient claim in question and is sent to the third-party payer after payment has been received and the provider feels that the reimbursement should be higher.

the primary insurance company has paid. Identified errors should be brought to the attention of the responsible individuals to improve the accuracy of outgoing claims and to avoid future problems.

There is a significant difference in the way problem claims are handled when filed by paper or filed electronically. Because most health insurance claims should be submitted electronically, the problems and solutions listed will focus mainly on electronic submission.

The following are specific claim problems and practical solutions.

Delinquent, Pending, or Suspense

PROBLEM: Delinquent claims are those which the insurance carrier has not made a determination on within a reasonable period of time. Typically, they are identified as beyond 30 to 45 days overdue on the aging report. Sometimes nonpayment is caused by a claim in review or in suspense because of an error or the need for additional information. The carrier may be investigating a claim because of preexisting conditions or because

the patient may have a work-related injury. If a service is not covered, the carrier may not respond, but a follow-up should be initiated to further investigate.

SOLUTION: Use claim management techniques to keep on top of delinquent claims so that follow-up can be accomplished in a timely manner. If the office handles a large volume of claims, divide the unpaid claims into four groups, one for each of the three largest insurers and the fourth for all others. Work on one group each week so that the work is spread out over the 4 weeks in each month. Routinely visit the online web portals to check for claims status and look for evidence of the claim being submitted while reconciling the electronic data interchange (EDI) clearinghouse acknowledgment report for up-to-date information. If the claim was submitted and confirmed as received, it is wise to look at how the claim was billed (e.g., accurate coding). If this information is correct and the dates on the claim are correct, contact the payer to find out what information is holding up the claim or why the claim was denied. If the claim was not successful in being received by the clearinghouse and there is no apparent reason on reports or on investigating the claim data showing exactly what information was amiss, then perhaps there was a problem with the format. For more insight as to why the claim was not successfully received or was rejected, contact the clearinghouse. The insurance billing specialist can contact the payer immediately after finding out that the claim is delinquent, or the payer can be contacted after initial steps of investigation take place, such as in-house editing and contacting the clearinghouse.

Lost Claims

PROBLEM: Lost claims are insurance claims that cannot be located after being sent to an insurance carrier. Lost claims are more common with paper claim submission; managing large volumes of claims leads to some getting lost from time to time. Paper claims can get lost in the mail, be sent to the incorrect address, or be mismanaged through the health insurance mail management system. It is important to track all claims, as some insurance contracts may have deadlines to file claims 30 days after the date of service.

SOLUTION: The insurance company should be contacted if there has been no response to a claim that has aged 30 to 45 days. The first step is to check the claim status through the online provider web portal or to place a phone call to the insurance carrier. If there is no record of the claim, all lost claims should be resubmitted. If a claim is determined to be lost, submit a copy of the original claim referencing it as "copy of the original claim submitted on (date)."

Always retain the electronic response or confirmation from the carrier saying it received the specific claim. Keep all clearinghouse reports confirming received transmissions and relay information regarding claim status. Medical billing software programs display the date of every claim submitted. Tamper-proof data recorded by the computer may be used as a legal form of proof that the claim was submitted to the third-party payer. Unfortunately, this does not "prove" that the payer received the claim, so some payers do not always accept this. Send a printed copy of electronic proof of timely filing to the third-party payer, along with a copy of the claim and a copy of the denial that was received for exceeding the timely filing limit.

Rejected Claims

A rejected claim is a submitted claim that does not follow specific third-party payer instructions or contains a technical error. Such claims may be disapproved or discarded by the insurance carrier prior to processing and returned to the biller. Technical errors consist of missing or incorrect information and are found through computer edits, screening processes for benefit provisions, and proofreading. Common reasons why health insurance claims are rejected can be found in Box 16.1.

PROBLEM: Paper or electronic claim rejections may occur as a result of one or more of the following:
- Transposed numbers
- Missing required Health Insurance Portability and Accountability Act (HIPAA) transaction code sets
- Missing subscriber date of birth
- Missing, invalid, or incorrect procedure codes and modifiers
- Missing or invalid place of service (POS)

BOX 16.1 Common Reasons Why Health Insurance Claims Are Rejected

Code description does not match services rendered
Duplicate charges
Duplicate dates of service
Incorrect dates of service
Incorrect electronic submission code
Incorrect number of days in the month (e.g., February)
Incorrect year of service
Incorrect, invalid, nonspecific, or missing diagnostic code numbers
Mismatch of POS to type of service
Missing NPI number for the provider and/or facility
Missing or invalid POS
Missing or invalid provider number when the patient was referred
Missing referring provider number when billing tests
Missing required HIPAA transaction code sets
Missing subscriber date of birth
Missing, invalid, or incorrect procedure codes and modifiers
Missing health care provider signature
Transposed numbers

HIPAA, Health Insurance Portability and Accountability Act; *NPI,* National Provider Identifier; *POS,* place of service.

- Mismatch of POS to type of service
- Missing referring provider number when billing tests
- Missing or invalid provider number when the patient was referred
- Incorrect, invalid, nonspecific, or missing diagnostic code numbers
- Incorrect dates of service
- Incorrect year of service
- Incorrect number of days in the month (e.g., February)
- Code description that does not match services rendered
- Duplicate dates of service
- Duplicate charges

SOLUTION: It is likely that an electronic claim will not make it into a batch to be transmitted to the payer if a series of computer edits have been performed before batching (i.e., grouping claims together). The billing system will flag this particular claim as needing edits and will not batch it with the rest. If the claim does go through to the payer and is reported as being rejected, review the rejection reason code, correct the field, and then resubmit the claim. Never send a corrected claim for review or appeal; instead, resubmit the claim with the correct information.

PROBLEM: A claim is submitted for several services. One line item is rejected for incomplete information, but the other services are paid.

SOLUTION: Generate a new claim for the rejected services online and note in Block 19 of the CMS-1500 claim form that it is a resubmission.

PROBLEM: A third-party payer requests further information or information about another insurance carrier.

Solution: A common mistake during the patient registration process is not obtaining the insurance subscriber's name, employer, and date of birth. It is important to verify insurance information with the patient (including confirmation of the patient's primary, and possibly secondary, insurance information), obtain a signed patient release of information form that follows HIPAA guidelines, and call or mail the information to the insurance company. Identify the subscriber, subscriber ID number, and date of service on all correspondence.

PROBLEM: A resubmitted claim is returned a second time.

PAPER CLAIM SOLUTION: Review the EOB statement to determine whether there is a denial code or narrative explanation. Examine the claim for missing, incomplete, or incorrect information, and if found, correct it. Evaluate the claim to determine whether it is a candidate for the appeal process. Determine whether a specific appeal form must be submitted. Submit chart notes, a detailed summary, or a copy of the operative or pathology report, as applicable, to clearly identify the procedure or service. Enclose a cover letter with the resubmitted data. The letter must specifically state what course of action is being requested (i.e., review) and it must have the name and signature of the person requesting the review.

A common claim denial reason is lack of medical necessity. *Medical necessity* refers to health care services that a health care provider, exercising their best clinical judgment, would provide to a patient for evaluating, diagnosing, or treating an illness, injury, disease, or its symptoms. Services are considered medically necessary if they are:

- in accordance with the generally accepted standards of medical practice;
- clinically appropriate in terms of type, frequency, extent, site, and duration, and considered effective for the patient's illness, injury, or disease;
- not primarily for the convenience of the patient or health care provider; and
- not costlier than an alternative service or sequence of services at least as likely to produce equivalent therapeutic or diagnostic results as to the diagnosis or treatment of that patient's illness, injury, or disease.

Claims that do not support medical necessity guidelines can be rejected through claim-editing programs. These rejections are sometimes caused by diagnosis and procedure code not matching. An example of this would be a denial for hammertoe surgery with a broken wrist diagnosis. Because these rejections can be related to lack of supporting documentation or errors in coding, they should be returned to the original coder to be corrected and resubmitted.

Denied Claims

Claims are often denied because they do not meet the criteria in a coverage policy. For example, a patient may have acupuncture services, but those services are listed as a noncovered service in the patient's insurance contract.

When a claim is denied, and the responsible party is indicated on the EOB to be the patient, transfer the entire balance to the patient's account. State laws require insurance companies to notify the insured of a denial and state why the claim was denied. However, if the insurance company has not contacted the patient, notify the patient by phone or mail as soon as possible to keep them informed. Always retain the correspondence from the insurance company so that it can be retrieved quickly in case a patient inquires or has additional questions.

When a claim is denied, simply changing information on the claim and resubmitting it will **not** resolve the problem. If it is determined that the claim was denied incorrectly, and the service meets the benefits requirements, the recourse is to challenge the insurance carrier's decision and file an appeal.

It stands to reason that insurance companies save money when a claim is denied, and only a small percentage of individuals pursue appeals. The appeals process for denied claims varies among third-party payers.

Common reasons why insurance claims are not paid because of denial include the following:

- Selected diagnoses not covered
- Frequency limitations or restrictions per benefit period
- Procedure performed by ineligible specialty provider (e.g., a podiatrist would not be paid for neurosurgery)
- Bundled with other services
- Payable only in certain locations (e.g., outpatient only)
- Prior approval needed and not obtained
- Service or procedure not justified by diagnosis
- Missing or incorrect POS code

Additional examples with suggested solutions are as follows:

PROBLEM: The medical service provided was not covered for the patient (e.g., routine physical examination, routine tests, routine foot care, routine dental care, cosmetic surgery, custodial care, eye or hearing examinations for glasses or hearing aids, and some immunizations). Plastic surgery and maternity care can be considered a general exclusion in many insurance policies.

SOLUTION: Send the patient a statement with a notation of the response from the insurance company. Before providing services, always verify coverage for routine physical examinations or tests and services by calling or checking the online provider web portal regarding whether the health insurance will accept financial responsibility. Discuss this with the patient before service is provided and advise of the likelihood of the claim being denied. In these instances, it may be appropriate to request payment at the time of service.

PROBLEM: Insurance coverage is canceled or temporarily lapsed before the date of service.

SOLUTION: It is a good practice to verify insurance coverage for each patient before their appointment for services by visiting the online web portal or by calling to verify coverage. If the claim is then denied after services were rendered, send the patient a statement with notation of the insurance determination on the bill.

PROBLEM: Upon processing of the claim, the health insurance company indicates that the provided service was not medically necessary, based on their coverage policies. "Medical necessity" has become the encompassing denial reason that indicates the insurance company does not agree with the services provided to the patient because they were not necessary. This makes clearing the medical necessity denial reason most challenging to overturn. The following are a few reasons why insurance companies deny medical necessity:

- The diagnosis code and the procedure code do not match
- The procedure code and the place or type of service do not match

- The procedure is performed by a physician of a different specialty
- The frequency of the same procedure rendered is more than authorized
- The procedure is experimental and has not yet been approved for reimbursement by the insurance company
- Supporting documentation is unclear or limited

SOLUTION: Determine under what circumstances the third-party payer considers the service to be medically necessary. It is vital that the service provider's documentation be specific enough to support the necessity of the services provided. If the service provider believes that the patient's condition supported the medical necessity for the service, send an appeal for review to the insurance company, explaining in detail the reasons why the service was necessary. Keep a list of codes that have been denied for medical necessity and what further determinations were made in the insurance company payment history. Check the insurance contract to determine whether the patient may be billed. Consider asking patients to sign an Advance Beneficiary Notice or Waiver of Liability form *before* treatment. Do not have every patient sign such documents because then these documents would be considered a blanket waiver if the claim is denied.

PROBLEM: Service was for an injury that is approved and covered under workers' compensation.

SOLUTION: Create a workers' compensation information sheet asking the employee and employer to fill out separate sections with space for the following: explanation of the injury, insurance information, claim adjuster's name and telephone number, and claim or case number. Because most workers' compensation insurance companies typically accept paper claims, all correspondence should be made directly with the claims adjuster via phone or mail. Locate the carrier for the industrial injury, request permission to treat, and send the carrier a report of the case with a bill. Notify the patient's health insurance carrier monthly about the status of the case.

PROBLEM: A service was not preauthorized for a surgery, hospitalization, or diagnostic procedure.

SOLUTION: Contact the insurance company or check the online web portal to determine whether preauthorization was necessary for the service or if any sanctions were imposed. The office may want to institute a standard procedure that all surgical procedures and durable medical equipment and supplies be confirmed with insurance companies before rendering services. Document the contact's name, date, and time of the call, or if using the online provider portal, print out the preauthorization information for the patient's chart. If there were problems or difficulties with the case leading to the reason that precertification was not obtained, write a letter of appeal noting the history. Insurance payers can change their policies on certain procedure codes throughout the year.

PROBLEM: The deductible was not met.

SOLUTION: Before rendering services to the patient, confirm with the insurance company the patient's current deductible and the amount for which the patient will be financially responsible for medical services. Inform the patient at the prescreening appointment that the deductible must be collected at that appointment or the procedure should be rescheduled.

PROBLEM: Elective surgery or procedures were billed that are not typically covered by health insurance.

SOLUTION: Inform the patient before scheduling the appointment that they are responsible for paying for services upfront, before the procedure.

PROBLEM: The claim is incomplete and denied because essential elements are missing and/or inaccurate.

SOLUTION: Prevention measures to avoid denied claims are as follows:

1. Be proactive and verify insurance coverage before the first patient encounter; this saves time and prevents surprises for everyone. Ensure that the demographic information is current at each subsequent encounter.
2. Include progress notes and orders for tests for extended hospital services.
3. Submit a letter from the prescribing health care provider documenting necessity when ambulance transportation is used.
4. Clarify the type of service (e.g., primary surgical services versus assist-at-surgery services).
5. Use modifiers to further describe and identify the exact service rendered.
6. Keep abreast of the latest policies for all contracted payers as well as for the federal programs by going to the Centers for Medicare and Medicaid Services (CMS) website to read currently posted Medicare Transmittals. For example, know the Medicare local coverage determinations (LCDs) and national coverage determinations (NCDs) that state which conditions and services are covered and the limitations on coverage. Read news releases from all insurance carriers.
7. Obtain current provider manuals for all contracted payers. When bulletins or pages are received from these programs during the year, keep the manuals up to date by inserting the current material.
8. Become familiar with the modifier descriptions and their appropriate use, and verify that the payer recognizes them.

Downcoding

PROBLEM: The insurance carrier has downcoded the claim. In these cases, the adjudicator or computer software determines that a lower level of procedure or service may have been warranted than was billed by the provider. Therefore, there is a reduction in reimbursement.

SOLUTION: Be sure to read through all procedure notes and provider orders to determine the most specific diagnosis code related to the patient's condition. If the patient experiences complications, these should be added to the code. If the service provider's notes are not specific enough to determine a more specific diagnosis, emphasize to the provider the importance of specificity, especially regarding diagnosis.

Payment Made to Patient

PROBLEM: An insurance payment sent to the patient instead of the provider can occur for two reasons: either the provider is considered out of network from the patient's health plan, or the assignment of benefits was not signed by the patient.

SOLUTION: Call the insurance company or visit the online web portal to verify whether the payment was made, to whom, for which dates of service, the amount, the check number, and the date of issue. If the provider has a participating agreement, the insurance company is obligated to pay the provider and must proceed by correcting the error. The following are two different courses of action to take after this has been verified:

1. Call the patient, explain that the insurance company sent payment to the patient in error, and ask when full payment can be expected. Document the commitment in the patient's financial record. If the patient cannot be reached by telephone, send a letter by certified mail to the patient. Document each effort that was made toward collection of the payment from the patient and the patient's responses.

2. Send a letter to the insurance company, including a copy of the claim with EOB indicating that payment was made to the patient, and a copy of the assignment of benefits. Demand payment from the insurance company, stating the need to honor the assignment and the signed participation agreement. The insurance company must recover the payment from the patient. If the insurance company admits that there is an assignment of benefits and that it inadvertently paid the patient, the insurance company must pay the service provider within 2 to 3 weeks and honor the assignment even before it recovers its money from the patient. The insurance company then files for payment from the patient.

Underpayment

Underpayments occur when the insurance carrier's payment is less than the negotiated contract rate. It is important that the insurance billing specialist performs random checks and monitors large claim payments made during the first 3 months of a new contract to ensure that the third-party payer's system has the contracted payment fee schedule correctly loaded into the software. Track the charge, allowable, deductible, and paid amount to determine whether the amounts are correct (Fig. 16.4).

PROBLEM: Claims are underpaid.

SOLUTION: Print the incorrectly paid claims and send them by mail to the third-party payer's contract negotiator to be resolved. Ask them to re-adjudicate the claims based on the agreed-upon contracted amount. Include a letter with the claims, clearly stating that they are not duplicate claims but do need to be reviewed for appropriate payment. Use codes or notations on the claims to indicate that they are updated.

Overpayment

An **overpayment** is a sum of money paid by the insurance company or patient to the provider of service. It may be more than the account balance or more than the allowed amount. Overpayments can happen for a variety of reasons, and handling them can be challenging.

The insurance payment poster usually discovers overpayments when payments are posted in patient accounts. It is wise to develop an overpayment policy and a procedure for each type of insurer, program, or managed care plan and for every type of overpayment situation that may occur.

PROBLEM: Overpayment scenarios that may occur are:

- Receiving payment twice for the same date of service. This often happens when a claim is rebilled.
- Receiving payment for a patient and date of service that do not exist.
- Receiving more than the contract rate from an insurance carrier.
- Receiving payments that should have been paid to the patient.
- Receiving duplicate payments from two or more insurance companies or from the patient and one or more third-party payers.
- Receiving payment made for someone who is not the provider's patient.

SOLUTION: When an overpayment occurs, post the activity to the appropriate patient account with an additional notation that it was received in error and a refund was made. Creating an account specifically for overpayments is advisable to track all funds in this category. In any type of overpayment situation, cash the third-party payer's check and make out a refund check payable to the originator of the overpayment. Keep a copy of the third-party payer's check before it is deposited. The refund check should always be brought to the attention of a specific person at the insurance company. In case of an audit, this establishes documentation showing that the problem has been resolved. Usually insurance companies process a credit of the overpayment amount to the next check voucher.

Refund checks should be given top priority and written as soon as reasonably possible. Ensure that the office policy is

Method for Calculating Over- and Underpayments						
Third-party payer: _____						
Patient name	Procedure/ service	Claims paid date	Provider charge	Allowed amount	Amount paid	Overpayment (+) Underpayment (−)
May Ito	Colonoscopy	5/2/20XX	$460	$400	$460	$60+

Fig. 16.4 Audit method used for calculating overpayments and underpayments. Subtract the allowed amount, which is the insurance contract's fee schedule amount minus any patient copayment or deductible from the amount paid. Any positive (+) number is an overpayment and any negative (−) number is an underpayment.

clearly stated and adhered to in all cases. If both the patient and a third-party pay and the overpayment must be refunded to the patient, always write a check—never refund in cash. Send the patient a letter with a check to explain the overpayment. If the patient pays by credit card, wait until the charges have cleared to draft a check, or preferably process a credit card refund to the credit card company.

If the patient cannot be located to return the money, send a check by registered mail to the patient's last known address. When it comes back marked "undeliverable," retain the document as legal proof that an honest effort was made to return the overpayment. The money should be listed as taxable income and put in the bank.

The Office of the Inspector General (OIG) strongly advises providers to return overpayments promptly. Not doing so can lead to severe fines and implicate fraudulent activity. Some states have laws or court decisions restricting insurance carriers from recovering payments made in error from health care providers. It is essential to research the law pertaining to the handling of overpayments in the state that the health care organization is located. First, determine whether an overpayment exists by reviewing the available financial documents on the case in question. Second, decide how to handle the overpayment. Be sure to get advice from the health care organization's attorney on the extent to which the demand for repayment can be challenged based on state law or court decisions.

Rebilling

If a claim has not been paid within a reasonable amount of time, do not automatically **rebill (resubmit)** the third-party payer without researching the reason why it is still outstanding. Simply rebilling claims can be considered duplicate claims, and the insurance company may audit the health care organization for trying to collect duplicate payment. Instead, follow up on the claim as indicated in the previous section. If it is discovered that an error has been made in completing the insurance claim form, make the changes and resubmit the form, indicating that the new claim is corrected.

Patient accounts with a balance should be billed monthly, even when an insurance payment is expected, so that patients understand what has been submitted and what is pending. The statement should clearly identify the claim that has been submitted and what action is expected from the patient. If collection becomes a problem, action can be referenced to the date of service if the patient has been billed consistently.

Some carriers do allow resubmission of claims with minor errors or omissions and have made special provisions. In fact, in December 2004, the CMS implemented a process that allows providers to resubmit corrected Medicare claims that have been rejected for minor errors or omissions rather than appealing those claims. For example, claims with missing or incorrect provider numbers, claims with incorrect modifiers, and claims with keying errors (incorrect date or POS) can be rebilled. These claims can be corrected through the clearinghouse and resubmitted electronically. Other insurance carriers may have similar resubmission processes.

🔨 **16.5 QUICK REVIEW**

Question: Explain why an insurance billing specialist would not simply rebill the insurance carrier for a claim that has not been paid within a reasonable amount of time.

REVIEW AND APPEAL PROCESS

An appeal is a request for review and reconsideration of a claim that has been underpaid, incorrectly paid, or denied by an insurance company. Some insurance carriers may refer to appeals as redeterminations. Before starting the appeals process, examine the insurance carrier's policy to determine whether there is a time limit for making an appeal. Most carriers have rather stringent time limits for filing an appeal after the original claim determination.

The first step in the appeals process is to carefully review the RA sent to the service provider. If the claim was paid, the insurance billing specialist should carefully check the reimbursement amount against the appropriate fee schedule for that insurance carrier. It is important to confirm that the insurance carrier has paid correctly. If payment was not made in accordance with the fee schedule, the reimbursement amount will need to be appealed.

If the claim was denied, the RA should be carefully reviewed to determine the reason the claim was denied. The decision to appeal a claim should be based on several factors. The health care provider should determine that there is sufficient information to back up the claim and the amount of money in question should be sufficient in the provider's opinion. Ultimately, the decision to appeal rests in the provider's hands, not the insurance billing specialist's. An appeal is filed in the following circumstances:

- Payment is denied and the reason for denial is not known.
- Service was denied as a noncovered service.
- Payment is received but the amount is incorrect. Verify that initially the correct amount was billed. Perhaps there was an excessive reduction in the allowed payment.
- The service provider disagrees with the decision by the third-party payer about a preexisting condition.
- Unusual circumstances warranted medical treatments that are not reflected in the payment.
- Precertification was not obtained within contract provisions because of extenuating circumstances and the claim was denied.
- Service was considered inclusive in a more comprehensive service performed on the same date of service.
- Service was considered inclusive in a global surgical period.
- Inadequate payment was received for a complicated procedure.
- "Not medically necessary" is stated as the reason for denial and the service provider disagrees.

Filing an Appeal

Appeals can be time consuming and costly. The insurance billing specialist should be well prepared for the appeals process and well versed in the basic guidelines for filing an appeal.

The process for filing appeals varies from insurance carrier to insurance carrier. Some require that the appeal be written, whereas others may allow telephone or online appeals. Some insurance carriers require completion of a specific form of appeals, whereas others request a written letter of appeals.

Most payers have a specific structure for appeals that moves through various stages, starting at the lowest level of appeals and moving to the highest level of the appeals process. The first step might simply consist of a simple request for reconsideration, and the highest level of appeals may involve a peer review or a medical director. A peer review is an evaluation done by a group of unbiased practicing physicians or other health care professionals to judge the effectiveness and efficiency of professional care rendered. This group determines the medical necessity and subsequent payment for the case in question.

When performing a telephone appeal, the insurance billing specialist should follow these basic guidelines:

- Assemble all documents needed (e.g., patient's medical record, copy of the insurance claim form, and EOB).

- Always remain courteous.
- Obtain the name and extension number of the insurance claims representative or adjuster and keep this with the telephone records. Oftentimes, the insurance billing specialist will develop a rapport with a claims representative who may be helpful with future claims. Ask for any toll-free numbers that the company may have and keep these for future reference.
- Listen carefully. Jot down the date and take notes of how to solve the problem. This may be of help if another problem of the same type occurs.

When performing written appeals, always send a copy of the original claim, EOB, and any other documents to justify the appeal. Refer to Procedure 16.1 at the end of this chapter for the procedure to follow when composing a letter of appeal (Fig. 16.5).

It is important to keep track of the status after inquiry or appeal until payment for the case is resolved. Use the insurance claims register or a separate active file labeled "Appeals Pending."

PHYSICIAN'S LETTERHEAD

January 2, 20XX

Committee on Physician's Services
Medicare
Street address of fiscal intermediary
City, State, ZIP Code

Dear Madam or Sir:

Re: Underpayment

Identification No.:	1910-2192283-101
Patient:	Mrs. Sarah C. Nile
Type of Service:	Exploratory laparotomy
Date of Service:	December 1, 20XX
Amount Paid:	$000.00
My Fees:	$0000.00

Herewith a request for a committee review of the above-named case, since I consider the allowance paid very low having in mind the patient's condition prior to surgery, the location, the extent, the type, and the necessary surgical procedure performed.

Enclosed are photocopies of the history and physical showing the grave status of the patient prior to surgery, operative report, pathology report, and discharge summary. The Medicare Remittance Advice and the Medicare CMS-1500 claim originally submitted are also enclosed.

Considering these points, I hope that you will authorize additional payment in order to bring the total fee to a more reasonable amount.

Sincerely,

Hugh R. Aged, MD
Hugh R. Aged, MD
NPI# 73542109XX

mf

Fig. 16.5 A cover letter signed by the health care provider appealing a claim.

If the appeal is won but copies of the same documents must be submitted each time this issue arises, ask the third-party payer how future claims with the same issue may be handled. Keep track of this information in a file.

If an appeal is denied, the service provider may want to proceed to the next step of the insurance carrier's appeal process.

Medicare Review and Redetermination Process

As noted previously, the appeals process can vary from insurance to insurance. CMS has its own appeals process for Medicare claims. The Medicare program has five levels of redetermination and special guidelines to follow:

- Level 1: Redetermination by the Medicare Administrative Contractor (MAC) that processed the original claim
- Level 2: Reconsideration by a Qualified Independent Contractor (QIC)
- Level 3: Disposition by Office of Medicare Hearings and Appeals (OMHA), also referred to as an Administrative Law Judge Hearing
- Level 4: Medicare Appeals Council review
- Level 5: Judicial review by a federal district court

Because Medicare guidelines change frequently, an internet resource has been provided at the end of this chapter to access the most current Medicare appeals process.

Redetermination (level 1). Redetermination is the first step in resolving a denied Medicare claim. Information about the denied claim is found on the Medicare RA. The request for redetermination must be made within 120 days of the initial determination. The insurance billing specialist should fill out a Redetermination Request Form and send it to the MAC. A written request for redetermination must include the following information:

- Beneficiary name;
- Medicare Beneficiary Identifier (MBI);
- Specific service and/or item(s) for which a redetermination is being requested;
- Specific date(s) of service; and
- Name and signature of the party or the representative of the party.

If the claim was denied because of a simple error made by the insurance billing specialist, such as omission of the National Provider Identifier (NPI) of the referring health care provider or failure to code a diagnosis, then complete a Medicare Redetermination Request form and resubmit a corrected claim (Fig. 16.6). Include only the denied services and indicate in Block 19 "resubmission, corrected claim." The MAC must respond within 60 days of receipt of a request for redetermination from a beneficiary or provider. It must include reasons for the decision, a summary of clinical or scientific evidence used in making the redetermination, a description of how to obtain additional information, a notification of the right to appeal, and instructions on how to appeal the decision at the next level. If requested, the Medicare intermediary must provide information about the policy, manual, or regulation used in making the redetermination decision. The decision must be written in language that the beneficiary can understand.

Reconsideration (level 2). The next step in the Medicare appeals process is a reconsideration request. A Qualified Independent Contractor (QIC) will conduct the reconsideration. QICs are independent contractors who did not take part in the level 1 appeals decision. When making reconsideration decisions, QICs are expected to give weight to local and national coverage policies and conduct a panel review of denials when necessary. The request must be made within 180 days of the date the Medicare redetermination notice was received. The CMS provides an online form (CMS-20033) that can be used to request reconsideration of a claim.

The request for reconsideration should clearly explain why there is a disagreement with the redetermination. Attach the following with the reconsideration request:
1. Copy of the original insurance claim
2. Copy of the RA showing the denial
3. Photocopy of other documents, such as operative or pathology report or detailed summary about the procedure, with appropriate words highlighted to help the reviewer
4. The reconsideration form with explanation of the procedure indicating justification for the services and the reason that the provider should receive more reimbursement

Mail the documents by certified mail with return receipt requested and retain copies of all documents sent to the carrier in the provider's pending file.

Generally, the QIC will send its decision to all parties within 60 days of receipt of the request for reconsideration. If the provider is not satisfied with the results of the review, move to the next level of appeals.

Disposition by Office of Medicare Hearings and Appeals (level 3). The third level of Medicare appeals is an OMHA review. OMHA is independent of CMS and is responsible for level 3 Medicare claims appeals. Either an Administrative Law Judge (ALJ) or an attorney adjudicator will make a decision based on evidence and the administrative record of the appeal. This level of appeals can be done via telephone, video teleconference, or occasionally in person. The hearing provides an opportunity to explain the request for appeal and supporting evidence of the claim to an ALJ.

To request a hearing by the ALJ, the amount remaining in controversy must meet the minimum threshold, which is updated annually. For calendar year 2020, the threshold amount was $170. Claims may be combined to meet the minimum threshold. The request must be made using the Department of Health and Human Services' form (OMHA-100) and must be filed within 60 days of receiving the reconsideration officer's decision. Because of the number of appeal requests, it may take up to 18 months to receive an ALJ assignment.

Proof that the claim represents an unusual case and warrants special consideration may lead to a successful conclusion. However, the decision might be reversed, it might allow partial adjustment of the carrier's payment, or payment might be denied. If the final judgment is not satisfactory, proceed to the next level.

Medicare Appeals Council (level 4). If the service provider is dissatisfied with the ALJ or attorney adjudicator's decision,

DEPARTMENT OF HEALTH AND HUMAN SERVICES
CENTERS FOR MEDICARE & MEDICAID SERVICES

OMB Exempt

MEDICARE REDETERMINATION REQUEST FORM — 1st LEVEL OF APPEAL

Beneficiary's name *(First, Middle, Last)*

Medicare number	Item or service you wish to appeal
Date the service or item was received *(mm/dd/yyyy)*	Date of the initial determination notice *(mm/dd/yyyy) (please include a copy of the notice with this request)*

If you received your initial determination notice more than 120 days ago, include your reason for the late filing:

Name of the Medicare contractor that made the determination *(not required)*	Does this appeal involve an overpayment? *(for providers and suppliers only)* ☐ Yes ☐ No

I do not agree with the determination decision on my claim because:

Additional information Medicare should consider:

☐ I have evidence to submit. Please attach the evidence to this form or attach a statement explaining what you intend to submit and when you intend to submit it. You may also submit additional evidence at a later time, but all evidence must be received prior to the issuance of the redetermination.	☐ I do not have evidence to submit.

Person appealing:
☐ Beneficiary   ☐ Provider/Supplier   ☐ Representative

Email of person appealing *(optional)*

Name of person appealing *(First, Middle, Last)*

Street address of person appealing

City	State	Zip code

Telephone number of person appealing *(include area code)*	Date of appeal *(mm/dd/yyyy) (optional)*

Privacy Act Statement: The legal authority for the collection of information on this form is authorized by section 1869 (a)(3) of the Social Security Act. The information provided will be used to further document your appeal. Submission of the information requested on this form is voluntary, but failure to provide all or any part of the requested information may affect the determination of your appeal. Information you furnish on this form may be disclosed by the Centers for Medicare & Medicaid Services to another person or government agency only with respect to the Medicare Program and to comply with Federal laws requiring or permitting the disclosure of information or the exchange of information between the Department of Health and Human Services and other agencies. Additional information about these disclosures can be found in the system of records notice for system no. 09-70-0566, as amended, available at 83 Fed. Reg. 6591 (2/14/2018) or at **https://www.hhs.gov/foia/privacy/sorns/cms-sorns.html**

Form CMS-20027 (01/20)

Fig. 16.6 Request for first level Medicare appeals. Redetermination by a Medicare Administrative Contractor (MAC). Form CMS-20027 (01/20).

the provider may request the fourth level of appeals, a review by the Medicare Appeals Council. The Medicare Appeals Council is part of the Department of Health and Human Services' Departmental Appeals Board. There are no requirements regarding the amount of money in controversy. A request must use the Department of Health and Human Services' form (DAB-101) and be filed within 60 days of the OMHA decision. If there is a question that the final judgment was not made in accordance with the law, the council by its own election may review the OMHA decision. Generally, the council issues a decision within 90 days from receipt of a request. If the council denies a review, the provider may file a civil action for a federal district court hearing.

Federal district court (level 5). To pursue the highest level of appeals, a judicial review in federal district court, the amount of the case must meet a minimum dollar amount. The minimum dollar amount changes annually; in 2020, the minimum dollar amount was $1670. It is acceptable to combine claims to meet this dollar amount. The hearing must be requested within 60 days from receipt of the level 4 appeals. There is no form provided by the Department of Health and Human Service; an attorney must be hired to represent the provider or manage the case. The attorney will file the case where the health care organization is located. There is no statutory lime limit as to when the decision must be made. The U.S. District Court makes the final decision.

Medigap Review and Appeal Process

Insurance companies that sell Medigap (MG) policies must be certified by the state insurance commissioner before being allowed to sell in each state. The certification can be lifted from any insurer that does not honor its contract agreements. If payment is slow in coming or is not received from an MG insurer, first try the paper or electronic claim solutions for delinquent claims mentioned previously in this chapter. As a last resort, tell the insurer, "If I do not receive payment, I will have no alternative but to contact the state insurance commissioner."

TRICARE Review and Appeal Process

Denials made by a TRICARE contractor can be appealed by the beneficiary or a participating provider. A provider who treats a TRICARE patient but is out of network is not able to obtain information from TRICARE. Contact the patient for their assistance.

In some cases, TRICARE may not have specialty providers available to treat patients. For example, an obstetrical patient may need to seek care from an out-of-network obstetrician if TRICARE does not have one available. In those cases, authorization from TRICARE must be obtained before the patient can receive care. There must be a reason the patient cannot go to a providing facility, and TRICARE determines whether it will approve the request. Otherwise, claims will be denied.

All TRICARE inquiries are done through the online portal or the automated phone system. TRICARE managed care contracts have been adopted throughout the United States, and the appeals procedures that TRICARE contractors use in these areas may vary. For information on how to file reviews and appeals for those contracts, ask the contracting insurance company for instructions and forms.

There are two types of TRICARE appeals: expedited and non-expedited. Expedited appeals must be filed within 3 days of the receipt of the initial denial. These appeals should include an expedited review of a prior authorization denial. This process varies slightly depending on the regional contractor, so research the appeals process with the local TRICARE contractor.

Non-expedited appeals must be filed no more than 90 days after the receipt of the initial denial. The steps to file a non-expedited appeal follow:

1. Send a letter to the regional TRICARE contractor at the address specified in the notice to appeal. The appeal letter must be submitted no more than 90 days after the date of the RA. Include in the appeal the RA stating the denial, along with a claim form and all medical documentation relating to the claim. If for some reason essential paperwork for the insurance claim is not available to be sent, include this reason in the appeal letter. Keep copies of all paperwork for future reference and follow-up.
2. The TRICARE contractor will review the case and make a decision. If the decision is not favorable, the next level of appeal is TRICARE Quality Monitoring Contractor (TQMC).
3. Send a letter to TQMC including all the documentation from the original appeal and the decision received from the regional TRICARE contractor. The letter must be received by TRICARE no more than 90 days after the date of the appeal decision. Again, if not all documentation is available to be sent along with the appeal, include the reasons why in the appeal letter. Keep all paperwork for future reference and follow-up.
4. The TQMC issues a second reconsideration decision. If the claim is for less than $300, the TQMC decision is final. If there is still a dispute about a claim that is more than $300, an independent hearing may be requested with the TRICARE Management Activity (TMA).

TRICARE Reconsideration. Participating providers may appeal certain decisions made by TRICARE and request reconsideration. Providers who do not participate may not appeal, but TRICARE patients and parents or guardians of patients under 18 years of age who seek care from nonparticipating providers may file appeals. Providers who do not participate may not receive any information about a claim without the signed authorization of the patient or the patient's parent or guardian.

Matters that can be appealed include the following:

1. Medical necessity disagreements (inappropriate care, level of care, investigational procedures)
2. Factual determinations (hospice care, foreign claims, provider sanction cases)
   a. Denials or partial denials of requests for preauthorization for certain services or supplies
   b. Coverage issues—notification that TRICARE will not pay for services before or after a certain date

Matters that cannot be appealed include the following:

1. Denial of services received from a provider not authorized to provide care under TRICARE
2. A specific exclusion of law or regulation
3. Allowable charges for particular services
4. Issues relating to the establishment and application of diagnosis-related groups
5. Decisions by the claims processor to ask for additional information on a case
6. A determination of a person's eligibility as a TRICARE beneficiary

The TRICARE department that handles appeals also collects and organizes all information necessary to review the case effectively. Usually, a determination decision is made within 60 days of receipt of the appeal. Disagreements about the amount allowed for a claim may be reviewed by the claims processor to determine whether it was calculated correctly. However, an individual cannot appeal the amount the TRICARE contractor determines to be the allowable charge for a certain medical service.

Requests must be sent to the claims processor of the state in which services were provided and must be postmarked within 90 days of the date the provider receives the Summary Payment Voucher (formerly referred to as an RA). Include photocopies of the claim, the Summary Payment Voucher, and other supporting documents with the request form or letter. The claim identification number assigned by the claims processor should be included in any inquiry concerning payment of the claim. If TRICARE denies the initial request, the other two levels of review—formal review and hearing—may be pursued.

 16.6   QUICK REVIEW

Question: What is the first step that an insurance billing specialist would take when requesting an appeal from any insurance carrier?

STATE INSURANCE COMMISSIONER

There is no federal regulatory agency that oversees insurance companies. Instead, insurance companies are regulated primarily by individual states. Insurance regulations vary widely from state to state. If a complaint arises about an insurance policy, medical claim, or insurance agent or broker, the insurance department of the state of residence or the state in which the insurance company's corporate office is headquartered should be contacted. This department is generally referred to as the state insurance commissioner. State insurance commissioners are public officials who regulate the insurance industry in their state.

State Insurance Department Objectives

State insurance departments usually have various objectives, including the following:

- To register insurance companies
- To establish standards and best practices
- To make certain that the financial strength of insurance companies is not unduly diminished

- To monitor the activities of insurance companies to ensure that the interests of the policyholders are protected
- To verify that all contracts are carried out in good faith
- To ensure that all organizations authorized to transact insurance, including agents and brokers, are in compliance with the insurance laws of that state
- To release information on how many complaints have been filed against a specific insurance company in a year
- To help explain correspondence related to insurance company bankruptcies and other financial difficulties
- To assist if a company funds its own insurance plan
- To help resolve insurance conflicts

The insurance commissioner can hold a hearing to determine whether licensed insurers, agents, or brokers are in compliance with the insurance laws of the state, but the commissioner does not have the authority vested in a court of law to order an insurance company to make payment on a specific claim.

The insurance commissioner reviews the policy to determine whether the denial of a claim by the insurance company was based on legal provisions of the insurance contract and advises the patient if there is an infraction of the law. If there is an infraction, the patient should consult an attorney to determine whether the claim should be submitted to a court of law.

Types of Problems

Problems that should be submitted to the insurance commissioner include the following:

1. Improper denial of a claim or settlement for an amount less than that indicated by the policy after proper appeal has been made
2. Delay in settlement of a claim after proper appeal has been made
3. Illegal cancellation or termination of an insurance policy
4. Misrepresentation by an insurance agent or broker
5. Misappropriation of premiums paid to an insurance agent or broker
6. Problems about insurance premium rates
7. Two companies that cannot determine which is primary

State Insurance Department Inquiries

An insurance billing specialist may not be in a position to know the particulars about a case and should never assume or accuse unless they are certain or have concrete evidence. Remember, "jump to conclusions, suffer contusions."

Requests to the insurance commissioner must be submitted online. In some states, the insurance commissioner requires that the complaint comes from the patient even if an assignment of benefits form has been signed. In such a case, a letter or form should be prepared for the patient to sign and then submit. Depending on the circumstances of the case, one may wish to send copies to the state medical association or an attorney. Mail may be sent certified, return receipt requested. The request should contain the following information:

1. The inquiring person's (patient) or policyholder's name—the commissioner's responsibility is to the patient (the consumer), not the health care organization

2. The policyholder's address
3. The policyholder's telephone number
4. The insured's name
5. Name, address, and title of the insurance agent or official of the insurance company
6. A statement of the complaint including, if possible, a copy of the policy, medical bills, unpaid medical insurance claim, canceled checks, and any correspondence from the company pertaining to the claim
7. The patient's signature
8. The name and address of the insurance company, agent, or broker, or the name and address of the finance company if the premium was financed
9. The policy or claim number
10. The date of loss
11. The date on which the patient signed the complaint form

If an insurance company is continually a slow payer, one method to speed up payments is to include a note to the carrier that reads, "Unless this claim is paid or denied within 30 to 45 days, a formal written complaint will be filed with the state insurance commissioner."

Another method is to send a letter to the insurance commissioner with a copy notation inserted at the end to the insurance company. It might read, "The attached claim has been submitted to the XYZ Insurance Company. It has not been paid or denied. Please accept this letter as a formal written complaint against the XYZ Insurance Company."

Insurance companies are rated according to the number of complaints received about them, so they do not want the insurance commissioner to be alerted to any problems. Some states have information available to the public on how many claims have been submitted against a company if this information is necessary.

> **🔨 16.7 QUICK REVIEW**
>
> Question: How can the state insurance commissioner assist health care providers with insurance carriers who are slow payers?

CLAIM DENIAL MANAGEMENT

Every health care organization will experience claim denials. Denied claims represent unpaid services, and failure to promptly work denials from insurance carriers results in lost revenue for the health care organization. Denials also present a significant burden on the health care organization from the perspective of staff time spent managing and working denials. Some organizations are unable to devote the needed manpower to the denied claim effort and eventually the denials are written off as bad debt. Health care organizations leave millions of dollars on the table because of inefficient claim denial management processes. Claim denial management is the process of identifying and reviewing specific reasons for claims denials, which is followed by development of a process for appealing denied claims. Claim denial management represents a significant opportunity for revenue cycle cash flow improvement and has become a critical component of any health care organization's strategic effort toward this goal.

Claim Denial Identification

Effective claim denial management starts with identifying the reason for denials. The insurance billing specialist will need to review RAs carefully to determine the specific reason for denial. The reason for the denial is usually identified on the RA with a reason code that translates to a specific denial description. If the denial description is unclear, it may be necessary for the insurance billing specialist to call the insurance carrier for additional information.

Claim Denial Review and Appeal

The health care organization should have a process in place to ensure that the denial will be reviewed and appealed within a week of receipt of the RA. Techniques for appealing the claim are outlined previously in this chapter. Creating a strong workflow for claim denied claims is key to the denial management process. To do this, a workflow must be established to track the claims as they enter and leave the organization's billing system. Keep in mind that many insurance carriers have time limits associated with how quickly a denial can be appealed.

Categorizing Claim Denials

In addition to working denials and appealing claims, the denials must be categorized by reason, source, and other pertinent factors. As the reasons for denials are identified, processes can be modified to reduce the number of denials. Examples of reasons for denial include:

- Registration errors such as incorrect payer, incorrect insurance identification number, and so on
- Charge entry errors
- Referral and preauthorization errors
- Duplicate claims incorrectly submitted
- Medical necessity
- Documentation
- Coding errors
- Bundled/noncovered services
- Incorrect/invalid modifier usage
- Credentialing issues

Measuring Claim Denials

Using medical billing software, the health care organization can track, report, and measure claim denials. The organization should compute denials as a percentage of all claims submitted to understand what the volume and reasons for denials reveal about the organization's revenue cycle. Gathering this type of data will provide important content to analyze your health care organization's processes and overall performance. It may be helpful to continue to drill down through the denial, based on even greater specificity. For example:

Step 1: The organization calculates a high percentage of denials for medical necessity.

Step 2: The next step would be to measure the amount of medical necessity denials per provider. In doing this, one provider is identified as having a higher percentage of medical necessity denials than other providers.

Step 3: The final step in this situation would be to measure the amount of medical necessity denials for this provider by procedure code. In doing this, it is identified that excision of benign lesions has the highest medical necessity denial rate of all procedures performed by this provider.

By doing this type of analysis, the organization is able to pinpoint the specific reason for the high percentage of denials and can now strategize how to correct the problem.

Developing Strategies to Prevent Future Denials

As denial categories are analyzed and measured, the organization will develop strategies to change processes, preventing future denials. Strategies might include adjusting workflows, retraining staff, assisting providers with documentation issues, reviewing medical necessity policies, implementing system alerts and notifications, researching coding issues, clarifying carrier guidelines and policies, implementing internal audit processes, and providing incentives for improving collection of patient information.

Denial management is a road map for change. Every time a denial is reduced, the health care organization will get paid correctly and will have eliminated all the rework required when a claim is denied. Denial management is key to improving any organization's cash flow.

16.8   QUICK REVIEW
Question: What are the five elements of claim denial management?

DISCUSSION POINT
Once claims have been successfully submitted to the insurance carrier, explain the importance of following up on unpaid claims. Describe important skills that an insurance billing specialist must develop to successfully resolve unpaid claims.

PROCEDURE 16.1   File an Appeal

Objective
To compose, format, key, proofread, and print a letter of appeal and attach photocopies of information to substantiate reimbursement requested

Directions
Follow these basic step-by-step procedures, which include rationales, to learn this skill.
1. Prepare to compose a letter of appeal. Start the appeal by placing the health care organization's name, address, and telephone number at the top of the letter.
2. Include the date the letter of appeals is being written.
3. Include the beneficiary's name, health insurance claim number, date of initial determination, date of service in question, items or services in question, name and address of the provider, and signature of the appellant.
4. Compose the letter with an introduction that stresses the service provider's qualifications, the provider's commitment to complying with regulations and providing appropriate services, and the importance of the health care organization to the payer's panel of health care professionals.

5. Provide a detailed account of the necessity of the treatment given and its relationship to the patient's problems and chief complaint. You might cross-reference the medical record and emphasize parts of it that the reviewer may have missed.
6. Explain the reason why the provider does not agree with the claim denial listed on the EOBs or RA.
7. Abstract excerpts from the coding resource book and attach a photocopy of the article or pertinent information showing the name of the article, coding resource, and date of publication.
8. Send copies of similar cases with increased reimbursement from the same insurance company if available from the insurance company payment history file.
9. Call the insurance company and speak to the individual responsible for appeals; explain what the resubmission is trying to accomplish. Direct the correspondence to this person.
10. Proofread the letter for spelling and grammar errors before sending.
11. Retain copies of all data sent for the health care organization's files.
12. Use a method that confirms the payer received the letter, such as a certified return receipt or signature using FedEx or Airborne Express services.

KEY POINTS

This is a brief chapter review, or summary, of the key issues presented. To further enhance your knowledge of the technical subject matter, review the key terms and key abbreviations for this chapter by locating the meaning for each in the Glossary at the end of this book, which appears in a section before the Index.
1. After the medical claim is submitted, the insurance carrier goes through a series of steps to determine their financial responsibility for payment of the claim. This process is referred to as adjudication.
2. Payment from a third-party payer after submission of a paper claim should occur within 4 to12 weeks, of an electronic claim should occur within 7 days. When a payment problem develops, and the insurance company is slow, ignores, denies, or exceeds time limits, contact the third-party payer.
3. An explanation of benefits (EOB) or electronic Medicare remittance advice (RA) should be read, interpreted line by line, and checked to establish whether the amount paid is correct. Amounts should then be posted to each patient's financial account.
4. Health care organizations need to manage the back-end office tasks associated with claims reimbursement such as oversight of unprocessed claims, payment posting, and handling of claim denials in an effort to quickly resolve claim reimbursement issues.
5. Routine periodic checks of the insurance claims electronic tracking report or insurance paper claims register (log) should be done to follow up on delinquent claims.
6. Aging reports are generated each month categorizing outstanding claims as current, 30 days, 60 days, 90 days, and

120 days. Proper follow-up on all outstanding accounts should be made.

7. The individual handling the front desk must collect insurance information accurately and update patient demographic information routinely to avoid future collection problems.

8. To avoid denied claims and assist in solving claim problems, keep abreast of the latest policies for all contracted payers as well as for the federal programs.

9. The Office of the Inspector General (OIG) strongly advises providers to return overpayments promptly. Failure to do so can lead to severe fines and implicate fraudulent activity.

10. A decision to appeal a claim should be based on whether there is ample information to back up the claim and if a substantial amount of money is in question.

11. The levels of a Medicare appeal are (1) redetermination by telephone, letter, or form; (2) reconsideration by a hearing officer; (3) disposition by Office of Medicare Hearings and Appeals (OMHA); (4) review by the Medicare Appeals Council; and (5) judicial review in the federal district court.

12. The types of a TRICARE appeal are expedited and non-expedited.

13. To complain about a problem with an insurance contract or a claim involving a private third-party payer or a MG supplemental plan, the state insurance commission must be contacted.

14. Always file the appropriate form or write a letter to begin the appeal process for resolving an insurance problem or complaint.

15. Denial management is critical to improving any organization's cash flow.

INTERNET RESOURCES

Medicare Appeals Process
- https://www.cms.gov/outreach-and-education/medicare-learning-network-mln/mlnproducts/downloads/medicare-appealsprocess.pdf

STUDENT ASSIGNMENT

- Study Chapter 16.
- Complete all exercises in the *Workbook* to reinforce the theory learned in this chapter.

- Turn to the Glossary at the end of this text for a further understanding of the key terms and key abbreviations used in this chapter.

17

Collection Strategies

Linda M. Smith

OBJECTIVES

After reading this chapter, you should be able to:

1. Explain the cash flow cycle in a health care organization.
2. Define *accounts receivable* and explain methods for management of it.
3. Describe procedures for collecting complete and accurate patient information.
4. Describe guidelines for missed appointments.
5. Recite and discuss types of fee adjustments available to patients.
6. List the proper ways to offer professional courtesy.
7. Discuss fees with patients.
8. Name and describe payment options available to patients.
9. Define how to use the aging accounts receivable report effectively in management of collections.
10. Discuss dun messages, electronic media, and manual and computer billing, as well as state the role of a billing service in the collection process.
11. List the names of the federal credit laws applicable to the healthcare setting.
12. Explain statutes of limitations of three kinds of financial accounts.
13. Perform oral and written communication collection techniques.
14. Describe insurance collection from the patient and from third-party payers.
15. State and discuss the role of a collection agency in the collection process.
16. Explain the purpose of small claims court in the collection process.
17. Name and discuss basic actions in tracing a debtor who has moved and left no forwarding address.
18. Identify and describe special collection issues.

KEY TERMS

accounts receivable	cycle billing	itemized statement
age analysis	debit card	lien
automatic stay	debt	netback
balance	debtor	no charge
bankruptcy	discount	nonexempt assets
bonding	dun messages	professional courtesy
cash flow	embezzlement	secured debt
collateral	estate administrator	skip
collection ratio	estate executor	statute of limitations
credit	fee schedule	unsecured debt
credit card	financial accounting record	write-off
creditor	garnishment	

KEY ABBREVIATIONS

A/R	FACT	FDCPA	NC
ATM	FCBA	FTC	NSF
e-check	FCRA	N/A	TILA
			W2

INSIGHTS FROM THE FIELD

Sue P.: Credentials: CPC (Certified Professional Coder)

I am employed by a large health care organization as a billing representative. My task is referred to as back-end billing. When patients receive bills they don't understand or think are inaccurate, they call me. It's important to remember that everyone is going through something. Listen to the patient. Don't talk over them. Don't interrupt them. Be understanding of their feelings. They are upset. Today, I helped a single mom with three children who had just gotten out of work and was feeling overwhelmed and frustrated when she received a bill. She didn't know how to handle her medical bills, but with my knowledge and experience, I was able to help her develop a plan. I was able to give her peace of mind so that she could go make dinner for her family. I bring the human touch to some very overwhelming and complex situations.

COLLECTION STRATEGIES

As discussed in earlier chapters, the insurance billing specialist's primary goal is to assist in management of the revenue cycle. *Revenue cycle management* refers to the processes a health care organization uses to collect unpaid bills, and it determines the organization's profitability. Collections of debts or unpaid bills from patients is the final component of revenue cycle management.

Billing practices for health care organizations have evolved from the barter system of days past. Since the Great Depression, the availability of credit and credit cards has become a common feature of the financial marketplace. The word *credit* comes from the Latin word *credere*, which means "to believe" or "to trust." This trust is based on the individual's integrity and their financial ability to meet obligations when they become due. For many, the idea of credit has changed and may simply mean to put off paying today what one can pay tomorrow.

Although a large percentage of reimbursement to health care organizations is generated from third-party payers (i.e., private insurance, government plans, managed care contracts, and workers' compensation), patients continue to take on more financial responsibility for their health care as a result of high-dollar-deductible health plans and rising copays and coinsurance.

The insurance billing specialist will need to be proficient in calculating patient balances, billing patients and in collection of balances due from patients. In today's environment, revenue cycle management requires focusing on collection strategies that will maximize cash collections as well as provide a positive patient experience.

Fig. 17.1 shows a flow chart and overview of a health care organization's billing procedures that illustrates the sequence from beginning to end.

Fig. 17.1 Flow chart showing a health care organization's billing procedures from scheduling the patient's appointment to producing accounts receivable management reports.

Accounts Receivable

Understanding the accounts receivable of the health care organization is essential to development of effective collection strategies. Accounts receivable (A/R) is the total amount of unpaid balances that are due to a health care organization, from patients and third-party payers, for services that have been rendered. A/R management is vital to a health care organization's financial stability, and each organization must start with a strong foundation of financial policies. The effectiveness of the policies (and enforcement of them) is reflected in the organization's cash flow. The cash flow is the ongoing availability of actual cash in the organization. The primary goal in management of an account receivable is to reduce the amount of time an account is outstanding and to ensure payment of all services. When payment is collected at the time of service, the number of days in A/R is zero. In an ideal situation, all outstanding balances are paid within 60 days; however, this is not possible for the following reasons:

1. Health care expenses have increased and exceed the expenses the patient pays for everyday living.
2. Laws have been enacted and health care organizations have instituted policies to ensure that all patients, regardless of their financial situations, receive the best possible health care. In many situations, care of the indigent becomes a nonreimbursable expense in the health care organization.
3. Legal proceedings often delay the payment of medical expenses.
4. Third-party payers do not always pay claims in a timely manner, resulting in further delays in the collection of patient copayments.

The best ways to keep A/R down is to verify insurance benefits before providing care to the patient (if possible), collect copayments and deductibles at the time of service, obtain authorizations when required, and monitor A/R weekly. Another recommendation is to set up automatic alerts when patients with an outstanding balance in their account want to schedule an appointment. This reminds the receptionist to ask for a copayment, deductible, or noncovered fee.

The collection ratio is the relationship of the amount of money owed to a health care organization and the amount of money collected on the A/R. A collection rate of 100% is obviously desirable, although unrealistic, and should always be sought as a goal for the person managing collections in the health care office. To calculate the collection ratio for a 1-month period, divide the amount of monies collected during the current month by the total amount of A/R.

17.1 QUICK REVIEW

Question: When payment is collected at the time of service, within how many days is the amount due in the account receivable?

When payment is *not* collected at the time of service, how many days does it typically take to collect the balance due in an ideal situation?

PATIENT EDUCATION

An important collection strategy for all health care organizations starts with patient education. Many Americans do not fully understand how health insurance works, so the burden of educating them falls on the health care organization's staff. Front-office medical staff should strive to educate the patient in the following aspects of health care:

- Plan benefits, including service limitations, copays, and deductibles
- The approximate out-of-pocket expense for patients after insurance has paid
- The cost of medications, medical equipment, and ambulatory services
- The difference between emergency and urgent care and the costs involved.

The Affordable Care Act of 2013 was enacted to allow more Americans access to quality health care. Some of the provisions include free preventive care, elimination of preexisting conditions, expanded Medicaid coverage, and discount medications for seniors.

The Affordable Care Act also provides subsidized health insurance for lower-income individuals and allows young adults up to age 26 to remain on their parent's health care plan. This Act does not affect how health care organizations are reimbursed; however, it has impacted how much revenue comes from the self-pay category. The number of self-pay patients has decreased due to there being a greater number of insurance options available to them; however, cost-sharing through higher deductibles, coinsurance, and copayments has increased the amount of self-pay balances for the patient to pay.

A new patient information packet containing information about payment policies should be provided to the patient on the initial encounter to the health care organization. This decreases the number of billing statements sent and increases collections. Never allow a patient to believe that he or she is not responsible for the bill; some medical offices prefer to post a sign stating the office policy (Fig. 17.2). Discuss copayment requirements with patients who are enrolled in managed care plans and convey the organization's policy of collecting this amount when registering the patient for services. A new patient information pamphlet or brochure and confirmation letter (Fig. 17.3)

Example for Calculating the Monthly Collection Rate:

Enter the total amount collected in 1 month: $187,000;

Divided by the Total amount of A/R: $236,000;

Equals the collection ratio for this 1-month period: 79%.

YOUR CO-PAY IS EXPECTED AT THE TIME OF SERVICE, UNLESS PRIOR FINANCIAL ARRANGEMENTS HAVE BEEN MADE.

Fig. 17.2 Signs for payment like this are commonly found in the health care organization.

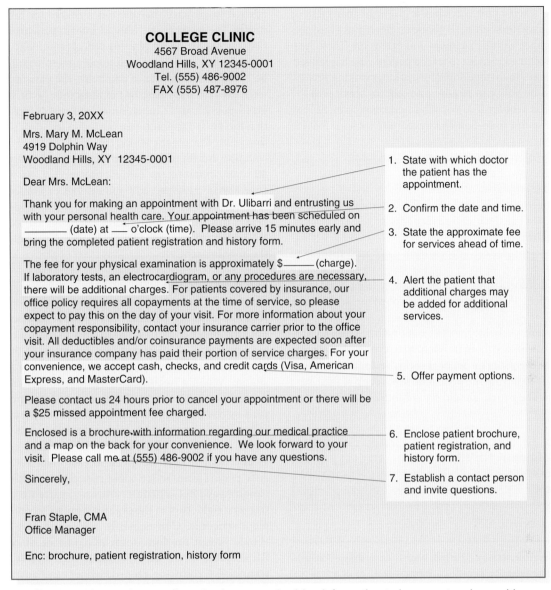

Fig. 17.3 New patient confirmation letter emphasizing information to incorporate when writing to a new patient.

may be e-mailed as an attachment or sent to welcome the new patient to the health care organization. This message or letter informs the patient about the organization, clearly outlines payment expectations, provides collection policies and procedures in printed form, includes a missed appointment clause, establishes a contact person, invites questions, and confirms all specific details discussed.

Patient Registration Form

There is no substitution for good information-gathering techniques at the time of initial patient registration because this assists later in billing and collection. Always obtain complete and accurate demographic and identifying information from the patient on their first encounter with the health care organization. Confirm the accuracy of that information on each subsequent encounter. For commercial insurance plans, have the guarantor agree in writing to pay for all medical treatment. By obtaining the guarantor's signature, he or she is then bound by contract to pay the bill.

Learn as much as possible about the patient before any services are provided. This is when the patient is likely to be the most cooperative. Information provided on the patient information sheet will prove critical to any billing and collection efforts. The patient should be instructed to answer all questions and indicate any spaces on the form that do not apply by marking N/A (not applicable). A helpful tip is to assist the patient to focus on vital information needed by using a yellow highlighter and blocking all necessary information. One field often overlooked is the subscriber information and date of birth, even though dependents may have insurance cards issued in their name. Reviewing the completed patient information sheet ensures that all blanks have been addressed and accurate information has been collected. It also alerts office staff of an account that may be a future problem. Items often overlooked are the street address, when a post office box is given; an apartment or mobile home park number; a cell phone number; and a business telephone number with department and extension. These help the insurance billing specialist to trace a patient who has moved. If a patient refuses to divulge any information, invoking privacy laws, it should be policy to require payment for services at the time that care is rendered. A potential nonpaying patient may be recognized at this time. Some indications to look for include the following:

- Incomplete information on the registration form
- Multiple changes of residence
- Questionable employment record
- No telephone numbers (business, cell, or home)
- Post office box listed with no street address
- A motel address
- Incomplete insurance information or no insurance coverage
- No referral information or authorization from a primary care provider (PCP) for patients enrolled in a managed care plan.

Employers are changing health plans with increasing frequency, and patients are more transient than ever, so update this form each time the patient is seen. This can be done by printing out a data sheet or having the patient review a copy of their registration form. The patient should sign or initial any changes or corrections.

 17.2   QUICK REVIEW

Question: List some of the fields that are often overlooked by the patient when completing a patient registration form.

FEES

Another collection strategy for all health care organizations is related to the fees the health care organization charges for the services they provide. Health care organizations operate with a set of fees that must be applied uniformly to all patients receiving services. Health care organizations set their own fees, and they are generally based on the Medicare fee schedule.

Fee Schedule

As discussed in previous chapters, a fee schedule is a listing of accepted charges or established allowances for specific medical procedures. Always quote fees and state policies about the collection of fees to the patient at the initial encounter. Under federal regulations, a list of the most common services the health care organization offers, including procedure code numbers with a description of each service and its price, must be available to all patients.

Missed Appointments

Missed appointments are expensive for health care organizations and patients should be informed of the importance of keeping appointments. There is no CPT code for missed appointments; however, patients can be billed for them as long as they are advised in advance that there is a charge for missed appointments. The medical staff should inform patients from the very first encounter about the missed appointment fee, which is typically $35 to $70. Missed appointment charges should not be billed to the insurance company; the patient is responsible for these fees regardless of the insurance he or she carries. To avoid possible discrimination or civil rights violations, ensure that the missed appointment fee is applied to all patients within the health care organization.

Some health care organizations hold a specific 24- to 48-hour appointment cancellation policy. As a professional courtesy to patients, staff should call or contact patients to remind them of the date and time of the appointment just before this cancellation period. The staff should also inform the patient of the cancellation fee if the patient were to miss the appointment.

Fee Adjustments
Discounted Fees

A health care organization may choose to discount its fees, but this practice is ill-advised and may be illegal in some circumstances. A discount is a reduction of the normal fee based on a specific amount of money or a percentage of the charge. When a health care organization offers a discount, it must apply to the total bill, not just the portion that is paid by the patient (copayment or coinsurance amount). By following this rule, the health care provider is giving a discount to both the patient and the insurance company. The same discount must be given to each member of the insurance plan. This practice could reduce the health care organization's payment schedule with the insurance company and trigger a reduction in the organization's allowable reimbursement schedule. Consequently, the health care organization should weigh the long-term outcome of discounting fees. All discounts must be electronically posted to the patient's financial accounting record (ledger) and any financial reasons or special circumstances should be documented in the patient's medical record. This ensures complete record keeping and safeguards any questions that may be asked during a financial audit.

Cash Discounts

Cash discounts may be offered to patients who pay the entire fee, in cash, at the time of service (Fig. 17.4). If a cash discount system is offered, this policy should be posted in the medical office and every active patient sent a notification. Research should be done on the applicable state laws because some states do not allow cash discounts; check the health care organization's insurance contracts to determine whether they are affected. Also, refer to the health care organization's compliance protocol to ensure that any such discounts do not implicate fraud.

Financial Hardship

Financial hardship cases are the most difficult for the health care organization to determine. The insurance billing specialist should never assume anything about a patient's financial status, nor judge a patient's ability to pay based on their appearance.

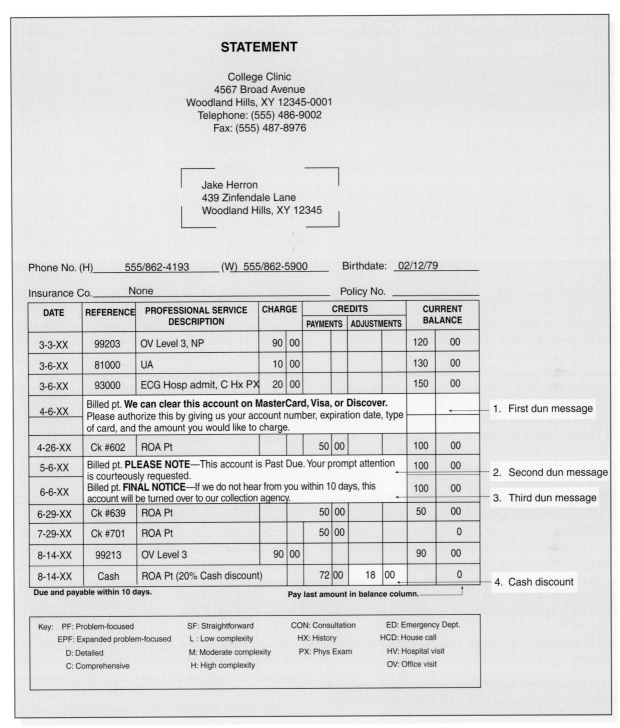

STATEMENT

College Clinic
4567 Broad Avenue
Woodland Hills, XY 12345-0001
Telephone: (555) 486-9002
Fax: (555) 487-8976

Jake Herron
439 Zinfendale Lane
Woodland Hills, XY 12345

Phone No. (H) ___555/862-4193___ (W) _555/862-5900_ Birthdate: _02/12/79_

Insurance Co. ___None___ Policy No. ___

DATE	REFERENCE	PROFESSIONAL SERVICE DESCRIPTION	CHARGE	CREDITS PAYMENTS	CREDITS ADJUSTMENTS	CURRENT BALANCE	
3-3-XX	99203	OV Level 3, NP	90 00			120	00
3-6-XX	81000	UA	10 00			130	00
3-6-XX	93000	ECG Hosp admit, C Hx PX	20 00			150	00
4-6-XX		Billed pt. **We can clear this account on MasterCard, Visa, or Discover.** Please authorize this by giving us your account number, expiration date, type of card, and the amount you would like to charge.						← 1. First dun message
4-26-XX	Ck #602	ROA Pt		50 00		100	00
5-6-XX		Billed pt. **PLEASE NOTE**—This account is Past Due. Your prompt attention is courteously requested.				100	00	← 2. Second dun message
6-6-XX		Billed pt. **FINAL NOTICE**—If we do not hear from you within 10 days, this account will be turned over to our collection agency.				100	00	← 3. Third dun message
6-29-XX	Ck #639	ROA Pt		50 00		50	00
7-29-XX	Ck #701	ROA Pt		50 00		0	
8-14-XX	99213	OV Level 3	90 00			90	00
8-14-XX	Cash	ROA Pt (20% Cash discount)		72 00	18 00	0	← 4. Cash discount

Due and payable within 10 days.   Pay last amount in balance column.

Key: PF: Problem-focused   SF: Straightforward   CON: Consultation   ED: Emergency Dept.
      EPF: Expanded problem-focused L : Low complexity   HX: History   HCD: House call
      D: Detailed   M: Moderate complexity   PX: Phys Exam   HV: Hospital visit
      C: Comprehensive   H: High complexity   OV: Office visit

Fig. 17.4 Electronic hard copy of a patient's financial accounting record showing dun messages, posted payments, and cash discount.

The Department of Health and Human Services (DHHS) annually publishes a guideline on poverty income (Table 17.1) which is used to determine eligibility for programs such as Head Start, the National School Lunch Program, and the Children's Health Insurance Program. Health care organizations may choose to follow these guidelines to direct patients to government-sponsored programs, obtain public assistance, and determine who is eligible for a hardship waiver. A hardship waiver can vary from 25% to 100% of the bill. Various financial forms are available to obtain this information; a copy of the patient's wage and tax statement (W2) or income tax return should be examined to make a reliable decision. The patient also should sign a written explanation to verify true financial hardship. This helps in the collection process and allows the health care organization to accept the insurance as payment in full, in certain circumstances, without being suspected of

TABLE 17.1	**Department of Health and Human Services Poverty Guidelines for 2020**		
Persons In Family Household	**Poverty Guidelines for the 48 Contiguous States and the District of Columbia**	**Poverty Guidelines for Alaska**	**Poverty Guidelines for Hawaii**
1	$12,760	$15,950	$14,680
2	$17,240	$21,550	$19,830
3	$21,720	$27,150	$24,980
4	$26,200	$32,750	$30,130
5	$30,680	$38,350	$35,280
6	$35,160	$43,950	$40,430
7	$39,640	$49,550	$45,580
8	$44,120	$55,150	$50,730

The 2020 poverty guidelines are in effect as of January 15, 2020.
Note that there are separate poverty guidelines for Alaska and Hawaii.
Department of Health and Human Services (DHHS). 2020. guidelines on poverty income. From Office of the Assistant Secretary for Planning and Evaluation. Available at: http://aspe.hhs.gov.

insurance fraud. The reason for a fee reduction must be documented in the patient's medical record. Large medical organizations or medical offices whose services may not be covered by insurance can create and use a sliding-scale fee schedule based on federal poverty levels, allowing according to their financial situation.

Be careful about giving a discount because it can be construed as discriminatory if not given to other patients consistently. To avoid problems, develop a written policy about what qualifies a patient for a financial hardship discount.

Write-Off

A write-off is a debt that has been determined to be uncollectible and is taken off (subtracted/credited) the accounting books. It is considered lost income but may not be claimed as a loss for tax purposes. The insurance billing specialist should obtain financial information on all patients who request a write-off. Office policies about adjustments and all discounts should be in writing, and all staff members should be informed. Write-off policies should clearly state who must approve all discounts, adjustments, and special payment arrangements, before the patient contract signature.

❗ COMPLIANCE ALERT

Compliance Guidelines for Deviations From Standard Collection Procedures

The Office of the Inspector General issued guidance to health care organizations that they are free to use whatever policy they want on charity care, discounts, write-offs, and collections, as long as it is done consistently and the reasons for granting these are documented in the organization's compliance manual. Ensure that these deviations from standard collection procedures are not tied to or conditional on referrals or use of the provider's services. The policy must also state the minimum effort in collection of debts, such as one or more letters or telephone calls. The health care organization that uses minimum collection efforts can waive the obligations of patients in financial need in accordance with office policy and try to collect more aggressively from other patients who are not financially needy.

The health care organization must appoint a designated individual to approve the portion of the charge to be credited to the financial record before the debt is forgiven. A write-off is possible in three circumstances:

- The first is as stated in the preceding discussion, when the patient has proved a financial hardship.
- The second is when it will cost more to bill the balance than what is owed. For example, the balance may be $1.05. It will cost the health care organization more than this amount to collect the balance. This type of write-off is known as a *small balance write-off.*
- The third situation is when the health care organization has made a good faith effort to collect the balance with no success. In this case the balance is written off and the account may or may not be sent to a professional collection agency depending on whether the agency accepts balances less than, for example, $35 for collection.

Professional Courtesy

Professional courtesy is a concept attributed to Hippocrates, but the foundations are derived from Thomas Percival's *Code of Medical Ethics,* written in 1803. The *American Medical Association (AMA) Code of Ethics,* formulated and adopted in 1847, closely mirrored Percival's code. The practice of professional courtesy served to build bonds between health care providers and reduce the incentive for providers to treat their own families. Most health care providers agree that one of the greatest honors and privileges in the practice of medicine is to be asked to care for another health care provider or a provider's family members. The practice of professional courtesy often was extended to others in the health care profession and members of the clergy. Now most health care providers have insurance coverage for medical expenses. Consequently, most hospitals and health care organizations have given up the practice of free care through professional courtesy.

Professional courtesy means either a discount or an exemption from charges that may be given to certain people at the discretion of the provider rendering the service.

An interim rule from the Centers for Medicare and Medicaid Services (CMS), effective September 5, 2007, identifies proper ways to offer professional courtesy:

1. The professional courtesy is offered to all health care providers on the entity's bona fide medical staff or in the entity's local community or service area, without regard to volume or value of referrals or other business generated between the parties.
2. The health care items and services provided are of a type routinely provided by the entity.
3. The entity's professional courtesy policy is written and approved in advance by the entity's governing body.
4. The professional courtesy is not offered to a health care provider (or immediate family member) who is a federal health care program beneficiary, unless there has been a good-faith showing of financial need.
5. If the professional courtesy involves any whole or partial reduction of any coinsurance obligation, the insurer is informed in writing of the reduction.
6. The arrangement does not violate the Anti-Kickback statute (section 1128B[b] of the Act) or any federal or state law or regulation governing billing or claims submission.

Health care organizations must examine their policies on professional courtesy to ensure that they do not violate the contractual terms in private, managed care, or government-sponsored insurance policies. If the treating provider does not bill the health care provider–patient for services rendered, the third-party payer is relieved of its contractual obligation. If the treating provider waives the deductible and copayment, he or she may be accused of not treating others with the same insurance coverage in an equal manner. Although there may be some situations in which it is defensible to not charge for services to health care professionals, the health care organization should ensure that this professional courtesy is not linked to patients who have been referred. Laws prohibit any inducement or kickbacks from health care organizations or providers that could influence the decision of a service provider to refer patients or that may affect a patient's decision to seek care.

> **! COMPLIANCE ALERT**
>
> ### Professional Courtesy Guidelines
>
> Professional courtesy may violate fraud and abuse laws, depending on how the recipients of the professional courtesy are selected and how the courtesy is extended. If selection depends on referral of individuals, it may implicate the Anti-Kickback statute. An insurance claim submitted as a result of such a professional courtesy may also be affected by the False Claims Act.

Copayment Waiver

Waiving copayments is another way that health care organizations have reduced the cost of medical care for patients in the past. In doing so, the organization accepts the insurance payment only. In most situations, both private insurers and the federal government ban waiving the copayment, so it is not recommended. Waiving copayments could violate the contract between the patient and third-party payer. If the health care

organization has contracted with a third-party payer, waiving the copayment may be a violation of the insurance contract. Some insurance companies look at this as a means of recouping its losses by undergoing litigation against the health care organization or demanding the return of all payments made to the service provider.

No Charge

No charge (NC) means waiving the entire fee for professional care. This is permitted as long as it is not part of a fraudulent scheme and is offered to all patients. All NC services must be fully documented in the clinical portion of the patient's medical record.

No charge situations may occur on a patient's account when follow-up visits are posted after a patient undergoes surgery and they are in the confinement of a global surgical package. When posting such charges in a medical billing system, *Current Procedural Terminology* (CPT) code 99024 (postoperative follow-up visit included in global fee) may be used.

Reduced Fee

Precautions should be taken before reducing the fee of a patient who dies. The health care organization's sympathy in this case could be misinterpreted and result in a malpractice suit. A fee reduction should never be based on a poor result in the treatment of a patient.

If a patient disputes a fee and the health care organization agrees to settle for a reduced fee, the agreement should be in writing inside the patient account file.

Discussing Fees

People have a difficult time asking each other for money and talking about financial obligations. Financial arrangements should be discussed up front and in great detail before any services are provided. Many health care organizations create their own collection problems by not being clear about how and when they expect to be paid. If patients are not told that payment is due at the time of service, most assume they can pay at a later time. The following are some guidelines to help communicate effectively about money:

- The patient's financial history is personal, so conversations about fees must be done in private so that other individuals cannot overhear.
- The patient should be made to feel comfortable so that they feel free to discuss any financial problems.
- Be courteous at all times, but express a firm, businesslike approach that will not offend the patient.
- Never badger or intimidate a patient into paying; merely state the payment policy and educate the patient.
- Inform patients of their full financial responsibility and balance due in a clear manner.
- Verify the patient's copayment listed on their insurance card and collect this amount before their encounter for services.
- Make it easier for patients to pay rather than to leave without making payment.
- Do not give patients an option by asking if they would like to pay now or have a bill sent.

- Motivate patients to pay by appealing to their honesty, integrity, and pride.

The following are examples of communicating in a positive manner and letting the patient know exactly what is expected:

- "Today's services are $62, Mrs. Smith. Would you like to pay by cash, check, credit card, or debit card?"
- "Your copayment for today's service is $20, Mr. Jones, and you can pay by cash, check, credit card, or debit card"
- "Your insurance policy shows a $100 deductible that is your responsibility and that currently has not been met, Miss Rodriguez. You must pay the full fee today, which is $100"
- "Mrs. Merryweather, I must collect $4.77 today for your vitamin B12 injection. The injection is not covered by your insurance policy"
- "We look forward to seeing you on Tuesday, March 3, at 10 AM, Mr. Gillespie. The consultation fee will be approximately $150 and payment is expected at the time of service. We accept cash, check, credit cards, or debit cards for your convenience."

 17.3 QUICK REVIEW

Question: Under what circumstances can a patient be billed for a missed appointment?

 17.4 QUICK REVIEW

Question: A health care organization may choose to discount its fees, but this practice can be illegal in some circumstances. Explain how a health care organization's policy should be developed to allow them to offer a discount.

COLLECTING FEES

Collecting applicable copayments and other amounts due from the patient at each health care encounter is strongly recommended. To avoid difficulties in collecting at a future date, ask for fixed copayments before the patient is seen by the provider. This will alleviate billing for small amounts. The importance of collecting outstanding bills, coinsurance amounts, and money from cash-paying patients up front should be communicated to office staff. One-on-one communication is the best way to motivate a debtor (someone owing money). Each patient's account balance (amount due) should be reviewed before their appointment. If the appointment schedule is on a computer system, print the account balance by each patient's name. If an appointment book is used, make a copy of the page showing the day's schedule. Write overdue balances by the patient's name after obtaining overdue amounts from each patient's financial accounting record. This information also should be recorded on the transaction slip for that day's encounter and may be "flagged" when the transaction slips are printed or written. Treat this information confidentially and keep it out of view of other patients. When a patient arrives whose name is flagged, alert the patient accounts manager.

To do effective preappointment collection counseling, the patient should be taken to a quiet area away from the general activity of the office. Sit down with the patient and discuss the situation. Use an understanding attitude and helpful nature while verbalizing phrases such as "I understand" and "I can help." Ask direct questions to learn exactly what problems the patient is facing. Answers to questions such as, "When do you expect your next paycheck?" and, "How much are you able to pay today?" help to determine the strategy. The goal should be to collect the full amount. If that is not possible, try to collect a portion of the balance. Get a promise to pay for the remaining balance by a specific date. If the patient is unable to comply, set up a payment plan. The chances of reaching a mutually satisfactory resolution are greatly improved when the two parties are face to face. Refer to Procedure 17.1 at the end of this chapter to create a financial agreement with the patient.

A face-to-face interview is better than a telephone interview because a financial agreement can be signed when the debtor is present (Fig. 17.5), resulting in a better follow-up response. Let the patient know that the health care organization is willing to help and that the debtor should inform the insurance billing specialist if he or she runs into further problems making the payment. This personal contact helps if a renegotiation of the agreement is necessary. A health care organization cannot refuse to let an established patient see the doctor because of a debt, but the office staff has every right to ask for payment while the patient is in the office.

Encounter Forms

Multipurpose billing forms are known by many names, including *encounter form*. These forms are helpful when collecting fees at the time of service. Encounter forms can be given to patients to bill their insurance companies, used to inform patients of current charges and outstanding balances, and used as receipts for payment (Fig. 17.6).

Patient Excuses for Nonpayments

Nonpayers tend to dismiss financial arrangements with curt remarks. Look directly at the patient, confidently expecting payment. Demonstrate to the patient the right to request payment. Be ready if excuses are offered. Table 17.2 shows examples of patients' excuses and possible responses.

When a patient chatters nervously, it may be a way of setting up reasons to rationalize not paying. Do not let this be distracting. Pause after asking for payment and do not say another word until the patient responds. Many people feel uncomfortable with silence, but pauses may be advantageous and help to complete a transaction. The cash flow and collection ratio are increased by taking this approach, while billing chores and collection costs are decreased. The quick identification of nonpayers may be obtained and the person responsible for collections notified.

Credit and Debit Cards

The current economic trend is heading toward the use of credit and debit cards. Patients find these easier to use and tend to always have them on hand. Accepting credit cards can have a positive impact on A/R management by improving cash flow, reducing billing costs, lowering overhead, and reducing the risk of bad debts.

Credit card payment is an option that provides patients with an alternative to clear their account balances. Credit cards are

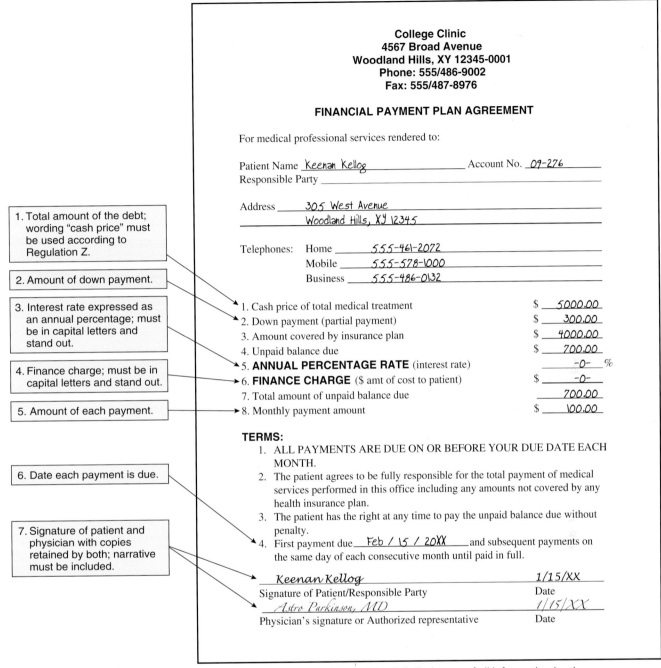

Fig. 17.5 Financial payment plan agreement that provides full disclosure of all information by the Truth in Lending Act, Regulation Z.

issued by organizations that entitle the cardholder to credit at their establishments. This method of payment may be most useful as a down payment on uninsured or elective procedures. It is estimated that approximately 35% of patients will use a credit card to pay for health care related expenses if the option were given. If a health care organization accepts credit cards, advise all patients in the following ways:

- Display a credit card acceptance sign.
- Include an insignia or message on the patient account statement.
- Include the credit card policy in the new patient brochure or new patient welcome letter.

- Have staff members verbalize to patients that this option is available.
- Patients may prefer to clear a debt immediately and make monthly payments to the credit card company instead of owing money to their service provider.

Verifying Credit Cards

The insurance billing specialist should check credit card warning bulletins to ensure that the card has not been canceled or stolen. Large health care organizations may have an electronic credit card machine that allows the insurance billing specialist to swipe the card through the machine, which is linked to

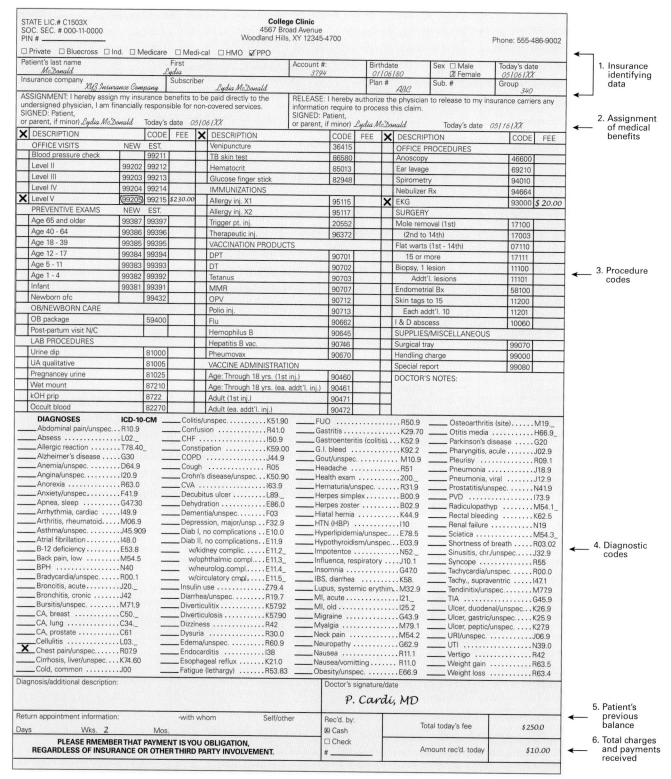

Fig. 17.6 Encounter form; diagnostic codes from *International Classification of Diseases, Tenth Revision, Clinical Modification* (ICD-10-CM) and procedural codes for professional services from *Current Procedural Terminology* (CPT). (Courtesy Bibbero Systems, Inc., Petaluma, Calif.; telephone: 800-242-2376; fax: 800-242-9330; www.bibbero.com.)

TABLE 17.2	Possible Responses to Patients' Excuses for Avoiding Payment
Excuse	**Response**
"Just bill me."	"As we explained when we made your appointment, Mr. Barkley, all copayments are to be paid at the time of the encounter. That will be $25 for today's service, please."
"I have insurance to cover this."	"We will be billing your insurance for you, Miss Butler, but your policy shows a deductible in the amount of $300 that still must be met. We must collect the full fee for today's visit, which is $150 to meet that deductible responsibility."
"I get paid on Friday; you know how it is."	"I understand. Why don't you write the check today and postdate it for Saturday? We will hold the check and deposit it on the next business day." (Depending on office policy.)
"If I pay for this, I won't be able to pay for the prescription."	"Our payment policy is very much like the pharmacy's: We expect payment at the time of service. Let me check and see if the doctor can dispense some medication samples to last until you can get your prescription filled."
"I don't have that much with me."	"How much can you pay, Mrs. Fish? I can accept $10 now and give you an envelope to send us the balance within the week or I can put it on your credit or debit card." (Get a commitment and write the balance due under the sealing flap of the envelope. Also write the date on a tickler calendar or the patient's financial accounting record while the patient is watching.)
"I'll take care of it."	"I know you will, Mr. Stone; I just need to know when that will be so that I can document your intentions for our bookkeeper." (Get a commitment and input the date in the patient's financial accounting record while the patient is watching. Hand him an envelope with the amount due written under the sealing flap.)
"I forgot my checkbook."	"We take Visa, MasterCard, and American Express, Mr. Storz." (If the patient still does not pay, provide him with a self-addressed envelope and write the patient's name, account number, date of service, amount due, and expected payment date under the sealing flap. Restate the expected payment date as you hand the patient the envelope. Input the date in the patient's financial accounting record while the patient is watching.)

the credit card company. Transactions are then approved, processed, and deposited in a bank account, usually in 2 working days. A receipt is generated for the patient.

Verifying Credit Card Holders

Always verify the cardholder by asking for photo identification, such as a driver's license. Examine the card carefully and observe the following guidelines:

- Accept a credit card only from the person whose name is on the card.
- Match the name on the card with the patient's other identification and ensure that the expiration date has not passed.
- Check the "hot list" for problem cards.
- Verify all charges regardless of the amount and get approval from the credit card company.
- Compare the signature on the credit card receipt against the signature on the card.

Credit Card Fees

Most banks directly deposit the amount on the credit card receipt and subtract the monthly fees from the health care organization's bank account. A statement from the bank indicates how much has been credited to the account. The fees can be negotiated on the basis of volume but usually range from 2% to 10% on each transaction. Some health care organizations charge patients a service fee for using credit cards. Do not issue cash or check refunds for any payments made by credit card. Patients who want to make payments may have their credit cards charged for each scheduled payment. Some health care organizations choose to impose a nominal fee (50 cents) for all credit and debit card transactions to recoup the fee charged by the credit card company. Simple credit card reader terminal devices attached to a smartphone or tablet are available (Fig. 17.7).

Fig. 17.7 Square device used with a tablet to collect credit card payments. (Photo copyright iStock.com.)

Credit Card Options

Online bill payment or e-payment, such as PayPal, is another way patients can pay their health care bills. It is done through the health care organization's secure website. Payment can be verified immediately and deposited directly into the organization's bank account.

Other cards are used for credit in a health care office. Automated teller machine (ATM) cards are sometimes accepted for medical care if the health care organization has a credit card scanner. An ATM card is a magnetically encoded bankcard used to make deposits and withdraw cash from checking or savings accounts. Private-label cards are credit vehicles that can be used only to pay for health care. Some large health care organizations offer their own private-label health cards. Smart cards also are used in some locations. They are small credit or debit cards that contain a computer chip that can store money in the form of electronic data. Special-use smart cards for telephone calls, gas stations, and fast food are now in use, as are common cards having multiple uses. These cards may also contain patient health care data.

Visa offers a credit card service unique to the health care market. It has a preauthorized health care form that allows patients to authorize the health care organization to bill their account directly for copayments and the balance not covered by insurance. Patients who need a series of treatments (e.g., allergy injections or chemotherapy) can fill out one form designating these services, which authorizes the staff to charge the patient's account directly.

Debit Cards

A debit card is a card that permits bank customers to withdraw cash at any hour from any affiliated ATM in the country. The holder may make cashless purchases from funds on deposit without incurring revolving finance charges for credit. Health care organizations that offer credit card payment may use the same electronic credit card machine to swipe the debit card for verification and approval. Separate debit card machines are also available for businesses that do not accept credit cards. Debit cards take the place of check writing; however, once the debit card is approved for a certain amount, the bank that issued the debit card is responsible for paying the funds that were approved. There are no returned checks for nonsufficient funds (NSF) with this method of payment.

Payment by Check

A personal check is a common method of payment in most medical offices, but it is not a personal guarantee of payment. Check verification requires the billing specialist to become familiar with the appearance of a good check. A driver's license and one other form of identification should always be required. Check these against existing records.

To verify all out-of-state and suspicious checks, find the bank name on the front of the check and call the bank to verify that funds are available. Tell the customer service representative that you would like to verify a check that the health care organization has received. Provide the bank account and routing numbers from the bottom on the front of the check.

A verification service (which is a private company with resources to identify patient information quickly over the telephone) or a check authorization system may be worthy of consideration for clinics and larger health care organizations.

E-Checks

Another payment option that is becoming popular is payment by e-check. With an e-check, the patient gives their checking account information to the health care organization, such as account number and bank routing number. A signature to confirm the electronic transaction is required and the check is deposited immediately.

Check Forgery

Forgery is false writing or alteration of a document to injure another person or with intent to deceive. An example of forgery is signing another person's name on a check to obtain money or pay off a debt without permission. To guard against forgery, always check that the endorsement on the back of the check matches the name on the front. Be suspicious if the beneficiary or provider states that he or she did not receive the check but the third-party payer shows it as being cashed, or if the payee of the check claims that the signature is not theirs.

Payment Disputes

Problem checks appear in many forms. One is the check for partial payment when the debtor (the patient) writes "payment in full" on the check. If the creditor (the health care organization) cashes the check, it may be argued that the debt is paid in full. A legal theory called *accord and satisfaction* may apply to this situation if the debt is truly disputed by the debtor. If the check is cashed by the health care organization, it can be considered "accord and satisfaction" and the organization cannot procure the balance from the patient. The operative words are *truly disputed*. If there is a legitimate, genuine dispute over the amount of the bill, and an amount less than the full amount of the bill is accepted, the health care organization could be precluded from seeking the balance. However, acceptance of payment does not necessarily mean acceptance of the "paid in full" remark. Even if a check marked "paid in full" is accidentally cashed, 90 days may be available to rectify the situation by returning the funds to the patient and informing them that the accord and satisfaction is not acceptable. A patient who is paying less may be dissatisfied with the health care organization in some way. This may help to defuse any lurking issues and to address the patient's underlying problem.

Postdated Checks

Checks dated to be payable 3 to 6 months in the future are not honored by the bank. Always read the date on every check. Federal collection law states that if a check dated more than 5 days in advance is accepted, the patient must be notified no more than 10 days and no less than 3 days before the check is deposited. State laws vary but some states have regulations in addition to federal laws.

Unsigned Checks

Another problem is unsigned checks. Ask the patient to come to the office and sign the check or send a new one. If the insurance billing specialist is unable to reach the patient or if there is a transportation or time limitation problem, they should write the word "over" or "see reverse" on the signature line on the front of the check. On the back of the check, where the endorsement should appear, write "lack of signature, guaranteed," the health care organization's name, and one's own name and title. This endorsement in effect is a guarantee that the health care organization will absorb the loss if the patient's bank or the patient does not honor the check.

Returned Checks

When the health care organization receives notice that a check was not honored, the reason should be stated on the back of the check. The most common reason for returned checks is non-sufficient funds (NSF); these are also referred to as "bounced checks" or "bad checks." In those cases, most health care organizations will repost the amount of the check to the patient's account. They will also add a charge for the service fee charged by the bank to the patient's account.

An NSF demand letter (Fig. 17.8) should be sent by certified mail with return receipt requested and include the following:
1. check date
2. check number
3. name of the bank where the check is drawn
4. name of the person the check was payable to
5. check amount
6. any allowable service charges
7. total amount due
8. number of days the check writer has to take action.

Future payments from patients who have issued an NSF check should be in the form of cash, money order, or a cashier's check. If the patient wants the check to be returned, it should be photocopied and kept in the financial record because it serves as an acknowledgment of the debt. The bad check may be returned to the patient after it has been replaced with a valid payment. A notation should be placed on the patient's record to this effect.

Payments Through Patient Portals

Many health care organizations offer patients access to their medical and financial records through a patient portal. By allowing patients to pay their medical bills online through a patient portal, most health care organizations see an improvement in revenue cycle management.

Health care organizations receive payment faster, in fuller amounts, and at a higher frequency.

Many patients prefer paying their bills online rather than by check. This online payment option makes it easy for patients to handle their financial responsibility and to access their account on any internet-supporting device. The patient can review their outstanding account and can pay it on their computer at work, during free time, or on their smartphone, anywhere.

COLLEGE CLINIC
4567 Broad Avenue
Woodland Hills, XY 12345-0001
Tel. (555) 486-9002
FAX (555) 487-8976

August 15, 20XX

Mrs. Maxine Holt
444 Labina Lane
Woodland Hills, XY 12345-0001

Dear Mrs. Holt:

The following check has been dishonored by the bank and returned without payment:

Date:	08/04/20XX
Check No.:	755
Amount:	$106.11
Payable to:	Perry Cardi, MD
Bank:	Woodland Hills National Bank
Reason:	Nonsufficient funds

This is a formal notice demanding payment in the amount of $106.11 within 15 days from today's date or your account will be considered for legal action.

Please make payment immediately by cash, cashier's check, or money order at the above address. Your immediate attention will be appreciated.

Sincerely,

Delores Yee, CMA-A

Patient Accounts Manager
for Perry Cardi, MD

Fig. 17.8 Demand letter for returned check. This letter serves as a formal notice to collect payment and notifies a patient of impending legal action.

In addition to allowing the patient to pay their outstanding balances more easily, patient portals can also securely hold credit card or bank information for repeat payments, if the patient chooses to use this feature.

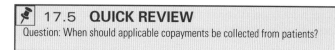

17.5 QUICK REVIEW

Question: When should applicable copayments be collected from patients?

SELF-PAY BILLING

Although collection of copayments and other amounts due from the patient at the health care encounter is strongly recommended, there are many instances in which a self-pay bill will need to be generated. And just as there are strategies for billing insurance carriers, there are strategies for self-pay billing.

Itemized Patient Statements

Every patient with an unpaid self-pay balance should receive an itemized statement (Fig. 17.9) of their account showing the dates of service, a list of detailed charges, copayments and deductibles paid, the date the insurance claim was filed, applicable adjustments, and the account balance. These items also are listed on the patient's account or financial accounting record card (see Fig. 17.4). Timeliness, accuracy, and consistency have a significant effect on the cash flow and collection process when sending itemized statements. A credit card option should be printed on the statement to encourage easier and faster payment.

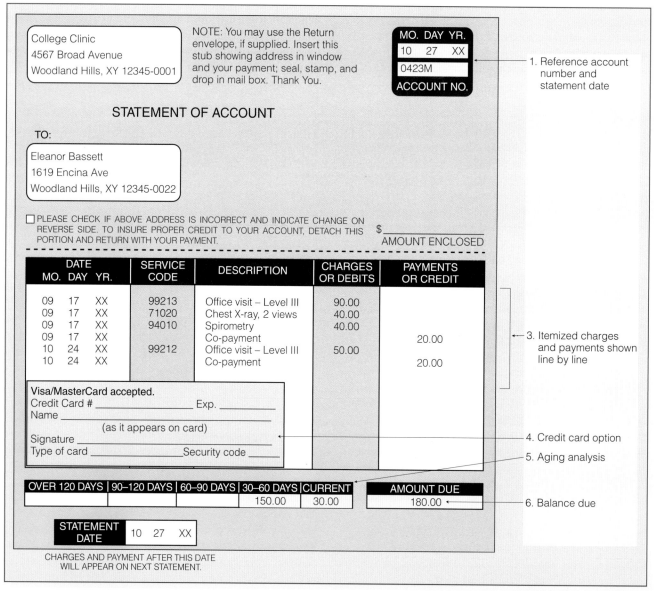

Fig. 17.9 Patient account statement. A credit card option should be printed near the bottom of the statement to encourage payment. (Form adapted courtesy Bibbero Systems, Inc., Petaluma, Calif.; telephone: 800-242-2376; fax: 800-242-9330; www.bibbero.com.)

Professional bills are a reflection of the health care organization. The billing statement should be patient-oriented and easy to read and understand. Avoid technical terms and abbreviations that might lead to misunderstandings and confusion. Enclose a return envelope with the address payments should be mailed to or that have a window that displays the health care organization's mailing address. Addressed envelopes should contain the statement "forwarding service requested" so that the postal service can forward the mail and provide the health care organization with a notice of the patient's new address. When this notice is received by the health care organization, it should be circulated to all necessary departments to record the new information.

Patients can be oriented to the billing process by having the insurance billing specialist electronically generate a printed statement as the patient leaves the service provider's office that explains pertinent information, such as account number, dates of service, payments, procedures, interest fees, copayments, and deductibles. Patients may choose to receive their statements electronically, so ask software providers for this component. If using standard mail, patient information pamphlets about common health concerns (such as blood pressure, cholesterol, or back pain) can be sent with the bill to convey a caring attitude.

The health care organization is likely to experience an increase in telephone calls from inquiring patients when statements go out in the mail. A patient account representative or department should handle all billing questions, ensuring a consistent response.

Accounts Receivable and Age Analysis by Aging Report

Age analysis is a term used for the procedure of systematically arranging the A/R by age based on the date of service. Accounts are usually aged in periods of 30, 60, 90, and 120 days and older. An aging report can be generated by the organization's medical billing system. This helps collection follow-up by providing easy recognition of overdue accounts, and allows the insurance billing specialist to determine which accounts need action in addition to a regular statement.

The formula for determining the A/R ratio is to divide the month-end A/R balance by the monthly average charges for the prior 12-month period. An average total A/R (all monies not collected at the time of service) should be no more than one-half to two times the charges for 1 month of services (Examples 17.1 and 17.2).

EXAMPLE 17.1 Formula for Calculating Accounts Receivable Ratio

Health Care Organization's Total Accounts Receivable:	Divided by Health Care Organization's Monthly Charge Total:	Equals the Accounts Receivable Ratio:
$75,000	$50,000	1.5

Total outstanding accounts receivable should range from $75,000 to $100,000. An accounts receivable higher than that would indicate a poor collection rate.

EXAMPLE 17.2 Calculation of Accounts Receivable Ratio

Annual gross charges	$150,000
Average monthly gross charges (150,000 ÷ 12 months)	$12,500
Current accounts receivable balance	$20,000
Accounts receivable ratio: 20,000 ÷ 12,500 = 1.60 months	

Accounts that are 90 days or older should not exceed 15% to 18% of the total A/R. To calculate this figure, divide the total amount of A/R by the amount of accounts that are 90 days old and older (Example 17.3). The medical billing system should calculate this automatically when an aging report is required.

A decision tree showing time frames for sending statements and making telephone calls is presented in Fig. 17.10.

EXAMPLE 17.3 Formula for Determining Percentage of Accounts over 90 Days

Amount of A/R over 90 days		A/R total	Percentage of A/R over 90 days
$12,000	÷	$75,000	= 16%

A/R, Accounts receivable.

Dun Messages

Dun messages are phrases printed on statements to inform or remind a patient about a delinquent account and to promote payment (see Fig. 17.4). The best and most effective collection statements include a handwritten note; however, this is seldom possible. Dun messages also can be printed by the computer system or applied with brightly colored labels. Examples of dun messages follow:

- "If there is a problem with your account, please call me at (555) 486-0000—Maralyn."
- "This bill is now 30 days past due. Please remit payment."
- "This bill is now 60 days past due. Please send payment immediately."
- "Your account is 90 days past due. Please remit payment now to avoid collection action."
- "FINAL NOTICE: If we do not hear from you within 10 days, this account will be turned over to our collection agency."

Do not send intimidating, impatient, or threatening statements. These serve only to antagonize patients. Dun messages should be printed in different languages and sent to patients who speak English as a second language.

Electronic Media

Health care organizations may receive e-mail messages about their bills, but it is advisable that a response is not given to patients via e-mail because of privacy concerns. An e-mail consent form must be signed and dated by the patient, and e-mail is then limited to appointment requests, prescription refills, requests for information, nonurgent health care questions, updates to information, or exchange of noncritical information, such as changes in office hours, holiday schedules, recalls or infectious diseases, immunizations,

Collection Decision Tree

Fig. 17.10 Collection decision tree. This is a quick reference used to help determine when to send statements, make telephone calls, and send accounts to a collection agency.

insurance changes, financial eligibility information, and so on. Furthermore, it is not advisable to send debt communications through social media, such as Twitter and Facebook. Too many people have access to social media over the internet.

Some organizations use their websites for live chat with patients because it is secure and similar to a telephone call. It is especially suitable for hearing impaired patients.

Computer Billing

Most health care organizations use the computer to generate billing statements. All charges, payments, and adjustments are reflected on hard copy and made readily available to mail to the patient (see Fig. 17.4) The computer program usually offers choices of billing types, including patient billing, insurance balance billing, billing according to types of adjustments, and no bill. The insurance billing specialist can instruct the computer to print all bills of a specific type. The computer also can be instructed to print bills according to specific accounts, dates, and insurance types. Accounts are automatically aged and standard messages can be printed on the statements for each of the aged dates (that is, 30, 60, 90, or 120 days). Some systems allow personalized messages to be inserted that override the standard messages.

Billing Services

Health care organizations can contract with billing services to reduce administrative paperwork by taking over the task of preparing, submitting, and following up for third-party health insurance companies and patients. They may provide data entry of patients' demographic and billing information, charges, receipts, and adjustments; tracking of payments from patients and third-party payers; production of management reports; purging of inactive accounts; and collection of accounts.

Some advantages of billing services are advanced technology, professional and understandable bills, experts answering all billing-related telephone inquiries, and no downtime caused by vacations, medical or personal leave. This service allows the health care organization to have fewer disruptions and freedom from worry about financial matters when trying to provide medical care.

The health care organization sends billing and receipt information to the billing service daily. This may be done in writing or through a computer system. The billing service then prepares the bills, mails them, and may also receive payments. Regular reports, whether weekly or monthly, are sent to the health care organization summarizing the transactions. Billing services may offer full revenue cycle management services and, in many cases, customize a service that meets the needs of the health care organization. Most medical billing services charge a percentage of every claim collected, typically 5% to 10%. Using a billing service company is most commonly referred to as *outsourcing*. When choosing a billing service, make a list of important questions and visit the facility. Also ask for references to obtain valuable feedback from other health care offices that have used the same billing service.

! COMPLIANCE ALERT

Guidelines When Contracting With a Billing Service

Have a written directive in place that gives the billing company permission to communicate directly with the insurance company and a Medicare administrative contractor (MAC) about denied or problem claims. When changing billing services, be sure to revoke such authorizations with each carrier and MAC.

Billing Guidelines

Billing procedures are determined by the size of the health care organization, the number of accounts, and the number of staff members assigned to the collection process. Adopt a specific method of handling accounts and decide which billing routine best fits the organization. Check insurance contracts carefully to determine which circumstances allow for patients to be billed. Be sure to conform to federal guidelines if there is a need to bill patients. See Procedure 17.2 at the end of this chapter for the procedure for seven-step billing and collection guidelines.

Payment Plans

Payment plans offer the patient a way of paying off an account by spreading out the amount due over time. Caution should be taken when offering patients a payment plan. The Truth in Lending Consumer Credit Cost Disclosure law (see the following section, Credit and Collection Laws), also referred to as *Regulation Z*, requires full written disclosure about the finance charges for large payment plans involving four or more installments, excluding a down payment. However, this regulation does not apply if the patient agrees to pay in one sum or in fewer than four payments and then decides independently to make drawn-out partial payments. Patients often think that if they make any amount of payment, the health care organization is required to accept that payment and not take any additional action. This is

incorrect. The health care organization can take action, including sending the account to a collection agency. Have a written payment plan schedule when working with accounts in which payment plans may be offered. Fig. 17.11 illustrates sample guidelines that may be used or revised according to the specific needs of a health care organization (Fig. 17.12).

When patients seek care from the health care organization but are honest about their financial status, it is necessary to develop a financial payment plan agreement. This agreement (see Fig. 17.5) provides the patient with a clear understanding of all fees, the agreed-upon monthly payment amount, and the monthly due date. It may be wise to set up an automatic monthly withdrawal from the patient's bank account or credit card to ensure receipt of the patient's payment. A statement that provides the account balance should be sent to the patient every month after a payment is made.

📌 17.6 QUICK REVIEW

Question: Age analysis is the procedure of systematically arranging the A/R from the date of service. When generating an aging report from the organization's medical billing system, what are the aged periods that accounts are typically separated into? Why is it helpful to separate the report in this manner?

PAYMENT PLAN SCHEDULE

Balance due amount	Minimum monthly payment	Time frame for full payment
$0 – $200	$35	6 months
$201 – $500	$50	1 year
$501 – $1000	$100	1 year
$1001 – $3000	$125	2 years
$3001 – $5000	$150	2 years
>$5001*	$200	5 years

*Accounts over $5000 must complete a credit card application to certify the minimum required payment and are subject to approval by the office manager.

Fig. 17.11 Payment plan schedule used in the health care organization to negotiate monthly payments shows balance due amounts, minimum monthly payment, and payment time frames.

Fig. 17.12 Insurance billing specialist setting up a payment plan with a patient.

CREDIT AND COLLECTION LAWS

The following laws are important because they provide the legal framework within which the insurance billing specialist must execute the health care organization's collection policy. Box 17.1 includes names and descriptions of the federal credit and collection laws that affect health care organizations.

! COMPLIANCE ALERT

Red Flags Rule

The Red Flags Rule is a set of Federal Trade Commission (**FTC**) requirements for businesses that have more than 20 employees and issue credit to their clients. This rule aims to prevent fraud and identity theft of a person's personal data for illegal use. A health care organization must create a plan to help recognize warning signs (or "red flags") associated with fraud and identity theft, or face civil penalties for violation. Medical identity theft occurs when someone uses a person's name and sometimes other parts of their identity, such as insurance information without that person's knowledge or consent. A health care organization must notify patients if their data have been stolen.

Statute of Limitations

A formal regulation or law setting time limits on legal action is known as a statute of limitations. Regarding collections, the statute of limitations is the maximum time during which a legal collection suit may be rendered against a debtor. However, for a lawsuit to be successful, a concerted effort should be made to collect on an account from the time services are rendered. The patient should receive regular statements indicating that if the insurer does not pay, the patient will be held responsible.

Statutes vary according to the following three kinds of accounts:

1. *Open book accounts* (also called *open accounts*) are open to charges made from time to time. Payment is expected within a specific period, but credit has been extended without a formal written contract. Patient accounts are usually open book accounts.
2. *Written contract accounts* have a formal written agreement in which a patient signs to pay their bill in more than four installments (see the Truth in Lending Act section in see Box 17.1).
3. *Single-entry accounts* have only one entry or charge, usually for a small amount.

 17.7 QUICK REVIEW

Question: Why is it important for the insurance billing specialist to become familiar with the Fair Credit Reporting Act, The Truth in Lending Act, the Fair Credit Billing Act, and other similar federal credit and collection laws?

BOX 17.1   Federal Credit and Collection Laws

Equal Credit Opportunity Act (ECOA)

Prohibits discrimination in all areas of granting credit. Detailed credit information should be obtained before performing services to prevent accusations of impartiality. New patients should be informed that payment is due at the time of service and that they should arrive 20 minutes early to fill out a credit application if they wish to establish credit for treatment. Data, such as the patient's address, previous addresses, length of residence, employment history, and approximate wage, can be verified with a credit bureau. The report will also contain the patient's name changes, the patient's bill-paying history, and any history of bankruptcy. If the patient has a poor credit rating, credit may be denied, and the patient then has 60 days to request the reason in writing. The law prohibits discrimination against any applicant for credit for the following reasons:

- age, color, marital status, national origin, race, religion, or sex
- whether the patient is receiving income from alimony or any public assistance program.

Fair Credit Reporting Act (FCRA)

Regulates agencies that either issue or use reports on consumers (patients) in connection with the approval of credit.

If credit is refused, the health care organization must provide the patient with a reason credit was denied and the name and address of the agency from which the report came. Specific information about what the report contains is not necessary and should not be given. The patient must have an opportunity to correct any inaccuracies if they occur.

Fair and Accurate Credit Transactions (FACT) Act (Public Law 108-159)

Establishes (as of December 4, 2003) medical privacy provisions as part of consumer credit law. The bill amends the FCRA to include improved medical privacy protections and protections against identity theft. Credit bureaus and creditors must comply with many medical privacy restrictions that ban the sharing of medical information. Title IV of the FACT Act limits the use and sharing of medical information in the financial system and provides an expanded definition of medical information. For military personnel, it provides an active-duty alert that can be placed on the credit file for a year at the three major credit bureaus. This means that a creditor cannot issue new credit or a card without first contacting the active-duty individual whose name is on the card.

Fair Credit Billing Act (FCBA)

Applies to "open end" credit accounts, such as credit cards. It does not cover installment contracts, such as loans or extensions of credit repaid on a fixed schedule. The FCBA settlement procedures apply only to disputes about "billing errors," such as unauthorized charges. Federal law limits the consumer's responsibility for unauthorized charges to $50; charges that list the wrong date or amount; charges for goods and services that the consumer did not accept or were not delivered as agreed; math errors; failure to post payments and other credits, such as returns; failure to send bills to the current address, provided the creditor receives the change of address, in writing, at least 20 days before the billing period ends; and charges for which an explanation or written proof of purchase along with a claimed error or request for clarification are requested. The consumer must write to the creditor at the address given for "billing inquiries," not the address for sending payments, and include one's name, address, account number, and a description of the billing error. Letters to creditors must be sent so that they reach the creditor within 60 days after the first bill was mailed that contained the error. The creditor must acknowledge the complaint in writing within 30 days after receiving it, unless the problem has been resolved. The creditor must resolve the dispute within two billing cycles (but not more than 90 days) after receiving the letter.

Electronic Fund Transfer Act (EFTA)

Limits consumers' liability if there has been an unauthorized use of an ATM card, debit card, or other electronic banking device.

BOX 17.1   Federal Credit and Collection Laws—cont'd

Truth in Lending Act (TILA)

Applies to anyone who charges interest or agrees to payment of a bill in more than four installments, excluding a down payment. When a specific agreement is reached between patient and health care organization, Regulation Z of this consumer protection act requires that a written disclosure of all pertinent information be made, regardless of the existence of a finance charge (see Fig. 17.5). This full disclosure must be discussed at the time the agreement is first reached between patient and health care organization and credit is extended.

It is essential to include the following items in the written agreement:

1. Total amount of the debt
2. Amount of down payment
3. Finance charge
4. Interest rate expressed as an annual percentage
5. Amount of each payment
6. Date each payment is due
7. Date final payment is due
8. Signature of patient and service provider with copies retained by both
9. Account balance with total interest and total amount paid by the patient at the end of the contract.

When a health care organization continues to treat a patient with an overdue account, the courts have viewed this as continuation of care and an extension of credit. Patients who fall into this delinquent status should be referred elsewhere.

After the patient has paid the overdue amount, the patient can be taken back and treated on a cash-only basis.

Truth in Lending Consumer Credit Cost Disclosure

Requires businesses to disclose all direct and indirect costs and conditions related to the granting of credit. All interest charges, late charges, collection fees, finance charges, and so forth must be explained up front, before the time of service. Include the following on all statements to charge interest and bill the patient monthly:

- Amount of each payment
- Due date
- Unpaid balance at the beginning of the billing period
- Finance charges
- Date balance is due

Fair Debt Collection Practices Act (FDCPA)

Addresses the collection practices of third-party debt collectors and attorneys who regularly collect debts for others. Although this Act does not apply directly to health care organizations collecting for themselves, a professional health care collector must avoid the actions that are prohibited for collection agencies. The main intent of the Act is to protect consumers from unfair, harassing, or deceptive collection practices. Refer to the guidelines in Box 17.2, which are taken from the FDCPA.

THE COLLECTION PROCESS

For collections to be handled effectively, staff members should be trained in collection techniques. Most insurance billing specialists can be trained to be efficient collectors when given the correct tools. New collectors need time to gain confidence, which is an important aspect of being a good collector.

Telephone Collection Procedures

Telephone collections are made easier if the insurance billing specialist is convinced that he or she *can* collect before trying to convince the patient to pay. Two important factors to consider are the insurance billing specialist's ability to contact the patient and the patient's ability to pay the bill. The following are helpful suggestions for using the telephone to address a collection problem:

- Contact the patient in a timely manner at the first sign of payment delay.
- Before contacting the patient, review the account carefully to ensure that the balance due is correct.
- Review the patient's registration information to determine where the patient is employed (or if unemployed).
- Decide what amount will be settled for if payment cannot be made in full.
- Make the first call count. Act in a calm, businesslike manner and combine empathy with diligence. Be positive and persuasive.
- Listen to what patients have to say, even if they get angry and raise their voice. Lower the volume of your own voice and respond in a composed manner. Try to pick up clues from what the patient is saying; the patient may be giving the real reason for nonpayment.
- Ask questions, show interest, and let the patient know that they are being listened to.

- Respond in a respectful manner and carefully word the reply; when patients are distressed, they do not always make sense. The goal is to encourage the patient to pay, not to agitate the patient.
- Use all resources and learn to negotiate.

Office Policy

The most organized approach to making collection calls is to print out the aging report and target accounts in the 60- to 90-day categories. The most effective results come from this group. Before making each call, review the patient's financial account in the medical billing system for notes on previous patient encounters. Start with the largest amount owed and work the accounts in decreasing amounts owed. After this category has been completed, move on to the 90- to 120-day accounts. Finally, go after accounts that are more than 120 days old.

Most state collection laws allow telephone calls to the debtor between 8 AM and 9 PM. Never call between 9 PM and 8 AM, because to do so may be considered harassment. According to collection experts, the best time to telephone is between 5:30 PM and 8:30 PM on Tuesdays and Thursdays, and between 9 AM and 1 PM on Saturdays. Regardless of when the call is made, track the times when the most patients are contacted and adjust the calling schedule accordingly. Perhaps the insurance billing specialist's hours should be increased to include one evening a week or Saturday mornings to make collection calls. Another option is the use of flex time, in which the employee can choose their own working hours from within a broad range of hours approved by management. Use a private telephone away from the busy operations of the office to eliminate interruptions. Patients may be embarrassed about not being able to pay their bills and patient confidentiality must be maintained. Follow the guidelines stated in the Fair Debt Collection Practices Act (Box 17.2).

BOX 17.2 Fair Debt Collection Practices Act Guidelines

1. Contact debtors only once a day; in some states, repeated calls in 1 day or the same week could be considered harassment.
2. Place calls after 8 AM and before 9 PM.
3. Do not contact debtors on Sunday or any other day that the debtor recognizes as a Sabbath.
4. Identify yourself and the health care organization represented; do not mislead the patient.
5. Contact the debtor at work only if unable to contact the debtor elsewhere; no contact should be made if the employer or debtor disapproves.
6. Contact the attorney if an attorney represents the debtor; contact the debtor only if the attorney does not respond.
7. Do not threaten or use obscene language.
8. Do not send postcards for collection purposes; keep all correspondence strictly private.
9. Do not call collect or cause additional expense to the patient.
10. Do not leave a message on an answering machine indicating that you are calling about a bill.
11. Do not contact a third party more than once unless requested to do so by the party, or the response was erroneous or incomplete.
12. Do not convey to a third party that the call is about a debt.
13. Do not contact the debtor when notified in writing that a debtor refuses to pay and would like contact to stop, except to notify the debtor in writing that there will be no further contact or that there will be legal action.
14. Stick to the facts; do not use false statements.
15. Do not prepare a list of "bad debtors" or "credit risks" to share with other health care providers.
16. Take action immediately when stating that a certain action will be taken (for example, filing a claim in small claims court or sending the patient's case to a collection agency).
17. Send the patient written verification of the name of the creditor and the amount of debt within 5 days of the initial contact.

Some health care organizations have found success in reaching patients by text messaging. The health care organization must receive permission to text the patient during the initial patient encounter before using this tool. There are many online companies that will text patients with appointment reminders. Be careful not to include any information that will violate the privacy of the patient, so keep the messages general, such as "The Mountain Valley Physical Therapy Associates has a message for you about your account; please call (888) 873-9472."

Be alert for new ideas or approaches to collection by watching how banks and other retailers implement sophisticated collection skills. Decide whether any of these could be used to the health care organization's advantage and present the techniques to the office manager. Keep abreast of improvements made to collection software that improve collection results and allow more collectors to work from their homes. Other advances such as call block, which is an expanded telephone service, have made it more difficult to make collection calls. This service was originally intended to screen out unwanted telemarketing calls by intercepting blocked, unlisted, or unknown numbers. Standard numbers are usually allowed to go through. The key to averting a block is to ensure that the number the call is being placed from is listed and within the patient's area.

For a step-by-step procedure on making telephone collection calls, see Procedure 17.3 at the end of this chapter.

Telephone "Don'ts"

Communication is important, especially when trying to work with a patient on difficulties in making payments. Remain professional at all times and treat the patient with respect. The following is a list of *don'ts* for telephone collections:

- Do not raise your voice and antagonize the patient.
- Do not accuse the patient of dishonesty or lying.
- Do not act like a "tough guy" or threaten a patient.
- Do not consent to partial payments until payment in full has been asked for, and do not agree to a long string of small partial payments.
- Do not engage in a debate.
- Do not report a disputed account to a collection agency or bureau until the patient's dispute is disclosed as part of the record.

Telephone collection calls are effective on the day before patients are due for their appointments. State the date and time of the appointment, and then remind the patient of the balance owed and ask whether they could please bring payment to the appointment.

Telephone Collection Scenarios

The most difficult part of one-on-one collections is preparing for the many situations that may be encountered and the various responses the patient may make. Table 17.3 lists some statements

TABLE 17.3 Telephone Collection Scenarios

Statement	Response
"I can't pay anything now."	"Are you employed? Are you receiving unemployment compensation, welfare, or Social Security benefits?" You are determining the patient's ability to pay.
"I can't pay the whole bill now."	"How long will it take you to pay this bill?" Ask this question instead of "How much can you pay?"
"I can pay but not until next month."	"When do you get paid?" Ask for payment the day after payday. "Do you have a checking account?" Ask for a postdated check.
"I have other bills."	"This is also one of your bills that should be paid now. Let's talk about exactly how you plan payment."
"How about $10 a month (on a $300 bill)?"	"I'd like to accept that but our accountant does not allow us to stretch out payments beyond 90 days, which would be $100 a month." This adheres to Truth in Lending law regulations for collecting payment in installments without a written agreement. If the patient tries to cooperate, then compromise. If not, turn the account over to a collection agency.

TABLE 17.3   Telephone Collection Scenarios—cont'd

Statement	Response
"I sent in the payment."	"When was the payment sent? To what address was it sent? Was it a check? On what bank was it drawn and for what amount? What is the canceled check number?" Investigate to determine whether the check was posted to a wrong account. If not, call the patient back and ask if he or she would call their bank to see if it cleared; if it has not cleared, the patient should stop payment. Ask the patient to call back and verify the status of the check. If the patient is not being truthful, he or she will not follow through. Ask for a new check and tell the patient that a refund will be made if the other one shows up.
"I cannot make a payment this month."	"The collection agency picks up all of our delinquent accounts next Monday. I don't want to include yours, but I need a check today."
"The check is in the mail."	"May I have the check number and date it was mailed?" Call back in 3 days if not received.
"I'm not going to pay the bill because the doctor didn't spend any time with me."	"May I confirm the doctor you saw, the date, and time? For what reason did you see the doctor? Do you still have the problem for which you saw the doctor?" Get as much information as possible and research the office schedule on the day the patient was seen. Let the doctor know about the patient's complaint and inquire how he or she would like to handle the complaint.
"I thought the insurance company was paying this."	"Your insurance paid most of the bill; now the balance is your responsibility. Please send your check before Friday to keep your account current." Explain why (deductible, copayment benefit) the service is not covered under the insurance plan.

that patients make about not paying an account and examples of responses that the insurance billing specialist can make.

Collection Letters

Collection letters are another method of reaching patients and reminding them of their debt. Knowledge of the patient base and of individual patients may help to determine the effectiveness of collection letters. Every health care organization is unique, and the type of service provided, the number of accounts, the geographic spread of patients, the staff size, and the amount of time collectors have to spend on individual accounts help determine which collection method best suits the organization.

The positive aspect of collection letters is that they can reach many patients rapidly and the cost is relatively low, especially if form letters are used (Fig. 17.13).

Collection letters have some negative aspects, such as the following:

- Letters usually take 2 or 3 days to reach the patient and may lie unopened for a week or more.
- Letters are one-way communication and thus lack the ability to provide the reason for nonpayment.
- Response and recovery through letters are relatively poor.
- Manual preparation takes time (especially if a decision must be made before sending each letter).
- The costs of postage and supplies are increasing.

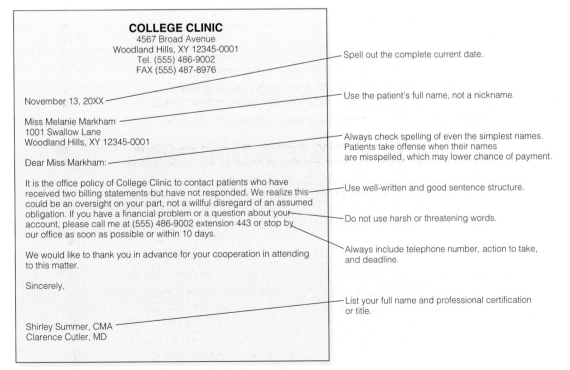

Fig. 17.13 Collection form letter sent to all patients who have not responded after two billing cycles.

The insurance billing specialist is often the one who composes collection letters and devises a plan for collection follow-up. A series of collection letters may be written using varying degrees of forcefulness, starting with a gentle reminder. When a collection letter is written, use a friendly tone and ask why payment has not been made. Imply that the patient has good intentions to pay. This may be done by suggesting that the patient has overlooked a previous statement. Communicate the health care organization's sincere interest in the patient. Always invite the patient to explain the reason for nonpayment in a letter, telephone call, or service encounter. It should sound as though the patient is eager to clear the debt.

When collection letters are sent toward the end of the year, include a statement letting the patient know that if the account is paid in full by the end of the year, the medical expense may be used as an income tax deduction. Another tactic is to send a notice advising the patient that he or she may skip December's payment because of increased expenses during the holidays. This tactic may be used as an opportunity to build patient relationships, but the collector must be firm and clear when offering such leeway. Collection letters sent after the first of the year can suggest that the patient clear the debt by using an income tax refund check.

Types of Collection Letters

A form letter saves time and can go out automatically at specific times during the billing cycle (Fig. 17.14).

Collection letters should contain the following information:
- Full amount owed
- Services performed

COLLEGE CLINIC
4567 Broad Avenue
Woodland Hills, XY 12345-0001
Tel. (555) 486-9002
FAX (555) 487-8976

March 16, 20XX

Mr. Frank Lincoln
3397 Westminster Avenue
Woodland Hills, XY 12345-0001

Account No.   593287
Amount Due: $ _____

Dear Mr. Lincoln:

The care of our patients is more important than writing letters about overdue accounts. Yet, as you must realize, the expense of furnishing care can only be met by payments from appreciative patients.

Your account is seriously past due and has been removed from our current files because of its delinquent status. Our office policy indicates that your account should be placed with a collection agency. However, we would prefer to hear from you regarding your preference in this matter.

Enclosed is a current statement of your account. Please indicate your payment choice.

☐ I would prefer to settle this account immediately. Please find payment in full enclosed.

☐ I would prefer to make monthly payments (up to six months). To exercise this option, please call and make arrangements to come into our office to sign a financial agreement.

☐ Please charge the full amount to my credit card. (We accept American Express, MasterCard, and Visa). To exercise this option, please telephone our office or fill in the enclosed form and return it with the envelope provided.

_____   _____
Signature   Date

Please select one of the three options above, sign the form, and return this notice within 10 days from the date indicated in the letter. A postmarked return envelope is provided. Failure to respond will result in an automatic referral to our collection agency. Please do not hesitate to call if you have any questions regarding this matter.

Sincerely,

Gil Steinberg
Office Manager

Enc. Envelope, Credit Card Agreement Form

Fig. 17.14 Multipurpose collection letter with checklist. This advises the patient of a seriously past due account, offers the patient three payment options, and warns the patient that failure to respond will result in a referral to a collection agency.

- What action the patient should take
- Time frame in which the patient should respond
- How the patient should take care of the bill
- Why the patient should take care of the bill
- Address to which the patient should send payment
- Telephone number to contact the office
- Contact person's name
- Signature, which can be listed as "Insurance Billing Specialist," or one's name and title with the health care organization's name below it.

When pursuing collection, the insurance billing specialist should stay within the authorization of the health care organization. All letters should be noted on the back of the financial accounting record, in the collection log, or in the computer comment area. Letters can be sent in brightly colored envelopes to attract attention. The envelope should include "address service requested" or "forwarding service requested" on the outside to ensure that the letter is forwarded if the patient has moved so that the office will be notified of the patient's new address. Always include a self-addressed stamped envelope.

After-Insurance Collections

Most patients carry some form of insurance; however, filing an insurance claim is only the first step in collecting fees owed. In many cases, the patient will have a balance due in the form of a copayment, coinsurance or deductible.

The first step to collecting patient balances after an insurance payment is to confirm that the insurance claim was paid accurately. Confirm that the amount of copayment, coinsurance or deductible due from the patient is correct by carefully reviewing the explanation of benefits (EOB). If the claim was denied, make sure that the balance is billable to the patient.

Use a letter or statement to collect from patients who have insurance coverage. Clearly indicate to the patient that the insurance billing specialist has submitted an insurance claim and advise the patient what action is expected. The status of the insurance claim should be noted on all statements. Notify patients promptly when an insurance payment has been received. Ask patients to get involved in the insurance process or to pay the bill within 10 days if a problem exists. The following are examples of notations on statements for patients with insurance coverage:

- "We have received payment from your insurance company. The balance of $_____ is now your responsibility."
- "Your insurance company has paid its share of your bill. This statement is for the amount payable directly by you."
- "Your insurance company has paid $_____ for the above services. The remaining portion of $_____ is now your responsibility."
- "The balance of this account is your share of the cost. Please remit today. For questions, call 486-9002."

Insurance Checks Sent to Patients

Send a letter immediately to notify patients who receive insurance checks. Advise such patients that they have received payment from their insurance company and that their account is due and payable within 10 days. Do not send continuous monthly bills; instead, speed up the collection process. If the patient refuses to pay and the health care organization does not want the patient to return, send a 10-day advance notification advising the patient that the account will go to a collection agency. If there is no response, refer to the health care organization's policy for discharging a patient and proceed accordingly.

Collection Agencies

Delinquent accounts should be turned over to a collection agency only after all reasonable attempts have been made to collect by the health care organization. Knowing when to turn accounts over helps determine the success of the collection agency. The longer the balance is unpaid, the less chance the agency has to collect the account, so the determination that an account is uncollectible should be made quickly. Following are some situations in which a health care organization should consider turning an account over to a collection agency:

- When a patient states that they will not pay or there is a denial of responsibility
- When a patient breaks a promise to pay
- When a patient makes partial payments and 60 days have lapsed without payment
- When a patient fails to respond to the health care organization's letters or telephone calls
- When payment terms fail for no valid reason
- When a check is returned by the bank because of NSF and the patient does not make an effort to rectify the situation within 1 week of notification
- When delinquency coexists with marital problems, divorce proceedings, or child support agreements
- When a patient is paid by the insurance company and does not forward the payment to the health care organization (This constitutes fraud and may be pursued with legal action.)
- When a patient gives false information
- When a patient moves, and the office has used all resources to locate the patient.

Many health care organizations prefer to adjust small bad debts off the books rather than increase administrative costs. All disputed accounts should be reviewed and approved by the individual designated by administration before they are sent to collection; to expedite the collection process, it is important for the health care organization and the office manager to establish a standard policy for deciding which accounts are sent to collections. There should be a systematized approach for turning accounts over to a collection agency that still allows room for exceptions.

Choosing an Agency

The collection agency is a reflection of the health care organization, so it is important to choose one wisely. Choose a reputable agency that is considerate and efficient, with a high standard of ethics. The agency should specialize in health care accounts and have an attitude toward debtors with which the organization agrees. Find out how long the agency has been in business and request a list of at least 10 references and statistics on their collection effectiveness. The average collection rate varies greatly but falls between 20% and 60% on assigned accounts. Ensure that the reported rate includes all accounts more than 1 year old and does not exclude accounts with small balances.

An agency's performance can be evaluated by the amount collected, less the agency's fees, which is called the netback. For instance, if a collector recovers 25% of $5000 ($1250) and takes a 50% commission, the health care organization's netback is $625. If a different collector recovers 25% of the $5000 ($1250) and charges a 30% commission, the netback is $375. Although the second agency collected the same amount, its lower commission afforded the health care organization more money.

When choosing a collection agency, make sure (1) to set up a separate post office box or lock box for the collection project; (2) to set up a separate bank account for the collection project; (3) that the contract stipulates that all correspondence be sent to the post office box (no correspondence is sent to the collection agency's physical or payment address); (4) that all e-checks and credit card receipts are deposited into the health care organization's bank account; and (5) that under no circumstance is the collection agency to receive any payments.

If collected funds go directly to the collection agency (whether insured, bonded, registered, or licensed), there is nothing to stop the agency from inappropriately handling the health care organization's money. The collection agency also could have a hidden lawsuit against it or an income tax lien and the organization may lose all its money if the money goes to the agency's bank account. Do not put "hold harmless" clauses in contracts. Hold the collection agency responsible for its actions. Many states do not regulate collection agencies and simply require that these agencies be registered. In addition to checking references, check with the state's Department of Corporations to determine whose name is on the collection agency's registration, if the tax identification number is correct and current, and if the address listed is different from the one the agency gave. Contact the circuit court to determine whether there are any lawsuits or judgments against the collection agency. Find out how many of the collection agency's employees will be assigned to the account, then monitor them once the contract is signed. They may have the best credentials and references and belong to all the correct organizations, but if they acquire an increasing number of accounts and the amount of recoupment remains constant each month, or is less than the national average, they may be picking and choosing the accounts. This is especially true when they are overanxious to receive a new file. If this happens, consider looking for another collection agency. Ensure that an account can be recalled without a penalty. The patient may have coverage with an insurance carrier that the health care organization has a contract with, so find out if the collection agency has the ability to resend a claim or if the billing company or office staff handles this. If so, does the contract have provisions for this and does the collection agency receive recoupment for obtaining insurance information?

The biggest key to the agency's effectiveness is the health care organization's own credit and collection policy. A comprehensive patient registration form, along with verifying employment, turning accounts over quickly when they qualify, and giving the agency all available information, helps the agency to pick up the paper trail and secure payment. A good collection agency has membership in a national collection society and the approval of the local medical society. Review the agency's financial statement and ensure that the agency is licensed, bonded, and carries "hold harmless clause" insurance. If a patient should sue because of harassment, this insurance will protect the health care organization from being sued as well. The local bar association and state licensing bureaus can be contacted to determine whether any complaints have been lodged against the agency or law firm. Find out if the agency reports uncollectable debtors ("deadbeats") to a credit bureau and investigate which one is used.

Types of Agencies

There are local, regional, and national agencies. National agencies and those that use the internet may have better results when tracing skips (patients who owe balances on their accounts and move without leaving a forwarding address). Local agencies are more aware of the socioeconomic status of patients. Some agencies pay their staff commissions and bonuses for high productivity and others are low-key and more customer-oriented. Find out the experience level of the staff and ensure that the agency values the health care organization's business.

Another option is to use an online collection service, such as CollectNet, which gives small and midsized facilities with limited budgets the collection capabilities of large collection systems by connecting to databases. The health care organization is able to make calling lists, print collection letters, search for telephone numbers and addresses, access patient credit reports, write and format reports, monitor collection progress, and set automatic callback reminders. Optional features include BankruptcyNet, SkipNet, LetterNet, and BureauNet. Collection agencies use this service, but it is also available to large groups and clinics.

Agency Operating Techniques

Collection agencies must follow all the laws stated in the Fair Debt Collection Practices Act. They may not "harass" the debtor or make false threats, and they may not use letters that appear to be legal documents. A provision should be included for the agency to seek permission from the health care organization's office before suing a debtor in municipal court and charging a percentage of the judgment. A progress report should be provided to the health care organization on a regular basis at least monthly. The agency also should return any uncollectible accounts within a reasonable time and not charge for these accounts. All procedures used to make collections should be shown to the health care organization, including collection letters and telephone scripts. The health care organization should be aware if the agency uses a personalized or standard approach. A personal visit to the premises of the collection agency can provide a firsthand view of its operating techniques.

Agency Charges

Agencies may be paid a flat rate on all accounts according to volume. Some agencies may leave the accounts in the control of the health care organization, where the staff speaks with the patient and posts all delinquent incoming monies. Other agencies charge a commission based on a percentage of an account and the health care organization refers all calls to the agency once the account is turned over to it. A standard rate needed for most agencies to break even is one-third of all monies collected and an average rate charged is 50%. Make sure the commission is based on how much is collected on the overdue accounts and not the total amount of overdue accounts turned over to the agency.

Agency Assigned Accounts

Patients' accounts turned over to a collection agency should have a letter of withdrawal sent by certified mail. Place a note on all financial accounting records indicating the date on which the account was assigned. Once an account has been given to a collection agency, it is illegal to send the patient a monthly statement. Revenue cycle management consultants usually recommend that the patient's balances be written off the A/R at the time the account is assigned. A portion of the account balance can be written back on if and when the agency collects on the debt. Accounts also should be listed in a separate journal to help track the effectiveness of the agency. Allow enough columns to show the future date, amount, and percentage of an account collected by the agency as well as the total account balance.

Each patient account that has been sent to collection should have an alert pop up every time the file is opened in the medical billing system. This will alert all medical staff of the situation if the patient calls on short notice or walks in to be seen. If the patient sends payment to the health care organization after the account has been turned over to an agency, notify the collection agency immediately. Any calls about accounts that have gone to collection should be referred to the agency.

Small Claims Court

Small claims court is a part of our legal system that allows lay-people access to a court system without the use of an attorney. Some advantages are a modest filing fee, minimal paperwork, exclusion of costly lawyers, and a short time frame from filing the action to trial date.

Most states have small claims courts (also called *conciliation courts, common pleas, general sessions, justice courts,* or *people's courts*). Each state has monetary limits on the amount that can be handled in small claims court and accounts should be reviewed for eligibility; the dollar amount varies from state to state and ranges from $2500 to $25,000. The link to the resource for dollar limits for small claims court by state is provided in the *Internet Resource* section at the end of this chapter.

When filing a claim, the health care organization filing the petition is referred to as the *plaintiff*, and the party being brought to suit (the patient) is called the *defendant*. It is generally recommended that the plaintiff send a written demand to the defendant before filing a lawsuit to give the defendant a final opportunity to resolve the claim.

For a step-by-step procedure on filing a claim in small claims court, see Procedure 17.4 at the end of this chapter.

After filing a claim, a trial date will be set and both plaintiff and defendant will be ordered to appear before the judge. Often a postcard is sent notifying the plaintiff when the defendant has been served. If the amount of delinquent debt is more than the monetary limit for small claims court, consider "cutting the claim to fit" the limit. For example, if the amount of debt is $2757 and the state limit is $2500, consider waiving (giving up) the $257 (difference) to bring the amount down to the limit. The claim cannot be divided into two different suits of $1378.50 and suing twice on the same claim is not allowed.

Claim Resolutions

The defendant has the following four options after he or she is served:

1. **Pay the claim.** The court clerk will receive the money and forward it to the health care organization, but the filing fee or service charges will not be refunded.
2. **Ignore the claim.** The judge may ask the health care organization's attorney or representative to state its case. The judgment will be awarded in the health care organization's favor, usually including court costs.
3. **Answer the petition.** A contested court hearing will be held. The health care organization has the burden of proving its claim to the court. A counterclaim may be filed by the patient at this time.
4. **Demand a jury trial.** The case will be taken out of small claims court and the health care organization will be notified by the county clerk to file a formal complaint in a higher court. An attorney must represent the health care organization if this occurs.

Trial Preparation

The plaintiff and defendant must both appear on the trial date or the claim will be dismissed and cannot be refiled. Instead of attending the trial in person, the health care organization may send a representative. If the claim is settled before trial, a dismissal form should be dated, signed, and filed with the clerk.

Preparation for the trial is essential and can mean the difference between success and failure. Decide what the judge should hear to conclude in the health care organization's favor. Although being represented in court by a lawyer is not allowed, a lawyer can be asked for advice before going to court. Recommendations to help prepare for trial are as follows:

1. Be on time; otherwise, the court may give a judgment in the defendant's favor.
2. Be ready to submit the basic data required by the court: the health care organization and service provider's name, address, and telephone number; the patient's name and address; the delinquent amount being claimed; and a brief summary of the claim.
3. Show all dates of service and amounts owed, the date on which the bill was due (if a series of treatments is involved), the last date service was provided, the date of the last payment (if any payment was made), and the amount still unpaid.
4. Include all attempts to collect the debt and organize all exhibits in chronologic order. Include documentation, such as copies of statements, letters, notes, receipts, contracts, dishonored checks, telephone calls, other discussions with the patient, and other evidence to present to the court. A timeline showing the sequence of events may be useful.

5. Speak slowly and clearly, present the case in a concise manner, and use a businesslike approach. Answer all questions accurately but briefly.
6. Present a witness if live testimony is relevant. A notarized statement from a witness is admissible but not as effective.
7. Try to anticipate the opposing party's evidence and arguments so that a rebuttal may be prepared. Keep in mind that a third party will be making the decision.

The judge will question the health care organization's representative and the patient, review the evidence, and then make a ruling. Winning the case gives the health care organization the right to attach a debtor's bank assets, salary, car, personal assets, or real property. The small claims office can advise on how to execute a judgment. Judgments are usually effective for many years. There is a small charge if the health care organization decides to execute against the patient's assets, but this charge is recoverable from the defendant.

A losing defendant may appeal and request a new trial in superior court. The defendant may ask the judge to make small installment payments, but not all judges order this alternative. If the defendant fails to pay, a writ of execution may be obtained from the clerk's office to enforce judgment. This writ of execution permits the marshal to obtain funds from a losing party's bank account or take items of the losing party's property to satisfy the judgment.

Federal Wage Garnishment Laws

Garnishment is a court order attaching a debtor's property or wages to pay off a debt. Federal wage garnishment laws provide a limit on the amount of employee earnings withheld in a work week or pay period when a debtor's future wage is seized to pay off a debt. They also protect the employee from being dismissed if their pay is garnished for only one debt, regardless of the number of levies that must be made to collect. This law is enforced by the compliance officers of the Wage and Hour Office of the US Department of Labor. The laws do not apply to federal government employees, court-ordered support of any person, court orders in personal bankruptcy cases, or state or federal tax levies. The patient's employer becomes involved as the "trustee" because the employer owes money to the debtor for wages earned.

Once a garnishment has been ordered by the court, an employer must honor it by satisfying the terms of garnishment before wages can be paid to the debtor. Only a percentage of the wage (usually 25%) is garnished and paid to the creditor. This amount is determined from the employee's disposable earnings. Disposable earnings are the amount left after Social Security and federal, state, and local taxes are deducted. The statute resulting in the smaller garnishment applies when state garnishment laws conflict with federal laws. This method of collection should be considered a last resort for a health care organization and used only with large bills.

Tracing a Skip

A patient who owes a balance on their account and moves but leaves no forwarding address is called a *skip*. In these cases, an unopened envelope is returned to the office marked "returned to sender, addressee unknown." Place the words "forwarding service requested" below the health care organization's return address on the envelope and the post office will make a search and forward the mail to the new address. The health care organization will be informed of this new address for a nominal fee. Complete a Freedom of Information Act form at the post office if the address is a rural delivery box number and the US Postal Service will provide the physical location of the person's residence. When patients send payments by mail, precautions must be taken to avoid discarding envelopes with a change of address. Always match the address on the envelope, along with the check, against the patient's account. One staff person should be responsible for updating all patients' addresses in all locations to prevent this problem.

Skip Tracing Techniques

Once it is determined that a patient is a skip, tracing should begin immediately. Office policies should be established stating how the skip will be traced and at what point the account will be sent to a collection agency. Some offices choose to make only one attempt, whereas others prefer to do most of the detective work themselves. Box 17.3 lists techniques that can be used to initiate the search for the debtor.

Never state one's business with the patient when trying to make any of these contacts. Keep all information confidential. A good skip tracer should have patience and the ability to pursue all necessary steps with tenacity and tact. A good imagination, a detective's instincts, and the ability to get along with people help in this tedious job.

BOX 17.3 Search Techniques Used to Trace a Debtor

1. Cross-check the address on the returned envelope with the patient registration form and account to ensure that it was mailed correctly.
2. Check the zip code directory to determine whether the zip code corresponds with the patient's street address or post office box.
3. File a request with the local post office to obtain a new or corrected address.
4. Call the primary care provider for updated information when investigating for a health care organization.
5. Determine whether the patient has been seen at the hospital; if so, speak to someone in the accounts department.
6. Inquire at the patient's place of employment. If the patient is no longer employed, ask to speak to the personnel department in an effort to locate the patient. Do not divulge the reason for the call.
7. Contact persons listed on the patient registration form, including personal referrals.
8. Request information from the Department of Motor Vehicles if a driver's license number is available.
9. Request information from utility companies.
10. Inquire at the patient's bank to determine whether he or she is still a customer.
11. Obtain the services of a local credit bureau to check reports and receive notification if the patient's Social Security number shows up under a different name or at a new address.
12. Check public records, such as tax records, voter registration, court records, death and probate records, hunting and fishing licenses, and marriage licenses.

Skip Tracing Services

There are several outside services from which to choose. Some agencies offer customized service with several levels of skip tracing available. Each level is more extensive and costly. The health care organization decides at which level it would like the search conducted. The first level usually involves verifying the patient's information and checking for typographic errors. The highest level uses every resource available to find the patient. The age of the account, the account balance, and the cost of the level of skip tracing service are all considerations when deciding which level to choose. A collection agency or credit bureau (as mentioned) may offer the services of skip tracing as well.

Search via Computer

Another method of skip tracing is to use electronic databases or online services. "Information wholesalers" also exist. They cater to bill collectors and similar interested parties. There are a number of bills pending in Congress aimed at restricting the flow of personal data in cyberspace. Perhaps in the future this information will not be so easy to obtain; however, conducting a successful electronic search is relatively easy at present. The following are several methods used to search electronic databases to locate a debtor's address and home telephone number:

- *Surname scan* can be done locally, regionally, or nationally using data banks that have been compiled from public source documents.
- *Address search* provides property search and any change of address from all suppliers of data to the database, including the US Postal Service. Names of other adults in the household who may have the debtor's telephone number listed under their name may be included.
- *Credit holder search* is used to establish occupation.
- *Phone number search* permits access to the names of other adults within the same household who have a telephone number.
- *Neighbor search* displays the names, addresses, and telephone numbers of the debtor's former neighbors.
- *Zip code search* provides the names, addresses, and telephone numbers of everyone within that zip code who has the same last name as the debtor.
- *City search* locates everyone with the same last and first name within a given city as well as all people who live in that city.
- *State search* finds all people with the same last name or same last and first name within the state and lists their addresses and telephone numbers.
- *National search* operates the same way as the state search. It is recommended for people with unusual last names.
- *Business search* lists all the names of the businesses in the neighborhood of the patient's last known residence. This search may help find where the patient has relocated or verify the patient's place of employment.

Explore several directories to cross-check results because data change frequently. Information is not secure when using the internet. The patient's right to privacy must never be violated.

17.8 QUICK REVIEW
Question: When placing telephone collection calls, what are the two important factors the insurance billing specialist should consider?

17.9 QUICK REVIEW
Question: When sending collection letters to patients, what is the most effective technique to ensure that the letter is forwarded if the patient has moved, and that the office will be notified of the patient's new address?

SPECIAL COLLECTION ISSUES

The insurance billing specialist must be aware that there will be special collection issues that will require special handling.

Bankruptcy

Bankruptcy is a condition under which a person or corporation is declared unable to pay debts. Bankruptcy laws are federal laws applicable in all states that ensure equal distribution of the assets of an individual among the individual's creditors. There are two kinds of bankruptcy petitions: voluntary and involuntary. A voluntary petition is one filed by a person asking for relief under the Bankruptcy Reform Act (the Code). An involuntary petition is one filed against a person by their creditors requesting that a person obtain relief under the Code.

When a patient files for bankruptcy, he or she becomes a ward of the court and has its protection. The patient is granted an automatic stay against creditors, which means that the health care organization may contact the patient only for the name, address, and telephone number of their attorney. The insurance billing specialist should no longer send statements, make telephone calls, or attempt to collect the account. A creditor can be fined for contempt of court if it continues to proceed against the debtor. If a collection agency has the account and has been notified of the bankruptcy, the situation is the same as if the health care organization has been notified. If the health care organization is notified first, the collection agency should be called and informed of the bankruptcy. Notification of bankruptcy does not have to be in writing; verbal communication is valid (for example, if a patient contacts the health care organization to inform it of the bankruptcy). Bankruptcy remains part of the debtor's permanent credit record for 10 years.

After a patient informs the health care organization of the bankruptcy, determine what type of bankruptcy the debtor has filed. Refer to Box 17.4 for a listing of the five types of bankruptcy cases.

Bankruptcy Rules

Under the bankruptcy rules effective October 17, 2005, debtors must meet an income test and must have insufficient assets to be eligible for filing a Chapter 7 bankruptcy. Otherwise they are forced into Chapter 13 bankruptcy, in which a debt repayment plan is ordered.

When filing a claim, the proper form may be obtained from the bankruptcy court. If a creditor fails to file a claim, the there must be a time lapse of 6 years before he or she can file again. The only exception to this is Chapter 13 bankruptcy.

Terminally Ill Patients

Although it may be difficult to collect from patients who are terminally ill, it is usually harder to collect from the estates after they have died. When a patient is too sick or scared to communicate necessary information, consult the health care provider about whether to obtain the patient's permission to speak to family members and stress the need for help. Usually, terminally ill patients want to do the right thing. Call the patient before he or she comes in to receive service. Ensure that the patient is aware of the existing balance and try to work with the patient to eliminate at least a portion of the balance before the next appointment. Estimate costs and prepare a plan that is agreeable to both the health care organization and the patient.

Estate Claims

Great care and sensitivity should be taken when trying to collect on a deceased patient's account. When the health care organization discovers that a patient has died, first pursue insurance coverage. The entire probate system was set up to help protect families from painful involvement in estate settlements. Do not offend the deceased's family by making contact during the time of bereavement. However, file a claim after the first or second week so that the health care organization's name can be added to the list of creditors.

Refer to Procedure 17.5 at the end of this chapter for filing an estate claim.

After filing, the claim is denied or accepted. If accepted, an acknowledgment of the debt is sent to the health care organization. Many delays arise because of the legal complications of settling an estate, but the debts are paid according to a priority system when the estate is settled. Usually funeral expenses are paid first; following in order are estate administration expenses, claims due for the deceased person's last illness, and taxes and other debts. Any amounts left are divided among family members. A lien or lawsuit may be filed against the estate in the rare case of a rejection of the claim.

Various state time limits and statutes govern the filing of a claim against an estate. Check with the county court in the applicable state to obtain filing deadlines. Deadlines may range from 2 months to 3 years but must be adhered to for successful collection from an estate.

Litigation

A difficult question arises when the health care organization is advised that a patient is involved in a pending litigation related to the services provided to the patient. It may not be necessary to wait until the litigation is resolved to pursue payment. Assess whether the patient has the ability to pay before possibly receiving a settlement in a lawsuit. Before withholding collection activity, the health care organization should get a guarantee that it will be paid in full before the patient (debtor) receives money from a settlement. The agreement must be guaranteed by the lawyer representing the patient. If the patient is working, regular payments should be required pending the settlement of the

creditor will lose the right to any proceeds from the bankruptcy. A plan for payment will be approved by the court. The trustee may be contacted from time to time to check the status of the claim and the payments that should be expected. Once a patient has obtained credit counseling and petitioned for bankruptcy, patient's litigation. It is always advisable to contact a malpractice attorney in such cases.

Liens

A lien is a claim on the property of another as security for a debt. This may include a claim on a future settlement of a lawsuit. The health care organization may be asked to accept a lien by a patient or the patient's attorney when the patient has been involved in an automobile accident and is awaiting a settlement (Fig. 17.15). In litigation cases, a lien is a legal promise to satisfy a debt owed by the patient to the health care organization out of any proceeds received on the case.

Patient Complaints

It is generally in the health care organization's best interest to resolve patient complaints and billing disputes quickly, accurately, and amicably. Always address collection complaints seriously. Listen to the patient with an open mind. Note specifically what the patient is saying and what the patient wants to do. Look beyond the complaint to determine what caused the problem. The source of the problem, not just the symptom of the problem, should be resolved. A patient complaint form may be adapted to prompt staff to pay close attention to positive customer relations. This form may help to screen poor collection techniques by staff members, pinpoint billing department

REQUEST FOR ALLOWANCE OF LIEN ASSIGNMENT AND AUTHORIZATION

WHEREAS, I have a right or cause of action out of personal injury, to wit:

I, _____ hereby authorize _____ ,
patient's name   physician's name

to furnish upon request, to my attorney, _____ , any and all medical records, or reports of examination, diagnosis, treatment, or prognosis but not necessarily limited to those items as set forth herein, in addition to an itemized statement of accounts for services rendered therefore or in connection therewith, which my attorney may from time to time request in connection with the injuries described above and sustained by me on the _____ day of _____ , 20XX.

I hereby irrevocably authorize and direct my said attorney set forth herein to pay to _____ all charges for attendance in court,
patient's name

if required as an expert witness whether he testifies or not; reports or other data supplied by him; depositions given by said doctor; medical services rendered or drugs supplied; and any other responsible and customary charges incurred by my attorney as submitted by _____ and in
physician's name

connection with said injury. Said payment or payments are to be made from any money or monies received by my attorney whether by judgment, decree, or settlement of this case, prior to disbursement to me and payment of the amount as herein directed shall be the same as if paid by me. This authorization to pay the aforementioned doctor shall constitute and be deemed as assignment of so much of my recovery I receive. It is agreed that nothing herein relieves me of the primary responsibility and obligation of paying my doctor for services rendered, and I shall at all times remain personally liable for such indebtedness unless released by the aforementioned doctor or by payment disbursed by my attorney. I accept the above assignment:

Dated: _____ Patient: _____

As the attorney of record for the above-named, I hereby agree to observe the terms of this agreement, and to withhold from any award in this case such sums as are required for the adequate protection of Dr. _____ ,

Date: _____ Attorney: _____

Fig. 17.15 A patient's authorization to release information to an attorney and grant lien to the health care organization against proceeds of settlement in connection with accident, industrial, or third-party litigation cases.

problems, and identify policies and procedures that need improvement.

The patient may refuse to pay the health care organization if the patient's complaint is not addressed. Some guidelines to follow when a patient calls or writes a letter complaining about medical care are:

1. Listen carefully (or read the letter carefully) and establish exactly what the patient complaint is and what the patient wants done about it.
2. Thank the person for calling (or writing); demonstrate appreciation of his or her input on the situation.
3. Apologize, regardless of whether the patient is right or wrong.
4. Answer the complaint. Explain what happened, if applicable, and state what is being done about it.
5. Use a professional and sincere approach. If the patient is wrong, state that the complaint is unjustified but first explain your interpretation of the situation and its resolution. Otherwise, the patient is likely to become quite upset. Do not be sarcastic, condescending, or insulting.
6. Take all complaints seriously. Do not respond in a light-hearted manner or use humor; it will only serve to upset the patient.
7. Respond in letter form. Whether the complaint has been received by telephone or by letter, take the time to write to answer the complaint. This indicates that the matter is not being taken lightly.
8. Be cordial and sincere. Express to the patient the hope of continuing a friendly relationship but that payment is necessary. Treat the patient with respect, good will, and sincere appreciation. Often, kindness can turn a negative into a positive. The complaint can be turned into a payment.
9. Follow up after the complaint has been resolved by looking at the root of the problem and taking the necessary time to communicate this to administration. This follow-up allows creation of a plan of action that can help to prevent the same type of problem from recurring.

> ⚖ **17.10 QUICK REVIEW**
> Question: When a patient files for bankruptcy, can the health care organization continue to bill them?

COLLECTION CONTROLS

All health care organizations should maintain certain collection controls to ensure that they are following collection laws and performing collections in an ethical manner. One of the primary collection controls is to make sure that there are written and well-defined collection policies for staff to follow. It is also important for the organization to implement a system of checks and balances for any task related to the organization's finances.

Bonding

Insurance billing specialists, claims assistance professionals, or anyone who handles checks or cash should be bonded or insured. When a health care organization carries a fidelity or honesty bond, it means that an insurance company will prosecute any employees found guilty of stealing. Bonding is an insurance contract by which a bonding agency guarantees payment of a certain sum to a health care organization in case of a financial loss caused by an employee or some contingency over which the payee has no control. Bonding methods for an organization with three or more office employees are:

- *Position-schedule bond* covers a designated job, such as a bookkeeper or nurse, rather than a named individual. If one employee in a category leaves, the replacement is automatically covered.
- *Blanket-position bond* provides coverage for all employees regardless of job title.
- *Personal bond* provides coverage for those who handle large sums of money. A thorough background investigation is required.

Such bonding contracts may be obtained from a casualty insurance agent or broker. Bond coverage should be reviewed periodically with the insurance agent to ensure that coverage is keeping pace with the expansion of the business.

Embezzlement

Embezzlement is stealing money that has been entrusted in one's care. In many cases of insurance claims embezzlement, the health care organization is held as the guilty party and must pay huge sums of money to the third-party payer when false claims are submitted by an employee. If an undiscovered embezzler leaves the organization, the employee who is hired to replace that person could be accused some months later of doing something that he or she did not do. Take precautions as an employee and to protect the health care organization.

Precautions for Financial Protection

To prevent the temptation to steal from a health care organization, the following policies should be routinely practiced. The organization must have a process by which management must approve all entries posted about adjustments, discounts, and write-offs. If a patient owes money that is uncollectible and adjusted off, seek management approval and confirm that the balance due has been brought to zero. Implement a process whereby an auditor or an outside consultant is occasionally brought in to check an entire day's records (the patient sign-in log and appointment schedule) with the daysheet, patients' financial accounting records, encounter forms, and cash receipt slips. A daily trail of the balance of A/R, including daily deposit of checks and cash, can assist in reviewing monthly income and aid in discovering embezzlement. Audit the daily collection and reconcile with the bank deposit (Fig. 17.16). If poor bookkeeping and record keeping are noticed, bring this to the management's attention immediately.

All insurance payment checks should be immediately stamped within the endorsement area on the back "For Deposit Only," called a *restrictive endorsement.* The bank should be given instructions never to cash a check made payable to the health care organization.

Encounter forms, transaction slips, and cash receipts should be prenumbered. If a mistake is made when completing one,

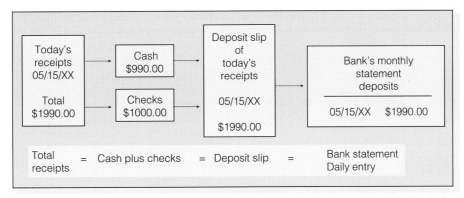

Fig. 17.16 Auditing the daily collection in the medical office to reconcile with the bank deposit.

void it and keep the slip as part of the financial records. It is imperative to have prenumbered insurance forms to eliminate the filing of fictitious insurance claims.

As a precautionary measure, insurance billing specialists should always type their initials at the bottom left or top right corner of the insurance claim forms that they submit. This will indicate to office personnel who did the work. Always retain the EOB or remittance advice (RA) documents that accompany checks from insurance companies.

Only a few of the many precautions for protection are mentioned here; embezzlement can occur in A/R, accounts payable, with petty cash, with the use of computers, and in various other aspects of a health care organization.

 17.11 QUICK REVIEW

Question: What method can be used to prevent insurance checks from being cashed by an unauthorized individual?

 DISCUSSION POINT

People have a difficult time asking others for money and talking about financial obligations. Explain tips or techniques that would be useful when asking patients for payment of balances.

COLLEGE CLINIC
4567 Broad Avenue
Woodland Hills, XY 12345-0001
Tel. (555) 486-9002
FAX (555) 487-8976

October 2, 20XX

Mr. Leonard Blabalot
981 McCort Circle
Woodland Hills, XY 12345-0001

Dear Mr. Blabalot:

I am glad we had an opportunity to discuss your outstanding balance with our practice during our phone conversation on October 1, 20XX. This will confirm and remind you that you agreed to pay $100 on your account on or before October 15, 20XX.

A return envelope is enclosed for your convenience.

Sincerely,

Charlotte Rose Routingham
Business Office

Enc. envelope

Fig. 17.17 Letter confirming telephone payment discussion sent to remind the patient of the payment terms agreed upon.

PROCEDURE 17.1 Create a Financial Agreement With a Patient

Objective
To assist the patient in making credit arrangements by completing and signing a Truth in Lending form

Equipment/Supplies
Patient's financial accounting record (ledger), calendar, Truth in Lending form, typewriter or computer, calculator, and quiet private room

Directions
Follow the step-by-step procedures, which include rationales, to learn this job skill:
1. Explain the patient's balance due and answer questions about credit.
2. Inform the patient of the health care organization's office policy about extending credit payments.
3. Discuss an installment plan concerning the amount of the total debt, the down payment, the amount and date of each installment, and the date of final payment.
4. Subtract the down payment from the total debt. Divide the remaining amount by the number of months the debt is being carried to determine the monthly installment amounts and the date of final payment.
5. Complete a Truth in Lending form after mutually agreeing on the terms if the payments require more than four installments. This procedure complies with Regulation Z.
6. Review the completed Truth in Lending form with the patient.
7. Ask the patient to sign the Truth in Lending form.
8. Make a photocopy of the Truth in Lending form for the patient to retain.
9. File the original Truth in Lending form in the patient's financial file in the office.

414	UNIT 5	Revenue Cycle Management

PROCEDURE 17.2   Seven-Step Billing and Collection Guidelines

Objective

To properly bill and collect payments for medical services rendered to patients

Equipment/Supplies

Patients' financial accounting statements, envelopes, calendar, and telephone

Directions

Follow these step-by-step procedures and guidelines, which include rationales, to learn this job skill:

1. Present the first statement at the time of service. This can be a formal statement or an encounter form (multipurpose billing form).
2. Mail the second itemized statement within 30 days of treatment. The phrase "due and payable within 10 days" should be printed on each statement. Local paycheck-issuing patterns should be considered before selecting a date for statements to be mailed. Choose which billing routine the office will use.
   a. Monthly billing. Using the monthly billing system, all statements are mailed at the same time during the month. Choose a mail-out day at the beginning of the month so that the patient will receive the bill near the 15th or send statements near the end of the month so that the patient receives the bill on the first.
   b. Cycle billing. Cycle billing is a system of billing accounts at spaced intervals during the month based on a breakdown of accounts by alphabet, account number, insurance type, or date of first service. This relieves the pressure of having to get all statements out at one time and allows collection at a faster, more organized rate than if accounts were collected at random. It also allows continuous cash flow throughout the month and distributes the influx of incoming calls from patients about

problem accounts. The number of cycles may be determined by how the collector wishes to divide the workload. Using two cycles per month, statements would be sent on the 25th to arrive by the first and on the 10th to arrive by the 15th of the month. Using four cycles per month, statements should be sent every Tuesday or Wednesday to arrive at the end of the week. If a cycle that was established by the first date of service is used and the patient was first seen on the 11th of the month, then he or she should receive a bill every month on the 11th.

3. Send the third statement 30 days after the second statement was sent. Indicate that the payment is past due.
4. If there is no response to the third statement, place the first telephone call to the patient depending on office policy (7–14 days). Ask if there is a problem. Ask for a payment commitment and set up a suspense file. Accounts are put in a suspense file for active follow-up. Action must be taken within the time frame mentioned, after the patient has been so advised.
5. Check for payment as promised. Allow 1 day for mail delay. Place the second telephone call to the patient and ask for payment. Set up a new payment date. Allow 5 days.
6. Check for payment as promised. Send a 10-day notice advising the patient that unless payment is received in 10 days, the account will be turned over for legal action.
7. Check for payment. Promptly surrender the account for collection or legal action. Fig. 17.10 shows a collection decision tree to be used when determining when to send statements, 10-day notices, and accounts to a collection agency and when to make telephone calls.

PROCEDURE 17.3   Telephone Collection Plan

Objective

To obtain payment of a delinquent account balance due by making the first collection telephone call

Equipment/Supplies

Telephone, pen or pencil, patient's financial accounting record, computerized account, or collection telephone log

Directions

Follow these step-by-step procedures and guidelines, which include rationales, to learn this job skill:

1. Set the mood of the call by the manner of speech and tone of voice. The first 30 s of the call sets the scene for the relationship with the patient. Follow the Fair Debt Collection Practices Act when making a telephone call.
2. State the name of the caller and the health care organization represented and identify the patient. Be certain the debtor is being spoken to before revealing the nature of the call.
3. Identify oneself and the health care organization.
4. Verify the debtor's address and any telephone numbers.
5. State the reason for the call by asking for full payment and stating the total amount owed. Ask for payment courteously but firmly.
6. Take control of the conversation and establish urgency by asking for full payment now. Speak slowly in a low voice; staying calm and polite prevents quarreling.
7. Ask when payment will be made, how it will be made, and if it will be sent by mail or in person.
8. Pause for effect. This turns the conversation back to the patient to respond to the demand or explain why payment has not been made. Never assume that if a patient does not respond, it means "no."
9. Find out if the patient needs clarification of the bill.

10. Inquire if the patient has a problem. Ask if the health care organization can be of assistance, especially when the patient is unable to give a reason for nonpayment.
11. If the patient is reluctant to agree to an amount, question him or her by asking one of the following: "How much are you willing to pay?"; "Do you have a regular paycheck?"; "Will payment be made through a checking account?"
12. Obtain a promise to pay with an agreeable amount and a due date; be clear how and when payment is expected but give the patient a choice of action. Set immediate deadlines for payment.
13. Ask for half of the amount if full payment is not possible.
14. Discuss a payment plan if the patient is not able to pay half of the balance owed. Be realistic and reasonable. It is self-defeating to set up payment arrangements the patient cannot afford. Advise the patient that the entire balance will become due and payable if the payment is even 1 day late. Ask the patient to please call before the due date with an explanation if any problems arise that prevent payment.
15. Restate the importance of the agreement.
16. Tell the patient to write down the amount and due date.
17. Document the agreement on the patient's financial accounting record by inserting the date of the call and abbreviated notations, in the computer system, or in a collection telephone log. Note the time the patient was spoken to.
18. Send confirmation of the agreement (Fig. 17.17) as a follow-up to the telephone call.
19. Check the account the day after the payment was due; allow 1 day for mail delay. If the patient fails to make a payment as promised, make another telephone call and ask the patient if there is still a problem. Get a new commitment to pay and confirm again. If the patient continues to avoid payment, advise the patient that the account will be turned over to a collection agency and follow through as stated.

PROCEDURE 17.4   File a Claim in Small Claims Court

Objective

To file a claim to obtain payment for a delinquent or uncollectable financial account in small claims court

Equipment/Supplies

Small claims court filing form, photocopy of the patient's financial accounting record, computer or typewriter, pen or pencil, envelope, and check for filing fee

Directions

Follow these step-by-step procedures and guidelines, which include rationales, to learn this job skill:

1. Obtain a Claim of Plaintiff or Plaintiff's Original Petition form to notify the patient that action is being filed. This can be obtained from the clerk's office located at the municipal or justice court. Obtain booklets and material to help guide the claimant through the process.

2. Complete and file the papers with the small claims court; make sure to have the patient's correct name and street address.

3. Make a photocopy of the small claims court form for the office files.

4. Pay the clerk the small filing fee. Filing fees vary by state, by county within some states, and by the amount of the claim.

5. Make arrangements to serve the defendant. The summons or citation can be served on the patient by a sheriff or court-appointed officer by paying a small fee plus mileage for the constable who serves it. The person serving the defendant must fill out a proof of service form.

6. After being served, a patient has one of four options:

   a. Pay the claim to the court clerk. This will be forwarded to the health care organization, but the filing fee or service charge will not be refunded.

   b. Ignore the claim. The health care organization will win by default. In some states, a judgment may be requested in writing, but in other states, the health care organization or its representative must appear on a specified date. If the patient does not appear, the judgment is granted in the health care organization's favor and usually court costs are included in the judgment.

   c. Request a small claims hearing. The court clerk will let both parties know when to appear. The patient may file a counterclaim against the health care organization at this time.

   d. Demand a jury trial. The case will be taken out of small claims court. The health care organization will be notified by the court clerk to file a formal complaint in a higher court and an attorney must represent the health care organization.

7. Appear in court (service provider or health care organization representative) on the specified date; otherwise, the claim will be dismissed and cannot be refiled.

8. Basic information required by the court follows:

   a. Health care organization and service provider's name, address, and telephone number

   b. Patient's name and address

   c. Delinquent amount

   d. Summary of the claim, including the date the health care organization's bill was due, date of the last encounter, date of the last payment, unpaid amount, and all records of telephone contacts and letters sent.

9. Determine what the judge needs to hear to decide a favorable case. Good preparation for the trial can make the difference between success and failure.

10. Organize all exhibits in a notebook, in chronologic order. A timeline showing the sequence of events can be useful.

11. Take a businesslike professional approach at the hearing by giving concise and accurate answers to the judge's questions, speaking slowly and clearly. The service provider or the health care organization's representative must bring any witnesses, statements, receipts, contracts, notes, dishonored checks, or other evidence to court. The judge will question the service provider or the health care organization's representative and the patient, review the evidence, and then make a ruling.

12. Put a lien on the debtor's wages, automobile, bank or personal assets, or real property if the judgment, which is usually effective for many years, is in the service provider's favor. This is the service provider's legal right. The small claims office will show the service provider or the health care organization's representative how to execute a judgment.

13. Pay a small fee if the health care organization decides to execute against the patient's assets. It is recoverable from the patient.

PROCEDURE 17.5   File an Estate Claim

Objective

To file a claim on an estate for a deceased patient who has an outstanding balance on his or her financial accounting record

Equipment/Supplies

Statement of Claim form, computer or typewriter, pen or pencil, photocopy machine, patient's financial accounting record, US Postal Service certified mail forms, and envelope

Directions

Follow these step-by-step procedures and guidelines, which include rationales, to learn this job skill:

1. Confirm the date and place of death with the hospital, nursing home, or funeral home.

2. Pursue payment from all third-party payers first.

3. Contact the Register of Wills office in the county where the patient lived or the probate department of the superior court, County Recorder's Office. Request a Statement of Claim form or the county's proper document to formally register a claim against an estate.

4. File the claim according to the instructions received with the claim form. When probate is filed, a notification will be sent advising the court of probate, the attorney representing the estate, and the **estate executor** or **estate administrator**. Perhaps a small fee should be included for court costs.

5. Send a photocopy of the patient's financial accounting record (itemized statement) by certified mail, return receipt, to the attorney, and copies to the executor and the court. If the health care organization treated the deceased patient's last illness, that fact should be clearly indicated on the statement.

6. Allow the legal system to take its course. A call to the executor can be made periodically to check on the status of the estate.

KEY POINTS

This is a brief chapter review, or summary, of the key issues presented. To further enhance your knowledge of the technical subject matter, review the key terms and key abbreviations for this chapter by locating the meaning for each in the Glossary at the end of this book, which appears in a section before the Index:

1. Although a large percentage of reimbursement to health care organizations is generated from third-party payers, patients continue to take on more financial responsibility for their health care as a result of high-dollar-deductible health plans and rising copays and coinsurance.

2. The insurance billing specialist must monitor the accounts receivable (A/R) weekly to determine the effectiveness of collection. An average A/R should be no more than one-half to two times the charges for 1 month of services.

3. Collect copayments and deductibles from patients at the time service is rendered. The health care organization can charge a missed appointment fee regardless of the health insurance the patient carries; the patient is responsible for paying the missed appointment fee.

4. According to the Office of Inspector General, health care organizations are free to use whatever policies they want on charity care, discounts, write-offs, and collections, but this must be done consistently and the reasons must be documented. Professional courtesy should be kept to a minimum.

5. When payments are made by check, require two forms of verification. Always take immediate action when the bank returns a check for nonsufficient funds (NSF). When payments are made by credit card, require picture ID verification.

6. Online services such as Square can be used to accept credit cards at any time. Fees vary depending on the amount of transactions for the health care organization. It is customary for the health care organization to impose a nominal fee on the patient for credit transactions.

7. Review overdue accounts to determine when to send dun messages on statements, make telephone calls, or send to a collection agency.

8. Use alternative payment methods to help cash flow and reduce collection costs such as credit card payments, debit cards, e-checks, patient portals, and payment plans.

9. Follow all federal and state laws that affect collection of delinquent accounts.

10. Contact the patient in a timely manner by telephone at the first sign of payment delay and then send a collection letter as a reminder.

11. Delinquent accounts should be turned over to a collection agency only after all reasonable attempts have been made to collect.

12. Learn and use all techniques in skip tracing a debtor.

13. It is in the health care organization's best interest to resolve patient complaints and billing disputes quickly, accurately, and amicably.

INTERNET RESOURCES

- Listing of dollar limits for small claims court by state: https://www.nolo.com/legal-encyclopedia/small-claims-suits-how-much-30031.html

- What you need to know about the Red Flag Rules: https://www.cms.org/uploads/red-flags-rule-edu.pdf

STUDENT ASSIGNMENT

- Study Chapter 17.
- Complete all exercises in the *Workbook* to reinforce the theory learned in this chapter.

- Turn to the Glossary at the end of this text for a further understanding of the key terms and key abbreviations used in the chapter.

Healthcare Facility Billing

18

Introduction to Health Care Facilities and Ambulatory Surgery Centers

Cheryl Fassett

OBJECTIVES

After reading this chapter, you should be able to:

1. Describe the various types of health care facilities.
2. Explain the difference between inpatient and outpatient services.
3. Understand the 72-hour rule and inpatient-only list.
4. Explain the revenue cycle of reimbursement systems for ambulatory surgical centers and hospital facility claims.
5. Describe the components of the inpatient prospective payment system.
6. Describe the components of the outpatient prospective payment and ambulatory surgical payment systems.
7. Describe other types of prospective payment systems.
8. Understand what a never event is.
9. Explain the Hospital Acquired Condition Reduction Program (HACRP).
10. Identify the Ambulatory Quality Reporting (ASCQR) measures and the effect on the ASC payment rates.
11. Explain the role of utilization management and the types of reviews.

KEY TERMS

72-hour rule
Accreditation
Accreditation Association for Ambulatory Health Care
Accreditation Association of Hospitals/Health Systems
activities of daily living
acute care facility
admission review
against medical advice
Ambulance Fee Schedule
ambulatory care
ambulatory payment classifications
ambulatory surgery center
Ambulatory Surgery Center Quality Reporting Program
ambulatory surgery units
American College of Surgeons
American Hospital Association
American Medical Association
American Osteopathic Association
Ambulatory Surgery Center Payment System
Capitation
case mix groups
chargemaster
clinic

complication/comorbidity
concurrent review
Consumer Assessment of Health Care Providers and Systems Outpatient and Ambulatory Surgery Survey
continued stay review
cost outlier
critical access hospital
discharge
discharge disposition
Discharge Not Final Billed
discounting
downcoding
DRG creep
Emergency Medical Treatment and Labor Act
Grouper
Healthcare Facilities Accreditation Program
Health Insurance Prospective Payment System Code Set
home health agency
Home Health Prospective Payment System
Hospice
Hospice Prospective Payment System
hospital

hospital-acquired conditions
Hospital Acquired Condition Reduction Program
Hospital Standardization Program
Hospital Value-Based Purchasing Program
inpatient
Inpatient Only List
Inpatient Psychiatric Facility Prospective Payment System
Inpatient Prospective Payment System
Inpatient Rehabilitation Facility Patient Assessment Instrument
Inpatient Rehabilitation Facility Prospective Payment System
long-term care facility
Long-Term Care Hospital Prospective Payment System
major complications/comorbidities
major diagnostic categories
Medicare Severity Diagnosis-Related Groups
national unadjusted payment
never event
nonpatient
observation

osteopathic medicine
outpatient
outpatient code editor
Outpatient Prospective Payment
    System
packaging
pass throughs
patient dumping
per diem
preadmission
preadmission testing

preauthorization
present on admission
prospective payment system
prospective reviews
Quality Improvement Organizations
rehabilitation impairment category
relative weight
Resident Assessment Instrument
retrospective review
revenue code
revenue cycle

skilled nursing facility
Skilled Nursing Facility Prospective
    Payment System
status (payment) indicator
swing bed
The Accreditation Association
The Joint Commission
Two Midnight Rule
Uniform Bill 04
utilization management
upcoding

KEY ABBREVIATIONS

AAAHC	CMGs	IRF PAI	PPS
ACS	DNFB	IRF PPS	QIO
ADLs	EMTALA	LTCH PPS	RAI
AHA	HACs	MCCs	RIC
AMA	HACRP	MDCs	SNF
AOA	HFAP	MS-DRGs	SNF PPS
APC	HHA	OAS CAHPS	TJC
ASCQR	HH PPS	OCE	UB-04
ASU	HIPPS	OPPS	UM
CAH	IPF PPS	PAT	VBP
CCs	IPPS	POA	

Justina V.: CPC (Certified Professional Coder),
CPMA (Certified Professional Medical Auditor),
CPC-I (Certified Professional Coder-Instructor)

I've worked in the health care field for 35 years. Currently, I am a Coding Manager (part-time) and Independent Healthcare Consultant. I think the most valuable skill a billing specialist can have is the ability to not only understand what your current tasks/responsibilities are, but also the ability to see the bigger picture. It's important to avoid tunnel vision. It will give you job satisfaction and make you a more valuable employee. Also, keep learning! Healthcare, guidelines, insurance rules are always changing and you'll do much better if you're not scared to challenge yourself.

HISTORY OF HEALTH CARE FACILITIES

Ancient Egyptian and Greek temples dedicated to healer gods were places to seek medical advice. Ancient Romans constructed buildings to care for sick and injured soldiers. The Middle Ages were marked by war and the spread of contagious diseases; hospitals became places to isolate the sick from the rest of the population. With the Renaissance, there came a new quest for scientific discovery. The first civilian hospitals were built in the 5th century.

In the United States, the expansion of the colonies brought spread of disease and population growth in cities. Early hospitals were primarily built to take care of the poor and isolate the sick. Early housing and living conditions were primitive

and lacked sanitation. Diseases such as malaria, smallpox and typhoid were rampant. Early medical practice consisted mainly of religious superstition and home cures.

The first hospital in the United States was a military hospital on Manhattan Island, New York. The first voluntary hospitals were founded in Pennsylvania, New York, and Massachusetts. These were funded by voluntary contributions from patients. Those who could not afford to pay for care volunteered their time cleaning or caring for others. Since, at this time, the cause of many illnesses was still unknown, many patients died at the hospitals and they were seen as a last resort.

Advances in medicine brought technological advances such as the microscope and diagnostic advances such as x-rays. A new understanding of sanitation and hygiene shed light on bacteria and disease processes. Hospitals became safe places to receive care.

In 1847, the American Medical Association (AMA) was formed. The mission of the founding members was to improve the standards of medical education. They introduced a process for ranking medical schools that is still used today.

The Association of Hospital Superintendents was formed in 1898. This acted as network where these professionals could share ideas. In 1906, they became the American Hospital Association (AHA). Their mission is to advance the health of individuals and communities through health policy development and regulation.

In 1913, the American College of Surgeons (ACS) was established. This organization promoted the highest standards of care through education and patient advocacy. They also promote standardization of medical care through the Hospital Standardization Program in 1918. This program established the minimal standards of patient care in hospital, and aimed at eliminating waste, inefficiency, and incompetence in the hospital system.

This program was later adopted by the Joint Commission on Accreditation of Healthcare Organizations (JCAHO) in 1951. This organization, later to become known as The Joint Commission (TJC) in 2007, focused their efforts on developing guidelines for hospitals and other health care facilities and organizations. These guidelines address standards in areas such as patient care, medication safety, and infection control.

🕊 18.1   QUICK REVIEW

Question: Name four organizations that help define quality patient care in the United States.

TYPES OF HEALTH CARE FACILITIES

Acute Care Facilities

The most common type of health care facility is a hospital. Hospitals services can vary greatly depending on their size and location. In general, hospitals treat a variety of illness and injury. They typically have an emergency department to treat immediate health threats. Emergency departments (ED) must be open 24 hours per day, 7 day per week to be considered an ED. They usually have a number of beds to accommodate extended stays, and have different departments that handle surgery, laboratory testing, radiology services, and childbirth. Specialized hospitals may focus on treatment of trauma, cancer and cardiac issues among others. They may also focus on a particular age group, such as children's hospitals. Sometimes referred to as an acute care facility, a general hospital offers both inpatient and outpatient services. They also offer rehabilitation services such as physical and occupational therapy.

Critical Access Hospital

In 1997, the Balanced Budget Act set up the Critical Access Hospital Program. A critical access hospital (CAH) is a small rural hospital set up to provide care to Medicare beneficiaries who would otherwise not have access to health care. They must have 25 or fewer beds and be 35 miles from another facility. Exceptions are made for areas with poor roads and difficult terrain. They must offer care 24 hours per day, 7 days per week and must have an RN on site and a physician on-call and able to be on-site within 60 minutes whenever there are patients admitted. They must have an average length of inpatient stay of 96 hours or less. A CAH must have all the equipment and medications on site for medical treatment and have a transfer agreement in place with a larger facility.

Ambulatory Surgery Centers

In the past, almost all surgery was performed in hospitals. Surgery was scheduled in advance, with preoperative tests, such as bloodwork and x-ray examinations, done during the initial inpatient stay. Surgery was done on the second inpatient day, and recovery added to the length of stay. Technologic advancements created a movement of specific types of high-volume surgeries, such as for cataracts and biopsies, to the outpatient setting, initiating an upsurge in the outpatient services for hospitals.

Ambulatory surgery centers, known as ASCs, are health care facilities specifically focused on providing same-day surgical care, including diagnostic and preventive procedures and services. ASCs allow patients greater access to care, a higher level of convenience, and more focused and cost-effective care when undergoing surgical procedures. ASCs are limited to perform only those surgeries that do not pose a significant safety risk and are not expected to require an overnight stay after the surgical procedure. CMS publishes a list of covered procedures for ASCs.

Over the past four decades, ambulatory surgery centers have seen significant growth due to reduced health care costs for patients, providers, and payers; expansion of types of surgeries and services performed; and the national technologic advancement of health care ambulatory surgery facilities.

The first freestanding ASC facility was launched in 1970 in Phoenix, Arizona, by two physicians who wanted to provide timely, convenient, and comfortable surgical services to patients in their community. Since that time, the number of ASCs has increased nationally. It is estimated that there are approximately 5,500 Medicare-certified ASCs in the United States. Fig. 18.1 displays the number of Medicare-certified ASCs by state. Common ASC specialties include Ophthalmology, Gastroenterology, Pain Management, Orthopedics and Dermatology. Fig. 18.2 identifies the specialties served in ASCs Ambulatory Surgery Center Association (ACSA).

There are two types of ASCs:
1. Independent ASCs are typically freestanding, and they are usually privately owned. They are not integrated as part of a hospital, they are not directly associated with a hospital, and they are not included in a hospital's cost report.
2. Hospital-based ASCs are affiliated with or owned by a hospital. They can be freestanding (but hospital based) or located within a hospital.

It is important for the medical billing specialist to understand the difference between a hospital-based ASC and an independent ASC because different billing and coding rules apply and reimbursement is based on different payment systems.

Clinics

A clinic is a facility for diagnosis and treatment of patients on an outpatient basis. They may be similar to an outpatient department in a larger hospital, but they do not offer the same inpatient options and emergency care as the general hospital does. The definition of a clinic includes private provider groups and multispecialty groups as well as those affiliated with larger hospital systems. It also includes walk-ins and other specialized types of health care services such as dental services.

Skilled Nursing Facilities

A skilled nursing facility (SNF) offers accommodations for patients who are not sick enough to be hospitalized but are too serious to be treated in their homes. They offer skilled nursing

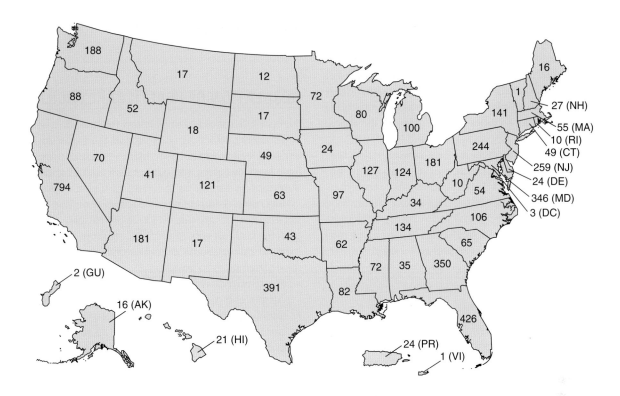

Fig. 18.1 Medicare-certified ambulatory surgery centers by state. (Copyright Ambulatory Surgery Center and ASCA Foundation. All rights reserved. https://www.ascassociation.org/advancingsurgicalcare/asc/numberofascsperstate, June 2018.)

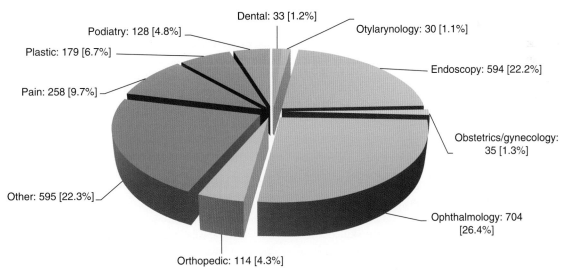

Fig. 18.2 Specialties served in ambulatory surgery centers (ASCs). (Copyright Ambulatory Surgery Center and ASCA Foundation. All rights reserved. https://www.ascassociation.org/advancingsurgicalcare/asc/whatisanasc, June 2017.)

care 24/7. Many patients spend a short period of time in an SNF as part of the recovery process from an illness, injury or surgery. While most people think of these facilities as nursing homes for the elderly, these facilities are for those who specifically require

skilled nursing care. Examples of skilled nursing services include wound care, catheter care, intravenous therapy, physical therapy and continuous monitoring of vital signs and medical equipment.

Long-Term Care Facilities

A long-term care facility provides custodial care to individuals who are chronically ill or disabled or are not able to live independently. Often referred to as *assisted living facilities*, they offer the type of services that help residents perform normal daily tasks or activities of daily living (ADLs) such as bathing, eating and getting dressed. These facilities provide medical care as well as personal care and services such as meals and laundry.

Some are set up to offer a home-like atmosphere where residents have their own apartment and have access to on-site nursing care as needed. Other facilities offer more therapeutic resources such as speech, occupational or physical therapy. Some facilities have specialized memory care units for patients with dementia and Alzheimer disease. Still others offer short-term respite care for frail or disabled patients when their family or caregivers require a break from providing care in the home.

Hospice

Hospice can be a confusing term. It is not a specific place, though hospice facilities do exist. Hospice is a care model for end-of-life care. Hospice is a coordinated care plan with the patient's primary provider, a hospice nurse, a palliative care team, and often a spiritual support person such as clergy. They focus specifically on comfort, dignity and pain control for patients who are dying. It focuses on the physical, emotional, and spiritual needs of the patient and their family. Once a patient has entered hospice care, whether it is in their own home or a long-term care facility, they are no longer seeking curative treatment, and care related to their terminal condition will not be reimbursed.

Home Health Agencies

A home health agency (HHA) provides part time skilled nursing services and therapeutic care in the patient's home. Examples of services offered through a home health agency include
- catheter care
- intravenous therapy
- wound care
- occupational therapy
- speech therapy
- physical therapy
- monitoring of vital signs or medical equipment
- non-skilled nursing services by a home health aide such as assistance in bathing and eating

Most insurance companies will only pay for the skilled nursing services offered by a home health agency. Any additional personal care services must be paid out of pocket.

18.2   QUICK REVIEW
Question: What are the types of ambulatory surgery centers?

18.3   QUICK REVIEW
Question: What is the difference between a skilled nursing facility and a long-term care facility?

18.4   QUICK REVIEW
Question: What is hospice?

REGULATION OF HEALTH CARE FACILITIES

All health care facilities must follow the statutes of various federal and state regulatory agencies such as the Department of Health and the Department of Labor. Many of these statutes and agencies have been discussed throughout this text. In addition to these, they must be licensed by the state in which they provide services.

Licensing requirements in each state outline standards that must be met to provide effective patient care. These generally pertain to all aspects of patient care from admission to treatment to billing. Some examples of licensing requirements in most states are as follows:
- an organized medical staff
- current and complete health records for each patient
- method of infection control
- a process to review patient care
- licensed health care providers

Accreditation

Accreditation is a voluntary assessment process that facilities use to assess their performance against national benchmarks and established standards of care. It is both a self-assessment and a peer review process. There are a number of accreditation organizations for different types of facilities.

The Joint Commission (TJC)

The Joint Commission provides accreditation to hospitals, laboratories, CAHs, home health agencies, ambulatory care facilities, and pharmacies. Their accreditation standards establish expectations for safe and effective patient care. Through the assessment process, hospitals identify gaps in compliance with the established standards and determine areas of improvement. Accreditation provides facilities with community confidence in the care they provide and enhances staff recruitment. TJC offers ongoing education and support as well as a method to continually improve patient care. It also helps facilities qualify for CMS certification without having to undergo a separate process.

Accreditation Association for Ambulatory Health Care (AAAHC)

The Accreditation Association for Ambulatory Health Care (AAAHC) has been designated by CMS as the accrediting body for ambulatory surgery centers. This voluntary organization was founded in 1979 to encourage and assist ambulatory health care organizations to provide the highest achievable level of care for recipients in the most efficient and economically sound manner. The organization provides ongoing consultative and education survey processes to ambulatory care facilities as they strive to set the highest of standards and to continuously advance patient care.

American Osteopathic Association (AOA)

The American Osteopathic Association (AOA) provides board certification for doctors of osteopathic medicine (DO).

Osteopathic medicine bases diagnosis and treatment on the philosophy that the body systems are interrelated; they treat the body as a whole instead of focusing on individual symptoms. The AOA also established the Healthcare Facilities Accreditation Program (HFAP) in 1945 to evaluate osteopathic hospitals, ambulatory surgery centers, CAHs, and laboratories and ensure quality patient care. Like TJC, this accreditation assists facilities in maintaining CMS certification without requiring a separate review. HFAP also offers specialty certification options for stroke, joint replacement, lithotripsy and wound care.

In 2012, the AOA sold the HFAP to the Accreditation Association of Hospitals/Health Systems (AAHHC) with the approval of CMS. This and the AAAHC are governed by an umbrella organization called The Accreditation Association.

Other Accreditation Organizations

There are a number of other health care accreditation organizations. Some examples are as follows:

- Accreditation Commission for Health Care (ACHC) (home health agencies, renal dialysis, durable medical equipment, hospice and home infusion therapy)
- American Association for Accreditation of Ambulatory Surgery Facilities (AAAASF) (outpatient facilities)
- American Board for Certification of Orthotics, Prosthetics, and Pedorthotics (orthotics, prosthetics and *pedorthotics* which are footwear to improve or prevent disabling conditions of the foot or ankle)
- Center for Improvement in Healthcare Quality (CIHQ) (acute care hospitals, free-standing emergency centers, congregate living health facilities and urgent care centers)
- The Compliance Team (durable medical equipment)
- Healthcare Quality Association on Accreditation (durable medical equipment)
- National Committee for Quality Assurance (NCQA) (individual providers, health plans and medical groups)

Emergency Medical Treatment and Labor Act

The Emergency Medical Treatment and Labor Act (EMTALA) was passed under the Consolidated Omnibus Budget Reconciliation Act (1985). This legislation applies to all hospitals except Shriner's Hospital for Children and some military hospitals. It states that hospitals must screen and stabilize patients presenting for emergency medical treatment or in active labor regardless of their ability to pay. They are only allowed to transfer care of that patient to another facility only if they are unable to provide appropriate treatment or once the patient is stable.

This act was passed to eliminate patient dumping where a hospital would refuse to treat patients without insurance or with potentially costly conditions. The law applies only to facilities equipped to treat emergencies such as acute care hospitals, and only applies to emergency conditions. A significant portion of emergency department visits are for non-emergent conditions. These do not fall under EMTALA. For example, a patient presenting without insurance or the ability to pay for a minor sinus infection would not be protected under this ruling.

The law also states that hospitals may not provide substandard care because a patient is unable to pay for services. They also may not delay services while they attempt to determine if the patient has the ability to pay. Hospitals, however, may refuse to provide additional outpatient services, drugs and supplies after discharge.

Medicare Certification of Ambulatory Surgery Centers

To provide services and bill as an ASC, a facility is required to be certified by CMS. Initial certification will involve a compliance survey to meet Medicare and state regulations. Certification and licensure must be maintained on an ongoing basis.

CMS defines Medicare-certified ASCs with the following criteria:

- An ASC must be certified and approved to enter into a written agreement with CMS. Participation as an ASC is limited to any facility that operates exclusively to provide surgical services to patients not requiring hospitalization. Patients are not expected to stay in the facility beyond 24 hours. An unanticipated medical circumstance may arise that would require an ASC patient to stay in the ASC longer than 24 hours but such situations should be rare.
- The ASC and another entity, such as an adjacent provider's office, are not allowed to mix functions and operations in a common space during concurrent or overlapping hours of operations.
- ASCs are not permitted to share space with a critical access hospital (CAH) outpatient surgery department or with a Medicare participating independent diagnostic testing facility. Specific radiology services that are reasonable, necessary, and integral to covered surgical procedures may be provided by an ACS.

It is expected that CMS will continue to look at ASC reform, specifically with regards to site neutrality and efficiency of care.

CMS also publishes an ASC exclusion list outlining procedures that are not reimbursable when done at an ASC. Medicare will not pay for surgical procedures in an ASC if the procedure meets any of the following criteria for exclusion:

- Is only approved to be done in an inpatient facility
- Poses a significant safety risk to the beneficiary
- Typically requires active medical monitoring and care past midnight
- Directly involves major blood vessels
- Requires major or prolonged invasion of body cavities
- Usually results in extensive blood loss
- Is emergent in nature
- Is life-threatening in nature
- Commonly requires systemic thrombolytic therapy
- Can only be reported using an unlisted surgical procedures code

The list of surgical procedures excluded from payment in the ASC can be found on the CMS website (Table 18.1).

TABLE 18.1   Surgical Procedures Excluded From Payment in the Ambulatory Surgery Center

CPT Code	Short Description
22857	Lumbar artif discectomy
22861	Revise cerv artific disc
22862	Revise lumbar artif disc
22864	Remove cerv artif disc
22865	Remove lumb artif disc
22899	Spine surgery procedure
22999	Abdomen surgery procedure
23200	Resect clavicle tumor
23210	Resect scapula tumor
23220	Resect prox humerus tumor
23335	Shoulder prosthesis removal
23470	Reconstruct shoulder joint

From CMS' List of Surgical Procedures to be Excluded from Payment in ASCs—Updated October 2018 (Addendum EE) Resource. (https://www.cms.gov/Medicare/Medicare-Fee-for-Service-Payment/ASCPayment/11_Addenda_Updates.html.)

18.5   QUICK REVIEW
Question: What is accreditation?

18.6   QUICK REVIEW
Question: What is EMTALA?

18.7   QUICK REVIEW
Question: What types of services will Medicare NOT allow to be done at an ASC?

INPATIENT, OUTPATIENT AND NONPATIENT SERVICES

To better understand the types of services that a billing specialist may encounter when working in a facility, it is important to differentiate between inpatient and outpatient services. The difference between inpatient and outpatient is not simply an overnight stay as is often assumed. It is also not dependent on the types of services a patient receives; there are many types of services such as radiology and laboratory services that are provided for both inpatient and outpatient admissions.

According to CMS, an inpatient stay begins when the provider writes the order admitting the patient to the hospital. An inpatient requires ongoing care for more than 24 hours. The provider must use their clinical judgement to determine if an inpatient admission is necessary for patient care.

It is important to understand that just because a patient stays overnight does not necessarily mean they are receiving inpatient services. When deciding to admit a patient, providers must consider the Two Midnight Rule. According to CMS, an inpatient admission is the benchmark in determining an inpatient or outpatient status. If the provider expects the patient will need care crossing two midnights, it is appropriate to admit them as an inpatient. If the care is expected to take less than the span of two midnights, it would be an outpatient service.

Most patients are admitted to inpatient status either through the emergency department or through their health care provider for preplanned surgery or treatment. Examples of inpatient services include complex surgeries, critical illness, and delivering a baby.

Sometimes a provider will admit a patient to observation. Observation status is for patients who are too sick to be discharged, but it has not yet been determined if they are sick enough to need inpatient services. A patient may be admitted to observation for up to three days. Despite spending the night in the hospital, observation is considered to be an outpatient service.

Outpatient hospital care is often called ambulatory care and covers various types of services that do not require an overnight hospital stay. In outpatient services, the patient is discharged within 24 hours of arrival. Some examples of outpatient services include colonoscopies, lab work, MRIs, minor surgeries and chemotherapy.

There are also nonpatient services. These services include test and procedures performed on a specimen. The patient is not present. These services are typically provided by the laboratory or pathology departments. Some insurance payers, including CMS, consider these types of services outpatient services.

Inpatient Only List

The Inpatient Only List is a list of over 1,700 procedures that CMS has determined should only be done in an inpatient hospital setting. These are chosen based on the nature of the procedure and the need to have more than 24 hours postoperative care. They are also chosen based on the typical underlying condition of patients who have the procedure. If a procedure on this list is performed in an outpatient hospital setting or ambulatory surgery center, CMS will not reimburse the facility for it. This list is updated annually. Some examples of procedures that are included in the Inpatient Only list are:

- Coronary artery bypass
- Gastric bypass
- Colectomy
- Radical Mastectomy
- Creation of an AV shunt
- Total abdominal hysterectomy

72-Hour Rule

The 72-hour rule, sometimes referred to as the 3-day payment window, states that if a patient receives any treatment related to the inpatient admission, such as diagnostic laboratory tests, x-ray examinations, medical equipment, or emergency services, or any outpatient services within 72 hours of admission to the same hospital, then all these services are bundled with the inpatient service claim. If the service is unrelated to the hospitalization, the rule does not apply. For example, routine preadmission blood work would be submitted to Medicare for payment as an outpatient service if it is completed within 72 hours of admission and if it is related to the reason for admission. If the patient was scheduled to be admitted to have a hysterectomy as an inpatient and the patient comes to the hospital to have routine blood work for a medication that was prescribed by her dermatologist for her acne, the outpatient claim can be submitted to Medicare.

There are exceptions to the 72-hour rule:

- Services provided by home health facilities, hospices, nursing facilities, and ambulance services
- Provider's professional portion of a diagnostic service (the technical portion of a diagnostic service must be included in the inpatient bill)
- Preadmission laboratory testing when the laboratory is not contracted with the hospital
- This rule does not apply to non-Medicare third-party payers.

 18.8 QUICK REVIEW
Question: What is the difference between inpatient and outpatient services?

 18.9 QUICK REVIEW
Question: What is the Inpatient Only List?

 18.10 QUICK REVIEW
Question: What is the 72-hour rule?

REVENUE CYCLE IN HEALTH CARE FACILITIES

Revenue cycle management is an important process that supports the financial strength of any health care facility. The revenue cycle of a health care facility is a complex process. The revenue cycle process begins with the scheduling of an appointment for services or when the patient arrives at the hospital for emergency services. The revenue cycle includes preadmission, preauthorization, admission, capture of charges, submission of claim, and receipt of reimbursement among others. This process can be divided into three periods: preadmission, patient care and postdischarge. Fig. 18.3 shows the key steps in the process.

Preadmission

For nonemergency hospital services, inpatient and outpatient, and ambulatory surgery centers, the patient goes through a preadmission process. Preadmission is the process of preparing for the patient's care by collecting demographic information and insurance information. These steps occur before the patient's arrival.

To obtain necessary diagnostic information and speed up patient care, a patient is often sent to the hospital for preadmission testing (PAT) a day or two before being admitted for surgery. These preadmission tests can include diagnostic studies, such as routine blood and urine tests, radiology imaging, and electrocardiogram. These tests generally fall within the 72-hour rule for Medicare beneficiaries having inpatient services and therefore are billed as part of the inpatient claim.

Some services require prior approval from the insurer before they can be performed. This is known as preauthorization. Common examples of services that require preauthorization are magnetic resonance imaging, colonoscopies, and inpatient hospitalizations. The services that require preauthorization vary by insurance carrier. The facility may appeal the need for preauthorization if the procedure/hospitalization is performed in a medical emergency.

Patient Care

This period of the revenue cycle are the stages that occur while the patient is receiving treatment at the facility. This may be as an inpatient, outpatient, or observation patient.

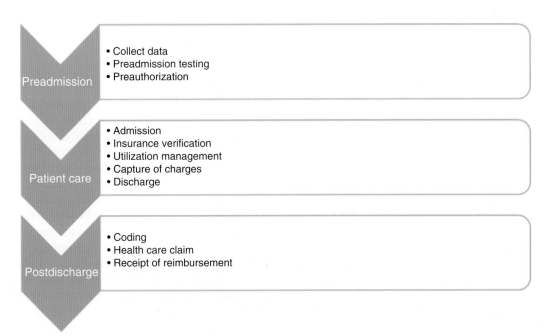

Fig. 18.3 Revenue cycle process in a facility.

The provider order must identify which patient type the patient should be.

During this admission process, additional information is collected, forms are completed and consents are signed. During either preadmission or admission, the patient's insurance is verified, meaning that the insurance carrier is contacted to ensure that the patient's insurance is in effect and to determine what the insurance covers, what the patient will pay, and if preauthorization is needed. A copy or scan of the insurance card is made and maintained by patient accounts department. If the patient is an inpatient or observation patient, the patient is assigned a room. The location depends on the provider's order. Locations can include regular nursing units, cardiac care unit, intensive care units, and more.

Charges for services rendered are posted, or entered, into the patient accounting system. These charges include supplies, procedures, room and board, equipment, medications, and much more. Many items have a barcode stamped on them to facilitate data entry and to improve data quality. The charges for all these items are recorded in the chargemaster.

A discharge occurs when the health care provider writes an order releasing the patient from the hospital. This order should include where the patient should go. Possible locations include home, home with home health, another acute care hospital, rehabilitation, and more. There are times when a patient wants to leave the hospital and the health care provider believes the patient needs continued hospitalization. If the patient insists, the patient leaves against medical advice. This should be documented in the health record. The location where the patient is being discharged to is known as the discharge disposition. This discharge disposition is entered in the hospital information system at the time of discharge for inclusion on the health care claim.

Chargemaster

The chargemaster, also called charge description master, is a list or database of all of the services, supplies, equipment, and so forth provided by the hospital and the charges that are associated with them. It is comparable to a fee schedule in a physician's office, but more complex. Other data elements in the chargemaster include a unique identifier for each item, the department providing the service, a revenue code, and the procedure code. Services that are provided by multiple departments have an entry for each department. A revenue code is a four-digit code used to group similar charges together, such as clinical laboratory services or room and board. See Table 18.2 for examples of revenue codes.

TABLE 18.2	Sample Revenue Codes
Revenue Code	Description
0270	Medical/Surgical Supplies
0305	Laboratory—Clinical Diagnostic: Hematology
0619	Magnetic Resonance Tech. (MRT): Other MRT
0720	Labor Room

Adapted from Centers for Medicare and Medicaid Services (2018A).

The chargemaster is used for laboratory, radiology, and other routine services. This prevents the coding specialists from having to manually assign the code for these routine services.

This chargemaster should be constantly monitored and updated as codes change, services are added or discontinued, and charges change. A chargemaster coordinator normally controls the day-to-day management of the chargemaster under the direction of the chargemaster committee. This chargemaster committee is responsible for the design and contents of the chargemaster. This committee should be made up of billing specialists, coding specialists, clinical staff, and others involved in the revenue cycle process.

Charges may include a professional charge and a technical charge. The hospital will charge a technical charge for its services such as a chest radiograph and pathologic testing. This technical charge would cover, for example, the costs of the x-ray examination itself, the radiology technician performing the procedure, supplies, and any other costs. The professional charge is for the health care provider's services. In the case of the radiology example, the professional charge for radiologist's services would reimburse the radiologist for reading and interpreting the radiology report. A professional charge would not be added for medications, supplies, room charges, and so forth. This professional charge will be billed by the hospital only if the physician or other health care professional is an employee of the hospital; otherwise, the professional charge is made by the health care professional's organization.

Postdischarge

The postdischarge phase includes all the steps that occur after the patient's discharge: coding, submission of the health care claim to the insurance carrier, receipt of reimbursement, hospital-acquired conditions, and the Discharge Not Final Billed report.

When the primary insurance carrier pays a claim, they notify the facility via remittance advice. The amount paid is documented in the patient's account and any adjustments are made. If there is a secondary insurance, the claim is forwarded to them and any payment is posted. The patient is billed for any remaining balance as appropriate.

The Discharge Not Final Billed (DNFB) report is a list of all facility (inpatient and outpatient) claims that have not been submitted to the insurance for payment. A claim may be on the DNFB for a number of reasons such as not being coded, missing data, still in window of time waiting for late charges, missing discharge disposition, and more. The DNFB is monitored to identify the claims that have issues preventing the claim from dropping and being sent to the insurance carrier.

One of the most common reasons that the claim remains on the DNFB is that the diagnosis and procedure codes have not been entered. The missing codes may be due to missing a health record in the paper environment, waiting on a health care provider for documentation, backlogs in coding, and so on. Administration typically monitors this report and may have a dollar threshold that they want the report to stay below. This threshold varies widely depending on the size of the hospital and other factors. For example, the threshold of a 60-bed community hospital may be $300,000, whereas a 900-bed hospital that provides transplants and trauma services, has a burn unit, and offers other advanced services may have a threshold of $2,000,000.

18.11 QUICK REVIEW
Question: What is the difference between preauthorization and insurance verification?

18.12 QUICK REVIEW
Question: What is a chargemaster?

18.13 QUICK REVIEW
Question: What are some reasons why a claim may be listed on the DNFB?

REIMBURSEMENT METHODOLOGIES

Medicare Prospective Payment Systems

Launched by Congress in 1965, the Medicare program was composed of both inpatient and outpatient services and based on hospital-specific, reasonable costs. As a result of the upsurge in demand for health care services, the fast-emerging presence of new technology, and the increased economic factors, national health care costs grew exponentially. This escalation prompted the Social Security Amendments of 1983, and the enactment of the prospective payment system for inpatient services in 1983. Implementation of this payment system for inpatient services proved to be successful in managing the increasing costs of health care. A prospective payment system (PPS) is one where insurance reimbursement is based on a predetermined payment regardless of the intensity of the actual service provided.

The Tax Equity and Fiscal Responsibility Act of 1982 (TEFRA) mandated the use of prospective payment systems for Medicare. TEFRA mandated the use of the PPS for acute care hospital's inpatient discharges. Today a number of PPS systems are in use for Medicare reimbursement of hospital services, including the following:

- Acute Inpatient Prospective Payment System
- Outpatient Prospective Payment System
- Ambulatory Surgery Center Payment System
- Long-Term Care Hospital Prospective Payment System
- Inpatient Rehabilitation Facility Prospective Payment System
- Psychiatric Prospective Payment System
- Skilled Nursing Facility Prospective Payment System
- Home Health Prospective Payment System
- Hospice Prospective Payment System
- Ambulance Fee Schedule

Changes to these reimbursement systems go into effect each October 1. These reimbursement systems apply to the traditional Medicare program but not Medicare Part C. Each of these reimbursement systems is discussed in the following sections.

Inpatient Prospective Payment System

The Inpatient Prospective Payment System (IPPS) is the prospective reimbursement system used for Medicare inpatient claims for acute care facilities. Reimbursement is made based on Medicare Severity Diagnosis-Related Groups (MS-DRGs). The MS-DRG system groups similar conditions that require similar resources and thus have similar costs together.

The MS-DRG system has a three-tiered system based on the severity of the patient's condition. Each MS-DRG is assigned a relative weight and a geometric mean length of stay. The geometric mean is a calculation that takes the average length of stay and adjusts for many factors such as outliers. Any patients who stay a much longer or shorter time than the majority will significantly affect the average. The geometric mean attempts to define a more appropriate average length of stay by accounting for these outliers.

Many, but not all, of the MS-DRGs have a structure in which the diagnosis and sometimes the diagnosis and procedure is linked to the following three-tiered structure:

- No complication or comorbidity
- A complication or comorbidity
- A major complication or comorbidity

A complication is a diagnosis or condition that arises during the patient's hospitalization that increases the patient's length of stay in 75% of the cases. A comorbidity is a condition that the patient has on admission that increases the patient's length of stay in 75% of the cases. Together these are known as complication/comorbidities (CCs). Medicare has identified some conditions as major complications/comorbidities (MCCs). These complications and comorbidities have a significant impact on the patient's care and therefore result in additional compensation for the acute care hospital. Example 18.1 shows how the MS-DRG would break this down.

EXAMPLE 18.1 Three-Tiered MS-DRG	
MS-DRG 037	Extracranial procedures with MCC
MS-DRG 038	Extracranial procedures with CC
MS-DRG 039	Extracranial procedures without CC/MCC

The MS-DRGs are grouped into major diagnostic categories (MDCs). Many of the MDCs are based on the body system, but others are based on factors such as injuries. See Table 18.3 for a breakdown of the MDCs.

TABLE 18.3 Major Diagnosis Categories	
MDC 01	Diseases & Disorders of the Nervous System
MDC 02	Diseases & Disorders of the Eye
MDC 03	Diseases & Disorders of the Ear, Nose, Mouth & Throat
MDC 04	Diseases & Disorders of the Respiratory System
MDC 05	Diseases & Disorders of the Circulatory System
MDC 06	Diseases & Disorders of the Digestive System
MDC 07	Diseases & Disorders of the Hepatobiliary System & Pancreas
MDC 08	Diseases & Disorders of the Musculoskeletal System & Connective Tissue
MDC 09	Diseases & Disorders of the Skin, Subcutaneous Tissue & Breast
MDC 10	Endocrine, Nutritional & Metabolic Diseases & Disorders

Continued

TABLE 18.3 Major Diagnosis Categories—cont'd

MDC 11	Diseases & Disorders of the Kidney & Urinary Tract
MDC 12	Diseases & Disorders of the Male Reproductive System
MDC 13	Diseases & Disorders of the Female Reproductive System
MDC 14	Pregnancy, Childbirth & the Puerperium
MDC 15	Newborns & Other Neonates with Conditions Originating in Perinatal Period
MDC 16	Diseases & Disorders of Blood, Blood Forming Organs, Immunologic Disorders
MDC 17	Myeloproliferative Diseases & Disorders, Poorly Differentiated Neoplasms
MDC 18	Infections & Parasitic Diseases, Systemic or Unspecified Sites
MDC 19	Mental Diseases & Disorders
MDC 20	Alcohol/Drug Use & Alcohol/Drug Induced Organic Mental Disorders
MDC 21	Injuries, Poisonings & Toxic Effects of Drugs
MDC 22	Burns
MDC 23	Factors Influencing Health Status & Other Contacts with Health Services
MDC 24	Multiple Significant Trauma
MDC 25	Human Immunodeficiency Virus Infections

Adapted from CMS ICD-10-CM/PCS MS-DRG v37.0 Definitions Manual (https://www.cms.gov/icd10m/version37-fullcode-cms/fullcode_cms/P0001.html.)

The hospital receives one MS-DRG payment as reimbursement for each inpatient admission. If the MS-DRG payment is more than the costs of providing care, the hospital has a profit; however, if the MS-DRG payment is less than the costs, the hospital has a loss unless the loss is significant enough to qualify as a cost outlier. When the cost of a patient's care is excessively large compared to the typical patient, it is called a cost outlier and the facility may receive additional reimbursement. Each MS-DRG is assigned a threshold for the that would qualify an admission as an outlier.

The amount of reimbursement for the assigned MS-DRG is based on the relative weight that CMS assigns the MS_DRG. The "average" relative weight is 1.0000 (all relative weights go four digits past the decimal point). Each hospital is assigned a base rate that covers salary and nonsalary costs. This base rate varies based on the cost of living in that area. The MS-DRG relative weight is multiplied by the base rate. Hospitals can also qualify for an add-ons for the following:

- teaching medical residents
- disproportionate number of indigent patients
- use of approved technologies
- cost outliers

There may also be adjustments to the IPPS in special circumstances. Fig. 18.4 shows an example of how a basic MS-DRG works.

MS-DRG 192

Base rate $4,567.00X Relative weight 0.7234 = MS-DRG Amount $3,303.77

MS-DRG Amount $3,303.77 + Add-on $765.00 = Reimbursement received $4068.77

Fig. 18.4 Calculating the basic Medicare Severity Diagnosis-Related Group *(MS-DRG)* reimbursement.

The MS-DRG payment is reduced under the following four circumstances:

- The length of stay is 1 or more days shorter than the geometric mean length of stay for the MS-DRG.
- The patient is transferred to another acute care hospital subject to the IPPS or in certain circumstances to a postacute setting. Postacute settings include rehabilitation hospitals and skilled nursing facilities, long-term care hospitals, and more.
- The patient is transferred to an acute care hospital not subject to the IPPS.
- The patient is transferred to a critical access hospital.

The MS-DRG is assigned by a software application known as a grouper. The grouper uses the principal diagnosis, procedures, discharge disposition, complications, comorbidities, major complications and comorbidities, and patient age to assign the MS-DRG.

> **! COMPLIANCE ALERT**
>
> Upcoding is assigning codes to increase reimbursement when the health record does not support the diagnosis and procedure codes. DRG creep is the result of upcoding. DRG creep results in increased reimbursement to a level that is not deserved by the hospital.
>
> Downcoding is coding a lower level of care when the health record would support a higher level. Some facilities practice this to not be accused of fraudulent claims. Downcoding results in poor data quality from the inappropriate codes as well as a smaller reimbursement amount.

Outpatient Prospective Payment System and Ambulatory Surgery Center Payment System

Because of the growth of outpatient surgeries that were being performed in hospital-based outpatient surgery departments, known as ambulatory surgery units (ASUs) and ASCs, federal legislation was further enacted in 1986 to segregate and pay for specific ambulatory surgical procedures performed at hospitals on an outpatient basis.

The Outpatient Prospective Payment System (OPPS) is used for hospital outpatient services, including surgical procedures; radiology, laboratory, and emergency services; observation; and more. Acute care hospitals are paid based on ambulatory payment classifications (APCs). APCs group similar services with similar costs together. A hospital can receive multiple APCs for services rendered. For example, if a patient came to the hospital to have a routine mammogram, a urinalysis and a chest radiograph, the hospital would receive three APCS, one for each service. The same ambulatory payment classifications are used in the Ambulatory Surgery Center (ASC) Payment System.

APCs use packaging, which means that all supplies, medications, and other components of a service are included in the APC. Because of this, the facility does not bill for these components separately. For example, if a patient has a cholecystectomy performed on an outpatient basis, the APC would include the surgery, anesthetic drugs, postoperative observation, medications, supplies, and more. CMS does pay separately for certain ancillary items and services when they are integral to surgical procedures. For example, CMS pays separately for corneal tissue acquisition, brachytherapy sources, certain radiology services, and many drugs.

In the OPPS and ASC payment system, every HCPCS and CPT code is given a status indicator. The status indicator provides information about the procedure, including whether or not it is covered under the payment system, if it is an inpatient-only procedure, if it is subject to discounting, and more. Discounting is when the APC reimbursement to the facility is reduced. Fig. 18.5 shows an example of status indicators that reflect discounting status. Discounting occurs in the following circumstances:

- The patient is prepared for surgery and is taken to the operating or procedure room before the surgery is cancelled. The anesthesia may or may not have been administered.
- Two or more surgical procedures are performed at the same operative session. When this occurs, the first surgical procedure is paid at 100% and the subsequent procedures are paid

at 50% of the APC amount. The logic behind this is that there is only one administration of anesthesia, one recovery, and so forth. The status indicator for the HCPCS codes associated with these procedures must indicate that they are subject to the discounting. Fig. 18.6 shows an example of two surgical procedures performed on the same day with sequencing and discounting. In determining the ranking of procedures for the assignment of the multiple procedure reduction, the surgical procedure with the highest fee schedule will have an allowance of 100%.

In both the OPPS and ASC payment systems, each APC receives a scaled relative payment weight that represents the average health care costs for the services included in the package. Then the weight is multiplied by a conversion factor (CF) to create a national unadjusted payment rate. That figure is then adjusted for the geographic location, including both labor and nonlabor costs. Fig. 18.7 is an example of an ASC payment.

APC	Status Indicator	Reimbursed at
1	T	This APC example is subject to discounting so the hospital would receive either 100% or 50% depending on whether APC 1 or APC 4 is reimbursed at a higher rate. The higher APC rate is reimbursed at 100% and the lower reimbursement APC is reimbursed at 50%.
2	S	100% as S payment indicators are not subject to discounting
3	J1	100% as J1 payment indicators are not subject to discounting
4	T	This APC example is subject to discounting so the hospital would receive either 100% or 50% depending on whether APC 1 or APC 4 is reimbursed at a higher rate. The higher APC rate is reimbursed at 100% and the lower reimbursement APC is reimbursed at 50%.

Fig. 18.5 Example of status indicators for discounting. Discounting is applied when the patient goes to surgery and has three procedures performed at the same time. *APC*, Ambulatory payment classification.

Service Sequence	CPT Code	Description	Fee	%
1st Service	13132	Repair, complex, 2.6 cm – 7.5 cm	$486.62	Higher code at 100%
2nd Service	15120	Split thickness autograft	$212.59	Lesser code at 50%
			Total	$699.21

Fig. 18.6 Example of surgical procedures performed together on the same day with discount. *CPT, Current Procedural Terminology.* (From Department of Health and Human Services, Office of Inspector General, https://oig.hhs.gov/oas/reports/region7/70302666.pdf.)

2016 APC CF	Wage index adjusted CF	Service/RW	Adjusted CF x RW	Total Payment
$74.17	(74.17 x .60 x .9444) + (74.17 x .40) 42.02 + 29.67 = 71.69	99282/1.5206	$71.69 x 1.5206	$109.01

Fig. 18.7 Example of ambulatory surgery center payment with relative weights (RW). *APC*, Ambulatory payment center; *CF*, conversion factor. (From Centers for Medicare and Medicaid Services, https://www.cms.gov/Medicare/Medicare-Fee-for-Service-Payment/HospitalOutpatientPPS/Addendum-A-and-Addendum-B-Updates.html.)

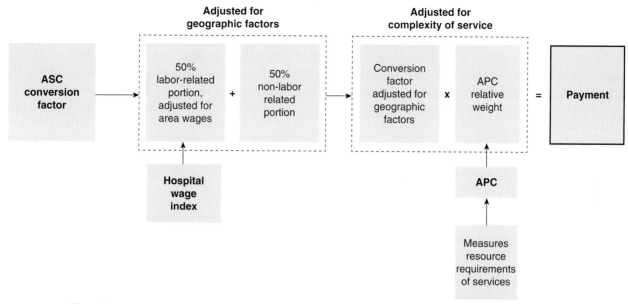

Fig. 18.8 MedPAC (Medicare Payment Advisory Committee) payment basics, 2018. *APC,* Ambulatory payment center; *ASC,* ambulatory surgery center. (From MedPAC, medpac.gov, Washington, DC.)

Although the relative weights of the ASC payment system are linked to the OPPS relative weights, the CF used to convert the relative weights into payment amounts are different. The ASC conversion factor is lower than the OPPS conversion factor, resulting in lower ASC payment rates for the same service. Fig. 18.8 describes the algorithm.

There are some outpatient services that do not fit into an APC, such as some diagnostic and nonsurgical therapeutic procedures, blood and blood products, clinic and emergency department visits, certain preventative services, and some drugs.

In the OPPS and ASC payment systems, facility services include all services and procedures provided in connection with covered surgical procedures furnished by nurses, technical personnel, and others involved in patient care. Payment under these systems include the following:

- Surgical supplies, nursing services and equipment;
- Use of the operating and recovery rooms, patient preparation areas, waiting room, and other areas used by the patient or offered for use by the patient's relatives, attendants, companions, or other person(s) accompanying the injured worker in connection with surgical services;
- Drugs, biologicals, intravenous fluids and tubing, surgical dressings, splints, casts, surgical supplies, and equipment required for both the patient and the facility personnel (for example, fiber-optic scopes and their associated supplies);
- Gowns, masks, drapes, case packs and their contents, and operating and recovery room equipment routinely furnished by the facility in connection with the surgical procedure;
- Simple diagnostic and preoperative testing performed by the facility in connection with the surgery, such as urinalysis, blood hemoglobin or hematocrit, blood glucose, or venipuncture to obtain specimens that are included in the facility charges; and
- Materials for conscious sedation and general anesthesia, including the anesthesia pharmaceuticals and any materials,

whether disposable or reusable, necessary for its administration.

In addition, some outpatient services related to the covered procedure receive a separate payment. Examples of these services are radiology services that are integral to the covered surgical procedure; brachytherapy sources implanted during a surgical procedure; pass-through and non–pass-through drugs that are paid for separately under the OPPS when provided as part of a covered surgical procedure; and devices with pass-through status under the OPPS.

Pass-through payments are for specific, new technology items that are used in the delivery of services. Facilities using the pass-through drugs and devices receive extra payments for these products. Congress established the pass-through provision in the Medicare law to encourage the distribution of new technologies.

These payment systems do not include professional services or medical services for which payment may be made under other Medicare provisions. For example, services of an independent laboratory located on the same site as the ASC, anesthetist professional services, or the independent surgeon's services will be covered under Fee for Service or other payment systems.

APCs are assigned using outpatient code editor (OCE) program. Claims are identified as OPPS or non-OPPS. The OCE targets individual errors and indicates what actions should be taken and the reasons why these actions are necessary. Some of the errors the OCE can flag are coding errors, questionable medical necessity, and gender-specific procedures that are inconsistent with the patient demographics.

CMS determines reimbursement rates for hospital outpatient departments and ASCs using two different measures of inflation, resulting in important cost differentials. For hospital outpatient departments, CMS uses the hospital market basket, which measures the cost of medical expenses. For ASCs, CMS uses the CPI-U, which measures the cost of consumer products.

The two payment systems also require different billing forms. Ambulatory surgical center claims are submitted to Medicare and Medicaid using the paper CMS-1500 claim form or the electronic format 837P. Hospital outpatient claims are filed with insurance carriers using the **Uniform Bill 04 (UB-04)** paper claim form or the 837I electronic format (Fig. 18.9). This form will be discussed in detail in Chapter 19.

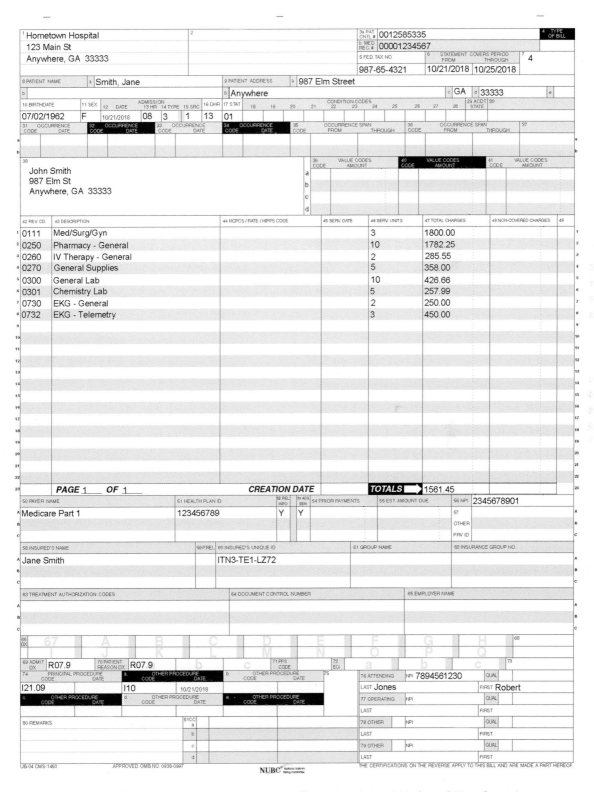

Fig. 18.9 Uniform Bill 04 (UB-04) or the 837I. (From the National Uniform Billing Committee, American Hospital Association, Chicago, Illinois.)

UB-04 NOTICE: THE SUBMITTER OF THIS FORM UNDERSTANDS THAT MISREPRESENTATION OR FALSIFICATION OF ESSENTIAL INFORMATION AS REQUESTED BY THIS FORM, MAY SERVE AS THE BASIS FOR CIVIL MONETARTY PENALTIES AND ASSESSMENTS AND MAY UPON CONVICTION INCLUDE FINES AND/OR IMPRISONMENT UNDER FEDERAL AND/OR STATE LAW(S).

Submission of this claim constitutes certification that the billing information as shown on the face hereof is true, accurate and complete. That the submitter did not knowingly or recklessly disregard or misrepresent or conceal material facts. The following certifications or verifications apply where pertinent to this Bill:

1. If third party benefits are indicated, the appropriate assignments by the insured /beneficiary and signature of the patient or parent or a legal guardian covering authorization to release information are on file. Determinations as to the release of medical and financial information should be guided by the patient or the patient's legal representative.

2. If patient occupied a private room or required private nursing for medical necessity, any required certifications are on file.

3. Physician's certifications and re-certifications, if required by contract or Federal regulations, are on file.

4. For Religious Non-Medical facilities, verifications and if necessary re-certifications of the patient's need for services are on file.

5. Signature of patient or his representative on certifications, authorization to release information, and payment request, as required by Federal Law and Regulations (42 USC 1935f, 42 CFR 424.36, 10 USC 1071 through 1086, 32 CFR 199) and any other applicable contract regulations, is on file.

6. The provider of care submitter acknowledges that the bill is in conformance with the Civil Rights Act of 1964 as amended. Records adequately describing services will be maintained and necessary information will be furnished to such governmental agencies as required by applicable law.

7. For Medicare Purposes: If the patient has indicated that other health insurance or a state medical assistance agency will pay part of his/her medical expenses and he/she wants information about his/her claim released to them upon request, necessary authorization is on file. The patient's signature on the provider's request to bill Medicare medical and non-medical information, including employment status, and whether the person has employer group health insurance which is responsible to pay for the services for which this Medicare claim is made.

8. For Medicaid purposes: The submitter understands that because payment and satisfaction of this claim will be from Federal and State funds, any false statements, documents, or concealment of a material fact are subject to prosecution under applicable Federal or State Laws.

9. For TRICARE Purposes:

    (a) The information on the face of this claim is true, accurate and complete to the best of the submitter's knowledge and belief, and services were medically necessary and appropriate for the health of the patient;

    (b) The patient has represented that by a reported residential address outside a military medical treatment facility catchment area he or she does not live within the catchment area of a U.S. military medical treatment facility, or if the patient resides within a catchment area of such a facility, a copy of Non-Availability Statement (DD Form 1251) is on file, or the physician has certified to a medical emergency in any instance where a copy of a Non-Availability Statement is not on file;

    (c) The patient or the patient's parent or guardian has responded directly to the provider's request to identify all health insurance coverage, and that all such coverage is identified on the face of the claim except that coverage which is exclusively supplemental payments to TRICARE-determined benefits;

    (d) The amount billed to TRICARE has been billed after all such coverage have been billed and paid excluding Medicaid, and the amount billed to TRICARE is that remaining claimed against TRICARE benefits;

    (e) The beneficiary's cost share has not been waived by consent or failure to exercise generally accepted billing and collection efforts; and,

    (f) Any hospital-based physician under contract, the cost of whose services are allocated in the charges included in this bill, is not an employee or member of the Uniformed Services. For purposes of this certification, an employee of the Uniformed Services is an employee, appointed in civil service (refer to 5 USC 2105), including part-time or intermittent employees, but excluding contract surgeons or other personal service contracts. Similarly, member of the Uniformed Services does not apply to reserve members of the Uniformed Services not on active duty.

    (g) Based on 42 United States Code 1395cc(a)(1)(j) all providers participating in Medicare must also participate in TRICARE for inpatient hospital services provided pursuant to admissions to hospitals occurring on or after January 1, 1987; and

    (h) If TRICARE benefits are to be paid in a participating status, the submitter of this claim agrees to submit this claim to the appropriate TRICARE claims processor. The provider of care submitter also agrees to accept the TRICARE determined reasonable charge as the total charge for the medical services or supplies listed on the claim form. The provider of care will accept the TRICARE-determined reasonable charge even if it is less than the billed amount, and also agrees to accept the amount paid by TRICARE combined with the cost-share amount and deductible amount, if any, paid by or on behalf of the patient as full payment for the listed medical services or supplies. The provider of care submitter will not attempt to collect from the patient (or his or her parent or guardian) amounts over the TRICARE determined reasonable charge. TRICARE will make any benefits payable directly to the provider of care, if the provider of care is a participating provider.

SEE http://www.nubc.org/ FOR MORE INFORMATION ON UB-04 DATA ELEMENT AND PRINTING SPECIFICATIONS

Fig. 18.9, cont'd.

Long-Term Care Hospital Prospective Payment System

Long-Term Care Hospital Prospective Payment System (LTCH PPS) is the prospective reimbursement system used by long-term care hospitals where the average length of stay must be at least 25 days. The LTCH PPS includes a subset of the same MS-DRGs used in the IPPS program. This subset used includes MS-DRGs for conditions that might require extended hospitalization, such as those where the patient is on mechanical ventilation. The relative weight of the LTCH DRGs is higher than those assigned to IPPS to accommodate the longer average length of stay.

The LTCH payment can be reduced in certain circumstances such as:

- Short stay outlier: When a patient is discharged before staying 5/6 of the length of stay given to each LTCH DRG, reimbursement is reduced.
- High-cost outlier: As discussed under the IPPS.
- Interrupted stay: This occurs if a patient leaves the LTCH and is then readmitted. This may be for continued care not provided by the LTCH or to go home. If the interruption is 3 days or less and the patient received care elsewhere, the LTCH is responsible for reimbursement of the other health care provider. If the interruption is more than 3 days and the patient was discharged to an acute care hospital, rehabilitation hospital, or skilled nursing facility and returns to the same LTCH, the LTCH hospitalization may be considered one hospitalization. The acute care hospital, rehabilitation hospital, and skilled nursing facility, including swing beds, are each assigned a range of days, known as fixed-day periods, that qualifies the LTCH for the greater than 3-day interruption. For example, if a patient is admitted to the acute care hospital between 4 and 9 days and then returns to the original LTCH during that period, it is considered to be the original LTCH hospitalization. A swing bed is a bed in an acute care hospital that can be used for acute care or for a skilled nursing facility depending on the needs at the time.

Inpatient Rehabilitation Facility Prospective Payment System

The Inpatient Rehabilitation Facility Prospective Payment System (IRF PPS) is the reimbursement system used for rehabilitation hospitals. To qualify for this reimbursement system, 60% of the hospital's inpatients must be treated for one of the following conditions:

- Stroke
- Spinal cord injury
- Congenital anomaly
- Amputation of limb
- Multiple trauma
- Fracture of femur
- Injury to the brain
- Specified neurologic disorders (for example, Parkinson disease)
- Burns
- Specific arthropathies causing difficulty with activities of daily living

- Systemic vasculitides with inflammation of the joints causing difficulty with activities of daily living
- Osteoarthritis (severe)
- Knee and/or hip replacement (procedure must be bilateral, patient obese, or patient 85 years of age or older)

The discharge is grouped into a rehabilitation impairment category (RIC) based on the patient's primary diagnosis or condition. Under each RIC are case mix groups (CMGs). CMGs are based on the patient's functional motor and cognitive scores as well as their age and comorbidities. These skills are evaluated using the Inpatient Rehabilitation Facility Patient Assessment Instrument (IRF PAI) which measures areas such as mobility, dexterity, mood, thought process, speech, vision and hearing. The CMGs are broken into four tiers based on the patient's comorbidities. The higher the tier, the higher the reimbursement.

Each year, Medicare sets a national base rate. This base rate is adjusted for local wages and nonlabor expenses. This rate is multiplied by the CMG weight. The CMG payment may be adjusted because of interrupted stays, short stays of less than 3 days, transfer to another facility, and cost outliers. There may also be adjustments as a result of location, number of indigent patients, and whether or not the facility is a teaching facility.

Inpatient Psychiatric Facility Prospective Payment System

The Inpatient Psychiatric Facility Prospective Payment System (IPF PPS) is the reimbursement system used for psychiatric hospitals and acute care hospitals' psychiatric units, which are exempt from the MS-DRG system. The provider must certify that the patient's condition justifies the need for inpatient hospitalization. A recertification of the patient's need for hospitalization is performed at day 12 and at least every 30 days thereafter. If the patient's condition changes significantly between recertifications, an additional evaluation would be needed when that significant change occurs.

Codes are assigned to patient claims using the health insurance prospective payment system (HIPPS) code set. These are five-character alpha-numeric codes that represent case mix groups.

The IPF PPS is based on a per diem rate. *Per diem* means that they are paid a specific rate for each day that the patient is hospitalized. This base rate, a dollar amount, is established each year by CMS. There are other factors that influence reimbursement, including the following:

- DRG
- Age
- Length of stay
- Emergency department
- Number of electroconvulsive shock treatments

In addition to these factors, the payment is adjusted based on the wage index for the area of the hospital, whether or not the facility is a teaching hospital, and additional funds if the facility a rural hospital. For an illustration of the structure of the IPF PPS payment, refer to Fig. 18.10.

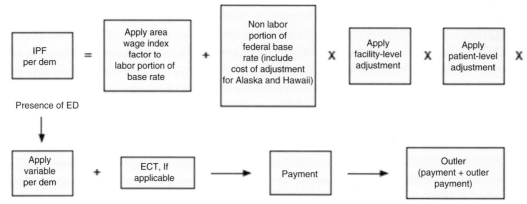

Fig. 18.10 Payment rates under the Inpatient Psychiatric Facility Prospective Payment System (IPF PPS). *ECT,* electroconvulsive therapy; *ED,* emergency department. (From Centers for Medicare and Medicaid Services. (2016d). *Inpatient Psychiatric Facility Prospective Payment System: Payment System Series.* Retrieved from https://www.cms.gov/Outreach-and-Education/Medicare-Learning-Network-MLN/MLNProducts/Downloads/Inpatient-Psychiatric-Facility-Prospective-Payment-System.pdf.)

Skilled Nursing Facility Prospective Payment System

Skilled nursing facilities are reimbursed under the Skilled Nursing Facility Prospective Payment System (SNF PPS). Payments are based on the case mix and the expected resources and care needs for each patient's condition. Like other PPS, adjustments are made for the cost of living and care within a geographic area.

A resident's conditions are identified through the Resident Assessment Instrument (RAI). SNFs are required to complete these assessments at regular intervals to adjust for changes in the patients' conditions. The RAI yields information about a resident's functional status, strengths, weaknesses, and preferences, and it offers guidance on further assessment.

Patients are grouped into one of the following classifications:
- Physical therapy
- Occupational therapy
- Speech language pathology
- Nursing
- Non-therapy ancillary

These categories, combined with the patient's case mix group, functional score and cognitive assessment, map to an overall score that will determine the patient's per diem rate. Claims are coded using the HIPPS code set.

Home Health Prospective Payment System

The Home Health Prospective Payment System (HH PPS) uses home health resource groups (HHRGs) to establish payment rates for every 2 months care is provided for a patient's condition. A 2-month (60 day) time frame is considered an episode of care in home health; there is no limit to the number of episodes of care a patient is eligible to receive.

Similar to case mix categories in other PPS, HHRGs classify patients based on the expected amount of resources their condition will require. HHRGs are reported to Medicare using a HIPPS code set. The codes are assigned following patient assessments.

Hospice Prospective Payment System

Under the Hospice PPS, Medicare pays a per diem rate for each day a patient is enrolled in hospice. The rate is the same regardless of the number of services the patient receives on a given day. Services covered under this PPS include the following:
- Hospice provider and nursing care
- Medical supplies
- Drugs for pain and symptom management
- Physical, speech and occupational therapy
- Dietary counseling
- Spiritual counseling
- Grief and loss counseling for the patient and the family before and after the patient's death
- Room and board if applicable

Payments are based on the level of care. These fall under four categories—routine home care, continuous home care, inpatient respite care and general inpatient care. Additional payment is made for services occurring within the last seven days of a patient's life. The per diem hospice rate is adjusted for wage differences within different geographic regions.

Ambulance Fee Schedule

Ambulance services are typically considered to be a professional service and not paid under a facility fee. However, some ambulance service providers are owned by hospital facilities, and these will be paid under a facility fee.

The Ambulance Fee Schedule is the reimbursement system used by Medicare to reimburse for ambulance services owned by hospital facilities. To pay for ambulance transport under this fee schedule, the services must meet the following criteria:
- It must be medically necessary.
- It must be used to bring a patient to or from a local destination.
- The patient must be covered by Medicare.

- The service must carry the patient to or from an appropriate health care facility.

The payment is a base rate plus mileage to the closest appropriate facility. This fee schedule includes both ground ambulance transport and air ambulance. Air ambulance is only covered in critical circumstances such as multiple traumas or when the patient requires specialized services not provided at all hospitals.

Self-Pay

As health care costs continue to rise, patients are taking on larger self-pay responsibilities. Many facilities are seeing a growing portion of their revenue coming from direct payments by patients. Collecting self-pay is a process that can require significant work and cost.

If possible, the facility's self-pay policy, including the fee and payment schedule, should be provided to the patient before services are provided. This will set the best practice for communication with the patient, moving forward through the encounters, including preoperative, postoperative, and follow-up for collections.

Capitation

Capitation is a fixed amount of money per patient per unit of time paid in advance to the hospital or ASC for the delivery of health care services. The amount paid is determined by the ranges of services provided, the number of patients treated in the facility, and the period during which the services are provided. Capitation rates are developed using local costs and average utilization of services and can vary nationally.

When the health care facility signs a capitation agreement, a list of specific services that must be provided to patients is included in the contract. The amount of the capitation will be determined in part by the number of services provided and will vary from health plan to health plan. This can include contractually agreed-on fee schedules that are discounted compared with the local usual and customary fees.

Capitation payments are used by insurance carriers to manage health care costs. Capitation payments control use of health care resources by putting the providers and health care organizations at financial risk for their services. To ensure that patients are not given suboptimal care as a way to cut costs, managed care organizations measure rates of resource utilization in health care organizations. These reports are made available to the public as a measure of health care quality and can be linked to financial rewards, such as bonuses.

Fee For Service

FFS is health care's most traditional payment model, in which health care facilities are reimbursed by third-party payers based on the number of services they provide or the number of procedures they order. Payments are unbundled and paid for separately each time patients have a procedure in the hospital or ASC. Box 18.1 is an example of the ASC calculation for Blue Cross/Blue Shield (BC/BS).

Medicare Part B covers provider-based outpatient and ASC services. Providers who furnish services in these facilities bill

---

> ### BOX 18.1 Ambulatory Surgery Center Fee Schedule Allowance Calculation Examples
>
> Amounts are displayed for illustrative purposes only. These examples demonstrate allowed amount calculations, not the Florida Blue payment because member deductible, coinsurance, and/or copayment liability have not been applied.
>
> For the below examples, the following sample contracted percentage is used:
>
> **Fee Schedule (FS) Surgery**
> The allowance is determined by:
>
> Fee schedule allowance × fee schedule percent = allowance
>
> 24515 $591 × 100% (1.0) = $591
>
> **Multiple Fee Schedule Surgery**
> The allowance is determined by:
> Surgical procedure with the highest fee schedule will have an allowance of 100% (1.0)
>
> Fee schedule allowance × fee schedule percent = allowance
>
> 24515 $591 × 100% (1.0) = $591
>
> Additional procedures will have an allowance of 50% (0.50) of the applicable fee schedule.
>
> 23650 $312 × 50% (0.50) = $156
>
> 12005 $419 × 50% (0.50) = $209.50
>
> Total allowance = $956.50

From Florida Blue, Manual for Physicians and Providers, 2018. Retrieved from https://www.floridablue.com/providers/tools-resources/provider-manual.

---

for and receive separate payment under Part B. For example, anesthesia providers and independent surgeons will be paid separately from the facility.

Medicare payment for provider services is based on the MPFS, a list of payment rates for services as described by HCPCS and CPT codes (Fig. 18.11). Unlike in the OPPS and ASC payment systems, payments for services are not packaged together as they are in the prospective payment systems. Providers generally receive a separate payment for each service provided.

Other Reimbursement Methodologies

Non-Medicare third party payers can use a variety of payment methodologies to reimburse facilities for their services. Some examples are listed here:

- Bed leasing. Some managed care plans lease beds from a facility and pay per bed regardless of whether they are used.
- Case rate. This method averages a flat rate on certain categories of procedures.
- Differential by day in hospital. This pays more for the first day of a hospitalization which tends to be more expensive than subsequent days.
- Differential by type of service. This method pays a set rate for the type of service (medicine, surgery, neonatal, obstetrics, intensive care) that the patient was admitted to receive.

CPT Code	Procedure Description	Allowed Amount
27060	Removal of ischial bursa	$181.20
27062	Remoe femur lesion/bursa	$181.20
27065	Remoe hip bone les super	$168.00
27066	Remoe hip bone les deep	$252.00
27067	Remoe/graft hip bone lesion	$545.10
27080	Removal of tail bone	$210.00
27086	Removal hip foreign body	$25.20

Physicians performing surgeries in an ASC will report the surgical code for their professional services and will be reimbursed under a Medicaid Physician Fee Schedule (PFS). This is an example of a Medicaid PFS from 2018; State of Rhode Island Medicaid Program.

Fig. 18.11 Medicaid physician provider fee schedule. *ASC*, Ambulatory surgery center. (From Executive Office of Health & Human Services, Cranston, Rhode Island. From Executive Office of Health & Human Services, Cranston, Rhode Island, http://www.eohhs.ri.gov/Portals/0/Uploads/ Documents/Fee%20Schedules/Medicaid%20Fee%20Schedule.pdf.)

18.14 QUICK REVIEW
Question: What is a prospective payment system?

18.15 QUICK REVIEW
Question: What is the main difference between the IPPS and OPPS/ASC systems?

18.16 QUICK REVIEW
Question: What is discounting in the OPPS and ASC systems?

QUALITY IN HEALTH CARE FACILITIES

Health care reimbursements under MACRA have been linked more and more to quality measures in patient care. Compliance with federal and state regulation and the standards of effective patient care are now mandatory. With the rising costs of health insurance, patients are becoming better-informed consumers when it comes to choosing their health care providers and organizations. Facilities are more invested in quality performance and positive patient outcomes than ever before.

Never Events

According to CMS, in 1999, 98,000 deaths per year were attributed to medical error. These errors, many of them never events, added up to $9000 per case to treatment costs. Another study showed that 18 types of medical events attributed to 2.4 million extra days in the hospital and over $9.3 billion in excess charges. CMS proposed that these deaths be decreased by 50% over 5 years.[a]

A never event in health care is an error in medical treatment that is preventable and has serious side effects for the patient. They indicate a breakdown in safety protocols and could have negative consequences in the credentialing of facilities and health care providers. To be considered a never event, the error must be serious, resulting in the loss of life or limb, disability or transient loss of bodily function. They must be clearly

identifiable as the cause of the resulting issue and also must be preventable. Examples of never events include the following:

- Instruments and other objects left in a patient during surgery
- Surgery performed on the wrong patient, or wrong body part of the right patient
- Intraoperative or immediate postoperative death of an otherwise healthy patient
- Death or serious disability related to contaminated drugs, devices or biologicals
- Death related to an air embolism or hypoglycemia while in the care of a facility
- Infant discharged to wrong person
- Serious surgical site infections following certain types of surgery
- Blood infections from a catheter
- Patient suicide or attempted suicide while in the care of the facility
- Medication errors, incorrect gas or incompatible blood products resulting in patient death or disability
- Maternal death or disability resulting from low-risk child birth
- Death or disability caused by spinal manipulation therapy
- Stage 3 or 4 pressure ulcers
- Death or disability related to a fall or use of restraints while in the care of the facility
- Death or disability related to electric shock or burn received while being treated
- Physical assault of a patient
- Patient being treated by someone impersonating a licensed health care provider

When a never event occurs, Medicare and other insurance carriers deny payment for the services. This is incentive to facilities and providers to address safety guidelines that were not followed to cause the event.

Surgical errors are reported with specific HCPCS Level II modifiers:

Surgical error modifiers for ASCs and hospital outpatient facilities:	
PA	Surgical or other invasive procedure on wrong body part
PB	Surgical or other invasive procedure on wrong patient
PC	Wrong surgery or other invasive procedure on patient

[a]https://www.cms.gov/newsroom/fact-sheets/eliminating-serious-preventable-and-costly-medical-errors-never-events.

Surgical error modifiers for inpatient hospital facilities:	
MX	Wrong surgery on patient
MY	Surgery on wrong body part
MZ	Surgery on wrong patient

Hospital Acquired Conditions

CMS identified a number of conditions that indicated a quality issue if the patient developed these conditions while an inpatient at an acute care hospital. These conditions are collectively known as hospital-acquired conditions (HACs). Some of these conditions include administration of wrong blood type, foreign body left in patient during surgery, trauma due to fall, and air embolism. For a full list, refer to Table 18.4.

The Hospital Acquired Condition Reduction Program (HACRP) began in 2014 aimed to reducing these avoidable occurrences by decreasing future payments to facilities with higher incidents of HACs. Documentation in the health record is key to determine if a condition was acquired at the facility or if the patient already had it and it was present on admission (POA). To identify whether or not the condition was POA or not, acute care hospitals are mandated to report a POA indicator for each diagnosis included on a Medicare inpatient claim. Table 18.5 shows the indicators that are assigned to each diagnosis on inpatient claims.

TABLE 18.4 Hospital-Acquired Conditions

Air embolism
Blood incompatibility
Catheter-associated urinary tract infection
Deep vein thrombosis and pulmonary embolism following specific orthopedic procedures
Falls and trauma
Foreign object left in patient after surgery
Iatrogenic pneumothorax with venous catheterization
Symptoms of poor glycemic control
Pressure ulcers (stages III and IV)
Surgical site infection following bariatric surgery for obesity
Surgical site infection following insertion of cardiac implantable electronic device
Surgical site infection following specified orthopedic procedures
Surgical site infection, mediastinitis, following a coronary artery bypass graft
Vascular catheter-associated infection

Adapted from Centers for Medicare and Medicaid Services. (n.d.). *FY 2013, FY 2014, and FY 2015 Final HAC List (no changes have been made).* (https://www.cms.gov/Medicare/Medicare-Fee-for-Service-Payment/HospitalAcqCond/Downloads/FY_2013_Final_HACsCodeList.pdf.)

TABLE 18.5 Present on Admission

Y: Diagnosis was present at time of admission.
N: Diagnosis was not present at time of admission.
U: Documentation in the health record is insufficient to determine whether the condition was POA.
W: The physician is unable to clinically determine whether the condition was POA.
1: The diagnosis is exempt from POA reporting.

Although mandated only for Medicare patients, facilities collect this information for all inpatient discharges. If a patient developed one of the conditions while in the hospital, the hospital is not reimbursed by Medicare for the higher weighted Medicare-severity diagnosis-related group that the HAC causes. If the condition was POA, then the hospital is reimbursed. Although the conditions affected are limited, not receiving reimbursement would have a serious impact on the hospital's reimbursement.

Utilization Management

Utilization management (UM) is a process that evaluates the effectiveness and appropriateness of medical treatment on a case-to-case basis. UM is performed to control costs and to ensure the patient's care is medically necessary.

Both facilities and health plans perform utilization management and case reviews. From a health care reimbursement perspective, because health care services are rendered prior to receiving payment, health care facilities need to evaluate each patient case to ensure future payment. CMS has zero tolerance for medical errors; they will not reimburse health care providers for mistakes in patient care. For this reason, utilization reviews are very important to the health care reimbursement process; it is the facility's responsibility to obtain the approved review of the case with the insurance carrier.

There are a few types of utilization reviews:

- An admission review is an evaluation for appropriateness and necessity of admission. The health record is reviewed and compared with utilization review criteria. This criterion is established by the insurer to identify when patients should be admitted to the hospital. This criterion generally evaluates the patient's "severity of illness" and "intensity of service"—in other words, how sick they are and what is being done for them.
- A continued stay review examines patients' health records to determine whether or not patients should stay in the hospital. If the documentation does not meet the criteria for admission or continued stay, the admission is referred to a provider advisor to conduct a medical review to determine whether the patient's hospitalization is appropriate.
- Prospective reviews are used to determine the medical necessity and appropriate setting for service before the service. *Appropriate setting* refers to whether the service should be performed as an outpatient or inpatient of the hospital or some other settings.
- A concurrent review is an evaluation of health care services to determine medical necessity and appropriateness of the care provided during the time services are being provided.
- A retrospective review is performed after the service is performed. An example of when a retrospective review occurs is when the patient is admitted and discharged before the review being performed, such as over a weekend or holiday.

Ambulatory Surgery Center Quality Reporting

The Affordable Care Act required the Secretary of Health and Human Services to develop a plan to implement a value-based purchasing (VBP) program for payments under the Medicare program for ASCs and other types of facilities.

The Ambulatory Surgery Center Quality Reporting Program (ASCQR), sponsored by CMS, began in 2014. This quality data program requires ASCs to report their quality of care data for standardized measures in order to receive the full ASC payment rate.

The ASC quality measures focus on the goals of quality improvement and accurate decision making. Efficiency and patient satisfaction are also evaluated. High-impact events, such as surgery performed on the wrong site, and safety issues, such as patient falls, are examples of the quality measures. Information is abstracted from the health record and assigned quality data codes on the claim form.

The ASC measures are updated annually. Examples of some recent measures for payment determination include the following:

- Patient Burn
- Patient Fall
- Wrong Site, Wrong Side, Wrong Patient, Wrong Procedure, Wrong Implant
- All-Cause Hospital Transfer/Admission
- Influenza Vaccination Coverage among Healthcare Personnel
- Appropriate Follow-Up Interval for Normal Colonoscopy in Average Risk Patients
- Colonoscopy Interval for Patients with a History of Adenomatous Polyps
- Improvement in Patient's Visual Function within 90 Days Following Cataract Surgery

ASCs that do not meet the reporting requirements will experience a 2% reduction to their payments. CMS has planned to look at intraoperative and postoperative measures in the future.

Hospital Value-Based Purchasing Program

The Hospital Value-Based Purchasing (VBP) Program pays incentives to acute care hospitals that report quality of care measures to CMS. These measures encourage hospitals to provide high quality, efficient and effective patient care while providing a better experience for the patients. Measures address the following types of issues:

- Reducing medical errors
- Reducing inappropriate care decisions
- Reducing mortality and complications
- Patient safety
- Reducing infections in the facility
- Adopting protocols to promote better health outcomes
- Develop processes that improve the patient's experience with the facility
- Providing higher quality care at lower cost to the insurance payer

Participating facilities who meet or exceed the expected quality measures are rewarded, not only with an increase in future payments, but with improved patient expectations. Patients who are satisfied with their care will return and send others through word of mouth.

Consumer Assessment of Health Care Providers and Systems Outpatient and Ambulatory Surgery Survey

CMS has developed the Consumer Assessment of Health Care Providers and Systems Outpatient and Ambulatory Surgery Survey (OAS CAHPS). This survey assesses the experience of care for patients who have surgery or a procedure in an outpatient hospital setting or ASC.

The survey measures patients' experiences on topics such as:

- communication and care provided by health care providers and office staff;
- preparation for the surgery or procedure;
- postoperative care coordination; and
- patient-reported outcomes.

Participating facilities can compare their patient responses against their state and the national averages. The program is currently voluntary.

Quality Improvement Organizations

Quality improvement organizations (QIOs) are hired by the CMS to improve patient care, ensure the medical necessity of care provided, review the appropriateness of the setting (inpatient vs. outpatient), and address beneficiary complaints.

Some of the reviews performed by QIOs in facilities include the following:

- Higher weighted DRG reviews evaluate whether or not the higher reimbursement Medicare severity DRG is justified by the health record.
- Readmission reviews are conducted when the patient is readmitted to the hospital for the same condition within a certain time frame. The purpose of the review is to determine whether or not the patient was discharged from the hospital too soon.
- Transfer reviews determine if patients were transferred appropriately following the rules established by EMTALA. The health record must support the need for transfer and that the patient is medically stable.

Whenever a problem is identified during a review, such as the patient's admission was not medically necessary, the QIO sends a denial letter to the hospital. The reimbursement that the hospital received for that hospitalization is returned to Medicare. To have the reimbursement returned, the hospital would need to appeal the decision. In this example, the hospital would need to request that the provider write the letter justifying the need for hospitalization.

18.17   QUICK REVIEW
Question: What is a never event?

18.18   QUICK REVIEW
Question: What is utilization management?

18.19   QUICK REVIEW
Question: What is the VBP program for ASC, outpatient and inpatient facilities?

18.20   QUICK REVIEW
Question: What is a QIO?

PROCEDURE 18.1 New Patient Admission and Insurance Verification

1. Interview the patient and obtain complete and accurate information during initial registration. If this is an emergency inpatient admission, the insurance carrier should be notified on the next working day or within 48 hours to obtain an authorization number.
2. Write down the information from the employee at the admitting provider's office who has telephoned for admittance of the patient.
3. Make photocopies of the front and back of all insurance cards.
4. Contact the insurance carrier to verify the type of health insurance, eligibility and benefits and to determine whether a prior authorization is necessary.
5. Collect any copayment or deductible.
6. Obtain information about the injured patient, workplace injury, workers' compensation carrier, and employer for a patient who was injured on the job.
7. Get an authorization for admission, length of stay and all surgical procedures for an elective admission.
8. Ask the patient to read and sign the necessary hospital admitting documents such as the Notice of Privacy Practices, consent for treatment and financial agreement.

KEY POINTS

1. There are many types of health care facilities. Acute care facilities are general hospitals that offer both inpatient and outpatient services. Critical access hospitals are small rural hospitals set up to provide care to Medicare beneficiaries who would otherwise not have access to health care. Ambulatory surgery centers are health care facilities specifically focused on providing same-day surgical care, including diagnostic and preventive procedures and services. A skilled nursing facility offers accommodation's for patients who are not sick enough to be hospitalized but are too serious to be treated in their homes. A long-term care facility provides custodial care to individuals who are chronically ill or disabled or are not able to live independently.

2. Accreditation is a voluntary assessment process that facilities use to assess their performance against national benchmarks and established standards of care. It is both a self-assessment and a peer review process. There are a number of accreditation organizations, such as The Joint Commission and the Accreditation Association for Ambulatory Health Care, for different types of facilities.

3. The Emergency Medical Treatment and Labor Act (EMTALA) states that hospitals must screen and stabilize patients presenting for emergency medical treatment or in active labor regardless of their ability to pay. They are only allowed to transfer care of that patient to another facility only if they are unable to provide appropriate treatment or once the patient is stable.

4. Inpatient admissions require a provider's order and involve an overnight stay. In outpatient services, the patient is typically discharged within 24 hours. However, an overnight stay does not automatically make it an inpatient service.

5. The Inpatient Only List is a list of procedures that CMS has determined should only be done in an inpatient hospital setting. These are chosen based on the nature of the procedure and the need to have more than 24 hours postoperative care. They are also chosen based on the typical underlying condition of patients who have the procedure. If a procedure on this list is performed in an outpatient hospital setting or ambulatory surgery center, CMS will not reimburse the facility for it.

6. The 72-hour rule states that if a patient receives any treatment related to the inpatient admission, such as diagnostic laboratory tests, x-ray examinations, medical equipment, or emergency services, or any outpatient services within 72 hours of admission to the same hospital, then all these services are bundled with the inpatient service claim.

7. The chargemaster, also called charge description master, is a list or database of all of the services, supplies, equipment, and so forth provided by the hospital and the charges that are associated with them.

8. A prospective payment system is one where insurance reimbursement is based on a predetermined payment regardless of the intensity of the actual service provided. CMS has established prospective payment systems for all types of facilities – inpatient, outpatient, ambulatory surgery centers, skilled nursing facilities and so on.

9. Discounting is when the APC reimbursement to the facility is reduced. Discounting occurs if the patient is prepared for surgery and is taken to the operating or procedure room before the surgery is cancelled or if two or more surgical procedures are performed at the same operative session.

10. A never event in health care is an error in medical treatment that is preventable and has serious side effects for the patient. They indicate a breakdown in safety protocols and could have negative consequences in the credentialing of facilities and health care providers. To be considered a never event, the error must be serious, resulting in the loss of life or limb, disability or transient loss of bodily function.

11. CMS identified a number of conditions that indicated a quality issue if the patient developed these conditions while an inpatient at an acute care hospital. These conditions are collectively known as hospital-acquired conditions (HACs). Some of these conditions include administration of wrong blood type, foreign body left in patient during surgery, trauma due to fall, and air embolism.

12. Utilization management (UM) is a process that evaluates the effectiveness and appropriateness of medical treatment on a case-to-case basis. UM is performed by both facilities and health care plans to control costs and to ensure the patient's care is medically necessary.

INTERNET RESOURCES

CMS Prospective Payment Systems
https://www.cms.gov/Medicare/Quality-Initiatives-Patient-Assessment-Instruments/Value-Based-Programs/HVBP/Hospital-Value-Based-Purchasing#:~:text=The%20Hospital%20VBP%20Program%20rewards%20acute%20care%20hospitals,they%20deliver.%20Why%27s%20the%20Hospital%20VBP%20Program%20important%3F

Ambulatory Surgical Center Payment System
https://www.cms.gov/Outreach-and-Education/Medicare-Learning-Network-MLN/MLNProducts/Downloads/AmbSurgCtrFeepymtfctsht508-09.pdf

CMS IPPS
https://www.cms.gov/Outreach-and-Education/Medicare-Learning-Network-MLN/MLNProducts/Downloads/AcutePaymtSysfctsht.pdf

CMS OPPS
https://www.cms.gov/Outreach-and-Education/Medicare-Learning-Network-MLN/MLNProducts/Downloads/HospitalOutpaysysfctsht.pdf

CMS SNF PPS
https://www.cms.gov/Outreach-and-Education/Medicare-Learning-Network-MLN/MLNProducts/Downloads/Skilled-Nursing-Facility-Prospective-Payment-System-Text-Only.pdf

CMS Hospice PPS
https://www.cms.gov/Outreach-and-Education/Medicare-Learning-Network-MLN/MLNProducts/downloads/hospice_pay_sys_fs.pdf

CMS LTCH PPS
https://www.cms.gov/Outreach-and-Education/Medicare-Learning-Network-MLN/MLNProducts/Downloads/Long-Term-Care-Hospital-PPS-Fact-Sheet-ICN006956.pdf

CMS HHA PPS
https://www.cms.gov/Outreach-and-Education/Medicare-Learning-Network-MLN/MLNMattersArticles/Downloads/MM11536.pdf

CMS Ambulance Fee Schedule
https://www.cms.gov/Outreach-and-Education/Medicare-Learning-Network-MLN/MLNProducts/Downloads/Medicare-Ambulance-Transports-Booklet-ICN903194.pdf

CMS ambulatory surgery payment rules
https://www.cms.gov/Regulations-and-Guidance/Guidance/Manuals/downloads/clm104c14.pdf.

A full list of status indicators
https://www.cms.gov/Medicare/Medicare-Fee-for-Service-Payment/HospitalOutpatientPPS/Addendum-A-and-Addendum-B-Updates.html

ASCQR program
http://www.qualitynet.org.

QIOs
https://www.cms.gov/Medicare/Quality-Initiatives-Patient-Assessment-Instruments/QualityImprovementOrgs

VBP Program
https://www.cms.gov/Medicare/Quality-Initiatives-Patient-Assessment-Instruments/Value-Based-Programs/HVBP/Hospital-Value-Based-Purchasing#:~:text=The%20Hospital%20VBP%20Program%20rewards%20acute%20care%20hospitals,they%20deliver.%20Why%27s%20the%20Hospital%20VBP%20Program%20important%3F

STUDENT ASSIGNMENT

- Study Chapter 18.
- Complete all assignments in the *Workbook* to reinforce the theory learned in this chapter.
- Turn to the Glossary at the end of this text for a further understanding of the key terms and key abbreviations used in this chapter.

19

Billing for Health Care Facilities

Cheryl Fassett

OBJECTIVES

After reading this chapter, you should be able to:

1. Explain the differences in professional, outpatient, and inpatient services.
2. Understand the different code sets and claim forms used in billing various types of services.
3. Understand the differences in diagnosis coding for outpatient and inpatient services.
4. Discuss guidelines for coding a principal diagnosis.
5. Understand how to code a principal procedure.
6. Explain the ICD-10-PCS code structure and what each character designates in the Medical and Surgical section.
7. Discuss how other sections differ in their character designations.
8. Explain how to code from the ICD-10-PCS code set.
9. Discuss various guidelines from the ICD-10-PCS Official Guidelines for Coding and Reporting.
10. Understand the five main sections of the CMS-1450 (UB-04) and what information is included in each of them.

KEY TERMS

Approach character
Body Part character
Body System character
Device character
First listed diagnosis
form locators
International Classification of Disease, Tenth Edition, Procedure Coding System

National Uniform Billing Committee
principal diagnosis
principal procedure
Qualifier character
reason for encounter
Root Operation character
Section character
Uniform Bill

KEY ABBREVIATIONS

CMS-1450
FL
ICD-10-PCS

NPI
NUBC
POA

PPS
UB-04

Reneé T.: Certified Professional Coder (CPC), Certified Professional Coding Instructor (CPC-I), Certified Professional Medical Auditor (CPMA), Certified Medical Billing Specialist (CMBS), ICD-10 Train the Trainer

I am a manager of professional coding and charge capture at a large facility.

My responsibilities changed drastically in March 2020 when we were asked to commit to the social-distancing practices that health officials said would help slow the spread of COVID-19. We were among the first departments to ramp up work plans for 100% of our staff to work remotely. During this time, it has become quite clear that flexibility is also a key component in keeping workers safe.

The greatest challenge for new people just coming into the health care field is its ever-changing nature. You never know what will be behind a door when it closes; for me it was an opportunity to give back all of the knowledge I have learned over my 20 years of experience.

INTRODUCTION TO FACILITIES BILLING

As discussed in Chapter 18, facility billing for inpatient, outpatient, or ambulatory surgery center services is different from billing for a provider's professional services. Facilities are reimbursed for the following types of services:

- use of the operating room and recovery room;
- medical and surgical supplies such as surgical instruments, bandages, and bed pans;
- medications;
- diagnostic and therapeutic services;
- various clinical services such as nurses and operating room technicians; and
- room and board for overnight stays.

Different types of services require different code sets and billing forms.

All diagnoses are coded from the ICD-10-CM as discussed in Chapter 12. However, differences exist in the guidelines for outpatient and inpatient coding. Procedures are coded for professional noninstitutional providers in an outpatient setting with CPT and HCPCS codes as discussed in Chapter 13. Those same code sets are also used for many types of outpatient

procedures when billing for the facility. Services such as radiology, laboratory, physical therapy, emergency room, observation, and ambulatory surgery also use CPT and HCPCS.

When patients are admitted to an inpatient facility, they receive different types of services that are not reflected in CPT codes. As such, inpatient facility billing requires a different code set (the ICD-10-PCS), which will be discussed in further detail later in this chapter. Facilities may also bill for professional services if they employ the physicians, radiologists, physical therapists, and so on.

Provider services are billed on a CMS-1500 claim form as discussed in Chapter 14. Some facility services are billed on the CMS-1500 as well, but many facility services are billed on a CMS-1450 (UB-04) claim form. Which will be explained in detail in this chapter. Table 19.1 illustrates the different types of coding involved in various types of health care services, the code sets used to represent them, and the claim forms used in billing for them.

 19.1 QUICK REVIEW
Question: Which code sets are used for professional services?

 19.2 QUICK REVIEW
Question: Which code sets are used for facilities services?

OUPATIENT AND INPATIENT DIAGNOSIS CODING GUIDELINES

The ICD-10-CM has guidelines specifically related to both outpatient and inpatient diagnosis coding.

First Listed Diagnosis

In outpatient and office encounters, the first listed diagnosis is used as the reason for the encounter. Sometimes the specific diagnosis is not known at the initial visit, and signs and symptoms are coded instead. The guidelines discussed in Chapter 12 apply to services performed in the outpatient setting as well as for the professional services.

TABLE 19.1 Code Sets and Claim Forms

Health Care Service	CLAIM FORM			CODE SETS				
	CMS-1500	CMS-1450 (UB-04)	ICD-10-CM	CPT	HCPCS	ICD-10-PCS	NDC
Provider professional Services	X			X	X	X		
Ambulatory surgery in a hospital outpatient setting		Xa		X	X	X		
Ambulatory surgery in an ASC	Xb			X	X	X		
ED Services		Xa		X	X	X		
Radiology, Laboratory		Xa		X	X	X		
PT/OT		Xa		X	X	X		
Hospital based clinic	X			X	X	X		
All inpatient services		X		X		X	X	
Nonpatient services		Xa		X			X	

aSome payers may require outpatient services be submitted on a CMS-1500.
bSome payers may require ASC charges be submitted on a CMS-1450 (UB-04).
NDC, National drug codes.

If a patient presents for outpatient surgery, a coding specialist should select the reason for the surgery as the diagnosis. This remains true even if the surgery is cancelled. If a patient is admitted to observation due to complications from outpatient surgery, the reason for the surgery is still treated as the first listed diagnosis. The codes for the complications are listed as secondary diagnoses.

As with coding for provider services, diagnoses that are listed as "probable" or "likely" are not coded in the outpatient setting.

If a patient receives routine diagnostic tests, such as lab work, and there is no underlying condition prompting the test, the code Z01.89, Encounter for other specified special examinations, should be assigned. Routine preoperative lab work and x-rays may be assigned the code Z01.81, Encounter for pre-procedural examinations.

Principal Diagnosis

There are several additional concepts outlined in the ICD-10-CM Official Guidelines that apply specifically to inpatient facility coding.

One of the key concepts in coding inpatient services is the definition of the **principal diagnosis**. It is the reason, after study, for admission to the hospital. This code is listed first on the health care claim. This is true even if the original treatment plan is not carried out. Two examples of how this definition is applied are as follows:

- A patient may come to the hospital with chest pain. After running tests, the physician determines that the chest pain is caused by an acute myocardial infarction. The acute myocardial infarction is the principal diagnosis, not the chest pain.
- A patient is admitted to the hospital for gastroenteritis. While in the hospital, the patient falls and fractures her arm. Surgery is required for the fracture. The principal diagnosis remains the gastroenteritis.

The concept of principal diagnosis selection differs from coding for an outpatient service or office visit. In outpatient coding, the reason for the encounter is the first-listed diagnosis. Unconfirmed or suspected diagnoses are not coded. Inpatient coding allows for an uncertain diagnosis in the absence of one that is confirmed. The principal diagnosis may or may not be the initial reason for the admission. Additional diagnosis codes are added to both inpatient and outpatient claims based on coding guidelines and health care facility policy.

Subsequent diagnostic codes should be used for any other condition that coexists with the principal condition, complicating the treatment and management of the principal disorder, and these are listed *after* the principal diagnosis. A secondary diagnosis is one that may contribute to the condition, treatment, or recovery of the principal diagnosis, and may also define the need for a higher level of care even though it is not related to the principal diagnosis. The diagnostic code sequence is important in billing of hospital inpatient cases because maximum reimbursement is based on the DRG system.

Additional ICD-10-CM Guidelines for Inpatient Coding

According to the ICD-10-CM Official Guidelines, Section II, the following rules and examples should be noted regarding the principal diagnosis:

- ICD-10-CM codes for signs and symptoms are not reported as principal diagnoses when a related definitive diagnosis has been established (Example 19.1).

EXAMPLE 19.1 Principal Diagnosis, Signs, and Symptoms

Mr. Brown was admitted to the hospital with fever, severe abdominal pain, nausea, and vomiting. Diagnosis is suspected acute appendicitis.

K35.9   Acute appendicitis, without generalized peritonitis

- When two or more conditions meet the definition of principal diagnosis, either condition may be sequenced first unless otherwise indicated by the circumstances of admission or the therapy provided (Example 19.2).

EXAMPLE 19.2 Two Medical Conditions

Mrs. Sanchez was admitted with acute congestive heart failure (CHF) and unstable angina. Both conditions are treated.

I50.9   Congestive heart failure NOS
I20.0   Unstable angina

- When two or more contrasting or comparative diagnoses are given, they are coded as though they are confirmed and sequenced based on the reason for the admission (Example 19.3).

EXAMPLE 19.3 Symptom as Principal Diagnosis, Followed by Conditional Diagnoses

Miss Chan was admitted with acute epigastric abdominal pain.
  Diagnosis was epigastric abdominal pain, acute pyelonephritis versus acute gastritis.

N10   Acute pyelonephritis
K29.00   Acute gastritis without bleeding

- For inpatient cases, code all "rule out," "suspected," "likely," "questionable," "possible," or "still to be ruled out" as if it existed. This is in direct contrast to the rules for outpatient coding in which these uncertain diagnosis codes are not included (Example 19.4).

EXAMPLE 19.4 Unconfirmed Diagnosis

Sally is not feeling well. The provider documents "upper abdominal pain, rule out cholecystitis."

K81.9   Cholecystitis, unspecified

If the patient is admitted with an inpatient status due to a complication from the surgery, assign the complication as the principal diagnosis. If no complication is documented, assign the reason for the outpatient surgery as the principal diagnosis. If the reason for admission is unrelated to the surgery, assign the unrelated condition as the principal diagnosis.

Additional diagnosis codes should be reported for all conditions that coexist at the time of admission, develop subsequent to the admission, or affect treatment received and/or length of stay. Conditions that were resolved prior to the admission should not be used as secondary diagnosis codes. Consider a personal history code, if appropriate, and if the condition has an impact on current care.

Abnormal findings in laboratory and other diagnostic tests are not reported unless the provider indicates there is a clinical significance. This is different from the coding concepts for outpatient diagnostic encounters that have been interpreted by the provider submitting the claim.

Institutional claims require that conditions present on admission (POA) be indicated in the CMS-1450 (UB-04). All inpatient facilities are required to collect data on conditions that were present on admission versus those that were acquired during the inpatient stay. A POA indicator is assigned to principal and secondary diagnoses. The ICD-10-CM Official Guidelines Appendix I outlines guidance for choosing a POA indicator for claims submission.

The principal diagnosis should be associated with the principal procedure. The principal procedure is the procedure code that is listed first on the health care claim. For example, an appendectomy would be a surgical treatment associated with the principal diagnosis of appendicitis. Additional significant procedure codes are added. Significant procedure codes have risk, require special training, and include both surgical (such as an appendectomy) and diagnostic procedures (such as cardiac catheterization). What is coded is determined by coding guidelines and the health care facility's policy.

 19.3   QUICK REVIEW

Question: How is the concept of a principal diagnosis different from one used in outpatient coding and billing?

 19.4   QUICK REVIEW

Question: How are uncertain diagnoses handled for inpatient claims?

 19.5   QUICK REVIEW

Question: How do the guidelines for diagnosis coding differ for a patient being admitted to observation due to a complication from outpatient surgery versus being admitted to an inpatient status?

INTRODUCTION TO INPATIENT FACILITY PROCEDURE CODING

The code sets used for outpatient and ambulatory surgery center procedure billing were covered in Chapter 13. Inpatient procedural coding, however, uses a different code set.

Inpatient procedures are coded using the International Classification of Disease, Tenth Edition, Procedure Coding System (ICD-10-PCS). The ICD-10-PCS was implemented in October 2015. ICD-10-PCS is maintained by CMS. The coding guidelines and codes are updated each October 1.

This coding system uses a table format to allow for unique identification of each procedure. ICD-10-PCS codes have a seven-character alphanumeric code structure that is multi-axial. In other words, the code set is divided by various sections and then further defined by smaller classifications.

ICD-10-PCS Code Structure

Each of the seven characters that make up an ICD-10-PCS code is assigned one of 34 possible alphanumeric values. To avoid confusion with digits 0 and 1, the letters O and I are not used. The ICD-10-PCS structure of codes is as follows:

Character:	1	2	3	4	5	6	7
	Section	Body System	Root Operation	Body Part	Approach	Device	Qualifier

Character 1: Section. The Section character is the largest classification in ICD-10-PCS; the Section defines the index of the medical specialty. The most expansive section is character 0 for Medical and Surgical Procedures; for inpatient hospital billing, coding specialists will most likely use Section 0. However, there are a number of other specialty sections such as Radiation Therapy and Obstetrics. A list of medical specialty sections is found in Table 19.2.

Character 2: Body System. The Body System character identifies the body system the procedure is being performed on, such as the cardiovascular or respiratory system. All complete ICD-10-PCS codes will have an assigned body system except the Rehabilitation and Mental Health sections.

Character 3: Root Operation. The Root Operation character identifies the objective of the procedure that was performed. It identifies whether the procedure removes the entire body part, a piece of the body part, restricts a body part, removes a foreign body, or other procedure. Root operations and their definitions are listed in Appendix A of the ICD-10-PCS. Not all root operations can be performed on every body

TABLE 19.2   ICD-10-PCS Character 1: Section Medical Specialties

Character	Section
0	Medical and Surgical
1	Obstetrics
2	Placement
3	Administration
4	Measurement and Monitoring
5	Extracorporeal Assistance and Performance
6	Extracorporeal or Systemic Therapies
7	Osteopathic
8	Other Procedure
9	Chiropractic
B	Imaging
C	Nuclear Medicine
D	Radiation Oncology
F	Physical Rehabilitation and Diagnostic Audiology
G	Mental Health
H	Substance Abuse Treatment
X	New Technology

Extracted from ICD-10-PCS, 2021.

system. For example, the root operation *fragmentation*, which involves breaking solid matter in a body part into pieces, cannot be performed on the nasal sinuses; therefore, a table cannot be found matching this body system with this root operation. See Table 19.3 for an example of some of the operations listed.

Character 4: Body Part. The Body Part character identifies the specific part in the body system the procedure was performed on. It may also be a region such as the trunk. For example, body parts can include right lower leg, gallbladder, or left lobe of the liver. The ICD-10-PCS does include laterality of the procedure as shown in the example in Table 19.4. Body parts are subsets of the body system; in other words, the trachea body part is not listed in the body system ear, nose, and sinus. For accurate coding, only body parts listed in the specific table can be used. If the coding specialist chooses body part characters that are not listed, the coding will be incorrect.

TABLE 19.3 Medical and Surgical Root Operations

Character	Root Operation	Explanation
0	Alteration	Modifying the anatomic structure of a body part without effecting the function of the body part Example: breast augmentation
1	Bypass	Altering the route of passage of the contents of a tubular body part Example: coronary artery bypass
2	Change	Taking out or off a device from a body part and putting back an identical or similar device in or on the same body part without cutting or puncturing the skin or a mucous membrane Example: catheter change
3	Control	Stopping, or attempting to stop, postprocedural or other acute bleeding Example: control of bleeding ulcer
4	Creation	Putting in or on biological or synthetic material to form a new body part that to the extent possible replicates the anatomic structure or function of an absent body part Example: creation of a vagina in a male
5	Destruction	Physical eradication of all or a portion of a body part by the direct use of energy force, or a destructive agent Example: fulguration of a polyp in the colon
6	Detachment	Cutting off all or a portion of the upper of lower extremities Example: below knee amputation
7	Dilation	Expanding an orifice or the lumen of a tubular body part Example: angioplasty
8	Division	Cutting into a body part, without draining fluids and/or gases from the body part, in order to separate or transect a body part Example: osteotomy
9	Drainage	Taking or letting out fluids and/or gases from a body part Example: arthrocentesis
B	Excision	Cutting out or off, without replacement, a portion of a body part Example: pancreatectomy
C	Extirpation	Taking or cutting out solid matter from a body part Example: thrombectomy
D	Extraction	Pulling out or stripping out all or a portion of a body part by use of force Example: vein stripping
F	Fragmentation	Breaking solid matter in a body part into pieces Example: lithotripsy
G	Fusion	Joining together portions of an articular body part rendering the articular body part immobile Example: arthrodesis
H	Insertion	Putting in a nonbiological appliance that monitors, assists, performs or prevents a physiological function but does not physically take the place of a body part Example: insertion of radioactive implant
J	Inspection	Visually and/or manually exploring a body part Example: exploratory laparotomy
K	Map	Locating the route of passage of electrical impulses and/or locating functional areas in a body part Example: cardiac mapping
L	Occlusion	Completely closing an orifice or the opening of a tubular body part Example: tubal ligation
M	Reattachment	Putting back in or on all or a portion of a separated body part to its normal location or other suitable location Example: reattachment of a finger
N	Release	Freeing a body part from an abnormal physical constraint by cutting or by the use of force Example: carpal tunnel release
P	Removal	Taking out or off a device from a body part Example: removal of a pacemaker

Continued

TABLE 19.3   Medical and Surgical Root Operations—cont'd

Character	Root Operation	Explanation
Q	Repair	Restoring, to the extent possible, a body part to its normal anatomic structure and function Example: colostomy takedown
R	Replacement	Putting in or on biological or synthetic material that physically takes the place and/or function of all or a portion of a body part Example: total joint replacement
S	Reposition	Moving to its normal location, or other suitable location, all or a portion of a body part Example: open reduction of a fracture
T	Resection	Cutting out or off, without replacement, all of a body part Example: total nephrectomy
U	Supplement	Putting in or on biological or synthetic material that physically reinforces and/or augments the function of a portion of a body part Example: hernia repair with mesh
V	Restriction	Partially closing an orifice or the lumen of a tubular body part Example: cervical cerclage
W	Revision	Correcting, to the extent possible, a portion of a malfunctioning device, or the position of a displaced device Example: repositioning a pacemaker lead
X	Transfer	Moving, without taking out, all or a portion of a body part to another location to take over the function of all or a portion of a body part Example: tendon transfer
Y	Transplantation	Putting in or on all or a portion of a living body part taken from another individual or animal to physically take the place and/or function of all or a portion of a similar body part Example: kidney transplant

Adapted from ICD-10-PCS, 2021.

TABLE 19.4   Section of ICD-10-PCS Table Showing Laterality of Body Part Characters

0	Medical and Surgical
8	Eye
5	Destruction
Body Part	
Character 4	
0	Eye, right
1	Eye, left
6	Sclera, right
7	Sclera, left
8	Cornea, right
9	Cornea, left
S	Conjunctiva, right
T	Conjunctiva, left

Extracted from ICD-10-PCS, 2021.

Character 5: Approach. The Approach character identifies the technique used to reach the site of the procedure. Some of the options are open (where the procedure is performed directly through an incision), laparoscopically (through small incisions using a camera), and endoscopically (through a natural or artificial opening). Table 19.5 shows a list of approaches and their character. For accurate coding, the documentation should clearly state how the procedure was performed. A placeholder character must be present even when there is no additional information provided.

Character 6: Device. The Device character is used to identify specific devices left in place after a procedure. Examples include artificial hip, pacemaker, tissue expanders,

TABLE 19.5   Examples of ICD-10-PCS Medical and Surgical Character 5: Approach

Open	Cutting through the skin or mucous membrane and any other layers necessary to expose the site of the procedure
Percutaneous	Entry, by puncture or minor incision, of instrumentation through the skin or mucous membrane and any other layers necessary to reach the site of the procedure
Percutaneous Endoscopic	Entry, by puncture or minor incision, of instrumentation through the skin or mucous membrane and any other layers necessary to reach and visualize the site of the procedure
Via Natural or Artificial Opening	Entry of instrumentation through a natural or artificial external opening to reach the site of the procedure
Via Natural or Artificial Opening Endoscopic	Entry of instrumentation through a natural or artificial external opening to reach and visualize the site of the procedure
Via Natural or Artificial Opening Endoscopic with Percutaneous Endoscopic Assistance	Entry of instrumentation through a natural or artificial external opening to reach and visualize the site of the procedure, and entry by puncture or minor incision, of instrumentation through the skin or mucous membrane and any other layers necessary to aid in the performance of the procedure
External	Procedures performed directly on the skin or mucous membrane and procedures performed indirectly by the application of external force through the skin or mucous membrane

Extracted from ICD-10-PCS, 2021.

drainage devices, radioactive elements, and so on. Most procedures do not include a device, thus a character "Z" is used to identify that no device was used. There are typically four types of devices:

- Biological or synthetic material that takes the place of all or a portion of a body part (i.e., skin graft, joint prosthesis)
- Biological or synthetic material that assists or prevents a physiological function (i.e., IUD)
- Therapeutic material that is not absorbed by, eliminated by, or incorporated into the body (i.e., radioactive implant)
- Mechanical or electronic appliances used to assist, monitor, take the place of, or prevent a physiological function (i.e., cardiac pacemaker, orthopedic pin)[a]

Character 7: Qualifier. The Qualifier character provides information for some codes that may not be identified elsewhere. This is used to provide additional information, such as origin of tissue for transplant, destination site of a bypass, or whether the removal of tissue was for diagnostic purposes. If there is no qualifier, this is indicated with the character "Z."

Obstetrics Character Designations

The Obstetrics Section allows only one value for a body system—Pregnancy (0). It offers 12 Root Operations including two unique to this Section:

1. Abortion (A). Artificially terminating a pregnancy. These procedures are broken down by the substance used or if it was done through a mechanical means, such as a vacuum.
2. Delivery (E). Assisting the passage of the products of conception from the genital canal. This root operation applies only to manually assisted vaginal deliveries. Cesarean deliveries are coded to the root operation *Extraction*.

There are only three valid body part characters allowed in this section:

- Products of conception
- Products of conception, retained
- Products of conception, ectopic

The qualifier character varies with the type of procedure. For example, in an assisted delivery, the qualifier may indicate the type of forceps.

Character Designations in Other Sections

Other sections may use some of the characters to designate other details of the procedure. For example, Section 5: Extracorporeal or Systemic Therapies designates the characters as shown as follows:

Character:	1	2	3	4	5	6	7
	Section	Body System	Root Operation	Body Part	Duration	Qualifier	Qualifier

Another example is Section 9: Chiropractic, where Character 6 represents method as opposed to device.

[a]Development of the ICD-10 Procedure Coding System (ICD-10-PCS), Averill, Mullin, Steinbeck, Goldfield, Grant and Butler; https://www.cms.gov/Medicare/Coding/ICD10/downloads/pcs_final_report2012.pdf.

Character:	1	2	3	4	5	6	7
	Section	Body System	Root Operation	Body Part	Approach	Method	Qualifier

A coding specialist will need to familiarize themselves with any nuances in each section.

The Administration Section uses the sixth character to designate substance. This can be a portion of blood such as whole blood, plasma, bone marrow, stem cells, and so on. It can also be a therapeutic substance such as anti-infective, anti-inflammatory, nutritional substance, and so on.

The Measurement and Monitoring Section uses the sixth character to define function/device. For example, the patient may be having pressure, temperature, electrical activity, metabolism, and so on, monitored or tested.

The Imaging Section uses the fifth character to specify contrast used.

In the Radiation Therapy Section, the third character represents Modality as opposed to Root Operation. Modalities include:

- Beam radiation
- Brachytherapy
- Stereotactic radiosurgery
- Other radiation

Characters four through six are also defined differently. Character four is for treatment site that is the focus of the therapy. Five is a modality qualifier that applies to brachytherapy only. Character six is for the isotope or chemical element that is introduced to the body. This, too, only applies to brachytherapy.

The Physical Rehabilitation and Diagnostic Audiology Section uses the fifth character to define type of therapy. Examples are muscle performance, therapeutic exercise, communication skills, various daily living skills such as bathing, feeding and grooming, or auditory processing. The sixth character designates equipment used in the therapy. Some examples here would be mechanical, aerobic, assistive, adaptive, cochlear implant, or audiometer.

ICD-10-PCS Coding Manual

As with the ICD-10-CM Coding Manual, there is both a tabular and alphabetic index in the ICD-10-PCS. The most effective way to code ICD-10-PCS is to use the Tabular Index. The Tabular Index is organized first by Section and then by Body Part. The tables are then presented by Root Operation characters. This method of coding prevents coding specialists from choosing erroneous codes; all acceptable codes are presented within each table. For an example of a complete section of an ICD-10-PCS table, see Table 19.6. Refer to Procedure 19.1 at the end of this chapter to learn how to look up a code in the ICD-10-PCS code set.

While the ICD-10-PCS does have an Alphabetic Index, it is not advisable to rely on this index alone for accurate coding. The alphabetic index is used to direct the coding specialist to the appropriate table, not to provide the complete code. The tables provide the only approved body parts, approaches, devises, and qualifiers. This information can be verified only by using the Section, Body System, and Root Operation tables to ensure accurate coding.

TABLE 19.6　ICD-10-PCS Table, Section 0, Body System C, Operation P

Section	0 Medical and Surgical
Body System	C Mouth and Throat
Root Operation	P Removal: Taking out or off a device from a body part

Body Part Character 4	Approach Character 5	Device Character 6	Qualifier Character 7
A Salivary Gland	0 Open 3 Percutaneous	0 Drainage Device C Extraluminal Device Y Other Device	Z No Qualifier
A Salivary Gland	7 Via Natural or Artificial Opening 8 Via Natural or Artificial Opening Endoscopic	Y Other Device	Z No Qualifier
S Larynx	0 Open 3 Percutaneous 7 Via Natural or Artificial Opening 8 Via Natural or Artificial Opening Endoscopic	0 Drainage Device 7 Autologous Tissue Substitute D Intraluminal Device J Synthetic Substitute K Nonautologous Tissue Substitute Y Other Device	Z No Qualifier
S Larynx	X External	0 Drainage Device 7 Autologous Tissue Substitute D Intraluminal Device J Synthetic Substitute K Nonautologous Tissue Substitute	Z No Qualifier
Y Mouth and Throat	0 Open 3 Percutaneous 7 Via Natural or Artificial Opening 8 Via Natural or Artificial Opening Endoscopic	0 Drainage Device 1 Radioactive Element 7 Autologous Tissue Substitute D Intraluminal Device J Synthetic Substitute K Nonautologous Tissue Substitute Y Other Device	Z No Qualifier
Y Mouth and Throat	X External	0 Drainage Device 1 Radioactive Element 7 Autologous Tissue Substitute D Intraluminal Device J Synthetic Substitute K Nonautologous Tissue Substitute	Z No Qualifier

Extracted from ICD-10-PCS, 2021.

ICD-10-PCS Official Guidelines

Just as the ICD-10-CM has Official Guidelines for coding and reporting, so does the ICD-10-PCS. These guidelines are approved by the AHA, AHIMA, CMS and the National Center for Health Statistics (NCHS). The guidelines establish general rules for choosing and applying the ICD-10-PCS code set. As with any coding system, documentation in the health record is the most important component in accurate code assignment.

It is not expected that a provider will dictate the exact definition of some of the terms used in PCS. For example, if the surgeon documents "partial excision," the coder may correlate that to the root operation "excision," without needing to query the provider.

Guidelines for Body Systems in the Medical and Surgical Section

Procedure codes in some anatomical regions (General, Upper Extremities, and Lower Extremities) may be used when the procedure is performed on an anatomical region as opposed to a specific body part. For example, suture repair of the abdominal wall is coded to the root operation "Repair in the body system Anatomical Regions, General."

When a general body part states "upper" or "lower" (e.g., Upper Arteries and Lower Arteries), the terms "upper" and "lower" refer to body parts located above or below the diaphragm.

Guidelines for Root Operations in the Medical and Surgical Section

There are many guidelines that address selection of root operations. Some examples are as follow:

- Components of a procedure specified in the root operation definition are integral to the root operation and are not coded separately. Procedural steps necessary to reach the site and close the site are not coded separately. For example, Resection of a joint as part of a joint replacement is not coded separately. However, in the case of a mastectomy, immediately followed by a breast reconstruction, both resection and replacement of breast are coded separately.
- If multiple procedures are performed during the same episode, they are coded separately if:

- the same root operation is performed on different body parts as defined by the distinct values in the character,
- the same root operation is repeated on multiple body parts that are separate and distinct,
- multiple root operations are performed on the same body part for different reasons, or
- the intended root operation is attempted with one approach and converts to another approach.

- If an intended procedure is discontinued, code the procedure to the root operation performed. If it is discontinued before any root operation is performed, code the root operation "Inspection."
- Biopsies are coded using root operations "Excision, Extraction," or "Drainage," with the qualifier "Diagnostic." If the biopsy is then followed by a more definitive procedure such as "Destruction, Excision or Resection," both the biopsy and the more definitive treatment are coded.
- If root operations are performed on overlapping layers of the musculoskeletal system, code the body part to the deepest layer.
- Bypasses indicate the body part bypassed *from*, with the body part character and the body part bypassed *to*, with the qualifier character. However, in the case of coronary artery bypass procedures, the body part character identifies the number of arteries bypassed, and the qualifier specifies the body part bypassed to. If multiple coronary arteries are bypassed, a separate code is used for each artery.
- If an attempt to stop bleeding (Control) is not successful, and another, more definitive root operation must be performed such as Bypass, Detachment, Replacement, and so on, the more definitive root operation is coded.
- If an anatomical subdivision of a body part is cut out or off, a Resection of that specific body part should be coded, as opposed to an Excision of a less specific body part. For example, if a let upper lung lobectomy is performed, code Resection of Upper Lung Lobe, left instead of Excision of Lung, Left.

Additional guidance in the root operation section is available for grafts, spinal fusions, inspection procedures, vessel embolization procedures, release procedures, fractures, transplants, and transfers.

Guidelines for Body Parts in the Medical and Surgical Section

There are many guidelines pertaining to the selection of the body part character. Some of them are explained here.

If a procedure is performed on a portion of a body part that is not listed in a table, a coding specialist should code the procedure to the whole body part. If the prefix "peri" is combined with a body part, and not listed specifically in the table, the procedure should be coded to the body part. For example, if a procedure is listed as periosteum, it should be coded to the corresponding bone body part.

If a specific branch of a body part does not have its own character designation, the closest branch is coded. When coding in the cardiovascular body system, it may be necessary to choose the general body part character if the closest branch would lead the coding specialist to assign a code from a different body part system. The example provided

in the official guidelines is for occlusion of the bronchial artery which would be coded to the body part character for Upper Artery in the body system "Upper Arteries" and not to the body part character for Thoracic Aorta, Descending in the body system Heart and Great Vessels.

In ICD-10-PCS, there are few characters to indicate bilateral body parts. If identical procedures are performed on bilateral body parts and no bilateral body part character is listed in the table, the coding specialist will code each procedure separately using the appropriate left and right characters.

Guidelines for Approach in the Medical and Surgical Section

There are four guidelines that pertain to selection of the Approach character. They are as follows:

- Procedures performed using an open approach with endoscopic assistance are coded as open (e.g., laparoscopic-assisted colectomy).
- External approach includes procedures performed within an orifice on structures that are visible without instrumentation (e.g., resection of tonsils).
- Procedures performed indirectly using external force, such as a closed reduction of a fracture, are coded as an external approach.
- Procedures performed via a percutaneous device are coded as a percutaneous approach (e.g., fragmentation of kidney stones via percutaneous nephrostomy).

Guidelines for Device in the Medical and Surgical Section

A device is coded only if the device remains after the procedure. If the device does not remain following the procedure, the device character for "No Device" is assigned. Occasionally, a coding specialist will find characters for Temporary or Intraoperative devices. If a device is intended to remain but is removed before the end of the procedure, both the procedure for the insertion and the procedure for removal are coded.

Sutures, radiological markers, and temporary drains are considered integral to the procedure and are not coded separately.

If a procedure is performed on a device and not a body part, the coding specialist should choose one of the following root operations:

- Change
- Irrigation
- Removal, or
- Revision

If a separate procedure is done to put in a drainage device as opposed to one being placed during another surgical procedure, the root operation Drainage with the device character for Drainage Device should be coded.

Obstetrics Guidelines

If a procedure is performed on the products of conception, it is coded to the Obstetrics section. However, if the procedure is performed on the pregnant female other than the products of conception, it is coded to the Medical and Surgical section. The official guidelines give the example that amniocentesis is coded to the product of conception body part in the Obstetrics section, while repair of obstetric laceration is coded to the appropriate body part in the Medical and Surgical section.

A dilation and curettage (d&c) following delivery or abortion, or evacuation of retained products of conception, are coded in the Obstetrics section. A d&c performed during times other than postpartum or post-abortion period are coded in the Medical and Surgical section.

Radiology Guidelines

If a radioactive brachytherapy source is left in the body after a procedure, it is coded separately as an Insertion with the device character for Radioactive Element. A procedure to place an applicator to deliver the brachytherapy is coded as Insertion with the device character for Other Device.

Principal Procedure Guidelines

The final section of the guidelines instructs the coding professional on how to choose a principal procedure. It states the following guidance:
- If more than one procedure is performed, the procedure performed for the definitive treatment of the principal diagnosis is the principal procedure and should be sequenced first.
- If there are also diagnostic procedures performed for the principal diagnosis, the principal procedure would still be the treatment.

- If a diagnostic procedure is done for the principal diagnosis and a definitive treatment is done for the secondary diagnosis, the diagnostic procedure for the principal diagnosis would be sequenced first as the primary procedure.
- If nothing was done for the principal diagnosis, and treatment and diagnostic procedures were performed for the secondary diagnosis, the definitive treatment of the secondary diagnosis would be the principal procedure.

 19.6 QUICK REVIEW
Question: What is the code structure in the Medical and Surgical section of the ICD-10-PCS?

 19.7 QUICK REVIEW
Question: When are multiple procedures coded separately?

 19.8 QUICK REVIEW
Question: What root operation is coded if a body part is cut out or off?

19.9 QUICK REVIEW
Question: How does a coding specialist determine the principal procedure?

CMS 1450/UNIFORM BILL UB-04

The Uniform Bill (CMS 1450 [UB-04]) claim form is used by facilities such as acute care hospitals, dialysis centers, skilled nursing facilities, and rehabilitation centers to submit charges for outpatient and inpatient services. When a patient receives care in a facility, there are generally two claims generated—one for the facility, and one for the professional services of the health care providers. The CMS-1500, which was discussed in Chapter 14, is used to report all professional and technical services such as provider services, laboratory, and radiology services. The CMS-1450 (UB-04) form is a summary document supported by an itemized or detailed bill in order to collect the facility fee.

Some facilities, such as critical access hospitals and rural health clinics, are required to submit a combined claim for Medicare patients. This claim includes both facility and professional services on the CMS 1450 (UB-04).

The National Uniform Billing Committee (NUBC) is responsible for the design and distribution of the printed CMS-1450 (UB-04). This paper claim form is printed in red ink on white paper for processing with optical scanning equipment.

The CMS-1450 (UB-04) has 81 form locators (FL) or fields and its five sections are divided as follows:

- Provider information (form locators 1 to 7)
- Patient information (form locators 8 to 38)
- Billing information (form locators 39 to 49 and claim line 23)
- Payer information (form locators 50 to 65)
- Diagnostic information (form locators 66 to 81)

Instructions for the completion of the CMS-1450 (UB-04) are the same for inpatient and outpatient claims unless otherwise noted.

Section 1: Provider Information

See Fig. 19.1 to understand the layout of Section 1.

FL 1—Billing Provider Name, Address, and Telephone Number

Required. At minimum, enter the provider name, city, state, and nine-digit ZIP code. The name should be entered exactly as it is on file with the payer to avoid delays in payment.

FL 2—Billing Provider's Designated Pay-to Name, Address, and Secondary Identification Fields

Not Required. If different from FL 1, enter the address in which payment is to be sent to.

FL 3a—Patient Control Number

Required by Medicare and some other third-party payers. Enter the patient's unique alphanumeric account number assigned by the provider's office.

FL 3b—Medical/Health Record Number

Situational. Enter the patient's medical/health record number assigned by the provider's office.

FL 4—Type of Bill

Required. Enter the appropriate four-digit alphanumeric code for type of bill. In general, the code is broken down as follows:

- First digit—zero, ignored by some carriers
- Second digit—type of facility (Table 19.7)
- Third digit—type of care (Table 19.8)

TABLE 19.7 CMS-14500 (UB-04), Type of Bill Code, Second Digit—Type of Facility

1	Hospital
2	Skilled Nursing Facility
3	Home Health
4	Religious Nonmedical Hospital
5	Religious Nonmedical Extended Care (discontinued)
6	Intermediate Care
7	Clinic or Hospital ESRD Facility
8	Special facility or Hospital (CAH or ASC)
9	Reserved for National Assignment

Extracted from https://med.noridianmedicare.com/web/jea/topics/claim-submission/bill-types#fouth.

TABLE 19.8 CMS-1450 (UB-04), Type of Bill Code, Third Digit—Type of Care

1	**Clinics:** Rural Health Center **Special Facilities:** Hospice (non-hospital based) **All Others:** Inpatient Part A
2	**Clinics:** Hospital or Independent Renal Dialysis Center **Special Facilities:** Hospice (hospital based) **All Others:** Inpatient Part B
3	**Clinics:** Free-Standing Provider-Based FQHC **Special Facilities:** ASC Services to Hospital Outpatient **All Others:** Outpatient
4	**Clinics:** Other Rehabilitation Facility **Special Facilities:** Free Standing Birthing Center **All Others:** Other (Part B)
5	**Clinics:** Comprehensive Outpatient Rehabilitation Facility **Special Facilities:** CAH **All Others:** Intermediate Care - Level I
6	**Clinics:** Community Mental Health Center **Special Facilities:** Residential Facility (not used for Medicare) **All Others:** Intermediate Care - Level II
7	**Clinics:** Reserved for National Assignment **Special Facilities:** Reserved for National Assignment **All Others:** Subacute Inpatient Eight Swing Bed
8	**Clinics:** Reserved for National Assignment **Special Facilities:** Reserved for National Assignment **All Others:** N/A
9	**Clinics:** Other **Special Facilities:** Other **All Others:** Reserved for National Assignment

Extracted from https://med.noridianmedicare.com/web/jea/topics/claim-submission/bill-types#fouth.

1 Hometown Hospital	2	3a PAT CNTL #	0012585335			4 TYPE OF BILL
123 Main St		b MED REC #	00001234567			
Anywhere, GA 33333		5 FED. TAX NO.	6 STATEMENT COVERS PERIOD FROM	THROUGH	7	4
		978-65-XXXX	10/21/2018	10/25/2018		

Fig. 19.1 CMS-1450 (UB0-04) Section 1: Provider Information (FL 1–7).

- Fourth digit—sequence of bill in this episode of care or frequency code (Table 19.9)

Some payers will require the first digit to be a zero, while others will not. Medicare prefers to not have a leading zero, instead having the other digits move up one space, the fourth digit being an "x." Other payers may do the same, but instead of an "x" in the fourth place, they require a "1" to indicate all dates of services are included in the claim, a "2" to indicate that this is the first claim and other claims will follow, or a "9" to indicate the last in a series of claims. For example, a hospital inpatient admit through discharge claim would be 0111, SNF initial claim would be 0212, and the final claim for home health services would be 0329.

TABLE 19.9 CMS-1450 (UB-04), Type of Bill Code, Fourth Digit—Frequency Code

0	**Non-payment/Zero Claim:** Use when it does not anticipate payment from payer for the bill, but is informing the payer about a period of non-payable confinement or termination of care. "Through" date of this bill (FL 6) is discharge date for this confinement, or termination of plan of care
1	**Admit Through Discharge:** Use for a bill encompassing an entire inpatient confinement or course of outpatient treatment for which it expects payment from payer or which will update deductible for inpatient or Part B claims when Medicare is secondary to an Employer Group Health Plan
2	**Interim— First Claim:** Use for first of an expected series of bills for which utilization is chargeable or which will update inpatient deductible for same confinement of course of treatment. For HHAs, used for submission of original or replacement RAPs
3	**Interim—Continuing Claims (Not valid for PPS Bills):** Use when a bill for which utilization is chargeable for same confinement or course of treatment has already been submitted and further bills are expected to be submitted later
4	**Interim—Last Claim (Not valid for PPS Bills):** Use for a bill for which utilization is chargeable, and which is last of a series for this confinement or course of treatment
5	**Late Charge Only:** These bills contain only additional charges; however, if a late charge is for: • Services on the same day as outpatient surgery subject to ASC limit; Services on same day as services subject to Outpatient PPS (OPPS); • ESRD services paid under composite rate; • Inpatient accommodation charges; • Services paid under HH PPS; and • Inpatient hospital or SNF PPS ancillaries It must be submitted as an adjustment request (xx7)
7	**Replacement of Prior Claim (See adjustment third digit):** Use to correct a previously submitted bill. Provider applies this code to corrected or "new" bill
8	**Void/Cancel of Prior Claim (See adjustment third digit):** Use to indicate this bill is an exact duplicate of an incorrect bill previously submitted. A code "7" (Replacement of Prior Claim) is being submitted showing corrected information
9	**Final claim for a Home Health PPS Episode:**
A	**Admission/Election Notice for Hospice:** Use when hospice or Religious Non-medical Health Care Institution is submitting Form CMS-1450 as an Admission Notice
B	**Hospice Termination/Revocation Notice:** Use when Form CMS-1450 is used as a notice of termination/revocation for a previously posted Hospice/Medicare Coordinated Care Demonstration/Religious Non-medical Health Care Institution election
C	**Hospice Change of Provider Notice:** Use when Form CMS-1450 is being used as a Notice of Change to Hospice provider
D	**Hospice Election Void/Cancel:** Use when Form CMS-1450 is used as a Notice of a Void/Cancel of Hospice/Medicare Coordinated Care Demonstration/Religious Non-medical Health Care Institution election
E	**Hospice Change of Ownership:** Use when Form CMS-1450 is used as a Notice of Change in Ownership for hospice
F	**Beneficiary Initiated Adjustment Claim:** Use to identify adjustments initiated by beneficiary. For FI use only
G	**CWF Initiated Adjustment Claim:** Use to identify adjustments initiated by CWF. For FI use only
H	**CMS Initiated Adjustment Claim:** Use to identify adjustments initiated by CMS. For FI use only
I	**FI Adjustment Claim (Other than QIO or Provider):** Use to identify adjustments initiated by FI. For FI use only

TABLE 19.9 CMS-1450 (UB-04), Type of Bill Code, Fourth Digit—Frequency Code—cont'd

J	**Initiated Adjustment Claim/Other:** Use to identify adjustments initiated by other entities. For FI use only
K	**OIG Initiated Adjustment Claim:** Use to identify adjustments initiated by OIG. For FI use only
M	**MSP Initiated Adjustment Claim:** Use to identify adjustments initiated by MSP. For FI use only. Note: MSP takes precedence for other adjustment sources
P	**QIO Adjustment Claim:** Use to identify adjustments initiated by QIO. For FI use only
Q	**Reopening/Adjustment:** Use when the submission falls outside of period to submit an adjustment bill

Extracted from https://med.noridianmedicare.com/web/jea/topics/claim-submission/bill-types#fouth.

FL 5—Federal Tax Number

Required. Enter the hospital/facility's federal tax or Employer ID number.

Format is NN-NNNNNNN.

FL 6—Statement Covers Period (From-Through)

Required. Enter the dates indicating when services were provided. (MMDDYY)

FL 7—Leave Blank. Reserved for future use.

Section 2: Patient Information

See Fig. 19.2 to understand the layout of Section 2.

FL 8—Patient's Name and Identifier

Required. Enter the patient ID number if is different than the policy holder's ID number in FL 60. Enter the patient's last name, first name, and middle initial, if any.

FL 9—Patient's Address

Required. Enter the patient's full mailing address.

FL 10—Patient's Birth Date

Required. Enter the patient's date of birth. If full date of birth is unknown, indicate zeros for all eight digits. Formatting may vary by payer as either MMDDYYYY or MM/DD/YYYY.

FL 11—Patient's Sex

Required. Enter the patient's sex. "M" for male, "F" for female, or "U" for unknown. The patient's sex is recorded at admission, outpatient service, or start of care.

FL 12—Admission/Start of Care Date

Required for Inpatient and Home Health. the hospital enters the date the patient was admitted for inpatient care (MMDDYY). The HHA enters the same date of admission that was submitted on the Request for Anticipated Payment for the episode.

FL 13—Admission Hour

Required by some third-party payers. Enter the two-digit code for the hour of the patient's admission be added here. These codes are as follows:

Code	AM (Midnight)	Code	PM (Noon)
00	12:00–12:59	12	12:00–12:59
01	01:00–01:59	13	01:00–01:59
02	02:00–02:59	14	02:00–02:59
03	03:00–03:59	13	03:00–03:59
04	04:00–04:59	14	04:00–04:59
05	05:00–05:59	15	05:00–05:59
06	06:00–06:59	16	06:00–06:59
07	07:00–07:59	17	07:00–07:59
08	08:00–08:59	18	08:00–08:59
09	09:00–09:59	19	09:00–09:59
10	10:00–10:59	20	10:00–10:59
11	11:00–11:59	21	11:00–11:59

FL 14—Priority (Type) of Admission or Visit

Required. Enter the code to indicate the priority of the patient encounter. These codes are as follows:

1	Emergency
2	Urgent
3	Elective
4	Newborn
5	Trauma
6	Information not available

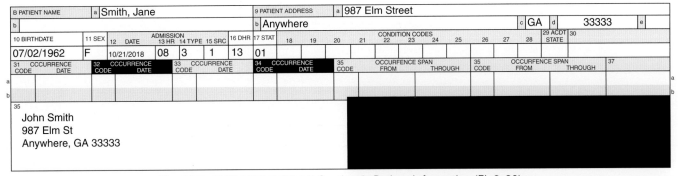

Fig. 19.2 CMS-1450 (UB0-04) Section 2: Patient Information (FL 8–30).

FL 15—Point of Origin for Admission or Visit

Required except for Bill Type 014X—Hospital Other Outpatient (Part B). Enter code to indicate the source of referral. Codes are as follows:

1	Non-health care facility point of origin
2	Clinic or physician's office
4	Transfer from other hospital
5	Transfer from skilled nursing facility, intermediate care facility or assisted living facility
6	Transfer from another health care facility
8	Court/law enforcement
9	Information not available
D	Transfer from one distinct unit of the hospital to another distinct unit of the same hospital, resulting in a separate claim
E	Transfer from ambulatory surgery center
F	Transfer from hospice facility

FL 16—Discharge Hour

Required by some third-party payers. Enter the two-digit code for the hour of the patient's discharge. Format and codes may be payer-specific. For example, some Medicaid payers require the minutes be dropped and the hour be entered in a 24-hour format (00–23). For example, 3 pm = 15.

FL 17—Patient Discharge Status

Required for inpatient, SNF, hospice, HHA and outpatient hospital services. This code indicates the patient's discharge status as of the "through" date of the billing period (FL 6). (Table 19.10)

FLs 18–28—Condition Codes

Situational. Enter the corresponding codes in numerical order to describe any of the following conditions or events that apply to his billing period. Some examples are as follows. (A full listing can be found on Medicare contractor sites.)

01	Military service related
02	Condition is employment related
03	Patient covered by insurance not reflected here
04	Information-only bill
05	Lien has been filed
06	ESRD patient in first 30 months of coverage by employer group health plan
07	Treatment of nonterminal condition for hospice patient
08	Beneficiary would not provide information concerning other insurance coverage
09	Neither patient nor spouse is employed
10	Patient and/or spouse is employed by no employer group health plan exists
17	Patient is homeless
30	Qualifying clinical trials
39	Private room medically necessary
50	Product replacement for known recall of a product
60	Day outlier
61	Cost outlier
AA	Abortion—rape
DR	Disaster related

FL 29—Accident State

Required for some third-party payers. Enter the appropriate two-digit state abbreviation where the auto accident occurred, if applicable to the claim.

TABLE 19.10 CMS-1450 (UB-04), Discharge Status Codes

01	Discharged to home or self-care (routine discharge)
02	Discharged/transferred to another short-term general hospital for inpatient care
03	Discharged/transferred to SNF in anticipation of covered skilled care
04	Discharged/transferred to a facility that provides custodial or supportive care
05	Discharged/transferred to a designated cancer center or children's hospital
06	Discharged/transferred to home health services in anticipation of covered skill care
07	Left against medical advice or discontinued care
09	Admitted as an inpatient to this hospital
20	Patient expired
21	Discharged/transferred to court/law enforcement
30	Still a patient or expected to return for outpatient services
43	Discharged/transferred to a federal health care facility such as a VA hospital or SNF
50	Discharged/transferred to hospice at home
51	Discharged/transferred to hospice in a medical facility
61	Discharged/transferred within this institution to a hospital-based Medicare-approved swing bed
62	Discharged/transferred to an IRF including day procedure units of a hospital
63	Discharged/transferred to long term care hospital
64	Discharged/transferred to Medicaid nursing facility (not Medicare certified)
65	Discharged/transferred to a psychiatric hospital or psychiatric day procedure unit of a hospital
66	Discharged/transferred to a Critical Access Hospital
70	Discharged/transferred to another type of health care institution not defined elsewhere in the code list

Extracted from https://medicare.fcso.com/Ub04/BillCodes.asp#tabs-5.

FL 30—Leave blank. Reserved for future use.

FLs 31–34—Occurrence Codes and Dates

Situational. Required when there is a condition code that applies to the claim. Occurrence codes can be found on the Medicare contractors' sites. Examples of reasons for occurrence codes are crime victim status, onset of symptoms/illness, dates of therapy beginning or ending, dates insurance denied coverage, date SNF bed became available and so on.

FLs 35–36—Occurrence Span Code/Date (From/Through)

Required for Inpatient. Enter codes and associated beginning and ending dates defining specific events relating to the billing period. Examples may be benefit eligibility periods, dates of respite care, and so on.

FL 37—Leave blank. Reserved for future use.

FL 38—Responsible Party Name and Address.

Required for some third-party payers. Enter the name and address of party responsible for the bill.

Section 3: Billing Information

See Fig. 19.3 to understand the layout of Section 3.

FLs 39–41—Value Codes and Amounts

Required. Codes and related dollar or unit amount(s) identify data of a monetary nature that are necessary for processing the claim. If more than one value code is shown, codes are

shown in ascending numeric sequence. A full listing of codes can be found on the Medicare contractor sites. Some examples are listed below.

01	Most common semi-private room rate
02	Hospital has no semi-private rooms
09	Coinsurance amount in the first calendar year
21	Catastrophic
31	Patient liability amount
50	Physical therapy visits
80	Covered days
A1	Deductible payer A
A2	Coinsurance payer A
D3	Patient estimated responsibility

FL 42—Revenue Code

Required. Enter the appropriate revenue code to identify specific accommodation and/or ancillary charges. Each department in the facility will typically have a related revenue code—anesthesia, pharmacy, radiology, laboratory, and so on. Examples of revenue codes are listed in Table 19.11.

FL 43—Revenue Description, IDE Number/Medicaid Drug Rebate

Required for some third-party payers. Enter the description or standard abbreviation for each revenue code. This information assists the clerical bill review. For home health services, enter the DME if applicable. If submitting drug rebate data, submit N4 followed by the 11-digit National Drug Code (NDC).

42 rev co.	43 DESCRIPTION	44 HCPCS /RATE /HPPS CODE	45 SEPT/ DATE	46 SEPT/ UNITS	47 TOTAL CHANGES	48 NON-COVERED CHANGES	49
1 0111	Med/Surg/Gyn			3	1800.00		1
2 0250	Pharmacy - General			10	1782.25		2
3 0260	IV Therapy - General			2	285.55		3
4 0270	General Supplies			5	358.00		4
5 0300	General Lab			10	426.66		5
6 0301	Chemistry Lab			5	257.99		6
7 0730	EKG - General			2	250.00		7
8 0732	EKG - Telemetry			3	450.00		8
9							9
10							10
11							11
12							12
13							13
14							14
15							15
16							16
17							17
18							18
19							19
20							20
21							21
22							22
23	PAGE 1 OF 1	CREATION DATE		TOTALS ▷	1561.45		23

(Value codes section top: 39 CODE / VALUE CODES AMOUNT | 40 CODE / VALUE CODES AMOUNT | 41 CODE / VALUE CODES AMOUNT — rows a, b, c, d)

Fig. 19.3 CMS-1450 (UB0-04) Section 3: Billing Information (FL 39–49 and claim line 23).

TABLE 19.11 Examples of Commonly Used Revenue Codes for Medicare Claims

011X	Room and board (private)
012X	Room and board (semiprivate room, two beds)
015X	Room and board (ward)
020X	Intensive Care Unit
021X	Coronary Care
025X	Pharmacy
026X	IV Therapy
027X	Medical/Surgical Supplies and Devices
028X	Oncology
029X	DME
030X	Laboratory
035X	CT Scan
036X	Operating Room Services
038X	Blood and Blood Components
041X	Respiratory Services
042X	Physical Therapy
043X	Occupational Therapy
054X	Ambulance Services
060X	Home Health Oxygen
065X	Hospice Services

Extracted from CMS.

FL 44—HCPCS/Rates/HIPPS Rate Codes

Required. When coding HCPCS (including CPT) for outpatient services, enter the code describing the procedure here. On inpatient hospital bills the accommodation rate is shown here. For SNFs and LTC facilities, HIPPS rate codes are entered.

FL 45—Service Date

Required for outpatient claims. Enter the applicable six-digit (MMDDYY) date for the service line item.

FL 46—Units of Service

Required. Generally, entries in this FL quantify services by revenue category. For example, it may quantify the number of days in a particular type of accommodation, the number of pints of blood, and so on. However, when HCPCS codes are required, the units are equal to the number of times the procedure/service was performed.

FL 47—Total Charges—Not Applicable for Electronic Billers

Required. Enter the sum of the total charges for each revenue code. The last revenue code entered in FL 42 is "0001" to indicate the grand total of all charges billed. The totals should include both covered and noncovered charges and depending on the payer, may include both inpatient and outpatient services.

FL 48—Noncovered Charges

Required. Enter the total non-covered charges pertaining to the related revenue codes.

FL 49—Leave blank. Reserved for future use.

Line 23: The 23rd line of the UB-04 contains an incrementing page and total number of pages for the claim, creation date of the claim on each page, and a claim total for covered and non-covered charges on the final claim page only indicated by using Revenue Code 0001.

Section 4: Payer Information

See Fig. 19.4 to understand the layout of Section 4.

FLs 50a–c—Payer Identification

A is required; B and C are situational. Enter the health plan(s).

FLs 51a–c—Health Plan ID

A is required; B and C are situational. Enter the health plan(s) ID number(s).

FLs 52a–c—Release of Information Certification Indicator

Required by some third-party payers. Enter a "Y" or "I" to indicate if provider has a signed statement on file from the patient or patient's legal representative allowing provider to release information to the payer.

FLs 53a–c—Assignment of Benefits

Required by some third-party payers. Enter a "Y," "N," or "W" to indicate if provider has a signed statement on file from the patient or patient's legal representative assigning payment to the provider for the primary(a), secondary(b) and/or tertiary(c) payer, if applicable.

FLs 54a–c—Prior Payments

Situational. Required when the indicated payer has paid an amount to the provider towards the bill. Enter the amount of payment the provider has received to date by the health plan toward payment of the claim.

Fig. 19.4 CMS-1450 (UB0-04) Section 4: Payer Information (FL 50–65).

FLs 55a–c—Estimated Amount Due
Required by some third-party payers. Enter the amount estimated by the provider to be due from the payer.

FL 56—Billing Provider National Provider ID (NPI)
Required. Enter the billing provider's 10-digit NPI Number.

FL 57—Other Provider Identifier
Required by some third-party payers such as Medicaid. Reserved for taxonomy code.

FLs 58a–c—Insured's Name
Required. Enter the name of the individual under whose name the insurance is carried for the primary (a), secondary (b), and tertiary (c) insurance, if applicable. Be sure to list the name exactly as it appears on the ID card of the insured to avoid delays in payment.

FLs 59a–c—Patient's Relationship to Insured
Required. Enter the appropriate two-digit code to describe the patient's relationship to the insured for the primary (a), secondary (b), and tertiary (c) insurance, if applicable. Examples of these codes are as follows.

01	Spouse
18	Self
19	Child
20	Employee
21	Unknown
53	Life partner
G8	Other relationship

FLs 60a–c—Insured's Unique Identifier
Required. Enter the insured's identification number for the primary (a), secondary (b), and tertiary (c) insurance, if applicable.

FLs 61a–c—Insured's Group Name
Required, if known. Enter the insured's employer group name for the primary (a), secondary (b), and tertiary (c) insurance, if applicable.

FLs 62a–c—Insured's Group Number
Required, if known. Enter the insured's employer group number for the primary (a), secondary (b), and tertiary (c) insurance, if applicable.

FL 63a–c—Treatment Authorization Code
Situational. Enter the pre-authorization for treatment code assigned by the primary (a), secondary (b), and tertiary (c) insurance, if applicable. Whenever QIO review is performed for outpatient preadmission, pre-procedure or home IV therapy services, the authorization number is required for all approved admissions or services.

FL 64a–c—Document Control Number (DCN)
Situational. Enter the control number assigned to the original bill by the health plan if this is a void or replacement bill.

FL 65a–c—Insured's Employer Name
Situational. Enter the employer name of the insured if the employer is believed to be involved with the payment of the claim (as in worker's compensation cases), or if it is an employer group health plan.

Section 5: Diagnostic Information
See Fig. 19.5 to understand the layout of Section 5.

FL 66—Diagnosis and Procedure Code Qualifier (ICD Version Indicator)
Required. Enter a "9" for ICD-9-CM, or a "0" of ICD-10-CM to indicate the ICD version based on the date of service.

FL 67—Principal Diagnosis Code
Required. Enter the principal diagnosis for the patient's condition. The decimal point is not necessary.

FL 67a–q Other Diagnosis Codes
Situational. Required when other condition(s) coexist or develop subsequently during the patient's treatment. A present on admission (POA) indicator applies to diagnosis codes for inpatient claims to acute care hospitals and other facilities. These are as follows:

Y	Condition was present at time of inpatient admission
N	Condition was not present at time of inpatient admission
U	Documentation is not sufficient to determine if condition was present at time of inpatient admission
W	Clinically undetermined. Provider unable to clinically determine whether the condition was present at the time of inpatient admission.
1	Unreported/Not used. Exempt from POA reporting.

Fig. 19.5 CMS-1450 (UB0-04) Section 5: Diagnostic Information (FL 66–81).

FL 68—Leave blank. Reserved for future use.

FL 69—Admitting Diagnosis Code
Required for inpatient claims.

FL 70—Patient's Reason for Visit
Situational. Required by some payers if certain bill types or revenue codes are reported. Refer to payer guidelines. If not required, it may be reported at the provider's discretion when this information substantiates the medical necessity of services.

FL 71—Prospective Payment System (PPS) Code
Required by some payers for inpatient claims. Enter the DRG based on software for inpatient claims when required under contract grouper with a payer.

FL 72—External Cause of Injury Code
Situational. Enter the cause of injury code or codes when injury, poisoning or adverse effect is the cause for seeking medical care.

FL 73—Principal Procedure Code and Date
Situational. Required on inpatient claims when a procedure was performed. Not used for outpatient claims.

FL 74a–e—Other Procedure Codes and Dates
Situational. Required on inpatient claims only when patient has undergone additional procedures.

FL 75—Leave blank. Reserved for future use.

FL 76—Attending Provider Name and Identifiers (including NPI)
Situational. Required when claim contains any services other than nonscheduled transportation services. The attending provider is the individual who has overall responsibility for the patient's medical care and treatment reported in the claim.

Secondary Identifier Qualifiers are as follows:

0B   State License Number
1G   Provider UPIN Number
G2   Provider Commercial Number

FL 77—Operating Provider Name and Identifiers (including NPI)
Situational. Required when a surgical procedure code is listed on the claim. Enter the name and identification number of the individual with the primary responsibility for performing the surgical procedure(s).

Secondary Identifier Qualifiers are as follows:

0B   State License Number
1G   Provider UPIN Number
G2   Provider Commercial Number

FLs 78–79—Other Provider Name and Identifiers (including NPI)
Situational. The name and ID number of the individual corresponding to the qualifier category indicated in this section of the claim.

Provider type qualifier codes are as follows:

DN   Referring Provider - the provider who sends the patient to another provider for services. Required on outpatient claims when referring provider is different than attending provider.
ZZ   Other Operating Provider—an individual performing a secondary surgical procedure or assisting the operating provider. Required when another operating provider is involved.
82   Rendering Provider—the health care professional who delivers or completes a particular medical service of non-surgical procedure. Report when state or federal regulatory requirements call for a combined claim such as a claim that includes both facility and professional fee components for a Medicaid clinic bill or CAH claim.

Secondary Identifier Qualifiers are as follows:

0B   State License Number
1G   Provider UPIN Number
G2   Provider Commercial Number

FL 80—Remarks
Situational. Enter any information that the provider deems appropriate to share that is not supported elsewhere. Examples for use:
- For DME billing, the provider shows the rental rate, cost, and anticipated months of usage.
- When Medicare is not primary because worker's compensation, no-fault, liability, or an employer group health plan is primary, there will be special notations here.
- For renal dialysis facilities, the provider enters the first month of the 30-month period during which Medicare benefits are secondary to benefits payable under an employer group health plan.

FL 81—Code-Code Field
Situational. To report additional codes related to a Form Locator or to report external code list approved by the NUBC for inclusion to the institutional data set.

Fig. 19.6 illustrates a completed CMS-1450 (UB-04) paper claim form for inpatient services. Colored blocks indicate data obtained by various departments within the facility. Job titles and exact data will vary from facility to facility. Form locator guidelines may vary by payer and may not always follow the visual guidelines presented here.

19.10   QUICK REVIEW
Question: What type of service is reported on a CMS 1450 (UB-04) claim form?

19.11   QUICK REVIEW
Question: What does each digit represent in the Type of Bill FL?

19.12   QUICK REVIEW
Question: What revenue code represents the grand total of all charges billed and what FL does it belong in?

❓ DISCUSSION POINT
Discuss…. the similarities and differences between coding and billing for professional services and for facilities.

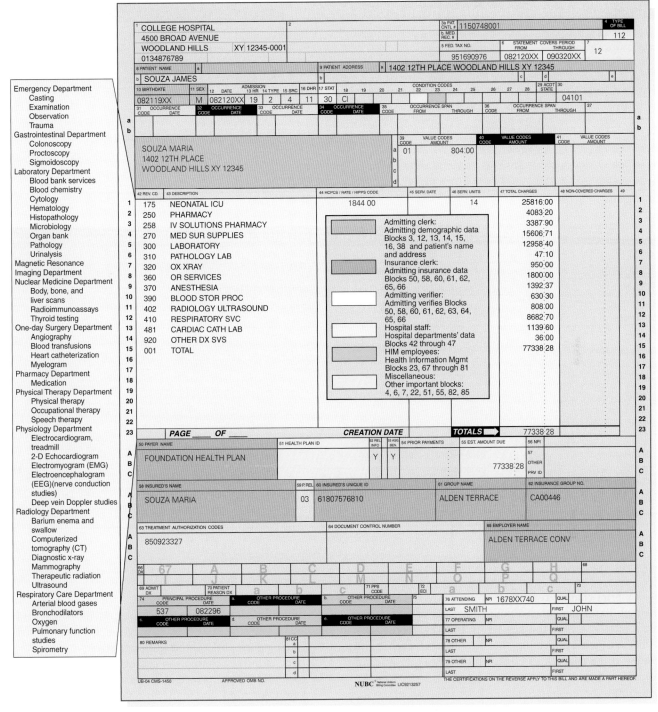

Emergency Department
  Casting
  Examination
  Observation
  Trauma
Gastrointestinal Department
  Colonoscopy
  Proctoscopy
  Sigmoidoscopy
Laboratory Department
  Blood bank services
  Blood chemistry
  Cytology
  Hematology
  Histopathology
  Microbiology
  Organ bank
  Pathology
  Urinalysis
Magnetic Resonance
Imaging Department
Nuclear Medicine Department
  Body, bone, and
    liver scans
  Radioimmunoassays
  Thyroid testing
One-day Surgery Department
  Angiography
  Blood transfusions
  Heart catheterization
  Myelogram
Pharmacy Department
  Medication
Physical Therapy Department
  Physical therapy
  Occupational therapy
  Speech therapy
Physiology Department
  Electrocardiogram,
    treadmill
  2-D Echocardiogram
  Electromyogram (EMG)
  Electroencephalogram
    (EEG)(nerve conduction
    studies)
  Deep vein Doppler studies
Radiology Department
  Barium enema and
    swallow
  Computerized
    tomography (CT)
  Diagnostic x-ray
  Mammography
  Therapeutic radiation
  Ultrasound
Respiratory Care Department
  Arterial blood gases
  Bronchodilators
  Oxygen
  Pulmonary function
    studies
  Spirometry

Fig. 19.6 Completed CMS-1450 (UB0-04).

PROCEDURE 19.1 Coding From an ICD-10-PCS Table

The basic steps in coding for a laparoscopic removal of the gallbladder (cholecystectomy) are as follows:

1. Locate the needed table from the index. Each table represents a three-character code for the Section, Body System, and Root Operation. Some entries in the Alphabetic Index will reference the fourth character for Body Part as well. In the case of coding for a laparoscopic cholecystectomy, the term *cholecystectomy* breaks down into two root operations—excision and resection. In the example, the entire gallbladder is being removed, which would be a resection. This entry in the Alphabetic Index directs the coding specialist to the table 0FT4. See Table 19.12 for a section of the appropriate table as a reference.

2. The body part, gallbladder (4), was indicated in the index entry.

3. The next character is *approach*. The information about the approach can be found in the operative report. Definitions of the approaches can be found in the official ICD-10-PCS guidelines. Since the example surgery states laparoscopic, the approach character will be 4 for percutaneous endoscopic.

4. The next character is for device. The table contains only one character for device, so the device character will be Z.

5. The final character is for qualifier. The table contains only one character for device, so the qualifier character will be Z.

6. The complete seven-digit ICD-10-PCS code for a laparoscopic cholecystectomy is 0FT44ZZ.
See Table 19.12.

TABLE 19.12 ICD-10-PCS Table, Section 0, Body System F, Root Operation B

Section	**0** Medical and Surgical		
Body System	**F** Hepatobiliary System and Pancreas		
Operation	**T** Resection: Cutting out or off, without replacement, all of a body part		
Body Part **Character 4**	**Approach** **Character 5**	**Device** **Character 6**	**Qualifier** **Character 7**
0 Liver 1 Liver, right lobe 2 Liver, left lobe 4 Gallbladder G Pancreas	0 Open 4 Percutaneous Endoscopic	Z No Device	**Z** No Qualifier
5 Hepatic duct, right 6 Hepatic duct, left 7 Hepatic duct, common 8 Cystic duct 9 Common bile duct C Ampulla of Vater D Pancreatic duct F Pancreatic duct, accessory	0 Open 4 Percutaneous Endoscopic 7 Via natural or Artificial Opening 8 Via natural or Artificial Opening Endoscopic	Z No Device	**Z** No Qualifier

Extracted from ID-10-PCS, 2021.

■ KEY POINTS

This is a brief chapter review, or summary, of the key issues presented. To further enhance your knowledge of the technical subject matter, review the key terms and key abbreviations for this chapter by locating the meaning for each in the Glossary at the end of this book, which appears in a section before the index.

1. Facilities are reimbursed for the following types of services:
   - use of the operating room and recovery room,
   - medical and surgical supplies such as surgical instruments, bandages and bed pans,
   - medications,
   - diagnostic and therapeutic services,
   - various clinical services such as nurses and operating room technicians, and
   - if the patient has an overnight stay, room and board.
   Different types of services require different code sets and billing forms.

2. When a patient is admitted as an inpatient to a facility, he/she receives different types of services that are not reflected in CPT codes. As such, inpatient facility billing requires a

different code set, the ICD-10-PCS, which will be discussed in further detail later in this chapter. Facilities may also bill for professional services if they employ the physicians, radiologists, physical therapists and so on.

3. One of the key concepts in coding inpatient services is the definition of the principal diagnosis. It is the reason, after study, for admission to the hospital. This code is listed first on the health care claim. This is true even if the original treatment plan is not carried out.

4. For inpatient cases, code all "rule out," "suspected," "likely," "questionable," "possible," or "still to be ruled out," as if it existed. This is in direct contrast to the rules for outpatient coding in which these uncertain diagnosis codes are not included.

5. If a patient is admitted to observation due to complications from outpatient surgery, the reason for the surgery is still treated as the first listed diagnosis. The codes for the complications are listed as secondary diagnoses.

6. If the patient is admitted to an inpatient status due to a complication from the surgery, assign the complication as the

principal diagnosis. If no complication is documented, assign the reason for the outpatient surgery as the principal diagnosis. If the reason for admission is unrelated to the surgery, assign the unrelated condition as the principal diagnosis.

7. Inpatient procedures are coded using the International Classification of Disease, Tenth Edition, Procedure Coding System (ICD-10-PCS). This coding system uses a table format to allow for unique identification of each procedure. ICD-10-PCS codes have a seven-character alphanumeric code structure that is multi-axial. In other words, the code set is divided by various sections and then further defined by smaller classifications.

8. The ICD-10-PCS structure for the largest Section, Medical and Surgical, is as follows:

Character:	1	2	3	4	5	6	7
	Section	Body System	Root Operation	Body Part	Approach	Device	Qualifier

9. The most effective way to code ICD-10-PCS is to use the Tabular Index. The Tabular Index is organized first by Section and then by Body Part. The tables are then presented by Root Operation characters. This method of coding prevents coding specialists from choosing erroneous codes; all acceptable codes are presented within each table.

10. Just as the ICD-10-CM has Official Guidelines for coding and reporting, so does the ICD-10-PCS. These guidelines are approved by the AHA, AHIMA, CMS, and the National Center for Health Statistics (NCHS). The guidelines establish general rules to choosing and applying the ICD-10-PCS code set. As with any coding system, documentation in the health record is that most important component in accurate code assignment.

11. The Uniform Bill (CMS 1450 [UB-04]) claim form is used by facilities such as acute care hospitals, dialysis centers, skilled nursing facilities and rehabilitation centers to submit charges for outpatient and inpatient services. When a patient receives care in a facility, there are generally two claims generated—one for the facility, and one for the professional services of the health care providers.

12. The CMS-1450 (UB-04) has 81 form locators or fields and its five sections are divided as follows:
   - Provider information (form locators 1 to 7)
   - Patient information (form locators 8 to 38)
   - Billing information (form locators 39 to 49 and claim line 23)
   - Payer information (form locators 50 to 65)
   - Diagnostic information (form locators 66 to 81)

INTERNET RESOURCES

CMS ICD-10-PCS Guidelines
- https://www.cms.gov/Medicare/Coding/ICD10/2020-ICD-10-PCS

CMS ICD-10-CM Guidelines
- https://www.cms.gov/files/document/2021-coding-guidelines.pdf

Novitas Guidance for UB-04 Completion
- https://www.novitas-solutions.com/webcenter/portal/MedicareJH/pagebyid?contentId=00103784

National Uniform Billing Committee (NUBC)
- https://www.nubc.org/

STUDENT ASSIGNMENT

- Study Chapter 19.
- Complete the assignments in the *Workbook* to reinforce the theory learned in this chapter.
- Turn to the Glossary at the end of this text for a further understanding of the key terms and key abbreviations used in this chapter.

Employment

20

Seeking a Job and Attaining Professional Advancement

Linda M. Smith

OBJECTIVES

After reading this chapter, you should be able to:

1. Prepare to find a position as an insurance billing specialist, claims assistance professional, or electronic claims processor.
2. Identify advanced job opportunities for insurance billing specialists.
3. List advantages of becoming affiliated with professional organizations.
4. State types of certifications available to insurance billers and coders.
5. State and discuss various actions to take when searching for a job.
6. Search online for employment opportunities and discuss job fairs.
7. List guidelines for completing job application forms.
8. Compose a letter of introduction to accompany the résumé.
9. Analyze education and experience to prepare a traditional or electronic résumé.
10. Prepare responses to common interview questions.
11. Identify illegal interview questions.
12. Name the items to assemble for a job portfolio and discuss follow-up letters.
13. Explore the business aspects of self-employment.
14. Discuss the importance of networking for professional advancement.

KEY TERMS

American Academy of Professional Coders (AAPC)
American Health Information Management Association (AHIMA)
application form
auditor
blind mailing
business associate agreement
certification
Certified Coding Specialist
Certified Coding Specialist–Physician
Certified Medical Assistant

Certified Medical Billing Specialist
Certified Professional Coder
chargemaster coordinator
chronologic résumé
clinical documentation improvement specialist
coding specialist
combination résumé
compliance specialist
continuing education
cover letter
employment agencies
functional résumé

interview
mentor
National Certified Insurance and Coding Specialist
networking
portfolio
Registered Medical Assistant
Registered Medical Coder
résumé
Revenue Cycle Manager
self-employment
service contract

KEY ABBREVIATIONS

AAPC	CECP	CPC-H	PAHCOM
AHIMA	CMA	ECP	RMA
CAP	CMBS	EEOC	RMC
CCAP	CMRS	FCS	USCIS
CCS	CPC	HRS	
CCS-P	CPC-A	NCICS	

INSIGHTS FROM THE FIELD

Cheryl F.: CPC, CRC, CPMA, CPPM, CPB, CDEO, CPC-I

I started in the field of medical billing 27 years ago, with no related knowledge or experience. After my first 5 years in billing, I transitioned to the position of practice manager for the anesthesia group I was working with. During that time, I saw the world of health care changing and many independent anesthesiology groups becoming employees of large health care facilities. I became concerned that my job could disappear tomorrow, and questioned if I would be able to transition to another type of practice. This fear encouraged me to look into certifications. I got my first coding certification (CPC), and 8 years later, I have obtained a total of seven varied certifications. Pursuing and achieving these certifications have not only expanded my knowledge base but made me a better practice manager. The journey has built discipline and confidence in myself and my abilities. I am more confident with the providers I work with, and in turn, they give me more respect. The journey has brought new opportunities to me, helped me mentor other people, and made me a better leader. And in the end, I am certain that there are *many* more possibilities for me.

EMPLOYMENT OPPORTUNITIES

Insurance Billing Specialist

Employment opportunities are available throughout the United States for insurance billing specialists who attain knowledge of insurance programs, develop coding skills, and display expertise in completing insurance claims accurately.

Because of the complexities of billing for health care services, there has been a corresponding increase in the need for insurance billing specialists. Health care organizations are looking for individuals who have knowledge of state and federal laws associated with the billing process, a firm understanding of Health Insurance Portability and Accountability Act (HIPAA) laws, and a solid foundation in fraud and abuse controls. They are also looking for individuals who have knowledge of the primary insurances that are routinely billed by health care organizations, such as Medicare, Medicaid, workers' compensation, and third-party payers. They are looking for insurance billing specialists who understand coding, the claims submission process, the reimbursement process, and revenue cycle management (Fig. 20.1).

The complexities of billing for health care services have also expanded the range of career titles the individual may see

Fig. 20.1 Staff conference discussing applicants for potential interviews.

advertised as available positions. A few of these job titles will be broad and cover the entire billing process, whereas others may be very specific and focused on a narrow set of job skills. Some of the job titles may be listed as follows:

- Electronic claims processor (ECP)
- Medicare or Medicaid billing specialist
- Workers' compensation specialist
- Reimbursement specialist
- Collection specialist
- Claims examiner
- Claims assistance professional (CAP)

Advanced Job Opportunities

As the insurance billing specialist gains experience and knowledge, there may be employment opportunities in more advanced roles. More advanced job opportunities might include the following positions.

Coding Specialist

Coding specialists are responsible for assigning the diagnosis and procedure codes that are included on the insurance claim. To assign the code, the medical coder must understand medical records, anatomy, diseases and conditions, procedures, pharmacology, medical terminology, and more. The coder must be able to identify key information in the medical record and assign the code based on the official coding guidelines and other resources.

The coder has a tremendous amount of responsibility because the health care organization's reimbursement is usually based on the diagnosis and procedure codes. Coding errors can cost the health care organization hundreds if not thousands of dollars and possibly result in accusations of fraud and abuse. As a result, coders are expected to code with a 95% to 98% accuracy rate. Coders are constantly learning about changes in the coding system, changes in procedures, and more.

Coders typically must earn a certificate in coding or an associate degree in health information management. Prospective students seeking a certificate in medical coding should look for a coding program that has been recognized as a Professional Certificate Approval Program. The two most widely known associations that award these certifications are the American Health Information Management Association (AHIMA) and the American Academy of Professional Coders (AAPC).

Clinical Documentation Improvement (CDI) Specialist

The clinical documentation improvement (CDI) specialist works with physicians and other health care professionals to ensure that the documentation in the medical record is complete and granular (at the appropriate level of detail). The CDI specialist must understand health care documentation, diseases, medical coding systems, and so forth, just as the coders do. Clinical documentation improvement is the process an organization undertakes to improve clinical specificity and documentation that will allow coding professionals to assign more concise disease classification codes.

Some of the ways that the CDI specialist improves clinical documentation include offering educational programs to physicians and other health care providers, writing articles for newsletters, and writing queries. The intent of CDI programs is to improve the quality of documentation available to the coders. For example, the health care provider may write that the patient has pneumonia but not provide the organism causing the pneumonia. In this case, the coder must assign the generic pneumonia code, though a more specific diagnosis code could be used if the organism was specified. Another example is a fracture of the tibia. The diagnostic statement does not provide the coder with information regarding which portion of the tibia is fractured, nor does it document laterality (right or left). Without detailed information, the specific code cannot be assigned, and a nonspecific code must be used. Both AHIMA and the AAPC offer certifications related to clinical documentation improvement.

Chargemaster Coordinator

The chargemaster coordinator manages the contents of the health care facility's listing of billable items. This listing, also referred to as the chargemaster, identifies all the services provided by the health care facility, the amounts charged for these services, and the corresponding codes. The chargemaster coordinator updates codes, adds new services, removes services that are no longer provided, and updates charge amounts as needed. The chargemaster coordinator must work with the clinical services, billers, financial department, and others to ensure the entries in the chargemaster meets their needs. Failure to maintain the chargemaster will result in overpayments and underpayments for services, submitting claims with invalid codes, and many other problems. This position is critical to the revenue cycle, as data in the chargemaster is used in the creation of health care claims.

Revenue Cycle Manager

Revenue cycle managers are responsible for overseeing billing accounts and helping departments resolve their revenue cycle problems. They oversee the billing teams that manage accounts, communication with insurance companies, collections, contract analysis, cash posting, billing transactions with clients, and create accounts receivable reports. Revenue cycle managers help ensure that these all aspects of the accounts receivable process run smoothly, and they must detect problems in the billing systems and correct them accordingly.

A revenue cycle manager must be an innovative person. As problems arise, they must find solutions. They must implement new processes and automations into various areas of the billing cycle. The revenue cycle manager may work in a medical facility or office setting, but also may move around the facility to communicate with various departments.

Auditor

Auditors monitor revenue cycle activities. The title varies according to what they are monitoring. Examples include diagnosis-related group (DRG) auditors and revenue cycle auditors. Auditors may be responsible for the ongoing auditing of health care claims, documentation, and other components of the revenue cycle. The auditor must have an overall understanding of the functions of the revenue cycle so that issues can be found. This includes understanding coding, documentation, revenue cycle, auditing, statistical analysis, federal and state laws, and more. The purpose of the audits is to identify and correct issues in the revenue cycle process before the Center for Medicare and

Medicaid Services or any other payer investigates the health care organization for fraud and abuse practices. Auditors ensure that policies and procedures are being followed. They also monitor the quality of billing, coding, and other revenue cycle steps to ensure the steps are being performed accurately. The auditor generates statistical reports that are then shared with management. These reports show the number of audits, error rates, types of errors, who is making the errors, and more.

Compliance Specialist

Compliance is a growing specialty in the health care field. Large and small health care organizations, including billing companies, are required to have an individual or a team of individuals who oversee compliance. A compliance specialist is responsible for the development and management of the health care organization's compliance program. These individuals assist in the development and monitoring of policies, procedures, and audit programs. They are responsible for identifying issues and for corrective action follow-up. The individual in this role must understand the compliance program, federal and state laws, data analysis, management of people, problem resolution, and much more.

An insurance billing specialist may be asked to be part of a compliance team. Even if a health care worker's job is not specifically focused on compliance, with training they can provide support and knowledge to the organization's efforts. There are several organizations that offer certification and training in compliance.

 20.1 QUICK REVIEW

Question: Because of the complexities of billing for health care services, health care organizations look for individuals with specific areas of knowledge and expertise. What are they?

PROFESSIONAL ORGANIZATIONS

Membership in professional organizations is an opportunity for the insurance billing specialist to surround themselves with others in their field to exchange information or services and help them keep up to date with current trends. Professional organizations offer continuing education opportunities through various types of publications, webinars, and conferences (local, regional, and national). Professional organizations can also assist with problem solving, provide reliable resources, and direct the insurance billing specialist to employment opportunities. Most of these associations have student (as well as active and associate) membership categories. In general, there are local chapters or state organizations affiliated with the national association. In addition to the professional organizations listed in Table 20.1, the Medical Association of Billers (MAB), the Healthcare Billing and Management Association (HBMA), AHIMA, and AAPC are some of the most popular professional organizations insurance billing specialists can be affiliated with.

Certification

An additional benefit to belonging to a professional organization is the opportunity to become certified. Certification is the process of earning a credential through a combination of advanced

TABLE 20.1 Certifications

Certification Title (Abbreviation)	Description to Obtain Certification or Registration	Professional Association Mailing Address	Website
• Advanced Coding Specialist (ACS) • Specialty Coding Professional (SCP) • Certified Compliance Professional–Physician (CCP-P)	2–3 years of experience and working knowledge of coding in the specialty	Board of Medical Specialty Coding 9737 Washington Blvd. Suite 200 Gaithersburg, MD 20878	www.medicalspecialtycoding.com
• Certified Billing and Coding Specialist (CBCS) • Certified Electronic Health Records Specialist (CEHRS)	Graduate of health care training program or 1 or more year(s) of full-time job experience; exam or home study certification program	National Healthcare Association 11161 Overbrook Rd. Leawood, KS 66211	www.nhanow.com
• Certified Bookkeeper (CB)	Self-study program and employment experience; pass three tests	American Institute of Professional Bookkeepers 6001 Montrose Rd. Suite 500 Rockville, MD 20852	www.aipb.org
• Certified Coding Associate (CCA) • Certified Coding Specialist (CCS) • Certified Coding Specialist–Physician (CCS-P) • Certified in Healthcare Privacy and Security (CHPS)	Self-study program; pass certification examination	American Health Information Management Association (AHIMA) 233 N. Michigan Ave. 21st Floor Chicago, IL 60601-5809	www.ahima.org
• Certified Specialist Accounting and Finance (CSAF)	2 or more years in health care	Healthcare Financial Management Association (HFMA) 3 Westbrook Corporate Center Suite 600 Westchester, IL 60154-5700	www.hfma.org
Claims assistant professional (CAP)	No formal certification process	Alliance of Claims Assistance Professionals (ACAP) 9600 Escarpment Suite 745-65 Austin, TX 78749	www.claims.org
Certified Healthcare Billing and Management Executive (CHBME)	Complete comprehensive program; pass proficiency test	Healthcare Billing and Management Association (HMBA) 2025 M St. NW Suite 800 Washington, D.C. 20036	www.hbma.com
Certified in Healthcare Compliance (CHC)	Have work experience and continuing education credits and pass examination	Health Care Compliance Association 6500 Barrie Rd. Suite 250 Minneapolis, MN 55435	www.hcca-info.org
Certified Medical Assistant (CMA)	Graduate from accredited medical assisting program; apply to take national certifying examination	American Association of Medical Assistants (AAMA) 20 North Wacker Dr. Suite 1575 Chicago, IL 60606	www.aama-ntl.org
Certified Medical Billing Specialist (CMBS)	Complete 6 courses and provide evaluation of billing performance by supervisor	Medical Association of Billers (MAB) 2620 Regatta Dr. Suite 102 Las Vegas, NV 89128	www.mabillers.com
Certified Medical Manager (CMM)	Examination for supervisors or managers of small-group and solo practices	Professional Association of Health Care Office Management (**PAHCOM**) 1576 Bella Cruz Dr. Suite 360 Lady Lake, FL 32159	www.pahcom.com
• Certified Medical Practice Executive (CMPE) • Nominee first level • Certification second level • Fellow third level	• First level—Eligible group managers join; membership/nominee • Second level—Complete 6- to 7-hour examination • Third level—Mentoring project of thesis	Medical Group Management Association (MGMA), American College of Medical Practice Executives (affiliate) 104 Inverness Terrace East Englewood, CO 80112-5306	www.mgma.com

Continued

TABLE 20.1 Certifications—cont'd

Certification Title (Abbreviation)	Description to Obtain Certification or Registration	Professional Association Mailing Address	Website
• Certified Medical Coder (CMC) • Certified Medical Insurance Specialist (CMIS) • Certified Medical Compliance Officer (CMCO)	Self-study program and successfully pass exam	Practice Management Institute 8242 Vicar Dr. San Antonio, TX 78218	www.pmimd.com
Certified Medical Reimbursement Specialist (CMRS)	Self-study program; successfully pass 18 sections of examination	American Medical Billing Association (AMBA) 2465 E. Main Davis, OK 73030	www.ambanet.net
Registered Healthcare Documentation Specialist (RHDS) Certified Healthcare Documentation Specialist (CHDS)	Self-study program and successfully pass written and practical examinations offered by Medical Transcription Certification Commission (MTCC)	Association for Healthcare Documentation Integrity (AHDI) 4120 Dale Rd. Suite J8-233 Modesto, CA 95356	www.ahdionline.org
• Certified Revenue Cycle Executive (CRCE) • Certified Revenue Cycle Professional (CCRCP) • Certified Revenue Integrity Professional (CRIP) • Certified Revenue Cycle Specialist (CRCS) • Certified Compliance Technician (CCT)	Complete self-study course; pass standard examination administered twice yearly	American Association of Healthcare Administrative Management (AAHAM) National Certification Examination Program 11240 Waples Mill Rd. Suite 200 Fairfax, VA 22030	www.aaham.org
• Certified Professional Coder (CPC) • Certified Outpatient Coder • Certified Inpatient Coder • Certified Professional Biller (CPB)	Independent study program; pass examination approximately 5 h (CPC) and 8 h (CPC-H) in length	American Academy of Professional Coders (AAPC) 2233 South Presidents Dr. Suite F Salt Lake City, UT 84120	www.aapc.com
National Certified Insurance and Coding Specialist (NCICS)	Graduate from an insurance program; sit for certification examination given by independent testing agency at many school sites across the nation	National Center for Competency Testing 7007 College Blvd. Suite 385 Overland Park, KS 66211	www.ncctinc.com
Registered Medical Assistant (RMA)	Sit for certification exam	American Medical Technologists (AMT) 10700 West Higgins Rd. Suite 150 Rosemont, IL 60018	www.americanmedtech.org
Compliance Certification Board (CCB)	Examination, work experience, and continuing education	Health Care Compliance Association 6500 Barrie Rd. Suite 250 Minneapolis, MN 55435	www.hcca-info.org

education and experience. Upon a person's satisfactory completion of requirements, the board or association will issue a certification statement verifying that the person meets the professional standards of that organization (see Table 20.1). Professional certifications identify experts in the field and can contribute to career advancement. Some certifications that an insurance billing specialist may want to explore include the following:
- Certified Medical Billing Specialist (CMBS)
- Certified Medical Reimbursement Specialist (CMRS)
- Certified Professional Coder (CPC)
- Certified Professional Coder–Apprentice (CPC-A)
- Certified Professional Coder–Hospital (CPC-H)
- Certified Coding Specialist (CCS)
- Certified Coding Specialist–Physician (CCS-P)

- Certified Electronic Claims Processor (CECP)
- Certified Claims Assistance Professional (CCAP)
- Facility Coding Specialist (FCS)
- Health Care Reimbursement Specialist (HRS)
- National Certified Insurance and Coding Specialist (NCICS)
- Registered Medical Coder (RMC)

Becoming certified is essential if one seeks career advancement. Credentials validate individuals' knowledge and expertise in the field and show their commitment in following the standards and code of ethics set by the professional organization they belong to. Credentials help insurance billing specialists advance their career, help health care organizations effectively manage their revenue cycle, ensure compliance, and prepare for future changes in health care.

Certified members of professional organizations must keep up to date by continuing to take educational sessions and earn continuing education credits to maintain their certification credential. Continuing education is intended to improve or maintain professional competence.

🎓 20.2 QUICK REVIEW

Question: Certification is the process of earning a credential through a combination of advanced education and experience. Why is professional certification important?

JOB SEARCH

In addition to possessing the skills necessary for the job, an insurance billing specialist should ask themselves the following questions to determine whether they need to sharpen their job-seeking techniques:

- Are you motivated and interested in finding a job?
- Can you communicate effectively in an interview?
- Are you prepared to market yourself and your skills?
- Do you present yourself in a knowledgeable and professional manner?

An insurance billing specialist can seek employment in several ways. Individuals may prefer to be employed by a physician, hospital, medical facility, insurance company, or managed care organization (MCO). The individual may choose to be self-employed if they have had a number of years of experience, or may even choose some type of combination situation. The following list suggests actions to take when searching for a job:

1. Explore the internet using a smartphone, tablet, or computer. Visit websites of professional billing and coding organizations. Make it easy to be found by being on LinkedIn, ExecuNet, or other professional networking sites. Resumes should be uploaded to as many databases as possible. Search names of local professional offices and hospitals to contact.
2. Join a professional organization to network with others in the same career field and hear about job openings (Fig. 20.2). Some chapters may have a newsletter that allows posting of available jobs.
3. Attend meetings and workshops in the career field to keep up-to-date and network with others.
4. For those who have just completed a course at a community college or trade school, a school placement office may be able to assist.
5. Spread the word to those who work in medical settings or might hear of openings in medical facilities, such as classmates, instructors, school counselors, relatives, and friends.
6. Contact pharmaceutical representatives who visit physicians' offices and hospitals for employment information or leads.
7. Visit public and private employment agencies, including temporary and temporary-to-permanent agencies. Before signing with an agency, ask whether the employer or applicant pays the agency fee.
8. Inquire at state and federal government offices and their employment agencies.
9. Look for part-time employment that might lead to a permanent full-time position.

Fig. 20.2 Student scanning a professional journal for job leads.

10. Check bulletin boards in the personnel offices of hospitals and clinics frequently for posted job offerings.
11. Check with a local medical society, which may be able to assist in offering job leads.
12. Send a blind mailing of the résumé and cover letter to possible prospects. A blind mailing means to send information to employers who have not advertised for a job opening.
13. Visit the local chamber of commerce to request some of their publications containing membership directories and names of major professional employers in specific areas.
14. Subscribe to an online principal newspaper from the city where employment is desired. Read help wanted advertisements in the classified section of the newspaper. Do not be discouraged by specific requirements in an advertisement; apply anyway. Send or transmit an email with a professional résumé and a cover letter the next day. Some employers give priority to candidates who respond within the first 3 or 4 days after a job announcement because they believe it is an indication that someone is truly interested in the position.
15. Email or telephone job hotlines of large medical clinics in the area.
16. Visit job locations unannounced (referred to as "cold calling").

Online Job Search

Because of the internet, newspaper and magazine classified advertisements may become resources of the past. An individual with internet access through a mobile device, tablet, or computer can locate potential employers who are offering jobs to health care workers on their websites. Typically, websites will provide detailed descriptions of positions that are available and allow individuals to respond to a specific job of interest by completing an online application or delivering an online résumé. Employers may use automated résumé scanning to sort emailed résumés for key words. Use standard typefaces and font sizes from 10 to 14 points. Keep text lines under 65 characters and use boldface for section headings.

To have a 95% to 100% key word match for the position, it is best to sprinkle the résumé and cover letter with the verbiage

Fig. 20.3 Student doing an online job search.

used in the job advertisement. Key words can be entered at the end of the document. To make them unnoticeable, select the words and make the font color white; they will not appear when printed or viewed on a monitor, but the electronic scan will see them when sorting.

Individuals without internet access may be able to use the campus internet. Many libraries have computers with free internet service (Fig. 20.3).

Helpful websites include www.jobsearch.about.com and www.indeed.com, which feature résumé templates and examples. Check out websites such as www.ziprecruiter.com, www.glassdoor.com, www.careerbuilder.com, and www.monster.com, which list job postings that can be browsed according to field, location, and career type. Many of these sites also allow job seekers to post their résumés at no cost.

Job Fairs

Annual community events feature job fairs at community colleges and technical trade schools. Some job fairs are sponsored by professional associations. Job recruiters set up booths with information about their companies and available positions; however, they do not have much time to spend with each job seeker. Thus, it is wise to go prepared and practice a 30-second introduction before attending. This introduction should consist of a quick overview of the applicant's career goals, experience, skills, training, education, and personal strengths. These are usually daylong events that allow applicants to investigate several participating employers' booths.

Individuals should prepare by dressing professionally and carrying a binder or folder of résumé copies to give to company representatives. Résumés should be neat, clean, and not folded,

wrinkled, or coffee stained. It is helpful to research which employers will be attending. Keep a positive attitude and approach each employer with confidence and enthusiasm.

Individuals should take home the business card and brochure of any potential employers they are genuinely interested in. After the fair, the individual should send the recruiter a follow-up letter or email message to reaffirm their interest.

Application

When visiting a potential employer, ask for an application form to complete and inquire whether the facility keeps potential job applicants on file and for how long (Fig. 20.4). Study each question on the application form carefully before answering and follow instructions. Furnish as much information as possible; if a question does not apply or cannot be answered, insert "no," "none," "NA" (not applicable), or "DNA" (does not apply). Some application forms may request information that could be considered discriminatory. If this occurs, it is important to use good judgment on whether to insert or omit an answer.

Follow these guidelines when completing an application form:

1. Read the whole application before completing; some instructions may appear on the last page or last line.
2. Read the fine print and instructions: "Please print," "Put last name first," or "Complete in your own handwriting." Responses indicate one's ability to follow instructions.
3. Abbreviate only when there is a lack of space.
4. Complete the application in black ink, unless pencil is specified.
5. Refer to data from a sample application form or résumé that has been checked for accuracy; copy this information onto each new application form. Be neat.
6. List correct dates of previous employment, in case the employer seeks verification. If a question asks for the applicant's reason for leaving a position, insert "to be discussed during the interview."
7. Name specific skills such as procedural coding, diagnostic coding, knowledge of insurance programs, ability to complete and/or transmit the CMS-1500 claim form, keyboarding (number of words per minute), fluency in a second language, knowledge of medical terminology, and knowledge and use of computer software.
8. When a question is asked about salary amount, write in "negotiable" or "flexible" and then discuss this during the interview.
9. Sign the application after completion.
10. Reread the entire form, word for word, to find any errors or omissions.

Letter of Introduction

Individuals spend days perfecting a résumé but throw together an email message or cover letter in minutes. This is a mistake. The main goal of the cover letter is to get the employer to take notice of the potential employee and résumé. A cover letter may be in the form of an email message, so make sure the subject line is clean and specific to the job being applied for (e.g., "Bilingual health insurance specialist seeks billing position"). Messages or

APPLICATION FOR POSITION / Medical or Dental Office
AN EQUAL OPPORTUNITY EMPLOYER

No employee, applicant, or candidate for promotion, training or other advantage shall be discriminated against (or given preference) because of race, color, religion, sex, age, physical handicap, veteran status, or national origin.

PLEASE READ CAREFULLY AND WRITE OR PRINT ANSWERS TO ALL QUESTIONS. DO NOT TYPE.

(In answering questions, use extra blank sheet if necessary)

Date of application: *7-2-20XX*

A. PERSONAL INFORMATION

Name - Last: *Valasquez*   First: *Jennifer*   Middle: *M*

Home Tel. (555) *439-4800*   Bus. Tel. (   )

E-mail (optional): *valasquezj@gmail.com*

Cell Phone (optional): *555-301-2612*

Present address: Street *1234 Martin Street*   (Apt.#)   City *Woodland Hills*   State *XY*   Zip *12345*

Person to notify in case of emergency or accident - name: *Elena Sanchez*

Address: *20 South M Street Woodland Hills, XY 12345*   Telephone: *555-261-0707*

B. EMPLOYMENT INFORMATION

Position desired: *insurance biller*

X Full-time   Part-time   Either

Date available for employment: *7-6-20XX*

Wage/salary expectations: *negotiable*

List hrs./days you prefer to work: *M-F   8-5 PM*

List any hrs./days you are not available: (Except for times required for religious practices or observances)

Can you work overtime, if necessary? X Yes   No

Are you employed now?: Yes X No

If so, may we inquire of your present employer?   No   Yes, if yes: Name of employer:

Phone number: (   )

Have you applied for a position with this office before? X No   Yes   If Yes, when?: Month and year _____   Location _____

Are you able to perform the essential functions of the job for which you are applying? .... X Yes   No

If no, describe the functions that cannot be performed. _____

Have you ever been convicted of a criminal offense (felony or serious misdemeanor)? *(Convictions for marijuana-related offenses that are more than two years old need not be listed.)*   Yes   No

If yes, state nature of the crime(s), when and where convicted and disposition of the case. _____

(Note: We comply with the ADA and consider reasonable accommodation measures that may be necessary for eligible applicants/employees to perform essential functions. Hire may be subject to passing a medical examination, and to skill and agility tests.)

(Note: No applicant will be denied employment solely on the grounds of conviction of a criminal offense. The nature of the offense, the date of the offense, the surrounding circumstances and the relevance of the offense to the position(s) applied for may, however, be considered.)

Referred by/or where did you learn of this job?   *Read advertisement in newspaper*

Can you, upon employment, submit verification of your legal right to work in the United States? X Yes   No

Submit proof that you meet legal age requirement for employment? X Yes   No

Language(s) applicant speaks or writes (if use of a language other than English is relevant to the job for which the applicant is applying: *Spanish*

C. EDUCATION HISTORY

	Name and address of schools attended (include current)	Number of months/ years attended	Highest grade/ level completed	Diploma/degree(s) obtained/areas of study
High school	*ABC High School, Woodland Hills, XY*	*2000-2004*	*12*	*Diploma*
College	*Vocational-Tech School, Woodland Hills, XY*	*2005*		Degree/major *Certificate*
Post graduate	*Montana State Univ., Woodland Hills, XY*	*2005-2007*		Degree/major *24 credits*
Business/trade/technical				Course/diploma/license/certificate
Other				Course/diploma/license/certificate

Specific training, skills, education, or experiences which will assist you in the job for which you have applied *See resume*

Membership/professional or civic organizations (excluding those that disclose race, color, religion or national origin) *Amer. Acad. of Professional Coders*

Future educational plans *Continuing education—preparing for certification in coding*

Military - did you serve in the armed forces? X No   Yes, if yes, branch? _____

Training relevant to position for which you are applying:

D. SPECIAL SKILLS (Check below the kinds of work you have done)

Front Office		Back Office	
X Accounts receivable	X Filing	Blood counts	Phlebotomy
Bookkeeping	X Medical terminology	Dental assistant	Urinalysis
X Collections	Medical transcription	Dental hygienist	X-ray
X Data entry	Receptionist	Injections	Other:
X Electronic/medical billing	Other:	Nursing/assisting	Other:

Other kinds of tasks performed or skills that may be applicable to position:

Office equipment/machines used: *computer, calculator, printer*

Keyboarding/typing speed: *65 wpm*

Computer programs used: *Word, Excel*

Fig. 20.4 Application for Position/Medical or Dental Office form. (Courtesy Bibiru Systems, Inc., Petaluma, CA. Telephone: [800] 242-2376; fax: [800] 242-9330; website: www.bibbero.com.)

E. EMPLOYMENT RECORD ☐ INFORMATION SUPPLIED ON ATTACHED RÉSUMÉ

LIST MOST RECENT EMPLOYMENT FIRST (Full or Part-Time) May we contact your previous employer(s) for a reference? ☒ Yes ☐ No

1) Employer/Company name *St. John's Outpatient Clinic*	Type of business: *Hospital outpatient medical clinic*
Address Street *24 Center St.* City *Woodland Hills, XY* State Zip code *12345*	Worked performed. Be specific:
Phone number *(555) 782-0155*	
Your position *Insurance billing specialist* Dates Mo. Yr. Mo. Yr. From *6* *07* To *6* *09*	
Supervisor's name *Candice Johnson* Hourly rate/salary Starting *$12/hr* Final *$15/hr*	
Reason for leaving *Professional advancement*	
2) Employer/Company name *Eastern Airlines*	Type of business: *Airline transportation*
Address Street City *Orlando* State *FL* Zip code	Worked performed. Be specific:
Phone number *(555) 350-7000*	
Your position *Receptionist* Dates Mo. Yr. Mo. Yr. From *1* *99* To *1* *2000*	
Supervisor's name *Gary Stevens* Hourly rate/salary Starting *$9/hr* Final *$11.50/hr*	
Reason for leaving *Career change*	
3) Employer/Company name	Type of business:
Address Street City State Zip code	Worked performed. Be specific:
Phone number ( )	
Your position Dates Mo. Yr. Mo. Yr. From To	
Supervisor's name Hourly rate/salary Starting Final	
Reason for leaving	

F. REFERENCES — List below two persons NOT related to you who have knowledge of your work performance within the last three years.

(1) _____ *Furnished upon request*
Name Address Telephone number (☐ Work ☐ Home) Occupation Years acquainted

(2) _____
Name Address Telephone number (☐ Work ☐ Home) Occupation Years acquainted

Please feel free to add any information which you feel will help us consider you for employment

DO NOT ANSWER ANY QUESTIONS IN THIS SECTION UNLESS THE BOXES ARE CHECKED - If the employer has checked the box next to the question, the information requested is needed for a legally permissible reason, including, without limitation, national security considerations, a legitimate occupational qualification or business necessity. The Civil Rights Act of 1964 prohibits discrimination in employment because of race, color, religion, sex or national origin. Federal law also prohibits discrimination based on age, citizenship and disability. The laws of most States also prohibit some or all of the above types of discrimination as well as some additional types such as discrimination based upon ancestry, marital status and sexual preference.

	Provide dates you attended school:	Elementary From To	☐ Number of dependents, including yourself
☐	High School From To	College From To	☐ Are you a Vietnam veteran? ☐ Yes ☐ No
	Other (give name and dates)		☐ Sex ☐ Male ☐ Female
☐	Marital status ☐ Single ☐ Engaged ☐ Married ☐ Separated ☐ Divorced ☐ Widowed	☐ Date of marriage	☐ Are you a U.S. citizen? ☐ Yes ☐ No
☐	What was your previous address?		☐ How long at previous address? _____ years
☐	State names of relatives and friends working for us, other that your spouse.		☐ How long at present address? _____ years
☐	Have you ever been bonded? ☐ Yes ☐ No If "Yes," with what employers?		☐ Are you over 18 years of age? ☐ Yes ☐ No If not, employment is subject to verification of age.

READ THE FOLLOWING CAREFULLY, THEN SIGN AND DATE THE APPLICATION

The information provided in this Application for Employment is true, correct, and complete. If employed, any misstatement or omission of fact on this application may result in my dismissal. I understand that acceptance of an offer of employment does not create a contractual obligation upon the employer to continue to employ me in the future. If you decide to engage an investigative consumer reporting agency to report on my credit and personal history I authorize you to do so. If a report is obtained you must provide, at my request, the name of the agency so I may obtain from them the nature and substance of the information contained in the report.

If requested, I hereby agree to submit to binding arbitration all disputes and claims arising out of the submission of this application. I further agree, in the event that I am hired by the company, that all disputes that cannot be resolved by informal internal resolution which might arise out of my employment with the company, whether during or after that employment, will be submitted to binding arbitration. I agree that such arbitration shall be conducted under the rules of the American Arbitration Association. This application contains the entire agreement between the parties with regard to dispute resolution, and there are no other agreements as to dispute resolution, either oral or written.

Date: *7-2-20XX* _____ Signature: _____ *Jennifer M. Valasquez*

Fig. 20.4, cont'd

letters should be typed, addressed to a specific person, and customized to each potential employer. If there is no specific contact person, address the email with "Dear Sir or Madam," "To Whom It May Concern," or a less formal "Hello," or "Good Morning."

When writing the letter of introduction, do not repeat everything in the résumé. Begin with an attention grabber and get right to the point. The message or letter should explain how your qualifications and skills would benefit the employer. Use

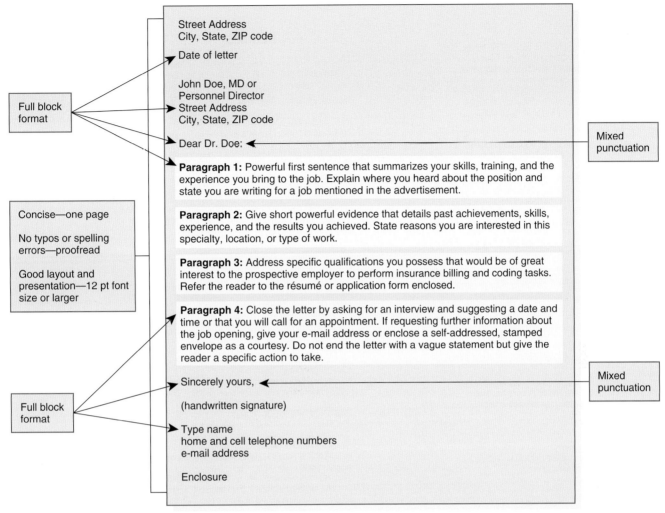

Fig. 20.5 Suggested content for a letter of introduction to accompany a résumé. Typed in full-block style with mixed punctuation.

key words that appear in the "position wanted" advertisement. Employers use applicant tracking systems (ATSs) to find and screen candidates, so include skill-oriented key words to boost the chance of being discovered. End the message or letter by requesting an interview and be sure to attach or enclose a résumé. Always include telephone numbers (home and cell) and the time of day when you are available.

Reread the message or letter to check for typos and errors in grammar, punctuation, and spelling. Avoid the use of "I" in the sentence structure (Fig. 20.5).

Résumé

A traditional **résumé** is a data sheet designed to sell job qualifications to prospective employers. A résumé should highlight information related to the position the applicant is trying to obtain; therefore, résumés will differ for each job. There are several formats from which to choose:

- A **chronologic résumé** gives recent experiences first, with dates and descriptive data for each job.
- A **functional résumé** states the qualifications or skills that an individual can perform.
- A **combination résumé** summarizes the applicant's job skills as well as educational and employment history. The combina-

tion style is the best choice for an insurance billing specialist (Fig. 20.6).

The ideal length for a résumé is one page. It can be typed on an 8½ × 14-inch page and reduced to letter size. The résumé should be keyed or typed, not handwritten, on high-quality off-white or white paper. It should be single-spaced internally, with double spacing between main headings and balanced spacing for all four margins. Laser-printed résumés give a professional appearance. The applicant may want to have a longer (two-page maximum) résumé on hand to offer during an interview.

Under the Civil Rights Act of 1964, enforced by the Equal Employment Opportunity Commission (EEOC), information about height, weight, birth date, marital status, Social Security number, and physical condition may be omitted. Additional items to omit are salary requirements, reason for leaving jobs, date of résumé preparation, date available to begin work, references, and vague references to time gaps. Questions about these items might be asked during an interview. If there are gaps of time between jobs, take a class, earn a new certification, or get involved in volunteer projects or consulting opportunities. These activities allow the individual to use or improve their skills and can be described further on the résumé. Hobbies and outside interests that relate to the profession might be included. Membership or leadership positions

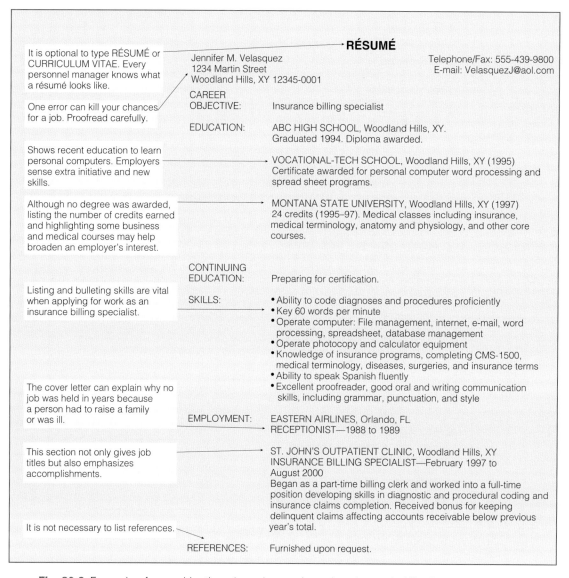

It is optional to type RÉSUMÉ or CURRICULUM VITAE. Every personnel manager knows what a résumé looks like.

One error can kill your chances for a job. Proofread carefully.

Shows recent education to learn personal computers. Employers sense extra initiative and new skills.

Although no degree was awarded, listing the number of credits earned and highlighting some business and medical courses may help broaden an employer's interest.

Listing and bulleting skills are vital when applying for work as an insurance billing specialist.

The cover letter can explain why no job was held in years because a person had to raise a family or was ill.

This section not only gives job titles but also emphasizes accomplishments.

It is not necessary to list references.

RÉSUMÉ

Jennifer M. Velasquez
1234 Martin Street
Woodland Hills, XY 12345-0001

Telephone/Fax: 555-439-9800
E-mail: VelasquezJ@aol.com

CAREER OBJECTIVE: Insurance billing specialist

EDUCATION: ABC HIGH SCHOOL, Woodland Hills, XY. Graduated 1994. Diploma awarded.

VOCATIONAL-TECH SCHOOL, Woodland Hills, XY (1995) Certificate awarded for personal computer word processing and spread sheet programs.

MONTANA STATE UNIVERSITY, Woodland Hills, XY (1997) 24 credits (1995–97). Medical classes including insurance, medical terminology, anatomy and physiology, and other core courses.

CONTINUING EDUCATION: Preparing for certification.

SKILLS:
• Ability to code diagnoses and procedures proficiently
• Key 60 words per minute
• Operate computer: File management, internet, e-mail, word processing, spreadsheet, database management
• Operate photocopy and calculator equipment
• Knowledge of insurance programs, completing CMS-1500, medical terminology, diseases, surgeries, and insurance terms
• Ability to speak Spanish fluently
• Excellent proofreader, good oral and writing communication skills, including grammar, punctuation, and style

EMPLOYMENT: EASTERN AIRLINES, Orlando, FL RECEPTIONIST—1988 to 1989

ST. JOHN'S OUTPATIENT CLINIC, Woodland Hills, XY INSURANCE BILLING SPECIALIST—February 1997 to August 2000 Began as a part-time billing clerk and worked into a full-time position developing skills in diagnostic and procedural coding and insurance claims completion. Received bonus for keeping delinquent claims affecting accounts receivable below previous year's total.

REFERENCES: Furnished upon request.

Fig. 20.6 Example of a combination résumé stressing education and skills. Personal data may be excluded as a result of the Civil Rights Act of 1964, enforced by the Equal Employment Opportunity Commission (EEOC).

held in professional organizations related to the medical field might be mentioned. A photograph is not necessary but might be included if it will be of value to the interviewer for recall purposes. The format may include the following:

- *Title.* Résumé, Personal Data Sheet, Biographic Sketch, or Curriculum Vitae.
- *Heading.* At the beginning of the résumé, list name, phone number, and email address. Mailing addresses are being phased out, so simply noting city and state is acceptable.
- *Summary.* This may be a statement as to why the employer should be interested in the applicant. Use action words as shown in Fig. 20.6 and avoid the personal pronoun.
- *Education.* Name high school, college, any business school attended, continuing education classes, city and state, degree, and date received. List in reverse chronologic order. Grade point average and awards or scholastic honors may be included.
- *Professional experience.* Name all employers in reverse chronologic order with addresses, telephone numbers, and dates of employment. Include summer, full-time, part-time, and

temporary jobs as well as externships and volunteer work. Detail achievements, not duties (for example, "possess strong communication, service to patients, and organizational skills" or "consistently surpassed collection goals by 10% or more each year").

- *Skills.* List keyboarding words per minute, experience with medical billing software programs, accurate procedure and diagnostic coding (including knowledge of modifiers), expertise in insurance claims completion and submission, knowledge of medical terminology and insurance terminology, bookkeeping (posting charges, payments, and adjustments to accounts receivable journal), experience in preparing appeals for denied claims, resubmittal of delinquent claims, ability to explain insurance programs and plans (e.g., benefits, requirements, and submission of claims), ability to abstract information from patients' medical and financial records, and ability to review insurance payments from explanation of benefits (EOB) documents. If you are fluent in another language, provide this information. Telephone and reception skills also

Fig. 20.7 Insurance billing student at an externship site.

might be mentioned. Skills might be placed near the top of the résumé, where they will catch a résumé screener's eye.
- *References.* Type in the phrase "Furnished on request." Prepare approximately five references on a separate sheet and be sure to contact the persons referenced before an interview.
- *Final details.* It is acceptable to email or fax a résumé to an employer who advertises a job opening but gives no guidelines on how to submit the résumé. It is wise to use every advantage possible in a competitive employment market where time is of the essence (Fig. 20.7).

Proofread the résumé carefully for spelling, punctuation, grammar, and typographic errors. Ask a friend or professional individual with excellent English skills to read and critique it. Remember that the résumé is a foot in the door.

Interview

After looking for a potential employer, preparing a résumé, and completing an application, the final step in landing a job is the interview. An **interview** is a formal consultation with questions from an employer, meant to evaluate the qualifications of a prospective job applicant (Fig. 20.8).

Phone Interviews

Many employers use telephone interviews as a first interview. This allows them to screen candidates and narrow the pool of applicants who will be invited for an in-person interview. It also

Fig. 20.8 Student being interviewed for an insurance billing position.

allows them to quickly, and with minimal effort and expense, determine if an applicant would be a suitable candidate for the position. In some situations, especially for remote positions, a phone interview may be the only option. As with all types of interviews, it is important for the applicant to prepare.
- Research the company you are interviewing with.
- Research the description of the job you are interviewing for.
- Compile and reference a list of your strengths and weaknesses during the interview.
- Compile and reference a list of questions you may have for the potential employer.
- Review your resume well and reference it during the interview.
- Before the phone call, confirm all details, including the date, time, and who you will be talking to. Use a quiet, comfortable, and private space with no distractions so you can focus on the interview. Standing during an interview helps you sound more energetic during the call.

Remote Interviews

Another interview option that potential employers will use is a remote interview. This may also be referred to as an online interview, video interview, or virtual interview. Some companies use this as their first-round interview, while others may use it as a second step after the phone interview. In some cases, the employer may use it as their only interview. In any case, it is essential that the applicant prepare for and pass this step.

Choose a location for the interview with a strong internet connection. Consider doing a practice run to determine if there is background noise that might interfere with the interview. A perfect video interview location is one without any distractions. Make sure that no family members, roommates, or pets will be joining the interview. If there are small children in the house, arrange for a caregiver to allow the quiet needed for the interview. The interview background can reveal a great deal about you to the interviewer.

It is important to join the remote call early and make sure the camera, the microphone, and all technology is working and ready for the call. Prepare for the interview in the same way one would prepare for a phone or in-person interview. Have your resume, questions, and lists of qualities nearby. Also keep in mind that you are using the eye of the camera to make a great impression on the interviewer. Kick off the interview with a great smile.

During the interview, use proper grammar, avoid using slang, slow down your speaking, and always maintain eye contact, even when it is through the lens of the camera. Employers want candidates who are well spoken and articulate.

In-Person Interviews

In an in-person interview, the applicant must make the best impression possible on their prospective employer as soon as they walk through the door. It is a well-known fact that the first 30 seconds makes either a positive or negative impression. Display a warm, positive, and interested attitude.

Good grooming is essential and starts with cleanliness. Applicants should dress conservatively in appropriate business attire and wear jewelry sparingly. Cosmetics should be minimal; avoid wearing fragrances. It has been found that when applicants have similar skills and education, the decision to hire is based on physical appearance at the interview.

Be poised and confident and focus on good posture. Eliminate nervous habits and do not smoke or chew gum. And above all, turn off your cell phone before the interview begins.

Do not be tempted to answer a call or send a text during the interview.

Fig. 20.9 is an example of an interview evaluation and reference investigation form. This form points out the areas an interviewer observes and how impressions are rated.

INTERVIEW EVALUATION AND REFERENCE INVESTIGATION FORM

SUMMARY OF EVALUATION	
POINTS FROM (21 CATEGORIES) APPLICATION AND INTERVIEW (FRONT)	
POINTS FROM REFERENCES (1 TO 3 CATEGORIES FROM BACK)	
TOTAL POINTS = (Front and Back)	
OVERALL IMPRESSION: Divide total points by number of categories rated (24 maximum categories).	

THIS IS: ☐ 1ST INTERVIEW ☐ 2ND INTERVIEW ☐ 3RD INTERVIEW

NAME OF APPLICANT: DATE

ADDRESS: PHONE

RATING: EXCELLENT – 3 POINTS / GOOD – 2 POINTS / FAIR – 1 POINT / POOR – 0 POINTS

POSITION APPLIED FOR:

FROM APPLICATION FOR POSITION, GAUGE APPLICANT IN FOLLOWING AREAS — EXC | GOOD | FAIR | POOR

APPLICATION SECTION REFERENCE:
1. NECESSARY SKILLS FOR THIS POSITION?
2. SUITABLE ADVANCEMENT HISTORY?
3. AN EMPLOYMENT HISTORY THAT POINTS TOWARD DEPENDABILITY?
4. STABILITY (REMAINED IN ONE PLACE OF RESIDENCE AND ONE JOB FOR A REASONABLE LENGTH OF TIME)?
5. THE PROPER EDUCATIONAL BACKGROUND TO FILL THE POSITION?
6. SALARY REQUIREMENT COMMENSURATE WITH POSITION?
7. LEGIBLE HANDWRITING?
8. LIMITATION ON WORKING HOURS?

FROM THE PERSONAL INTERVIEW – (SHOULD BE SPECIFIC QUALITIES – OBJECTIVE)
9. SUFFICIENT CAPABILITY TO HANDLE ANY SITUATION THAT MAY ARISE WHEN ALONE IN OFFICE?
10. AN APPROPRIATE ATTITUDE TOWARD WORK?
11. APPROPRIATE DICTION, GRAMMAR, ARTICULATION?
12. POISE?
13. SELF CONFIDENCE (NOT OVER-CONFIDENCE)?
14. TACT?
15. SUFFICIENT MATURITY FOR JOB?
16. AN ABILITY TO EXPRESS ONESELF WELL?
17. AN INITIATIVE OR INTEREST IN LEARNING?
18. ABILITY TO WORK WITH OTHERS IN OFFICE?
19. APPROPRIATE APPEARANCE (NEAT, CLEAN; SUITABLE TO BUSINESS)?
20. ENERGY, VITALITY, AND PERCEIVED ABILITY TO HANDLE PRESSURE OF POSITION?
21. EAGERNESS TO OBTAIN THE POSITION IN QUESTION?

NOTES: COLUMNAR TOTALS

TOTAL POINTS THIS PAGE

DIRECTIONS FOR USE OF FORM:
1. Look over your ratings. A zero score on any one VITAL question should automatically eliminate applicant. Add up the total rating points and enter in the SUMMARY OF EVALUATION BLOCK in the upper right-hand corner of this page.
2. After finishing all interviews, choose the "best bets" and check their references using the reverse side of this form.
3. Enter, as above, the results of your reference check and then your overall impression (E – Excellent, G – Good, F – Fair, P – Poor).

ORDER # 72-120 • BIBBERO SYSTEMS, INC. • PETALUMA, CA. • (REV.07/03)
TO REORDER CALL TOLL FREE: (800) BIBBERO (800-242-2376) OR FAX (800) 242-9330 MFG IN U.S.A.   (PLEASE TURN OVER)

Fig. 20.9 Example of an interview evaluation and reference investigation form. (Courtesy Bibbero Systems, Inc., Petaluma, Calif. Telephone: [800] 242-2376; fax: [800] 242-9330; website: www.bibbero.com.)

NOTES:

RATING: 0 - POOR, 1 - FAIR, 2 - GOOD, 3 - EXCELLENT

	REFERENCE INVESTIGATION	
1.	OFFICE CONTACTED	PHONE: ( ) DATE
	PERSON CONTACTED	TITLE OR POSITION:
	HOW LONG HAVE YOU KNOWN THIS PERSON?	TITLE/POSITION THIS PERSON HELD?
	BETWEEN WHAT DATES WAS THIS PERSON EMPLOYED BY YOU?	FROM TO
	RESPONSIBILITIES?	SATISFACTORILY COMPLETED?
	WAS THIS PERSON CONSISTENTLY COOPERATIVE?	WHAT WERE SHORTCOMINGS?
	DID THIS PERSON GET ALONG WELL WITH OTHERS?	
	WAS THIS PERSON TRUSTWORTHY/DEPENDABLE?	ATTENDANCE RECORD:
	REASON FOR LEAVING?	SALARY LEVEL:
	WOULD YOU REHIRE THIS PERSON?	
	NOTES:	
		RATING:
2.	OFFICE CONTACTED	PHONE: ( ) DATE
	PERSON CONTACTED	TITLE OR POSITION:
	HOW LONG HAVE YOU KNOWN THIS PERSON?	TITLE/POSITION THIS PERSON HELD?
	BETWEEN WHAT DATES WAS THIS PERSON EMPLOYED BY YOU?	
	RESPONSIBILITIES?	
	WAS THIS PERSON CONSISTENTLY COOPERATIVE?	
	DID THIS PERSON GET ALONG WELL WITH OTHERS?	
	WAS THIS PERSON TRUSTWORTHY/DEPENDABLE?	ATTENDANCE RECORD:
	REASON FOR LEAVING?	SALARY LEVEL:
	WOULD YOU REHIRE THIS PERSON?	
	NOTES:	
		RATING:
3.	OFFICE CONTACTED	PHONE: ( ) DATE
	PERSON CONTACTED	TITLE OR POSITION:
	HOW LONG HAVE YOU KNOWN THIS PERSON?	TITLE/POSITION THIS PERSON HELD?
	BETWEEN WHAT DATES WAS THIS PERSON EMPLOYED BY YOU?	
	RESPONSIBILITIES?	
	WAS THIS PERSON CONSISTENTLY COOPERATIVE?	
	DID THIS PERSON GET ALONG WELL WITH OTHERS?	
	WAS THIS PERSON TRUSTWORTHY/DEPENDABLE?	ATTENDANCE RECORD:
	REASON FOR LEAVING?	SALARY LEVEL:
	WOULD YOU REHIRE THIS PERSON?	
	NOTES:	
		RATING:
INTERVIEWER _____ DATE: _____		TOTAL POINTS THIS PAGE:

Fig. 20.9, cont'd

Fig. 20.10 Job applicant concluding an interview with an office manager.

Do research before the interview to know whether the salary (when offered) is acceptable. If you want to ask questions about benefits, do not appear overly interested in them.

If you are given a choice, avoid scheduling interviews for Mondays or Fridays. Mondays are usually catch-up, heavily scheduled days, while Fridays are getaway days, which means the interviewer may be rushed. Arrive promptly for the interview. Carry something in your hand (e.g., a notepad, résumé, and other documents) to avoid showing nervousness or anxiety.

Role-playing is a good method to prepare for any type of interview. Give a friend a list of questions to ask you and then try to answer the questions spontaneously without stumbling. Videotape or audiotape the session, if possible, to see or hear what the employer will experience.

Questions an interviewer might ask about personal life (marital status), family planning, pregnancy, provision for child care, religious preference, club memberships, height, weight, dependents, age (birth date), ethnic background, maiden name, native language, physical or psychiatric problems, spouse's employment and earnings, credit rating, and home and automobile ownership are illegal and do not have to be answered. (It is not considered discriminatory if an employer wants to know whether an applicant smokes.) Three suggestions for handling an illegal question follow:

1. Answer the question and ignore the fact that you know it is illegal.
2. Ask "Is this question relevant to the requirements of this position?"
3. Refuse to answer and contact the nearest EEOC office.

Shake the interviewer's hand at the conclusion of the meeting (Fig. 20.10). Ask how long it will be before a job offer or denial is forthcoming and then leave with a "thank you." If the job is offered at the interview and you are not sure about accepting, ask, "How soon do you need to know?" This will allow time to think and compare job offers before making a commitment.

Portfolio

Prepare in advance for the interview by organizing a **portfolio**. A portfolio is a compilation of items that represents a job applicant's skills. Include letters of recommendation (from former employers, teachers, family physicians, professional friends, or community leaders), school diplomas or degrees, transcripts, certificates, names and addresses of references, a résumé, timed keyboarding test certified by an instructor, insurance claim forms you may have completed with evidence of coding skills, and any other items related to prior education and work experience. A web-based portfolio can also be created by scanning the recommended documents and inserting a link to the portfolio for online job applications.

Proof of Citizenship

Within 3 days of being hired, an employee must provide their employer with proof of citizenship by completing an Employment Eligibility Verification Form I-9. The employee must also show proof of citizenship by providing appropriate documentation, which may consist of a single document or combination of driver's license, Social Security card, birth certificate, US passport, naturalization certification, or authorization card. The specific documentation requirements can be found on the US Citizenship and Immigration Services (**USCIS**) website (www.uscis.gov). Assemble your proof of citizenship documents and have them available in the event that they are requested by the prospective employer during the interview.

Follow-Up Letter

Write a follow-up letter or send an email message within 24 hours of the interview. Thank the person for the interview and restate your interest in the position (Fig. 20.11). This keeps your name before the potential employer. Telephone to express continued interest in the position if no response is heard within the time frame given.

Street Address
City, State, ZIP code
Date of letter

John Doe, MD or
Personnel Director
Street Address
City, State, ZIP code

Dear Dr. Doe:

Thank you for spending your valuable time yesterday to interview me for the insurance billing specialist position in your clinic.

I am confident that my training and experience will allow me to perform the tasks associated with this position with expertise. It was a pleasure to meet with your staff and it would be my pleasure to be part of the team.

I am looking forward to hearing from you in the near future.

Sincerely yours,

(handwritten signature)

Type name

Fig. 20.11 Example of a thank-you letter sent after an interview.

20.3 QUICK REVIEW
Question: What are the 3 different types of interviews?

 20.4 QUICK REVIEW
Question: What steps should an individual do to prepare for any type of interview?

SELF-EMPLOYMENT

When an individual wants to be their own boss (**self-employment**), it is usually wise to become well-educated and have experience in the chosen career before undertaking this task. Having a positive and effective rapport with the public, as well as a strong background in insurance, is desirable for the individual who wants to work independently as an insurance billing specialist. Outpatient hospital and physician billing experience in several specialties is important if you choose to focus on professional billing and coding services. If you specialize in facility billing and coding services, experience is necessary, especially because it is not common for a hospital to outsource these services to a small billing company. If coding services are to be part of the billing company's offerings, the coding professional should be certified by a reputable professional organization, such as the AAPC or AHIMA.

! COMPLIANCE ALERT

Security Policies When Working From Home
The Health Insurance Portability and Accountability Act (HIPAA) security rules indicate that working from home requires the same security policies and practices as working in the office. However, no specific policies are given. It is up to each covered entity to establish these documents based on its security risk assessment. Security measures should address the technical setup. For example, a typical security policy might stipulate that the telecommuter use a dedicated computer with a virtual private network solution, antivirus software, and firewall. Privacy compliance policies apply at home just as they do when working in an office. All oral, written and electronic information should be protected from family members and visitors.

One must have something to offer clients when marketing and selling one's services and skills. This knowledge and expertise can be gained only with years of experience and persistence. Full-time commitment, hard work, dedication, and many long hours obtaining clients are encountered when beginning a business. Be cautious when purchasing billing service software and obtain a complete picture of what hardware is necessary, how the programs work, and the benefits they offer to your clients.

Networking is extremely important when starting and growing a successful business. Contacts that you have met in previous jobs may lead to future business partners. Many times, it is the people the individual knows who may get a foot in the potential client's door.

An insurance billing specialist can work as an independent contractor to have flexible hours, work from home, and reduce a health care organization's overhead. Working at home requires self-discipline, and one must develop a schedule and stick to it. Good time management is essential. It takes additional hours to advertise, obtain clients, bill, and perform bookkeeping tasks. Box 20.1 is a checklist of tasks that must be done to establish a new business.

Planning Your Business

Every successful business endeavor begins with a smart business plan. This is a road map that can guide your financial and business strategies from start-up to continuous success. A business plan addresses facts and figures pertinent to your business and financial abilities and assesses your objectives and goals. It would be wise to meet with an accountant, an attorney, or a business consultant to help get your company started in the right direction.

For more information about business planning, visit the US Small Business Association (SBA) website at www.sba.gov.

Professional Mailing Address

No doubt you will receive mail, so it is important to establish a professional address. Opting to rent a post office box creates a business-oriented mailing address, helps maintain confidentiality in mailings you receive about clients and patient accounts, and protects you from unwanted visitors to your home. Visit the website of the Internal Revenue Service (IRS) at www.irs.gov/Businesses/Small-Businesses-&-Self-Employed for self-employed and small business resources.

Finances to Consider
Taxes

You must decide what form of business entity you will be (i.e., sole proprietor, partnership, or corporation). It is advisable to seek the services of a lawyer, accountant, or both before legally establishing a business and making appropriate selection of the tax options involved. Set up detailed financial records using the services of an accountant and simplified bookkeeping software for use on the computer. Expert advice is essential and helps develop a successful business.

Establishing a business in a home may result in some deductions, so obtain all the information you can from your accountant and the IRS regarding important laws concerning small business and self-employment taxes. Keep receipts and complete records of income and expenses. Retain records for the period stipulated by the IRS. The following is a sample record retention schedule for a small business:

- Bank statements and canceled checks: 7 years
- Expired contracts: 7 years
- Financial statements: permanently
- General correspondence: 1 to 5 years
- Payroll records and summaries: 7 years
- Income tax returns: permanently
- Worksheets and supporting documents: 7 years
- Business travel expenses and documentation of mileage: 7 years

BOX 20.1 New Business Checklist

The following is a checklist to help you in starting a new home business. This is neither a complete list of items to consider nor the exact order to accomplish them in; however, important points are covered in this list.

- Define your services and construct a business plan. Make sure you forecast for success. Will this business be viable? Can you accomplish the services you will promise to carry out? Can you financially afford this endeavor?
- Research whether you need to obtain a business license from the business license section of your city hall. Regulations vary in each city licensing office. If you are renting, you might have to obtain a home occupation permit from the planning department and have it signed by your landlord. The city may have guidelines on hours of business, pedestrian and vehicular activity, noise, and so on in residential areas. Determine whether your county has rules on operating a small business from home.
- Consider a name for your business. File a fictitious business name (doing business as [DBA]) at the county clerk's office by obtaining the proper form for completion. If you use your given name, you do not have to file a fictitious business name.
- Decide what address to use. You may want to obtain a post office box number instead of using your home address. This will provide a professional mailing address as well as protect you from unexpected visitors to your home.
- Consult with an accountant for advice on the tax structure of your company (e.g., sole proprietor, corporation). Learn what expenses are deductible. Depending on how you set up your business, some possible tax breaks may include depreciation of office equipment, declaring a room of your home as an office, subscriptions to professional publications, dues to professional associations, expenses associated with your automobile, telephone, photocopying, and office supplies, promotion and advertising, and any expenses pertaining to meetings, conventions, workshops, or seminars.

- Obtain the insurance you need: health insurance, disability insurance, life insurance, liability insurance, workers' compensation (if you have employees), and so on. Insurance called "release of information insurance" or "errors and omissions insurance" with a "hold harmless" clause is available to protect you against loss of material. Consider a retirement plan, such as an individual retirement account.
- Obtain a separate telephone number and possibly a fax number to separate "home" from "business."
- Create a website advertising your services, incorporating a video clip and web-based portfolio with other visuals as well as links to LinkedIn, Facebook, and Twitter.
- Open a bank account. Many banks offer small business accounts with nominal monthly fees.
- Create a professional image through business cards, stationery, and invoice billing forms. You can find resources on the internet or in software programs to print your own.
- Stay current in the industry with up-to-date reference books. Begin to assemble a library that includes a good medical dictionary, procedural and diagnostic code books, compliance handbooks, trade journals, and so on.
- Start a contact database and begin to advertise your business using some of the following methods: visiting offices, mailing flyers, advertising in trade journals or your local newspaper, sending announcements, and sending personalized letters to prospects (hospitals, clinics, and physician's offices).
- If you have opened an office at a location outside of your home, make sure you have reviewed a proper lease before signing it and consider the finances needed for items such as utility deposits (i.e., water, gas, and electricity). Rent, renovation, and janitorial or trash services must also be considered.

Some contracts include a statement of confidentiality assuring the contracting facility that all patient data are handled in a confidential manner.

Start-Up Expenses

Money is necessary for equipment, computer software, overhead, taxes, stationery, preprinted statements and forms, and myriad other expenses. It is vital that you accrue sufficient funds to run the business for a period of 1 year or more before vacating a full-time job. This will help eliminate a lot of fear and anxiety associated with business start-up. A common reason for business failure is running out of the money necessary to keep the business going. It may take a year or more to begin seeing a profit, so one must be patient. This is where the business plan becomes a useful resource!

If an individual has no business management experience, courses may be taken to gain knowledge and instill confidence in these areas before beginning a business. Attend workshops and lectures on starting a business that are offered by financial institutions, universities, community colleges, or private institutions.

Bank Account

Open a bank account that is separate from your own personal accounts. This smart approach saves a lot of time in the future when it comes to sorting out expenses and working on taxes. Also, think about the professional image that a business check will convey. Most banks have small business account services, including those for the self-employed.

Business Name and License

Some towns or counties require a license to operate a business. This may include working from your home office. Check with

your local offices to determine whether an application or fee is required. This is the time to choose an appropriate business name and obtain applicable town and county licenses.

A business name should be easy to remember and explain what your company does. For example, "ABC's #1 Medical Billing Service" tells potential clients that the company works with health care related to billing and insurance claims.

Insurance

Business owners should protect income and property from unexpected losses. The following are types of insurance to investigate:

- Professional liability/errors and omissions protects you and your company from claims if your client holds you responsible for errors or a failure to perform as promised in your service contract. Coverage can include legal costs and may pay for resulting judgments against you.
- Business interruption insurance and property insurance in case of fire, theft, or disaster protects your assets and may help you in the recovery of data.
- Disability insurance, if one becomes unable to work because of illness or injury, can include yourself and/or an employee.
- Health and life insurance covers health care for you and/or employees as well as providing life insurance.

Business Associate Under the Health Insurance Portability and Accountability Act

HIPAA rules apply to most billing, coding, or consulting companies because they are considered business associates.

If your billing, coding, or consulting company gets personal health information from a covered entity to perform a function or activity on behalf of that covered entity, your relationship is likely that of a business associate, and your responsibilities must be defined with a business associate agreement.

The **business associate agreement** must give "satisfactory assurances" to the covered entity on whose behalf the business associate performs services and must include, according to HIPAA rules, the following terms as set forth in the regulation:

- Business Associate agrees to not use or disclose protected health information (PHI) other than as permitted or required by the Agreement or as required by law.
- Business Associate agrees to use appropriate safeguards to prevent use or disclosure of the PHI other than as provided for by this Agreement.
- Business Associate agrees to mitigate, to the extent practicable, any harmful effect that is known to Business Associate of a use or disclosure of PHI by Business Associate in violation of the requirements of this Agreement.
- Business Associate agrees to report to Covered Entity any use or disclosure of the PHI not provided for by this Agreement of which it becomes aware.
- Business Associate agrees to ensure that any agent including a subcontractor, to whom it provides PHI received from, or created or received by Business Associate on behalf of, Covered Entity agrees to the same restrictions and conditions that apply through this Agreement to Business Associate with respect to such information.
- Business Associate agrees to provide access, at the request of Covered Entity, and in the time and manner [insert negotiated terms], to PHI in a Designated Record Set, to Covered Entity or, as directed by Covered Entity, to an Individual to meet the requirements under 45 CFR § 164.524. (Not necessary if business associate does not have PHI in a designated record set.)
- Business Associate agrees to make any amendment(s) to PHI in a Designated Record Set that the Covered Entity directs or agrees to pursuant to 45 CFR § 164.526 at the request of Covered Entity or an Individual, and in the time and manner [insert negotiated terms]. (Not necessary if business associate does not have PHI in a designated record set.)
- Business Associate agrees to make internal practices, books, and records, including policies and procedures and PHI, relating to the use and disclosure of PHI received from, or created or received by Business Associate on behalf of, Covered Entity available [to the Covered Entity, or] to the Secretary, in a time and manner [insert negotiated terms] or designated by the Secretary, for purposes of the Secretary determining Covered Entity's compliance with the Privacy Rule.
- Business Associate agrees to document such disclosures of PHI and information related to such disclosures as would be required for Covered Entity to respond to a request by an Individual for an accounting of disclosures of PHI in accordance with 45 CFR § 164.528.
- Business Associate agrees to provide to Covered Entity or an Individual, in time and manner [insert negotiated terms], information collected in accordance with Section [insert

section number in contract where provision (i) appears] of this Agreement, to permit Covered Entity to respond to a request by an Individual for an accounting of disclosures of PHI in accordance with 45 CFR § 164.528.2.

Service Contract

The service contract is a separate document from the business associate agreement. The **service contract** is a necessary document that defines the duties and obligations of each party involved in the business relationship. Contracts or agreements should be made in writing, signed, and notarized. For example, a contract should define the following:

- Who is responsible for the coding (the health care organization or the billing service)?
- What will be the routine for claim submission?
- Is there a per-claim processing fee or a flat monthly fee?
- Who is responsible for follow-up on collection procedures (telephone calls or letters)?
- Who pays for rebilling, photocopying of records, mailing fees, and clearinghouse charges? Is this included in a flat monthly service fee?
- Under whose name will bills be sent to patients (the health care organization or the billing service)?
- Will the billing service telephone number appear on the statement, or will a toll-free or local number be used?
- How will the telephone be answered?
- What are the charges for coding consultation services?
- What are the coverage arrangements for absence or illness?
- How will information be protected and handled between the client and billing company?

If there is any change in the terms of the agreements, write an addendum to the original agreement and have both parties sign to acknowledge the change. Be sure that all agreements and contracts have proper effective and termination dates. Remember that renegotiation is possible when the contract expires.

Pricing Your Services

Define your services and work out a structured fee schedule. It is imperative that you get legal advice when creating contracts and agreements.

A variety of methods are used to price services, such as a percentage of reimbursement or an annual, hourly, or per-claim fee. Review state laws regarding percentage billing, which is illegal in some states. Deciding on which method to use depends on the type of client being served and the work to be done. For example, a coding specialist may bill a per-claim service, whereas a CAP may bill in 15-minute increments. Contact other billing and insurance services to learn what they are charging.

Security and Equipment

The most important consideration when starting your business is privacy and security of the health information and business documents that you will handle and be responsible for.

An initial equipment checklist may include the following:

- Computer
- Laser or ink jet printer
- Paper

- Current billing and coding manuals and books
- Desk supplies such as stapler, paper clips, and self-adhesive notes
- Locking file cabinets
- Copy and fax machine

Also consider using separate computer backup protection (e.g., a surge protector with battery power) to guard against faulty wiring or power failure. This gives you more than ten minutes to back up your current project and then shut down.

Shop smart. Research upcoming sales and lease programs, rebates, upgrade trade-ins, and service plans.

Research the various medical billing software programs and ask for demonstration software before purchasing. Also look for a reputable clearinghouse. Compare functionality, customer service, technical support, and prices.

Marketing, Advertising, Promotion, and Public Relations

Marketing refers to how a business is presented or advertised to promote sales. Marketing strategies vary depending on the section of the public that is targeted. When promoting a medical billing service, develop a well-organized marketing plan and follow basic guidelines to reach a specific target audience.

Ways to market a business and the reasons behind these marketing strategies are presented in Table 20.2.

At this point, you should be ready to start marketing your business. If you are creative, you can design your own business cards and have them printed. A classic white card with black print conveys professionalism. When creating business brochures, obtain financial data to help convince clients that the service you are offering is better and can do more for their businesses than what they presently have. Save them time and money! Stress being honest, reliable, committed, efficient, and professional and offer them something they cannot do for themselves.

Put yourself in front of office managers and health care providers to advertise your services. Consider visiting the health care offices in your area, being cognizant of offices that have a sign stating, "No Soliciting." If you see this sign, respect it and jot down the address to mail them literature instead. Also note that solicitation by fax is illegal according to the Federal Communications Commission.

Marketing can be tough and intimidating. Persistence and networking with colleagues and professionals will pay off.

Business Incubator

Another way to develop a business and obtain management assistance is to seek the services of a business incubator. A *business incubator* is an environment that grows and nurtures small businesses through their early years of existence by offering an array of business assistance services, shared resources, and networking. An incubator facility can be an actual building that has several small business tenants. It is run by managers and staff who offer tenants business advice, referral services, and many other services, such as high-speed internet, conference rooms, secretarial, mail, and courier service, fax, copier, printer, TV, DVD, and VCR, a break room, and free parking.

Reassess and Continue With Success

Once your business is underway, you will find it necessary to routinely assess its overall health. Review your business plans and make sure you are following the guidelines. Make changes

TABLE 20.2   Business Marketing and Strategies

Strategy	Reason
Obtain professionally printed stationery and business cards.	Enhances professional image.
Pass out business cards at professional meetings.	Advertises availability and services. Helps with networking.
Develop a business name and logo for the company.	Enables potential clients to identify that you are in business.
Ensure accuracy of all printed materials.	When items are not professionally assembled or proofread to eliminate typographical errors, a potential client receives a doubtful or negative image of the company.
Develop a professional flyer and distribute it to medical facilities and physicians' offices.	Introduces company name, advertises services, and describes benefits.
Follow up with a personal visit or telephone call.	A friendly voice and professional image offer services that are personal and let potential clients know that you are available and interested.
Advertise in the journal or newsletter of the county medical society and state medical association.	Potential clients read such publications, and advertisements of this nature lend to your credibility.
Join a local chamber of commerce to network with members and network using social media, such as LinkedIn.	Networking and advertising can be the best public relations tools.
Promote your business with a professionally developed website.	Search engines will help find you. Websites deliver immediate, detailed information about your company.
Check with established businesses to determine whether they are overloaded with work, the owner needs a vacation, or they need help with a temporary situation because of illness.	Present your services as a help, not a threat to current office staff.

where applicable and revise your strategies and goals. Running your own successful business is challenging and highly rewarding both emotionally and financially.

 20.5 QUICK REVIEW
Question: What is a business plan and why is it important for an individual who wants to start their own business?

ATTAINING PROFESSIONAL ADVANCEMENT

Whether you become the employee of a health care organization or strike out as a self-employed contractor, advancing your skills and your career is essential to a successful and long-term career. As stated earlier in this chapter, it is important to join professional organizations and seek certifications as part of your professional advancement. To be an expert in the ever-changing field of health care will require continuous learning and education on the part of the insurance billing specialist.

Networking

Networking is a core principle for success in developing any career. Networking is the exchange of information or services among individuals, groups, or institutions and making use of professional contacts. Networking has many benefits and can open the door to long-term friendships, business opportunities, advice, and positive influences.

As you develop your network, you are creating a community of people who provide information and emotional support to each other. You will learn of new developments in your field, new tools, and new processes, training programs, products, and services. You will identify the leaders in your network that you aspire to follow and mirror their image. And as you develop your career, you may have the satisfaction of providing support or a key piece of information that makes a difference in the life of a member of your network.

Find a Mentor

A valuable vehicle for career development is finding a mentor in the business. A mentor is a guide or teacher who offers advice, criticism, wisdom, guidance, and perspective to an inexperienced but promising protégé to help reach a life goal. Decide what kind of help you want (e.g., technical, general feedback, or managerial) and then look for a mentor whose background, values, and style are similar to yours. Be willing to face criticism with a positive attitude and express gratitude when excellence is praised.

 20.6 QUICK REVIEW
Question: What is networking and why is it important in the advancement of the insurance billing specialist?

 DISCUSSION POINT
Becoming certified through a professional organization is an essential goal for an insurance billing specialist who seeks to advance their career. Explain which professional organization you would be interested in exploring to advance your knowledge and become certified.

PROCEDURE 20.1 Creating an Electronic Résumé

Once a medical position has been identified, a résumé may be emailed or a hard copy may be faxed. The basic steps for creating a résumé are as follows:
1. Compose a résumé using computer software with accurate spelling features. Be sure to keep it simple. Each line should be no more than 65 characters in length.
2. Discard traditional résumé-writing techniques, such as focusing on action verbs. Instead, think of descriptive key words, such as *medical biller, education, work experience, skills, knowledge,* and *abilities.* To catch a résumé screener's eye, you might insert a "skills" section at the top of the résumé.
3. Avoid the use of decorative graphics, complex typefaces, bulleted lists, complicated page formatting, symbols, underlining, and italics. These features may not appear the same on an employer's computer online.
4. When applying for an entry-level position, use only one page (two-page maximum). Save your résumé using a file name such as medical biller, medical coding specialist, or insurance biller, because in some tracking systems this will help get you past the filters more effectively than "myrésumé"
5. Proofread the electronic résumé and save it in a job search file.
6. Study the potential employer's online guides presenting special procedures for sending email and files.
7. Use the computer's "copy and paste" feature to enter the information into an email. Alternatively, if you save the résumé as an electronic file, it can be transmitted as an attachment to an email message.
8. Do not post a letter of introduction when posting a résumé to a bulletin board. Upload the résumé to post online using the file transfer feature.
9. After you send a résumé electronically, mail a hard copy and call the hiring manager directly to follow up. Be assertive.

PROCEDURE 20.2 Compose, Format, Key, Proofread, and Print a Cover Letter

1. Assemble materials: computer, printer, letterhead paper, envelopes, attachments, thesaurus, English dictionary, medical dictionary, and pen or pencil.
2. Obtain recipient's name, address, and title and choose letterhead style (modified or full block format with mixed punctuation). Refer to see Fig. 20.5.
3. Turn computer on and select the word processing software program (e.g., Microsoft Word). Open a blank document.
4. Key the date line beginning three lines below letterhead and format in the location for the chosen style.
5. Double space down and insert the recipient's title, name, and address. If necessary, double space down for an attention line.
6. Double space down and key the salutation. Use open or mixed punctuation.
7. Double space down and key the reference line ("Re" or "Subject") in the location for chosen letter style.
8. Double space down and key the body (content) of the letter in single-spaced format. Paragraphs should match the chosen format. Always double space down between paragraphs.
9. Proofread the letter on screen for typos, spelling, grammar, and auto-correction errors.
10. If a second page is needed, key that page with a heading (name, page number, and date) in vertical or horizontal format.
11. Key a complimentary close, making sure it is in the correct location for the chosen style.
12. Drop four spaces down and key the sender's name and title with credentials as shown on the letterhead.
13. If enclosures or attachments accompany the letter, single or double space down to insert "CC" for copy or "Enc" for enclosures or attachments.
14. If necessary to insert a postscript, double space down to insert "P.S."
15. Save the file to the hard drive before proofreading the letter, making final corrections.
16. Print two copies, one to be sent and one to be retained in the files.
17. Prepare an envelope. If the letter is to be sent registered or certified, insert mailing instructions on the envelope.
18. Sign the letter, fold it, and insert it with enclosures into the envelope for mailing.

PROCEDURE 20.3 Complete a Job Application Form

1. Assemble materials: job application form, notes of previous employment, pen or pencil.
2. Read the entire application before beginning.
3. If instructions say, "please print," "use pen only," or "put last name first," follow these directions precisely.
4. Complete the application in ink unless directed to use a pencil.
5. Block print if handwriting is illegible and abbreviate words only if there is a lack of space.
6. Insert data on the application form, stressing clarity and neatness.
7. Record dates of previous employment accurately, as these data may be used for verification purposes. If there is a question asking you to state the reason you left a position, insert "To be discussed during the interview."
8. Specifically list all job skills that pertain to the position for which you are applying.
9. If salary expectation is requested, insert hourly wage or salary amount expected followed by "negotiable" or "flexible" for further discussion during the interview.
10. Sign and date the completed application.

KEY POINTS

This is a brief chapter review of the key issues presented. To further enhance your knowledge of the technical subject matter, review the key terms and key abbreviations for this chapter using the Glossary at the end of this book, which appears in a section before the Index.

1. Use many paths to search for a job as an insurance billing specialist.
2. Access the internet to locate job offers by potential employers.
3. Prepare for and attend job fairs to make contact and network with potential employers.
4. Visit potential employers and complete job application forms.
5. Compose a letter of introduction and an updated résumé focusing on the type of job you wish to obtain.
6. Prepare yourself for an interview so that you make a positive impression.
7. Organize a job portfolio of documents relating to education, prior work experience, and skills.
8. Research thoroughly and begin the steps to establish a billing service.
9. Know all Health Insurance Portability and Accountability Act (HIPAA) security and confidentiality policy and practice requirements when working from a home-based business.
10. Pursue becoming certified or registered to convey a higher level of professionalism.
11. Become a member of a professional organization to network and keep current on technical data and federal regulations.

INTERNET RESOURCES

American Academy of Professional Coders (AAPC)
- www.aapc.com

American Association of Medical Assistants (AAMA)
- www.aama-ntl.org

American Health Information Management Association (AHIMA)
- www.ahima.org

American Medical Billing Association (AMBA)
- www.americanmedicalbillingassociation.com

STUDENT ASSIGNMENT

- Study Chapter 20.
- Complete all exercises in the *Workbook* to reinforce the theories learned in this chapter.

- Turn to the Glossary at the end of this text for a further understanding of the key terms and key abbreviations used in this chapter.

REFERENCES

Federal Register; Department of Health and Human Services; Title 45, Section 164.528. https://www.usa.gov/federal-agencies/u-s-department-of-health-and-human-services.

Health Information Portability and Accountability Act of 1996, §160.103. https://www.hhs.gov/hipaa/index.html.

KEY ABBREVIATIONS

Chapter number(s) is (are) shown in parentheses after each term.

AAAHC   Accreditation Association for Ambulatory Health Care (18)

AAPC   American Academy of Professional Coders (20)

ABN   Advance Beneficiary Notice of Noncoverage (6)

ACA   Affordable Care Act (4)

ACS   American College of Surgeons (18)

ADL   activities of daily living (18)

ADSM   active duty service member (8)

AHA   American Hospital Association (12, 18)

AHIMA   American Health Information Management Association (12, 20)

ALJ   administrative law judge (16)

AMA   American Medical Association (1, 18)

AME   agreed medical evaluator (9)

ANSI   American National Standards Institute (15)

AOA   American Osteopathic Association (18)

APC   ambulatory payment classification (18)

APM   Advanced Alternative Payment Model (6)

A/R   accounts receivable (4, 17)

ARRA   American Recovery and Reinvestment Act (2, 11)

ASC   ambulatory surgery category (18)

ASC X12   Accredited Standards Committee X12 (15)

ASCA   Administrative Simplification Compliance Act (14)

ASCQR   Ambulatory Surgery Center Quality Reporting (18)

ASET   Administrative Simplification Enforcement Tool (15)

ASHD   arteriosclerotic heart disease (1)

ASP   application service provider (15)

ASU   ambulatory surgery units (18)

ATM   automatic teller machine (15, 17)

BCBSA   Blue Cross/Blue Shield Association (5)

C and R   compromise and release (9)

CAC   computer-assisted coding (12)

CAH   critical access hospital (18)

CAP   claims assistance professional (1, 20)

CC   chief complaint (11, 12)

CCs   complication/comorbidity (18)

CCAP   Certified Claims Assistance Professional (20)

CCI   Correct Coding Initiative (6)

CCS   Certified Coding Specialist (20)

CCS-P   Certified Coding Specialist–Physician (20)

CCU   coronary care unit (11)

CDHP   Consumer Directed Health Plan (4, 5)

CDI   clinical documentation improvement (11)

CE   consultative examiner (10)

CECP   Certified Electronic Claims Processor (20)

CERT   Comprehensive Error Rate Testing (3)

CF   conversion factor (13)

CHAMPUS   Civilian Health and Medical Program of the Uniformed Services (8)

CHAMPVA   Civilian Health and Medical Program of the Department of Veterans Affairs (4, 8)

CHIP   Children's Health Insurance Program (7)

CLIA   Clinical Laboratory Improvement Amendments (3)

CMA   Certified Medical Assistant (20)

CMBS   Certified Medical Billing Specialist (20)

CMGs   case mix groups (18)

CMP   Civil Monetary Penalty (3)

CMRS   Certified Medical Reimbursement Specialist (20)

CMS   Centers for Medicare and Medicaid Services (2, 3, 6, 16)

CMS-1450   Center for Medicare and Medicaid Services Health Insurance Claim Form 1450 (19)

CMS-1500   Centers for Medicare and Medicaid Services Health Insurance Claim Form 1500 (14)

COB   coordination of benefits (4, 8)

COBRA   Consolidated Omnibus Budget Reconciliation Act (4)

COLA   cost-of-living adjustment (10)

copay   copayment (4, 5)

CPC   Certified Professional Coder (20)

CPC-A   Certified Professional Coder–Apprentice (20)

CPC-H   Certified Professional Coder–Hospital (20)

CPT   Current Procedural Terminology (12, 13)

CSRS   Civil Service Retirement System (10)

CT   Computed Tomography (11)

DDE   direct data entry (15)

DDS   Disability Determination Services (10)

DEERS   Defense Enrollment Eligibility Reporting System (8)

DEFRA   Deficit Reduction Act (7)

DHHS   Department of Health and Human Services (2, 3, 6, 15)

DM   diabetes mellitus (12)

DME   durable medical equipment (6, 13, 14)

DNA   does not apply (14)

DNFB   discharge not final billed (18)

DoD   Department of Defense (10)

DOJ   Department of Justice (3)

DOS   date of service (4)

DRG   diagnosis-related group (18)

DSL   digital subscriber line (15)

dx or Dx   diagnosis (11)

ECG   electrocardiogram (13)

e-check   electronic check (17)

ECP   electronic claims processor (20)

ED or ER   emergency department or emergency room (11, 13)

EDI   electronic data interchange (15)

EEOC   Equal Employment Opportunity Commission (20)

EFT   electronic funds transfer (15)

EHR   electronic health record (11, 15)

EIN   employer identification number (2, 14)

E/M   evaluation and management (11, 13)

e-mail   electronic mail (1)

EMC   electronic medical claim (15)

EMG   emergency (14)

EMR   electronic medical record (11)

EMTALA   Emergency Medical Treatment and Active Labor Act (3, 18)

EOB   explanation of benefits (8, 13, 16)

EOMB   explanation of Medicare benefits (15)

ePHI   electronic protected health information (2)

EPO   exclusive provider organization (4, 5)

EPSDT   Early and Periodic Screening, Diagnosis, and Treatment (7, 14)

ERA   electronic remittance advice (6, 15)

ERISA   Employee Retirement Income Security Act (9)

ESRD   end-stage renal disease (6)

FACT   Fair and Accurate Credit Transactions (17)

FBI   Federal Bureau of Investigation (2)

FCA   False Claims Act (3)

FCBA   Fair Credit Billing Act (17)

FCRA   Fair Credit Reporting Act (17)

FCS   Facility Coding Specialist (20)

FDCPA   Fair Debt Collection Practices Act (17)

FDIC   Federal Deposit Insurance Corporation (3)

FECA   Federal Employees' Compensation Act (9)

FERA   Federal Enforcement and Recovery Act of 2009 (3)

FERS   Federal Employees Retirement System (10)

FFS   fee-for-service (5)

FH   family history (11)

FI   fiscal intermediary (8)

FL   form locators (19)

FMLA   Family and Medical Leave Act (10)

FPL   federal poverty level (7)

FSA   flexible spending account (4)

FTC   Federal Trade Commission (13, 17)

FTP   file transfer protocol (2)

GAF   geographic adjustment factor (13)

GPCIs   geographic practice cost indices (6, 13)

HACs   Health Administration Centers (18)

HACRP   The Hospital Acquired Condition Reduction Program (18)

HBA   health benefits advisor (8)

HCERA   Health Care and Education Reconciliation Act (4)

HCF   health care finder (8)

HCFAC   Health Care Fraud and Abuse Control [program] (3)

HCPCS   Healthcare Common Procedure Coding System (13)

HDHP   high-deductible health plan (4)

HEAT   Health Care Fraud Prevention and Enforcement Action Team (3)

HFAP   Healthcare Facilities Accreditation Program (18)

HHA   home health agency (18)

HHS (2)   Health and Human Services

HH PPS   Home Health Prospective Payment System (18)

HIM   health information management (11)

HIPAA Health Insurance Portability and Accountability Act (2, 16)

HIPPS health insurance prospective payment system (18)

HITECH Health Information Technology for Economic and Clinical Health [Act] (2)

HIV human immunodeficiency virus (11, 12)

HMO health maintenance organization (4, 5)

HPI history of present illness (11)

HPID health plan identifier (15)

HRA health reimbursement account (4)

HRS Health Care Reimbursement Specialist (20)

HSA health savings account (4)

ICD-10-CM *International Classification of Diseases,* Tenth Revision, Clinical Modifications (12)

ICD-10-PCS *International Classification of Diseases,* Tenth Revision, Procedure Coding System (12, 19)

ICD-11 *International Classification of Diseases,* Eleventh Revision (12)

ICR intelligent character recognition or image copy recognition (14)

ICU intensive care unit (6, 11)

IIHI individually identifiable health information (2)

IME independent medical evaluator (9)

IPA independent [or individual] practice association (4, 5)

IPF PPS Inpatient Psychiatric Facility Prospective Payment System (18)

IPPS Inpatient Prospective Payment System (18)

IRF PAI Inpatient Rehabilitation Facility Patient Assessment Instrument (18)

IRF PPS Inpatient Rehabilitation Facility Prospective Payment System (18)

IRS Internal Revenue Service (15)

LCD local coverage determination (6)

LGHP large group health plan (6)

LHWCA Longshore and Harbor Workers' Compensation Act (9)

LLQ left lower quadrant (11)

LMP last menstrual period (14)

LTCH PPS long-term care hospital prospective payment system (18)

LUQ left upper quadrant (11)

MA Plan Medicare Advantage Plan (6)

MAC Medicare administrative contractor (3, 6, 15)

MACRA Medicare Access and CHIP Reauthorization Act of 2015 (6)

MBI Medicare Beneficiary Identifier (6)

MCCs major complication/comorbidity (18)

MCHP Maternal and Child Health Program (4)

MCO managed care organization (5)

MDCs major diagnostic category (18)

MDM medical decision making (11)

Medi-Medi Medicare/Medicaid (4, 6)

MFS Medicare fee schedule (6)

MG Medigap (6)

MHS Military Health System (8)

MIP Medicare Integrity Program (3)

MIPPA Medicare Improvements for Patients and Providers Act (6)

MIPS Merit-based Incentive Payment System (6)

MLN Medicare Learning Network (6)

MMA Medicare Prescription Drug, Improvement, and Modernization Act (6)

MN medically needy (7)

MRI magnetic resonance imaging (11, 12)

MSA medical savings account (4, 6)

MS-DRGs Medicare Severity Diagnosis-Related Groups (18)

MSN Medicare Summary Notice (6)

MSO management services organization (1)

MSP Medicare secondary payer (6, 7, 14)

MTF Military Treatment Facility (8)

NA or N/A not applicable (14, 17)

NC no charge (17)

NCCI National Correct Coding Initiative (13)

NCD national coverage determination (6)

NCHS National Center for Health Statistics (12)

NCICS National Certified Insurance and Coding Specialist (20)

NCQA National Committee for Quality Assurance (5)

ND Nondisability claim (9)

NDC National Drug Code (15)

NEC not elsewhere classifiable (12)

NF nursing facility (6)

nonpar nonparticipating [provider or physician] (4, 6, 8)

NOS not otherwise specified (12)

NPI National Provider Identifier (2, 6, 14, 16, 19)

NPP non-physician practitioner (1, 4)

NPP Notice of Privacy Practices (2)

NSF National Standard Format (15, 17)

NSF nonsufficient funds or not sufficient funds (17)

NUBC National Uniform Billing Committee (19)

NUCC National Uniform Claim Committee (14)

OAS CAHPS Consumer Assessment of Health Care Providers and Systems Outpatient and Ambulatory Surgery Survey (18)

OBRA Omnibus Budget Reconciliation Act (7)

OCE outpatient code editor (18)

OCR Office of Civil Rights (2, 14)

OHI other health insurance (8)

OIG Office of the Inspector General (2, 3)

OOY over-one-year [claims] (7)

OPPS Outpatient Prospective Payment System (18)

ORT Operation Restore Trust (3)

OSHA Occupational Safety and Health Administration (3, 9)

OWCP Office of Workers' Compensation Programs (9)

PACU post-anesthesia care unit (11)

P&P policies and procedures (2, 3)

P and S permanent and stationary (9)

PACU post-anesthesia care unit (11)

PAHCOM Professional Association of Health Care Office Management (20)

par participating [physician or provider] (4, 6, 8)

PAT preadmission testing (18)

PC professional component (13)

PCM primary care manager (8)

PCP primary care provider (5, 11)

PD permanent disability (9)

PE or PX physical examination (11)

PFFS private fee-for-service [plan] (6)

PFML Paid Family and Medical Leave (10)

PFSH past, family, or social history (11)

PH past history (11)

PHI protected health information (2)

PMPM per member, per month (5)

PMS practice management software or practice management system (4)

PO privacy officer or privacy official (2)

POA present on admission (18, 19)

POMR system problem-oriented medical record system (11)

POR physician of record (9)

POS place-of-service (8)

POS machine point of service machine (7)

POS plan point-of-service (4, 5)

Postop post-operative (11)

PPACA Patient Protection and Affordable Care Act (2, 3, 4)

PPO preferred provider organization (4, 5)

PPS prospective payment system (6, 18, 19)

Preop pre-operative (11)

PS physical status (13)

PSA Prime Service Area (8)

PSO provider-sponsored organization (5, 6)

QC qualifying circumstances (13)

QI Qualifying Individuals [program] (7)

QIC Qualified Independent Contractor (16)

QIO Quality Improvement Organization (6, 18)

QMB qualified Medicare beneficiary (7)

QME qualified medical evaluator (9)

RA remittance advice (6, 7, 16)

RAC Recovery Audit Contractor (3)

RAC Initiative Recovery Audit Contractor Initiative (6)

RAI Resident Assessment Instrument (18)

RBRVS resource-based relative value scale (6, 13)

RCM revenue cycle management (16)

RCU respiratory care unit (11)

RICs Rehabilitation Impairment Category (18)

RLQ right lower quadrant (11)

RMA Registered Medical Assistant (20)

RMC Registered Medical Coder (20)

ROA received on account (4)

ROM range-of-motion (9)

ROS review of systems (11)

RUQ right upper quadrant (11)

RVS relative value studies or scale (13)

RVU relative value unit (13)

SCHIP State Children's Health Insurance Program (4)

SCIF State Compensation Insurance Fund (9)

SDHP Self-Directed Health Plan (4)

SDI State Disability Insurance (4, 10)

SDP Self-Disclosure Protocol (3)

SH social history (11)

SHCP Supplemental Health Care Program (8)

SHOP Small Business Health Options Program (4)

SIF subsequent-injury fund (9)

SLMB Specified Low-Income Medicare Beneficiary (7)

SNF skilled nursing facility (18)

SNF PPS skilled nursing facility prospective payment system (18)

SNOMED CT Systematized Nomenclature of Medicine – Clinical Terms (12)

SOAP subjective objective assessment plan (11)
SOF signature on file (4, 14)
SOR source-oriented record [system] (11)
SSA Social Security Administration (10)
SSDI Social Security Disability Insurance (10)
SSI Supplemental Security Income (7, 10)
SSN Social Security number (14)
TAMP Transitional Assistance Management Program (8)
TANF Temporary Assistance to Needy Families (7)
TC technical component (13)
TCS Transaction and Code Set [rule] (15)

TD temporary disability (9, 10)
TDI temporary disability insurance (10)
TFL TRICARE for Life (8)
TILA Truth in Lending Act (17)
TJC The Joint Commission (18)
TMA TRICARE Management Activity (8)
TPO treatment, payment, or health care operations (2)
TPR TRICARE Prime Remote (8)
TSC TRICARE service center (8)
UB-04 Uniform Bill–04 (18, 19)
UCD Unemployment Compensation Disability (4, 10)
UCR usual, customary, and reasonable (5,13)

UM utilization management (18)
UR utilization review (5)
U/S ultrasound (11)
USCIS US Citizenship and Immigration Services (20)
USPSTF United States Preventive Service Task Force (6)
VA Veterans Affairs (4, 8, 10)
VBP value-based purchasing (18)
W2 wage and tax statement (17)
WC Workers' Compensation (4)
WHO World Health Organization (12)
WNL within normal limits (11)
WP waiting period (9, 10)
ZPIC Zone Program Integrity Contractor (3)

GLOSSARY

Chapter number(s) is (are) shown in parentheses after each term.

72-hour rule (18) Medicare policy that states if a patient receives diagnostic tests and hospital outpatient services within 72 hours of admission to a hospital, all such tests and services are combined (bundled) with inpatient services only if services are related to the admission. Also called the 3-day payment window because it is 3 calendar days rather than 72 hours. Sometimes referred to as the 72/24-hour rule.

Abuse (3) Incidents or business practices, not usually considered fraudulent, that are inconsistent with accepted sound medical business or fiscal practices.

Accident (9) An unexpected happening, causing injury traceable to a definite time and place.

Accidental death and dismemberment (10) An insurance policy provision that protects the insured if he or she suffers loss of sight, loss of limb(s), or death by accident.

Accounts receivable (A/R) (1, 17) The total amount of money owed to a health care organization for services rendered or goods provided.

Accounts receivable management (4) The process of ensuring that a health care organization collects appropriate reimbursement for services or goods provided.

Accreditation (18) A voluntary assessment process that facilities use to assess their performance against national benchmarks and established standards of care. It is both a self-assessment and a peer review process.

Accreditation Association for Ambulatory Health Care (18) The accrediting body designated by CMS for ambulatory surgery centers.

Accreditation Association of Hospitals/Health Systems (18) The accrediting body designated by CMS for hospital and health systems.

Accredited Standards Committee X12 (ASC X12) (15) The United States standards body formed by the American National Standards Institute (ANSI) for cross-industry development, maintenance, and publication of electronic data exchange standards.

Accredited Standards Committee X12 Version 5010 (15) System developed by the American National Standards Institute (ANSI) that meets Health Insurance Portability and Accountability Act (HIPAA) standards for the transmission of either ICD-9 or ICD-10 diagnostic code data.

Active duty service member (ADSM) (8) An active member of the United States government military services (e.g., Army, Navy, Air Force, Marines, Coast Guard).

Activities of daily living (ADL) (18) Normal daily tasks performed by individuals, such as bathing, eating, and getting dressed.

Acute (11) A medical condition that runs a short but relatively severe course.

Acute care facility (18) A general hospital that provides inpatient and outpatient medical care.

Adjudication (6, 9, 16) (1) The process of paying claims submitted or denying them after comparing the claim to benefit and coverage requirements; also known as a claim settlement. (2) In workers' compensation cases, final determination of the issues involving settlement of a work-related accident and the rating of a case.

Adjustments (6) An adjustment refers to any change to the balance due of an account such as additional payment, partial payment, courtesy adjustment, write-off, discount, or change made to correct an error in billing or processing of a claim (overpayment or underpayment) or as a result of a retroactive rate change (late charges for a previously submitted bill).

Administrative Law Judge (ALJ) (16) The attorney involved in a third level of Medicare appeals a health care provider may use if they disagree with a claims reconsideration decision. The hearing provides an opportunity to explain your position to an Administrative Law Judge.

Administrative Safeguards (2) Management controls used to guard patient data integrity, confidentiality, and availability though development, implementation, and maintenance of policies and procedures.

Administrative Simplification Compliance Act (ASCA) (14) Legislation enacted by Congress to improve administration of the Medicare program by increasing efficiencies gained through electronic claim submission. The Act required all claims sent to the Medicare program to be submitted electronically.

Administrative Simplification Enforcement Tool (ASET) (15) A web-based tool implemented by the federal government to address issues of noncompliance with the HIPAA by enabling health care providers, payers, clearinghouses, and others to submit complaints against a covered entity that fails to adopt and follow the HIPAA rules for transactions and code sets.

Admission review (18) A review for appropriateness and necessity of formal acceptance into the hospital for care.

Advance Beneficiary Notice of Noncoverage (ABN) (6) An agreement given to the patient to read and sign before rendering a service if the participating physician thinks it may be denied for payment because of medical necessity or limitation of liability by Medicare. The patient agrees to pay for the service; also known as a waiver of liability agreement or responsibility statement.

Advanced Alternative Payment Model (APM) (6) A system for medical reimbursement that provides additional compensation as an incentive for the delivery of high-quality and more cost-efficient health care by providers.

Adverse effect (12) An unfavorable, detrimental, or pathologic reaction to a drug that occurs when appropriate doses are given to humans for prophylaxis (prevention of disease), diagnosis, and therapy.

Affordable Care Act (ACA) (Obamacare) (4) Health insurance reform signed into law in 2010 to make health care available and affordable to Americans who did not have health insurance.

Against medical advice (AMA) (18) Situations when a patient insists upon leaving the hospital and the physician recommends that the patient needs continued hospitalization.

Age analysis (17) The procedure of systematically arranging the accounts receivable by age, from the date of service.

Aging report (16) Document that reports the status of insurance claims to the provider of the medical services and identifies individual transactions that need to be followed up (e.g., appeal or resubmit a corrected claim).

Allowable charge (8) An amount on which TRICARE figures the patient's cost share for covered care. This is based on 75% to 80% of the allowable charge.

Ambulance Fee Schedule (18) The reimbursement system used by Medicare to reimburse for ambulance services.

Ambulatory care (18) Also referred to as Outpatient hospital care; covers various types of services that do not require an overnight hospital stay. The patient is discharged within 24 hours of arrival.

Ambulatory payment classification (APC) (18) A system of outpatient hospital reimbursement based on procedures rather than diagnoses.

Ambulatory Surgery Center payment system (18) The payment system used by CMS for services provided in an ambulatory surgery center which uses packaging; all supplies, medications, and other components of a service are included in the payment package.

Ambulatory Surgery Center Quality Reporting Program (ASCQR) (18) A data quality program sponsored by CMS that requires ASCs to report their quality-of-care data for standardized measures in order to receive the full ASC payment rate.

Ambulatory Surgery Units (ASU) (18) Hospital-based outpatient surgery departments.

American Academy of Professional Coders (AAPC) (20) A national professional organization that provides training programs and award certifications in the areas of medical billing and coding.

American College of Surgeons (ACS) (18) An association of surgeons that promotes the highest standards of care through education, patient advocacy, and standardization of care.

American College of Surgeons (ACS) (18) An association of surgeons that promotes the highest standards of care through education, patient advocacy, and standardization of care.

489

American Health Information Management Association (AHIMA) (20) A national professional organization that promotes the art and science of medical record management and improves the quality of comprehensive health information for the welfare of the public.

American Hospital Association (AHA) (18) An association of hospitals whose mission is to advance the health of individuals and communities through health policy development and regulation.

American Medical Association (AMA) (1, 18) A national professional society of physicians.

American National Standards Institute (ANSI) (15) A private, nonprofit organization that oversees development of voluntary consensus standards for products, services, processes, systems, and personnel in the United States.

American Osteopathic Association (AOA) (18) An association that provides board certification for doctors of osteopathic medicine.

American Recovery and Reinvestment Act (ARRA) (2) A fiscal stimulus package that ended the Great Recession and was signed into law by President Obama in 2009. Included in ARRA legislation is the Health Information Technology for Economic and Clinical Health (HITECH) Act that contained incentives for adopting health care information technology designed to speed up the adoption of electronic health record systems in health care organizations.

Ancillary services (5) Supportive services other than routine hospital services provided by the facility, such as x-ray films and laboratory tests.

Anti-Kickback Law (3) Legislation enacted in 1972 that made kickbacks (paying for referrals) a crime. A kickback may include any type of gift, reward, or inducement for facilitating a transaction or appointment.

Appeal (16) A request for a review of an insurance claim that has been underpaid or denied by an insurance company in an effort to receive additional payment.

Application form (20) A request form to be completed with pertinent data when applying for employment.

Application service provider (ASP) (15) A practice management system available over the internet in which data are housed on the server of the ASP but the accounts are managed by the health care provider's staff.

Approach character (19) An ICD-10-PCS character that identifies the technique used to reach the site of the procedure. Some of the options are open, laparoscopically, and endoscopically.

Approved charges (6) A fee determined by an insurance carrier as to what a medical service is worth, which may or may not be the same as the amount billed. The patient may or may not be responsible for the difference.

ASC X12 Version 5010 (15) The electronic data interchange claim form developed by the Accredited Standards Committee X12 (ASC X12). Providers, payers, and clearinghouses were required to implement and start using this standard on January 1, 2012. Version 5010 allows providers and payers to transmit either ICD-9 or ICD-10 data.

Assignment (4, 6) In health care, this is an agreement signed by the patient to allow the insurance carrier to send payment directly to the service provider.

Assumption coding (3) Inappropriate assignment of diagnosis or procedure codes based on a review of clinical evidence in a patient's record rather than basing it on information specifically documented by the provider of services.

Attending physician (11) A medical staff member who is legally responsible for the care and treatment given to a patient.

Auditing (3) A systemic and objective review of a transaction.

Auditor (20) An individual authorized to review and verify the accuracy of business records; auditing titles vary according to what they are monitoring (coding auditor, revenue cycle auditor, compliance auditor).

Audit trail (15) Chronologic record of submitted data that can be traced to the source to determine the place or origin. Also referred to as audit log.

Authorization (2) Under the Health Insurance Portability and Accountability Act (HIPAA) Privacy Rule, an individual's formal, written permission to use or disclose his or her personally identifiable health information for purposes other than treatment, payment, or health care operations.

Authorization form (2) A document signed by the patient that is needed for use and disclosure of protected health information that is not included in any existing consent form agreements.

Authorized provider (8) A physician or other individual authorized provider of care, or a hospital or supplier approved by TRICARE to provide medical care and supplies.

Automatic stay (17) A court order that goes into effect once a bankruptcy petition is filed; all other legal actions, such as attachments and foreclosures, are halted.

Back-up (11) The process of saving data entered into a computer system on a regular basis.

Balance (17) An amount owed on a credit transaction; also known as the outstanding or unpaid balance.

Bankruptcy (17) A condition under which a person or corporation is declared unable to pay debts.

Batch (15) A group of claims for different patients from one office submitted in one computer transmission.

Beneficiary (6, 8) An individual entitled to receive insurance policy or government program health care benefits. Also known as participant, subscriber, dependent, enrollee, or member.

Benefit period (6, 10) (1) A period of time during which payments for Medicare inpatient hospital benefits are available. A benefit period begins on the first day an enrollee is given inpatient hospital care (nursing care or rehabilitation services) by a qualified provider and ends when the enrollee has not been an inpatient for 60 consecutive days. (2) In workers' compensation cases, the maximum amount of time that benefits will be paid to the injured or ill person

for the disability. (3) For disability insurance, the maximum amount of time that benefits will be paid to the injured or ill person for a disability.

Benign tumor (12) An abnormal growth that does not have the properties of invasion and metastasis and is usually surrounded by a fibrous capsule; also called a neoplasm.

Bilateral (13) When coding surgical procedures, this term refers to both sides of the body.

Birthday rule (4) An informal rule that the health insurance industry has adopted for the coordination of benefits when children are listed as dependents on two parents' health plans. Under the birthday rule, the health plan of the parent whose birthday comes first in the calendar year is designated as the primary plan.

Blanket contract (4) Comprehensive group insurance coverage through plans sponsored by professional associations for their members.

Blind mailing (20) To send a résumé with a cover letter to possible prospects whom the individual does not know personally and who have not advertised for a job opening.

Blue Cross/Blue Shield Association (5) A national association of approximately 36 independent, community-based, and locally operated Blue Cross/Blue Shield companies providing some form of health insurance in every state within the U.S. and a program for U.S. federal employees, retirees, and their families.

Body Part character (19) The ICD-10-PCS character that identifies the specific part in the body system the procedure was performed on. For example, body parts can include right lower leg, gallbladder, or left lobe of the liver.

Body System character (19) The ICD-10-PCS character that identifies the specific organ system the procedure was performed on. Examples of a body system would be respiratory or cardiovascular.

Bonding (17) An insurance contract by which, in return for a stated fee, a bonding agency guarantees payment of a certain sum to an employer in the event of a financial loss to the employer by the act of a specified employee or by some contingency over which the employer has no control.

Breach (2) Breach means "breaking or violation of a law or agreement." In the context of the medical office, it means the unauthorized release of information about the patient.

Bundled codes (13) To group more than one component (service or procedure) into one Current Procedural Terminology (CPT) code.

Business associate (2) A person who, on behalf of the covered entity, performs or assists in the performance of a function or activity involving the use or disclosure of individually identifiable health information, including claims processing or administration, data analysis, process or administration, utilization review, quality assurance, billing, benefit management, practice management, and repricing.

Business associate agreement (20) Contract between the provider and a clearinghouse that submits the electronic claims on behalf of the provider.

Cable modem (15) A modem used to connect a computer to a cable television system that offers online services.

Cancelable (4) A renewal provision in an insurance agreement that grants the insurer the right to cancel the policy at any time and for any reason.

Capitation (4, 5, 18) A system of payment used by managed care plans in which physicians and hospitals are paid a fixed per capita amount for each patient enrolled over a stated period of time, regardless of the type and number of services provided; reimbursement to the hospital on a per-member/per-month basis to cover costs for the members of the plan. Capitation can also mean a set amount to be paid per claim.

Carcinoma in situ (12) Cancer confined to the site of origin without invasion of neighboring tissues.

Carrier-direct system (15) A method for submission of claims, in which data is transmitted electronically directly to the payer's system, without the need for a clearinghouse.

Carve outs (5) Medical services not included within the capitation rate as benefits of a managed care contract and that may be contracted for separately.

Case mix groups (CMG) (18) A patient classification system to group together patients with similar characteristics (such as functional motor and cognitive scores and age) as a basis for describing the types of patients a hospital or other health care provider treats.

Cash flow (1, 17) In a health care organization or medical practice, the amount of actual cash generated and available for use within a given period of time.

Catastrophic cap (8) The maximum dollar amount that a member has to pay under TRI-CARE or CHAMPVA in any fiscal year or enrollment period for covered medical bills.

Catchment area (8) In the TRICARE program, an area, defined by zip codes, that is approximately 40 miles in radius surrounding each United States military treatment facility.

Categorically needy (7) Aged, blind, or disabled individuals or families and children who meet financial eligibility requirements for Aid to Families with Dependent Children (AFDC), Supplemental Security Income (SSI), or an optional state supplement.

Centers for Medicare and Medicaid Services (CMS) (6) A federal agency within the U.S. Department of Health and Human Services (DHHS) that administers the Medicare program. It is responsible for implementation of all rules, regulations, and health-related policies governing the Medicare program.

Certification (20) A statement issued by a board or association verifying that a person meets professional standards.

Certified Coding Specialist (CCS) (20) A title received by a person after appropriate training and by passing a certification examination administered by the American Health Information Management Association (AHIMA) for hospital-based coding.

Certified Coding Specialist–Physician (CCS-P) (20) A title received by a person after appropriate training and by passing a certification examination administered by the American Health Information Management Association (AHIMA) for physician-based coding.

Certified Medical Assistant (CMA) (20) A title received by a person after appropriate training and by passing a certification examination administered by the American Association of Medical Assistants (AAMA).

Certified Medical Billing Specialist (CMBS) (20) A title received by a person after appropriate training and by passing a certification examination administered by either the American Association of Medical Billers (AAMB) or the Medical Association of Billers (MAB).

Certified Professional Coder (CPC) (20) A title received by a person after appropriate training and the passing of a certification examination administered by the American Academy of Professional Coders (AAPC).

CHAMPVA (4, 8) See Veterans Health Administration.

Chapter 11 (5) Chapter 11 refers to the U.S. bankruptcy code 11 which is a form of bankruptcy that involves reorganization of a debtor's business affairs, debts, and assets.

Chargemaster (18) A list or database of all the services, supplies, equipment, and so forth provided by the hospital and the charge that is associated with it. Other data elements in the chargemaster include a unique identifier for each item, the department providing the service, a revenue code, and the procedure codes (discussed later in this section). Also called a charge description master.

Chargemaster Coordinator (20) An individual who oversees managing the contents of the chargemaster including tasks such as updating codes, adding new services, deleting services no longer provided, updating charges, and working with the clinical services, billers, financial department, and others to ensure the entries in the chargemaster meet their needs.

Chief complaint (CC) (11, 12) A patient's statement describing symptoms, problems, or conditions as the reason for seeking health care services from a physician.

Children's Health Insurance Program (CHIP) (7) A partnership between the federal and state governments that provides low-cost health coverage to children in families that earn too much money to qualify for Medicaid. In some states, CHIP also covers care for pregnant women.

Chronic (11) A medical condition persisting over a long period of time.

Chronologic résumé (20) A data sheet that outlines experience and education by dates.

Civil False Claims Act (3) Legislation authorizing the United Stated federal government to recover monetary damages from people who file fraudulent claims for payment with the federal government.

Civilian Health and Medical Program of the Department of Veterans Affairs (CHAMP-VA) (8) See Veterans Health Administration.

Civilian Health and Medical Program of the Uniformed Services (CHAMPUS) (8) The program created by the US Congress in 1966 under Public Law 89-614. The purpose of the law was to assist individuals in the military who were finding it increasingly difficult to pay for the medical care required by their families. In January 1994, TRICARE became the new title for CHAMPUS.

Civil Monetary Penalty (CMP) (3) Federal statute that imposes fines and sanctions to combat health care fraud and abuse and is imposed on individuals or health care facilities that do not comply with the Centers for Medicare and Medicaid Services (CMS) regulations.

Civil Service Retirement System (CSRS) (10) A program for federal employees who work in civil service and become totally disabled.

Claim (4) A bill sent to an insurance carrier requesting payment for services rendered; also known as encounter record.

Claim attachments (15) Documents that contain information, hard copy or electronic, related to a completed insurance claim that assists in validating the medical necessity or explains the medical service or procedure for payment (for example, operative report, discharge summary, invoice).

Claim denial management (16) The process of identifying and reviewing specific reasons for claim denials, followed by development of a process for appealing denied claims when appropriate.

Claims assistance professional (CAP) (1) A practitioner who works for the consumer and helps patients to organize, complete, file, and negotiate health insurance claims of all types to obtain maximum benefits as well as tells patients what checks to write to providers to eliminate overpayment.

Claims examiner (1, 9) A representative of the insurer who authorizes treatment and investigates, evaluates, and negotiates the patient's insurance claim and acts for the company in the settlement of claims; also known as claims adjuster, claims representative, and claims administrator.

Clean claim (14) A completed insurance claim form submitted within the program time limit that contains all necessary information without deficiencies so that it can be processed and paid promptly.

Clearinghouse (2, 15) An independent organization that receives insurance claims from a health care organization or a physician's office, performs software edits, and redistributes the claims electronically to various insurance carriers.

Clinic (18) A facility for diagnosis and treatment of patients on an outpatient basis; includes private provider groups and multispecialty groups as well as those affiliated with larger hospital systems. It also includes walk-ins and other specialized types of health care services such as dental services.

Clinical documentation improvement (11) The process of creating accurate and effective patient health records in an effort to improve patient outcomes, provide accurate data for quality measurement reporting, and ensure proper reimbursement.

Clinical Documentation Improvement Specialist (20) An individual who works with physicians and other health care professionals to ensure that the documentation in the health record is complete and granular (at the appropriate level of detail).

Clinical Laboratory Improvement Amendments (CLIA) (3) Legislation that ensures quality lab testing through certification requirements for health care laboratories.

Cloned note (11) (1) Entry in a patient's medical record worded exactly like or similar to the previous entries. (2) Medical documentation that is worded exactly the same from patient to patient. Cloned notes are considered a misrepresentation of the medical necessity requirements for insurance coverage of medical services and can trigger audits.

Clustering (3) Reporting one level of service for all patient visits, regardless of the patient's presenting problem or the amount of work or time spent with the patient.

Code sets (15) Any set of codes with their descriptions used to encode data elements, such as tables of terms, medical concepts, medical diagnostic codes, or medical procedure codes.

Coding Specialist (20) An individual trained to review health record documentation and extract the appropriate diagnosis and procedure codes that will be reported on the insurance claim.

Coinsurance (4, 5, 7) A cost-sharing requirement under a health insurance policy in which the insured will assume a percentage of the costs for covered services.

Collateral (17) Any possession, such as an automobile, furniture, stocks, or bonds, that secures or guarantees the discharge of an obligation.

Collection rate (5) The collection rate is the percentage of money that will be received on each service dollar charged to an insurance company.

Collection ratio (17) The relationship between the amount of money owed and the amount of money collected in reference to the doctor's accounts receivable.

Combination code (12) A code from one section of the procedural code book combined with a code from another section that is used to completely describe a procedure performed; in diagnostic coding, a single five-digit code used to identify etiology and secondary process (manifestation) or complication of a disease.

Combination résumé (20) A data sheet that combines specific dates or work experience with educational skills.

Comorbidity (13, 18) An ongoing condition that exists along with the condition for which the patient is receiving treatment; regarding diagnosis-related groups (DRGs), a preexisting condition that, because of its presence with a certain principal diagnosis, causes an increase in length of stay by at least 1 day in approximately 75% of cases. Also known as substantial comorbidity.

Compliance (3) A process of meeting regulations, recommendations, and expectations of federal and state agencies that pay for health care services and regulate the industry.

Compliance plan (3) A management plan composed of policies and procedures to accomplish uniformity, consistency, and conformity in medical record keeping that fulfills official requirements.

Compliance Specialist (20) An individual who is responsible for the development and management of the health care organization's compliance with federal and state laws. Tasks include development of policies and procedures, auditing and monitoring, ensuring the programs are being followed, identifying risk areas and compliance issues, and developing corrective actions to be taken.

Complication/comorbidity (CC) (12, 18) A disease or condition arising during the course of or as a result of another disease modifying medical care requirements; for diagnosis-related groups (DRGs), a condition that arises during the hospital stay that prolongs the length of stay by at least 1 day in approximately 75% of cases. Also known as substantial complication. Also see Comorbidity.

Comprehensive code (13) A single procedural code that describes or covers two or more CPT component codes that are bundled together as one unit.

Comprehensive Error Rate Testing (CERT) (3) An audit program implemented by CMS to measure the accuracy of payments made by Medicare Administrative Contractors (MACs) and to identify OIG target issues.

Compromise and release (C and R) (9) An agreement arrived at, whether in or out of court, for settling a workers' compensation case after the patient has been declared permanent and stationary.

Computed tomography (11) A type of radiography that uses a series of X-rays to visualize a cross-section of the body.

Computer-assisted coding (CAC) (12) Use of computer software that automatically generates a set of medical codes for review, validation, and use based on clinical documentation provided by health care practitioners. CAC uses two technology options: natural language processing (NLP) and structured input.

Concurrent care (11) The provision of similar services (for example, hospital visits) to the same patient by more than one physician on the same day. Usually a separate physical disorder is present.

Concurrent review (5, 11, 18) An evaluation of health care services to determine medical necessity and appropriateness of the care provided during the time services are being provided.

Conditionally renewable (4) An insurance policy renewal provision that grants the insurer a limited right to refuse to renew a health insurance policy at the end of a premium payment period.

Confidential communication (2) A privileged communication that may be disclosed only with the patient's permission.

Confidentiality (2) The state of treating privately or secretly, and not disclosing to other in-dividuals or for public knowledge, the patient's conversations or medical records.

Consent (2) Verbal or written agreement that gives approval to some action, situation, or statement.

Consultation (11) Services rendered by a physician whose opinion or advice is requested by another physician or agency in the evaluation or treatment of a patient's illness or suspected problem.

Consultative examiner (CE) (10) A physician who is paid a fee to examine or test a person for disability under either the Social Security Disability Insurance (SSDI) or Supplemental Security Income (SSI) program.

Consulting physician (11) A provider whose opinion or advice about evaluation or management of a specific problem is requested by another physician.

Consumer Assessment of Health Care Providers and Systems Outpatient and Ambulatory Surgery Survey (18) A survey developed by CMS to assess the experience of care for patients who have surgery or a procedure in an outpatient hospital setting or ASC.

Consumer Directed Health Plan (CDHP) (4, 5) Type of health insurance that allows the consumer to design and customize the plan based on their specific needs and circumstances. Also referred to as Self-Directed Health Plan (SDHP).

Continued stay review (18) Examination of a patient's health records to determine whether or not the patient should stay in the hospital.

Continuing education (CE) (20) Formal education pursued by a working professional and intended to improve or maintain professional competence.

Continuity of care (11) When a physician sees a patient who has received treatment for a condition and is referred by the previous doctor for treatment of the same condition.

Contract (4) A legally enforceable agreement when relating to an insurance policy; for workers' compensation cases, an agreement involving two or more parties in which each is obligated to the other to fulfill promises made. (The contract exists between the physician and the insurance carrier.)

Conventions (12) Rules or principles for determining a diagnostic code when using diagnostic code books, such as each space, typefaces, indentations, punctuation marks, instructional notes, abbreviations, cross-reference notes, and specific usage of the words "and," "with," and "due to." These rules assist in the selection of correct codes for the diagnoses encountered.

Conversion factor (9, 13) The dollars and cents amount that is established for one unit as applied to a procedure or service rendered. This unit is then used to convert various procedures into fee-schedule payment amounts by multiplying the relative value unit by the conversion factor.

Conversion privilege (4) An element of some group insurance policies that allows an insured to continue coverage under an individual policy if they are leaving the employer or organization or if the group contract is terminated.

Cooperative care (8) A term used when a patient is seen by a civilian physician or hospital for services cost-shared by TRICARE.

Coordination of benefits (COB) (4, 8) Two insurance carriers working together and coordinating the payment of their benefits so that there is no duplication of benefits paid between the primary and secondary insurance carriers.

Copayment (copay) (4, 5) A type of cost-sharing that requires the patient to pay a predetermined fee to the health care provider at the time the service is rendered.

Correct Coding Initiative (CCI) (6) Federal legislation that attempts to eliminate unbundling or other inappropriate reporting of procedural codes for professional medical services rendered to patients.

Corrective action plan (3) A step-by-step plan of action that is developed to achieve resolution to errors or offenses that have been identified in a health care organization.

Cost-of-living adjustment (10) A disability insurance provision to increase monthly benefits.

Cost outlier (18) A typical case that has an extraordinarily high cost when compared with most discharges classified to the same diagnostic cost group (DCG).

Cost report (3) A summary of information CMS requires institutional health care providers to submit annually which identify operating costs.

Cost share (4, 8) A requirement by most insurance plans in which the patient is responsible for a portion of the covered service. Examples include copays, deductible, and coinsurance amounts payable by the patient.

Counseling (11) A discussion between the physician and a patient, family, or both concerning the diagnosis, recommended studies or tests, prognosis, risks, and benefits of treatment, treatment options, patient and family education, and so on.

Covered entity (2, 15) An entity that transmits health information in electronic form in connection with a transaction covered by the Health Insurance Portability and Accountability Act (HIPAA). The covered entity may be (1) a health care coverage carrier such as Blue Cross/Blue Shield, (2) a health care clearinghouse through which claims are submitted, or (3) a health care provider, such as a primary care physician (PCP), a hospital, or nursing home.

Covered services (7) Specific services and supplies for which Medicaid will provide reimbursement; these consist of a combination of mandatory and optional services as stated in the state's Medicaid plan.

Cover letter (20) A letter of introduction prepared to accompany a résumé when seeking a job.

Credit (17) (1) From the Latin *credere*, meaning "to believe" or "to trust"; trust regarding financial obligation. (2) Accounting entry reflecting payment by a debtor (patient) of a sum received on his or her account.

Credit card (17) A card issued by an organization and devised for the purpose of obtaining money, property, labor, or services on credit.

Creditor (17) A person to whom money is owed.

Criminal False Claims Act (3) Legislation enacted stating that anyone who knowingly makes or presents a false or fraudulent claim to any department or agency of the United States shall be imprisoned up to 5 years and shall be subject to a fine.

Critical access hospital (CAH) (18) A small rural hospital set up to provide care to Medicare beneficiaries who would otherwise not have access to health care. They must have 25 or fewer beds, and be 35 miles from another facility. They must offer care 24 hours per day, 7 days per week and must have an RN on site and a physician on call and able to be on site within 60 minutes whenever there are patients admitted. They must have an average length of inpatient stay of 96 hours or less. A CAH must have all the equipment and medications on site for medical treatment and have a transfer agreement in place with a larger facility.

Critical care (11) In reference to coding professional services, this phrase relates to intensive care provided in a variety of acute life-threatening conditions requiring constant bedside attention by a physician.

Crossover claim (6) A bill for services rendered to a patient receiving benefits simultaneously from Medicare and Medicaid or from Medicare and a Medigap plan. Medicare pays first and then determines the amount of unmet Medicare deductible and coinsurance to be paid by the secondary insurance carrier. The claim is automatically transferred (electronically) to the secondary insurance carrier for additional payment. Also known as claims transfer.

Current Procedural Terminology (CPT) (13) A reference procedural code book using a five-digit numeric system to identify and code procedures established by the American Medical Association (AMA).

Custodial services (6) Assistance to patients with personal needs (e.g., dressing, eating, bathing, and getting in and out of bed).

Customary fee (13) The amount a physician usually charges most of her or his patients.

Cycle (1) A complete set of events that are repeated on a regular basis.

Cycle billing (17) A system of billing accounts at spaced intervals during the month based on a breakdown of accounts by alphabet, account number, insurance type, or date of first service.

Data elements (15) Medical code sets used uniformly to document why patients are seen (diagnosis, ICD-10-CM) and what is done to them during their encounter (procedure, CPT-4, HCPCS).

Daysheet (4) A register for recording daily business transactions (charges, payments, or adjustments); also known as daybook, daily log, or daily record sheet.

Debit card (17) A card permitting bank customers to withdraw from any affiliated automated teller machine (ATM) and make cashless purchases from funds on deposit without incurring revolving finance charges for credit.

Debt (17) A legal obligation to pay money.

Debtor (17) A person owing money.

Deductible (4, 5) A type of cost-sharing that requires a specific dollar amount to be paid by the insured before a medical insurance plan or government program begins covering health care costs.

Deep (11) A surgical term used to identify a location that is internal or closer to the center of the body; the opposite of superficial.

Defense Enrollment Eligibility Reporting System (DEERS) (8) An electronic database used to verify beneficiary eligibility for individuals in the TRICARE programs.

Degaussing (11) Method to dispose of confidential or sensitive information by use of electromagnetic fields to erase data.

Deleted claim (14) Insurance claim that has been canceled, deleted, or voided by a Medicare fiscal intermediary for the following reasons: CMS-1500 (08-05) or current CMS-1450 is not used, itemized charges are not provided, more than six line items are submitted on the CMS-1500 (08-05) claim form, patient's address is missing, internal clerical error was made, Certificate of Medical Necessity (CMN) was not with the Part B claim or was incomplete or invalid, and name of the store is not on the receipt that includes the price of the item.

Delinquent claim (16) An insurance claim submitted to an insurance company, for which payment is overdue.

Denied claim (16) An insurance claim submitted to an insurance company in which payment has been rejected owing to a technical error or because of medical coverage policy issues.

Department of Defense Disability (10) Military disability benefits provided by the Department of Defense to all active duty service members and reservists who leave the military with service-connected medical conditions that make the service member unfit for duty.

Department of Veterans Affairs (8) The federal agency that oversees health care services to military veterans and determines eligibility of beneficiaries.

Dependent (4) The term that refers to the spouse and children of the insured. Under some contracts, dependents may also include parents, other family members, and domestic partners of the insured.

Deposition (9) The process of taking sworn testimony from a witness out of court. This is usually done by an attorney.

Designated record sets (2) A specific set of information that is maintained by a health care organization on behalf of a patient, which may include health records, billing and claim records, and health plan enrollment records. This information is used to make decisions about a patient.

Determination (16) The insurance carrier's decision as to whether they will pay the claim in full, deny the claim, or reduce the amount they will pay.

Device character (19) An ICD-10-PCS character that is used to identify specific devices left in place after a procedure. Examples include artificial hip, pacemaker, tissue expanders, drainage devices, radioactive elements, and so on.

Diagnostic creep (DRG creep) (3, 18) Coding that is inappropriately altered to obtain a higher payment rate; also known as coding creep, DRG creep, or upcoding.

Digital subscriber line (DSL) (15) A high-speed connection through a telephone line jack; usually a means of accessing the internet.

Direct data entry (DDE) (15) Keying claim information directly into the payer system by accessing over modem, dial-up, or digital subscriber line (DSL). This is a technology to directly enter the information into the payer system via the access, whether it is dial-up or DSL.

Direct contract model HMO (5) An HMO plan that contracts directly with private health care providers in the community to furnish services to their members. The plan offers a broad panel of service providers, including primary care and specialty providers.

Direct referral (5) Certain services in a managed care plan may not require preauthorization. The authorization request form is completed and signed by the physician and handed to the patient (for example, obstetric care or dermatology) to be done directly.

Dirty claim (14) A claim submitted with errors or one that requires manual processing to resolve problems or is rejected for payment.

Disability (6, 10) A disability is defined by the Social Security Administration (SSA) as the inability to engage in any substantial employment due to physical or mental impairment that can be expected to last for 12 continuous months or result in death.

Disability Determination Services (DDS) (10) A state Social Security division office that assesses a case for disability benefits.

Disability income insurance (4, 10) A form of health insurance that provides periodic payments to replace income when the insured is unable to work as a result of illness, injury, or disease and not as a result of a work-related accident or condition.

Discharge (18) Occurs when the physician writes an order releasing the patient from the hospital. This order should include where the patient should go. Possible locations include home, home with home health, another acute care hospital, rehabilitation, and more.

Discharge disposition (18) The location where the patient is being discharged to (home, nursing facility, etc.).

Discharge not final billed (DNCB) (18) A list of all hospital (inpatient and outpatient) claims that have not been submitted to the insurer due to a number of reasons such as: not coded, missing data, still in window of time waiting for late charges, missing discharge disposition, and more.

Disclosure (2) The release, transfer, provision of access to, or divulging in any other manner of information outside the entity holding the information.

Discount (17) A reduction of a normal charge based on a specific amount of money or a percentage of the charge.

Discounting (18) The reduction of APC reimbursement to the hospital occurring for a number of reasons such as surgery is cancelled or more than one surgery is performed at an operative session.

Disenrollment (5) A member's voluntary cancellation of membership in a managed care plan.

Documentation (11) (1) A chronologic detailed recording of pertinent facts and observations about a patient's health as seen in chart notes and medical reports; entries in the medical record, such as prescription refills, telephone calls, and other pertinent data. (2) For computer software, a user's guide to a program or piece of equipment.

Donut hole (6) A temporary limit on what a Medicare drug will pay. The coverage gap begins after the patient and the drug plan together have spent a certain amount for covered drugs.

Double indemnity (10) A feature in some life and disability insurance policies that provides for twice the face amount of the policy to be paid if death results to the insured from accidental causes.

Downcoding (13, 18) The practice of reporting a code for a lower level of care when the health record would support a higher level. This also occurs when the insurance carrier processing the claim converts the code submitted to a lower level of service, generating decreased payment.

Dress code (1) A set of guidelines identifying what is appropriate for the employee to wear to work

DRG creep (3, 18) Slang expression for diagnostic creep. See Diagnostic creep.

Dual eligible (6) Patients who qualify for both Medicare and Medicaid

Dun message (17) A message or phrase to inform or remind a patient about a delinquent account.

Durable medical equipment (DME) (6, 13, 14) Any equipment that provides therapeutic benefits to a patient in need because of certain medical conditions and/or illnesses.

Early and Periodic Screening, Diagnosis, and Treatment (EPSDT) (7) The EPSDT program covers screening and diagnostic services to determine physical or mental defects in recipients younger than 21 years of age and health care, treatment, and other measures to correct or ameliorate any defects and chronic conditions discovered. In New York, this is called the Child Health Assurance Program (CHAP).

Electronic claim (14) Digital files that are not printed on paper claim forms when submitted to the payer; instead, claims are submitted using a central processing unit (CPU), tape, diskette, direct data entry, direct wire, dial-in telephone, digital fax, or personal computer download or upload.

Electronic data interchange (EDI) (15) The process by which understandable data items are sent back and forth via computer linkages between two or more entities that function alternatively as sender and receiver.

Electronic funds transfer (EFT) (15) A paperless computerized system that enables funds to be debited, credited, or transferred, eliminating the need for personal handling of checks.

Electronic health record (EHR) (11) A patient record that is created using a computer with software. A template is brought up and by answering a series of questions, data are entered.

Electronic mail (1) Electronic message that is transmitted, received, stored, or forwarded text, voice messages, attachments, or images by computer from one person to another or from one person to a defined group or all users on a system.

Electronic protected health information (ePHI) (2). Any protected health information that is produced, saved, transferred, or received in an electronic form.

Electronic remittance advice (ERA) (15) An online transaction about the status of a claim.

Electronic signature (4) An electronic signature is digital data attached to a computerized document as verification of the provider's intent to sign the document.

Emancipated minor (4) A person younger than 18 years of age who lives independently, is totally self-supporting, and possesses decision-making rights.

Embezzlement (3, 17) A willful act by an employee of taking possession of an employer's money.

Emergency (8) A sudden and unexpected medical condition, or the worsening of a condition, that poses a threat to life, limb, or sight and requires immediate treatment to alleviate suffering (for example, shortness of breath, chest pain, drug overdose).

Emergency care (11) Health care services provided to prevent serious impairment of bodily functions or serious dysfunction to any body organ or part. Advanced life support may be necessary. Not all care provided in an emergency department of a hospital can be termed "emergency care."

Emergency department (13) Defined by CPT as an organized hospital-based facility, open 24 hours day, 7 days per week; for the provision of unscheduled episodic services to patients who present for immediate medical attention.

Emergency Medical Treatment and Labor Act (EMTALA) (3, 18) Legislation requiring that anyone who comes to an emergency room, or is in active labor, be evaluated and stabilized regardless of their ability to pay.

Emoticons (1) A short sequence of keyboard letters and symbols used to convey emotion, gestures, or expressions (e.g., "smiley" [(; :–)]).

Employer identification number (EIN) (2, 14) An individual's federal tax identification number issued by the Internal Revenue Service (IRS) for income tax purposes.

Employment agency (20) A business organization that refers job applicants to potential employers.

Encoder (15) An add-on software program to practice management systems that can reduce the time it takes to build or review insurance claims before batch transmission to the carrier.

Encounter (1) An interaction between a patient and a health care provider for the purpose of providing health care services or assessing the patient's health status.

Encounter form (4) Also referred to as a charge slip, multipurpose billing form, patient service slip, routing form, superbill, or transaction slip.

Used to record the patient's name, the date, the procedural and diagnostic codes, and the date the patient should return for a follow-up appointment.

Encryption (15) To assign a code to represent data. This is done for security purposes.

End-stage renal disease (ESRD) (6) End-stage renal disease occurs when a patient who has chronic kidney disease has gradual loss of kidney function and reaches an advanced state; the kidneys are no longer able to work as they should to meet the body's needs.

Eponym (11, 12) The name of a disease, anatomic structure, operation, or procedure, usually derived from the name of a place where it first occurred or a person who discovered or first described it.

Ergonomic (9) Science and technology that seek to fit the anatomic and physical needs of the worker to the workplace.

Errors and omissions insurance (1) A type of insurance that provides protection against loss of money caused by failure through error or unintentional omission on the part of the individual or service involved in any aspect of preparation or submission of an insurance claim.

Essential modifiers (12) In ICD-10-CM, subterms that are indented two spaces to the right under main terms. They are referred to as essential modifiers because their presence changes the diagnostic code assignment.

Established patient (11) An individual who has received professional services within the past 3 years from the physician or another physician of the same specialty who belongs to the same group practice.

Estate administrator (17) One who takes possession of the assets of a decedent, pays the expenses of administration and the claims of creditors, and disposes of the balance of an estate in accordance with the statutes governing the distribution of decedent's estates.

Estate executor (17) One who takes possession of the assets of a decedent, pays the expenses of administration and the claims of creditors, and disposes of the balance of an estate in accordance with the decedent's will.

Ethics (1) Standards of conduct generally accepted as a moral guide for behavior by which an insurance billing or coding specialist may determine the appropriateness of his or her conduct in a relationship with patients, the physician, co-workers, the government, and insurance companies.

Etiology (12) The cause of disease; the study of the cause of a disease.

Etiquette (1) Customs, rules of conduct, courtesy, and manners of the medical profession.

Exacerbation (12) An acute increase in the severity of an illness. Acute respiratory infection such as bronchitis or pneumonia would be an example of an exacerbation.

Excludes 1 (12) Word with number that is one of the conventions used in the diagnostic code book titled *International Classification of Diseases,* Tenth Revision, Clinical Modification (ICD-10-CM). This indicates that the code excluded should never be used at the same time as the code above the Excludes 1 note. An Excludes 1 is when two conditions cannot occur together (for example, congenital form versus acquired form of a condition). A note instructs the reader to go to another code for the excluded condition.

Excludes 2 (12) Word with number that is one of the conventions used in the diagnostic code book titled *International Classification of Diseases,* Tenth Revision, Clinical Modification (ICD-10-CM). This note represents "Not included here" and indicates that the condition excluded is not part of the condition represented by the code, but a patient may have both conditions at the same time. When an Excludes 2 note appears under a code, it is acceptable to use both the code and the excluded code together.

Exclusion(s) (4, 10) Provisions written into the insurance contract denying coverage or limiting the scope of coverage.

Exclusion Statute (3) Federal law in that the OIG is required to exclude individuals, health care providers, and health care organizations who commit criminal offenses from participation in any federal health care programs. Offenses that can earn exclusion from these programs range from Medicare fraud to patient abuse to financial misconduct.

Exclusive provider organization (EPO) (4, 5) A type of managed health care plan that combines features of health maintenance organizations (HMOs) and preferred provider organizations (PPOs). It is referred to as "exclusive" because it is offered to large employers who agree not to contract with any other plan. EPOs are regulated under state health insurance laws.

Explanation of benefits (EOB) (8, 16) A document detailing services billed and describing payment determinations; also known in Medicare, Medicaid, and some other programs as a remittance advice (RA). In the TRICARE program, it is called a summary payment voucher.

Expressed contract (4) A verbal or written agreement.

External audit (11) A review done after claims have been submitted (retrospective review) of medical and financial records by an insurance company or Medicare representative to investigate suspected fraud or abusive billing practices.

External causes of morbidity (12) Classification of codes used for external causes of injury rather than disease. The code description refers to the circumstances that caused an injury rather than the nature of the injury. The codes are also used in coding adverse reactions to medications.

Extraterritorial (9) State laws effective outside the state by either specific provision or court decision. In workers' compensation cases, benefits under the state law that apply to a compensable injury of an employee hired in one state but injured outside that state.

Facility billing (1) Charging for services done in hospitals, acute care hospitals, skilled nursing or long-term care facilities, rehabilitation centers, or ambulatory surgical centers.

Facility provider number (14) A facility's (hospital, laboratory, radiology office, or nursing facility) provider number to be used by the facility to bill for services, or by the performing physician to report services done at that location.

Family and Medical Leave Act (10) A federal law that gives eligible employees the right to take time off work, *unpaid,* to recover from serious medical conditions and care for ailing family members, among other things.

Family history (FH) (11) A review of medical events in the patient's family, including diseases that may be hereditary or place the patient at risk.

Federal Deposit Insurance Corporation (FDIC) (3) Fraud and abuse laws associated with mailing and wiring of money or property.

Federal Employees' Compensation Act (FECA) (9) An Act instituted in 1908 providing benefits for on-the-job injuries to all federal employees.

Federal Employees Retirement System (FERS) (10) A retirement program for federal employees hired after 1984 or those hired before 1984 who switched from Civil Service Retirement System (CSRS) to FERS.

Federal poverty level (FPL) (7) A measure of income issued every year by the Department of Health and Human Services found in the *Federal Register;* used to determine eligibility for certain Medicaid programs.

Fee-for-service (FFS) (4, 5) A method of payment in which the patient pays the health care organization or provider for service performed from an established schedule of fees.

Fee schedule (13, 17) A list of charges or established allowances for specific medical services and procedures. See also Relative value studies (RVS).

Financial accounting record (17) An individual record indicating charges, payments, adjustments, and balances owed for services rendered; also known as a ledger.

First listed diagnosis (19) The reason for outpatient and office encounters. If the specific diagnosis is not known at the visit, signs and symptoms are coded instead.

Fiscal agent or fiscal intermediary (7, 8) An organization under contract to the federal or state government to process claims for a health care program.

Flexible Spending Account (4) An employee-sponsored health plan that allows individuals to put aside a certain amount of wages for qualified medical expenses and dependent care. The amount is not subject to payroll taxes.

Form locators (19) The 81 fields in the CMS-1450 (UB-04) claim form, used to provide provider information, patient information, and information related to the services provided.

Formal referral (5) An authorization request (telephone, fax, or completed form) required by the managed care organization contract to determine medical necessity and grant permission before services are rendered or procedures performed.

Formulary (6) List of drugs that a health insurance plan covers as a benefit.

Fraud (3) An intentional misrepresentation of the facts to deceive or mislead another.

Intoxication (12) A diagnostic coding term that relates to an adverse effect rather than a poisoning when drugs, such as digitalis, steroid agents, and so on, are involved.

Invalid claim (14) A claim that contains complete, necessary information but is illogical or incorrect (for example, listing an incorrect provider number for a referring physician). Invalid claims are identified to the provider and may be resubmitted.

Itemized statement (17) A detailed summary of all transactions of a patient's account: dates of service, detailed charges, payments (copayments and deductibles), date on which the insurance claim was submitted, adjustments, and account balance.

Jurisdiction (6) A defined geographical area over which a Medicare Administrative Contractor oversees processing of claims.

Kickback (3) Any type of gift, reward, or inducement for facilitating a transaction or appointment.

Laboratory service (11) Medical tests performed for diagnosis, treatment, and prevention of disease.

Late effect (12) An inactive residual effect or condition produced after the acute phase of an illness or injury has ended.

Lateral/Laterality (11, 12) Defines the side of the body affected.

Legible (11) Pertaining to a health record, data that is easily recognizable by individuals outside of a medical practice who are unfamiliar with the particular handwriting.

Lien (9, 17) A claim on the property of another as security for a debt. In litigation cases, it is a legal promise to satisfy a debt owed by the patient to the physician out of any proceeds received on the case.

Life cycle of a claim (4) Also referred to as the revenue cycle of an insurance claim, which includes the administrative and clinical functions that are required to capture and collect payment for services provided by a health care organization.

Limiting charge (6) A percentage limit on fees, specified by legislation, that nonparticipating physicians may bill Medicare beneficiaries above the fee schedule amount.

Local coverage determination (LCD) (6) Decisions made by a Medicare contractor that are developed to decide whether to cover a particular service in accordance with CMS' definition of what is medically necessary and to provide coverage information for medical services. LCDs are only applicable to that Medicare contractor's jurisdiction.

Long-term care facility (18) A facility that provides custodial care to individuals who are chronically ill or disabled or are not able to live independently. Often referred to as *assisted living facilities*, they offer the type of services that help residents perform normal daily tasks or activities of daily living (ADLs) such as bathing, eating, and getting dressed. These facilities provide medical care as well as personal care and services such as meals and laundry.

Long-term care hospital prospective payment system (LTCH PPS) (18) The prospective reimbursement system used by long-term care

hospitals that provide services to patients who no longer need acute care but their level of care is still significant. Long-term care hospitals must provide an average length of stay of at least 25 days.

Long-term disability insurance (10) A provision to pay benefits to a covered disabled person to age 65.

Lost claim (16) An insurance claim that cannot be located after sending it to an insurer.

Magnetic resonance imaging (MRI) (11) A type of radiography that uses a magnetic field and protons in the body to produce a cross section image of ligaments, the brain, spinal cord, heart, and other internal

Major complication/comorbidity (MCC) (18) Main underlying condition or other condition that arises or exists along with the condition for which the patient is receiving treatment. Used in diagnostic-related group (DRG) reimbursement.

Major diagnostic category (MDC) (18) A broad classification of diagnoses. There are 83 coding system–oriented MDCs in the original diagnosis-related groups (DRGs) and 23 body system–oriented MDCs in the revised set of DRGs.

Major medical (4) A health insurance policy designed to offset heavy medical expenses resulting from catastrophic or prolonged illness or injury.

Malignant tumor (12) An abnormal growth that has the properties of invasion and metastasis (for example, transfer of diseases from one organ to another). The word "carcinoma" refers to a cancerous or malignant tumor.

Managed care (5) Refers to a group of techniques intended to reduce the cost of providing health care while improving the access to care and the quality of care.

Managed Care Organization (5) A generic term applied to an insurance plan that utilizes techniques to keep down medical costs by reducing unnecessary hospitalizations, forcing providers to discount their rates, and causing the health care industry to become more efficient and competitive.

Management Service Organization (1) A business that performs a variety of administrative and business functions, such as accounting, billing, coding, clinical documentation improvement, collections, computer support, compliance oversight, legal advice, marketing, payroll, and management expertise.

Mandated benefit (4) Health service (treatment or procedure) required by state and/or federal law that may be given to a patient for a specific health condition. This health service may be delivered by certain types of health care providers for some categories of dependents, such as children placed for adoption. Also referred to as mandated services.

Manifestation (12) An associated secondary process or disease.

Maternal and Child Health Program (MCHP) (4) A state service organization to assist children younger than 21 years of age who have conditions leading to health problems.

Medial (11) A positional term that means toward the center.

Medicaid (4, 6, 7) A federally aided, state-operated, and state-administered program that provides medical benefits for certain low-income persons in need of health and medical care.

Medi-Cal (7) California's version of the nationwide program known as Medicaid.

Medical billing representative (1) See Insurance billing specialist.

Medical decision making (MDM) (11) Health care management process done after performing a history and physical examination on a patient that results in a plan of treatment. It is based on establishing one or more diagnoses and/or selecting a management or treatment option, amount of data or complexity of data reviewed, and complications and/or morbidity or mortality.

Medical necessity (3, 4, 6, 11, 12, 16) The performance of services and procedures that are consistent with the diagnosis in accordance with standards of good medical practice, performed at the proper level, and provided in the most appropriate setting. Medical necessity must be established (via diagnostic or other information presented on the individual claim under consideration) before the carrier may make payment.

Medical record (1) Refers to patient charts that include notes and information collected by and for the clinicians in that specific health care provider's office or organization.

Medical Savings Account (MSA) (4) A type of tax-free savings account that allows individuals and their employers to set aside money to pay for health care expenses.

Medical service order (9) An authorization given to the physician, either written or verbal, to treat the injured or ill employee.

Medically necessary (4) See Medical necessity.

Medically needy (MN) (7) Persons in need of financial assistance or whose income and resources will not allow them to pay for the costs of medical care; also called medically indigent in some states.

Medically (or psychologically) necessary (8) Medical or psychological services considered appropriate care and generally accepted by qualified professionals to be reasonable and adequate for the diagnosis and treatment of illness, injury, pregnancy, and mental disorders or that are reasonable and adequate for well-baby care.

Medicare (4, 6) A nationwide health insurance program for people age 65 years of age and older and certain disabled or blind persons regardless of income, administered by Centers for Medicare and Medicaid Services (CMS).

Medicare Access and CHIP Reauthorization Act of 2015 (MACRA) (6) Legislation enacted to establish quality payment programs as a new way to pay providers by giving incentives for high-quality and high-value care.

Medicare Administrative Contractors (MAC) (3, 6) A private insurance carrier that has been contracted by CMS to process Medicare Part A and Part B medical claims for Medicare fee-for-service (FFS) beneficiaries.

Medicare Advantage Plan (6) Private insurance companies who have been approved by

Qualifier character (19) The ICD-10-PCS character that provides information for some codes that may not be identified elsewhere. This is used to provide additional information, such as origin of tissue for transplant, destination site of a bypass, or whether the removal of tissue was for diagnostic purposes.

Qualifying circumstance modifiers (QC) (13) Add-on codes for anesthesia services used when a patient's age or status has a significant effect on the service provided.

Quality Improvement Organization (QIO) (6, 18) A program that replaces the peer review organization program and is designed to monitor and improve the usage and quality of care for Medicare beneficiaries.

Query (11) A tool used by a clinical documentation improvement specialist to request additional clarification from the provider of services.

Qui tam (3) A provision under the FCA that offers financial incentives to private citizens who act as informants and report suspected fraud on behalf of the federal government.

Real time (15) Online interactive communication between two computer systems allowing instant transfer of information.

Reasonable fee (13) A charge is considered reasonable if it is deemed acceptable after peer review even though it does not meet the customary or prevailing criteria. This includes unusual circumstances or complications requiring additional time, skill, or experience in connection with a particular service or procedure. In Medicare, the amount on which payment is based for participating physicians.

Reason for the encounter (19) First diagnosis stated or listed for an outpatient insurance claim.

Reassess (16) A review. For example, an appeal is a documented request to the insurance company to review (reassess) a claim and reconsider for payment.

Rebill (resubmit) (16) To send another request for payment for an overdue bill to either the insurance company or the patient.

Recipient (7) A person certified by the local welfare department to receive the benefits of Medicaid under one of the specific aid categories; an individual certified to receive Medicare benefits.

Reconsideration (10) The first level of appeal process for an individual applying for Social Security Disability Insurance (SSDI) or Supplemental Security Income (SSI). It is a complete review of the claim by a medical or psychological consultant or disability examiner team who did not take part in the original disability determination.

Recovery Audit Contractor (RAC) (3) A company that contracts with Medicare to recoup money from inappropriately paid claims.

Recovery Audit Contractor (RAC) Initiative (6) Legislation enacted allowing CMS to contract with audit companies for identification of Medicare underpayments and overpayments and recover overpayments using automated review and complex review. An automated review

is done electro… and complex r… view of the med…

Reexamination r… report sent to … the status of a … who has made … to 4 weeks of tre…

Referral (11) Th… care of a patient… In managed care… a specific service…

Referring provide… the patient for te…

Regional contrac… CHAMPVA, the… dles the claims f… ular state or cou… cessor and forme… carrier, or fiscal i… Medicare admin…

Registered Medic… title earned by c… and passing a r… tered by the An… (AMT).

Registered Medic… istered title awar… work given by t… tute (MMI) with…

Rehabilitation in… (18) Categories… based on patient… for which a patie…

Reimbursement … provided.

Reimbursement s… billing specialist…

Rejected claim (14… mitted to an insur… the system becaus… or erroneous info… follow carrier ins… provider for corr… be processed prop…

Relative value stu… A list of procedu… vices and procedu… ues that indicate t… dure over anothe…

Relative value un… value assigned to… the amount of ph… es, and cost of p… These three RVU… to geographic are… termine Medicare…

Relative weight (1… DRGs based on t… treat Medicare pa… used to determin… ment for the assig… relative weight is …

Remittance advice… sent by an insuran… vices, detailing ser… ment determinatio… programs as an ex…

Medicare to offer Medicare Part C coverage to patients eligible for Medicare benefits, as an alternative to traditional Medicare.

Medicare Beneficiary Identifier (MBI) (6) The 11-character beneficiary identifier used on Medicare insurance cards.

Medicare Claims Processing Manual—Internet Only Manual (6) The publication that provides Medicare's general billing requirements for various health care professionals and suppliers, as well as claims submission information.

Medicare fee schedule (6) A comprehensive listing of accepted charges or established allowances for specific medical procedures identified by procedural codes developed by CMS for health care professionals, physicians, ambulance services, clinical laboratory services, and durable medical equipment.

Medicare Improvements for Patients and Providers Act (MIPPA) (6) A multi-faceted piece of legislation containing provisions and funding to states to help older adults, individuals with disabilities, and their caregivers for special assistance. It also required CMS to implement quality incentives into the ESRD bundled payment system to promote high-quality services to outpatient dialysis facilities treating patients with ESRD.

Medicare Integrity Program (MIP) (3) A program designed to promote the integrity of the Medicare program through a series of audits and reviews of health care organizations' claims and cost report data.

Medicare Learning Network (6) A Medicare resource that offers free educational materials for health care professionals on programs, policies, and initiatives.

Medicare/Medicaid (Medi-Medi) (4, 6) Refers to an individual who receives medical or disability benefits from both Medicare and Medicaid programs; sometimes referred to as a Medi-Medi case or a crossover.

Medicare Part A (6) Hospital benefits of a nationwide health insurance program for persons age 65 years of age and older and certain disabled individuals regardless of income, administered by Centers for Medicare and Medicaid Services (CMS).

Medicare Part B (6) Medical insurance of a nationwide health insurance program for persons age 65 years of age and older and certain disabled individuals regardless of income, administered by Centers for Medicare and Medicaid Services (CMS). Local Social Security offices take applications and supply information about the program.

Medicare Part C (6) Medicare Plus (+) Choice plans offer a number of health care options in addition to those available under Medicare Part A and Part B. Plans may include health maintenance organizations (HMOs), fee-for-service plans, provider-sponsored organizations, religious fraternal benefit societies (RFBSs), and Medicare medical savings accounts.

Medicare Part D (6) Stand-alone prescription drug plan, presented by insurance and other private companies, that offers drug coverage that meets the standards established by Medicare.

Other names for these plans are Part D private prescription drug plans (PDPs) or Medicare Advantage prescription drug plans (MA-PDs).

Medicare savings program (MSP) (7) Programs developed by state Medicaid programs designed to help low-income individuals with out-of-pocket costs for Medicare, including Medicare Part A and B premiums, deductibles, copayments, and coinsurance.

Medicare secondary payer (MSP) (6) The primary insurance plan of a Medicare beneficiary that must pay for any medical care or services first before Medicare is sent a claim.

Medicare select (6) A supplementary Medigap policy that limits the patient's coverage to a network of doctors and hospitals that charge less for the services they provide to members.

Medicare Severity Diagnosis-Related Groups (18) Groups of similar conditions that require similar resources and have similar costs; used in The Inpatient Prospective Payment System (IPPS) as the prospective reimbursement system used for Medicare inpatient claims for acute care facilities.

Medicare Summary Notice (MSN) (6) A document received by the patient explaining amount charged, Medicare approved, deductible, and coinsurance for medical services rendered.

Medigap (MG) (6) A specialized supplemental insurance policy devised for the Medicare beneficiary that covers the deductible and copayment amounts typically not covered under the main Medicare policy written by a nongovernmental third-party payer.

Mentor (20) Guide or teacher who offers advice, criticism, wisdom, guidance, and perspective to an inexperienced but promising protégé to help reach a life goal.

Merit-Based Incentive Payment System (MIPS) (6) A quality payment program established under MACRA that will determine Medicare payment adjustments to providers.

Metastasis (12) Process in which tumor cells spread and transfer from one organ to another site.

Microscopy (11) A **laboratory service** performed for diagnosis, treatment, and prevention of disease in which the specimen is examined under the microscope.

Military Health System (8) A federated system of uniformed, civilian, and contract personnel and additional civilian partners at all levels of the Department of Defense and beyond. The mission of the MHS is to ensure that **active duty service members (ADSMs)** of the United States military (Army, Navy, Air Force, Marines, Coast Guard) are healthy and able to complete their missions, are trained to provide medical care to operational forces around the world and to provide them, their families, and retirees with medical benefits.

Military Treatment Facility (MTF) (8) All uniformed service hospitals or health clinics; also known as military hospitals or uniformed service hospitals.

Minimum necessary rule (2) A requirement of the HIPAA privacy rule for covered entities to

take reasonable steps to limit the use or disclosure of protected health information to only what is necessary to accomplish the intended purpose.

Mitigation (2) For a breach of privacy under the Health Insurance Portability and Accountability Act (HIPAA), this means to alleviate the severity, reduce, or make mild any harmful effects of such violation.

Modality (3) A modality is defined in the CPT as any physical agent applied to produce therapeutic changes to biological tissue. Examples of modalities used in therapy services include heat, ice, traction, infrared, ultraviolet light, electrical stimulation, and massage.

Modifiers (13) In Current Procedural Terminology (CPT) coding, a two-digit add-on number placed after the usual procedure code number to indicate a procedure or service has been altered by specific circumstances. The two-digit modifier may be separated by a hyphen. In HCPCS Level II coding, one-digit or two-digit add-on alpha characters, placed after the usual procedure code number (Example 27372-51).

Monitoring (3) A spot check for quality control; less structured than an audit.

Morbidity (11, 12) A diseased condition or state.

Mortality (11, 12) Death.

Mutually exclusive code edits (13) National Correct Coding Initiative (NCCI) edits that relate to procedures that are code combinations restricted by the guidelines outlined in CPT, procedures that represent two methods of performing the same service, procedures that cannot reasonably be done during the same session, and procedures that represent medically impossible or improbable code combinations.

National Certified Insurance and Coding Specialist (NCICS) (20) An insurance and coding certification that is awarded by an independent testing agency, the National Center for Competency Testing (NCCT).

National Committee for Quality Assurance (5) A not-for-profit organization that accredits managed care health plans through adherence to a rigorous set of standards to which health plans must attest and adhere.

National Correct Coding Initiative (NCCI) (13) A code editing system implemented into the Medicare program in 1996, consistent with Medicare policies to eliminate unbundling or other inappropriate reporting of CPT codes.

National coverage determination (NCD) (6) Guidelines mandated by CMS at the federal level that all Medicare contractors must follow that are developed to decide whether to cover a particular service in accordance with CMS' definition of what is medically necessary and to provide coverage information for medical services.

National health insurance (6) A legally enforced system of health insurance that insures a countries' population against the costs of health care. It is usually established by national legislation, but may be administered by the public sector, the private sector, or a combination of both.

National Provider Identifier (NPI) (2, 6, 14) A lifetime number issued to health care organizations and providers and used to identify them on claim forms.